DIFFICULT PROBLEMS IN
HAND SURGERY

DIFFICULT PROBLEMS IN
HAND SURGERY

JAMES W. STRICKLAND, M.D.

Clinical Professor of Orthopaedic Surgery, and
Chief of Hand Surgery Service, Department of Orthopaedic Surgery,
Indiana University School of Medicine;
Chief of Hand Surgery Section, Department of Orthopaedic Surgery,
St. Vincent Hospital and Health Care Center, Indianapolis, Indiana

JAMES B. STEICHEN, M.D.

Clinical Associate Professor of Orthopaedic Surgery,
Department of Orthopaedic Surgery,
Indiana University School of Medicine;
Attending Hand Surgeon, St. Vincent Hospital and Health Care Center,
Indianapolis, Indiana

With **792** illustrations

The C. V. MOSBY COMPANY

SAINT LOUIS • TORONTO • LONDON   1982

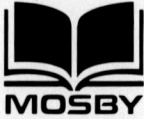

A TRADITION OF PUBLISHING EXCELLENCE

Editor: Eugenia A. Klein
Assistant editor: Kathryn H. Falk
Manuscript editor: Susan K. Hume
Book design: Nancy Steinmeyer
Cover design: Suzanne Oberholtzer
Production: Mary Stueck, Linda R. Stalnaker

Copyright © 1982 by The C.V. Mosby Company

All rights reserved. No part of this book may be reproduced in any manner without written permission of the publisher.

Printed in the United States of America

The C.V. Mosby Company
11830 Westline Industrial Drive, St. Louis, Missouri 63141

Library of Congress Cataloging in Publication Data

Main entry under title:

Difficult problems in hand surgery.

   "Much of the material was presented at symposia . . . held in Indianapolis in 1978 and 1981 and sponsored by the American Society for Surgery of the Hand."—Pref.
   Bibliography: p.
   Includes index.
   1. Hand—Surgery—Congresses. I. Strickland, James W., 1936-   . II. Steichen, James B. III. American Society for Surgery of the Hand.
[DNLM: 1. Hand, Surgery—Congresses. WE 830 D569 1978-81]
RD559.D53   617'.575059   82-2230
ISBN 0-8016-4851-3   AACR2

AC/CB/B 9 8 7 6 5 4 3 2 1   02/B/275

Contributors

PETER C. AMADIO, M.D.

Assistant Professor of Clinical Orthopaedics,
S.U.N.Y.–Stony Brook Hand Surgery Service,
University Hospital, Stony Brook, New York

JAMES L. BECTON, M.D.

Associate Professor of Orthopaedic Surgery,
Department of Surgery, Medical College of Georgia,
Augusta, Georgia

JOHN L. BELL, M.D.

Professor of Clinical Surgery, Department of Surgery,
Northwestern University Medical School, Chicago, Illinois

JAMES E. BENNETT, M.D., F.A.C.S.

W.D. Gatch Professor of Surgery, Director of Plastic Surgery,
Department of Surgery, Indiana University Medical Center,
Indianapolis, Indiana

HARRY J. BUNCKE, M.D.

Clinical Professor of Surgery, Division of Plastic Surgery,
University of California, San Francisco, California

WARREN B. BURROWS, M.D.

The Western Hand Center, Downey, California;
Former Hand Fellow, St. Vincent Hospital and
Health Care Center, Indianapolis, Indiana

WILLIAM H. CALL, M.D.

Orthopaedic Surgeon, St. Paul, Minnesota;
Former Hand Fellow, St. Vincent Hospital and
Health Care Center, Indianapolis, Indiana

MARK L. CLAYTON, M.D.

Clinical Professor of Surgery (Hand Surgery),
University of Colorado School of Medicine; Staff,
Denver Orthopedic Clinic, Denver, Colorado

JOHN F. COOK, Jr., M.D.

Hand Surgeon and Orthopedic Surgeon,
Newport Beach, California

ROBERT J. DURAN, M.D.

Clinical Professor of Surgery and Co-director of the
Hand Service, Division of Plastic Surgery,
Ohio State University College of Medicine, Columbus, Ohio

J. ANTHONY DUSTMAN, M.D.

Orthopaedic Surgeon, Bloomington; Adjunct Associate
Professor of Medical Sciences and Sports Medicine,
Department of Health, Physical Education, Recreation,
and Dance, Illinois State University, Normal, Illinois;
Former Hand Fellow, St. Vincent Hospital and
Health Care Center, Indianapolis, Indiana

DONALD C. FERLIC, M.D.

Assistant Clinical Professor, Orthopedic Surgery,
University of Colorado Medical Center, Denver, Colorado

NOREEN FLYNN, M.L.S.

Research Associate, Strickland, Steichen, Kleinman,
Hastings, MD's, Inc., Indianapolis, Indiana

THOMAS L. GREENE, M.D.

Instructor, Section of Orthopaedic Surgery, University of
Michigan, Ann Arbor, Michigan; Former Hand Fellow,
St. Vincent Hospital and Health Care Center,
Indianapolis, Indiana

GERALD D. HARRIS, M.D.

Associate Professor, Department of Surgery, Northwestern
University, Chicago, Illinois

ROBERT H. HARTWIG, M.D.

Clinical Assistant Professor of Surgery, Department of
Orthopaedic Surgery, Medical College of Ohio,
Toledo, Ohio; Former Hand Fellow, St. Vincent Hospital
and Health Care Center, Indianapolis, Indiana

HILL HASTINGS II, M.D.

Clinical Assistant Professor of Orthopaedic Surgery,
Department of Orthopaedic Surgery, Indiana University
School of Medicine; Chief, Division of Orthopaedic Hand
Surgery, Wishard Memorial Hospital, Indianapolis, Indiana

CONTRIBUTORS

JAMES H. HOUSE, M.D.

Professor of Orthopaedic Surgery, Department of Orthopaedic Surgery, University of Minnesota, Minneapolis, Minnesota

ROBERT G. HOUSER, M.D.

Clinical Assistant Professor of Surgery, Division of Plastic Surgery, Ohio State University College of Medicine, Columbus, Ohio

JAMES M. HUNTER, M.D.

Clinical Professor of Orthopaedic Surgery, Department of Orthopaedics, Jefferson Medical College of Thomas Jefferson University, Philadelphia, Pennsylvania

HAROLD E. KLEINERT, M.D.

Clinical Professor of Surgery, Indiana University School of Medicine, Indianapolis, Indiana; Clinical Professor of Surgery, University of Louisville, Louisville, Kentucky

WILLIAM B. KLEINMAN, M.D.

Clinical Assistant Professor, Department of Orthopaedic Surgery, Indiana University Medical Center; Attending Hand Surgeon, St. Vincent Hospital and Health Care Center, Indianapolis, Indiana

L. ANDREW KOMAN, M.D.

Assistant Professor of Orthopaedic Surgery, Bowman Gray School of Medicine, Winston Salem, and Duke University Medical Center, Durham, North Carolina

WILLIAM B. LaSALLE, M.D.

Orthopaedic Surgeon, Department of Orthopaedics, Parkview Hospital, Fort Wayne; Former Hand Fellow, St. Vincent Hospital and Health Care Center, Indianapolis, Indiana

IAN LEITCH, F.R.A.C.S.

Plastic Surgeon and Hand Surgeon, Adelaide, South Australia

RONALD L. LINSCHEID, M.D.

Professor of Orthopaedic Surgery, Department of Orthopaedics and Hand Surgery, Mayo Medical School, Rochester, Minnesota

LAWRENCE M. LUBBERS, M.D.

Clinical Instructor, Division of Orthopaedic Surgery, Ohio State University School of Medicine, Columbus, Ohio

ROBERT M. McFARLAND, M.D.

Professor of Surgery and Chief of the Division of Plastic Surgery, University of Western Ontario, London, Ontario, Canada

EVELYN J. MACKIN, L.P.T.

Director of Hand Therapy, Hand Rehabilitation Center, Philadelphia, Pennsylvania

GEORGE E. OMER, Jr., M.D.

Professor and Chairman, Department of Orthopaedics and Rehabilitation; Professor of Surgery and Chief, Division of Hand Surgery; Professor of Anatomy, University of New Mexico School of Medicine, Albuquerque, New Mexico

STEPHEN G. POWELL, M.D

Surgeon, Missoula Orthopaedic Clinic, Missoula, Montana; Former Hand Fellow, St. Vincent Hospital and Health Care Center, Indianapolis, Indiana

ELLIOTT H. ROSE, M.D.

Clinical Instructor, Department of Surgery (Plastic and Reconstructive), Stanford University Medical Center, Burlingame, California

LAWRENCE H. SCHNEIDER, M.D.

Associate Clinical Professor of Orthopaedic Surgery, Department of Orthopaedic Surgery, Jefferson Medical College of Thomas Jefferson University, Philadelphia, Pennsylvania

FRANK SEINSHEIMER III, M.D.

Greater Washington Orthopaedic Group, Silver Spring, Maryland

DAVID J. SMITH, Jr., M.D.

Assistant Professor of Surgery, Department of Surgery, Plastic Surgery Division, Indiana University, Indianapolis, Indiana

RICHARD J. SMITH, M.D.

Clinical Professor of Orthopaedic Surgery, Harvard Medical School; Chief of Hand Surgery, Department of Orthopaedic Surgery, Massachusetts General Hospital, Boston, Massachusetts

GRAEME J. SOUTHWICK, F.R.A.C.S.

Plastic Surgeon to the Cancer Institute, The Royal Southern Memorial Hospital, and The Alfred Hospital, Melbourne, Victoria, Australia

JAMES B. STEICHEN, M.D.

Clinical Associate Professor of Orthopaedic Surgery, Department of Orthopaedic Surgery, Indiana University School of Medicine; Attending Hand Surgeon, St. Vincent Hospital and Health Care Center, Indianapolis, Indiana

LEO STELZER, M.D.

Orthopaedic Surgeon, Alamosa Community Hospital, Alamosa; Consultant, Colorado Handicapped Children's Program, Denver, Colorado; Former Hand Fellow, St. Vincent Hospital and Health Care Center, Indianapolis, Indiana

JAMES W. STRICKLAND, M.D.

Clinical Professor of Orthopaedic Surgery, and Chief of Hand Surgery Service, Department of Orthopaedic Surgery, Indiana University School of Medicine; Chief of Hand Surgery Section, Department of Orthopaedic Surgery, St. Vincent Hospital and Health Care Center, Indianapolis, Indiana

WILLIAM B. STROMBERG, Jr., M.D.

Associate Clinical Professor, Department of Surgery, Northwestern University Medical School, Chicago, Illinois

JULIO TALEISNIK, M.D.

Assistant Clinical Professor of Surgery, Orthopaedic Surgery, University of California at Irvine, Irvine, California

R. FRED TORSTRICK, M.D.

Clinical Instructor in Orthopaedics and Rehabilitation, Department of Orthopaedics, Vanderbilt University, Nashville, Tennessee; Former Hand Fellow, St. Vincent Hospital and Health Care Center, Indianapolis Indiana

JAMES R. URBANIAK, M.D.

Professor of Orthopaedic Surgery, Duke University Medical Center, Durham, North Carolina

H. KIRK WATSON, M.D.

Chief of Connecticut Combined Hand Surgery Service, Hartford Hospital, Hartford, University of Connecticut, Farmington, Yale University, and Newington Children's Hospital, Newington, Connecticut

ELVIN G. ZOOK, M.D.

Professor and Chairman, Division of Plastic Surgery, Department of Surgery, Southern Illinois University School of Medicine, Springfield, Illinois

Preface

This volume contains 50 essays by experienced hand surgeons addressing difficult clinical problems. Much of the material was presented at symposia on "Difficult Problems in Hand Surgery" held in Indianapolis in 1978 and 1981 and sponsored by the American Society for Surgery of the Hand.

No attempt has been made to make these proceedings an all-inclusive course; rather, this book concentrates on challenging clinical situations in 13 different subject areas. Although most chapters are concisely written, with the identification of a particular problem followed by a description of the author's preferred technique for management, the approach to each subject varies somewhat according to the individual style of the contributor. It must be emphasized that these chapters represent the highly personal views and preferences of the authors and in certain instances may vary somewhat from more traditional views.

We believe that this book transmits meaningful information gleaned from the experience of leading hand surgeons, and we hope that readers will find it to be of considerable clinical value.

James W. Strickland
James B. Steichen

Contents

SECTION ONE
SKIN PROBLEMS

1 Abrasion injuries of the hand, 3
   James E. Bennett

2 Skin coverage for challenging hand injuries, 10
   Harry J. Buncke and **Gerald D. Harris**

3 Fingernail injuries, 22
   Elvin G. Zook

4 Reconstruction of the contracted first web space, 28
   James W. Strickland

5 The coverage of difficult digital defects with local rotation flaps, 38
   James W. Strickland

SECTION TWO
EXTENSOR TENDON PROBLEMS

6 Reconstruction in chronic extensor tendon problems, 47
   Lawrence H. Schneider

7 Boutonniere deformity, 54
   Julio Taleisnik

8 Results of surgical treatment of chronic boutonniere deformity: an analysis of prognostic factors, 62
   James B. Steichen, James W. Strickland, William H. Call, and **Stephen G. Powell**

SECTION THREE
FLEXOR TENDON PROBLEMS

9 Functional recovery after flexor tendon severance in the finger: the state of the art, 73
   James W. Strickland

10 Problems in the management of flexor tendon injuries in zones I and II, 86
   Robert J. Duran and **Robert G. Houser**

11 The pulley system: rationale for reconstruction, 94
   James M. Hunter and **John F. Cook, Jr.**

SECTION FOUR
BONE PROBLEMS

12 Scaphoid fractures, 105
   Donald C. Ferlic

13 Articular fractures: beware of the "unseen" forces, 107
   James H. House

14 Complex fractures of the finger metacarpals, 114
   James L. Becton

15 Factors influencing digital performance after phalangeal fracture, 126
   James W. Strickland, James B. Steichen, William B. Kleinman, and **Noreen Flynn**

16 The role of tenolysis after phalangeal fractures, 140
   Warren B. Burrows, Robert H. Hartwig, William B. Kleinman, and **James W. Strickland**

SECTION FIVE
INFECTION PROBLEMS

17 The management of difficult infections of the hand, 147
   Thomas L. Greene and **James W. Strickland**

18 Difficult infections of the hand, 156
   Lawrence H. Schneider

SECTION SIX
JOINT PROBLEMS

19 The thumb axis joints: a biomechanical model, 169

Ronald L. Linscheid

20 Management of posttraumatic arthritis of the proximal interphalangeal joint with silicone implant arthroplasty, 173

James W. Strickland, J. Anthony Dustman, Leo Steizer, William B. Stromberg, Jr., James B. Steichen, and John L. Bell

21 Controversies in hand surgery: resection arthroplasty versus silicone replacement arthroplasty for trapeziometacarpal osteoarthritis, 183

Richard J. Smith and Peter C. Amadio

22 Carpometacarpal dislocations (excluding the thumb), 189

Thomas L. Greene and James W. Strickland

SECTION SEVEN
RHEUMATOID ARTHRITIS PROBLEMS

23 The caput ulnae syndrome: update, 199

Mack L. Clayton

24 Flexor tenosynovitis in the rheumatoid hand, 203

Donald C. Ferlic and Mack L. Clayton

25 Complex arthritic disabilities of the thumb, 205

James W. Strickland and William B. LaSalle

26 Rheumatoid arthritis of the wrist, 216

Julio Taleisnik

27 The surgical management of multiple-level deformities of the rheumatoid hand: a practical approach, 224

James W. Strickland and William B. LaSalle

SECTION EIGHT
MICROVASCULAR PROBLEMS

28 A rationale for digital salvage, 243

James W. Strickland

29 Ulnar artery thrombosis: a rationale for management, 253

James R. Urbaniak and L. Andrew Koman

30 Traction avulsion amputations of the upper extremity replanted by microvascular anastomosis, 264

Harry J. Buncke and Elliott H. Rose

SECTION NINE
TENDON TRANSFER PROBLEMS

31 Restoration of lateral pinch in quadriplegia secondary to spinal cord injury: surgery selection by functional level, 275

James H. House

32 Low ulnar nerve palsy: evaluation and treatment considerations, 285

Hill Hastings II

33 Hand reconstruction and tendon transfer problems, 300

H. Kirk Watson

SECTION TEN
PAIN PROBLEMS

34 Reflex sympathetic dystrophy, 305

Harold E. Kleinert and Graeme J. Southwick

35 Tenolysis: pain control and rehabilitation, 312

James M. Hunter, Frank Seinsheimer III, and Evelyn J. Mackin

36 The painful neuroma, 319

George E. Omer, Jr.

37 The surgical management of painful neuromas in the hand, 324

Thomas L. Greene and James B. Steichen

SECTION ELEVEN
WRIST PROBLEMS

38 Limited wrist arthrodesis, 335

H. Kirk Watson

39 Scapholunate dissociation, 341

Julio Taleisnik

40 Static and dynamic forces on the multiple-linked carpus as an explanation for wrist deformity, 349

Ronald L. Linscheid

41 Arthrodesis of the wrist (position and technique), 352
Mack L. Clayton

42 Management of the radial clubhand, 355
William B. Kleinman

SECTION TWELVE
NERVE PROBLEMS

43 The neuroma-in-continuity, 369
George E. Omer, Jr.

44 The ulnar nerve at the elbow, 374
George E. Omer, Jr.

45 Selection of type of peripheral nerve repair, 379
James R. Urbaniak

SECTION THIRTEEN
DUPUYTREN'S CONTRACTURE

46 Persistent contracture of the little finger in Dupuytren's disease, 389
Robert M. McFarlane

47 Treatment of Dupuytren's contracture by extensive fasciectomy through multiple Y-V–plasty incisions: short-term evaluation of 170 consecutive operations, 399
H. Kirk Watson

48 Problems of Dupuytren's contracture, 402
Harold E. Kleinert, Ian Leitch, David J. Smith, Jr., and Lawrence M. Lubbers

49 Dupuytren's contracture: treatment by the open-palm technique, 409
William B. Kleinman

50 The proximal interphalangeal joint in Dupuytren's contracture, 414
Thomas L. Greene, James W. Strickland, and R. Fred Torstrick

SECTION ONE   SKIN PROBLEMS

Chapter 1 Abrasion injuries of the hand

James E. Bennett

Abrasions of the hand are common. Fortunately most are superficial and heal without sequelae. A few, however, are more harmful to the skin and may expose or damage deeper tissues. Heat generated by friction may increase tissue loss, but it is difficult to assess its impact on the injury. Patients I have treated for serious hand or forearm abrasions usually have had an element of avulsion in the injured area. The mechanism of injury is either contact of the part with a moving object (e.g., bench grinder, rope or cable, or conveyer belt) or projection of the victim from or by a moving vehicle onto a dirt, gravel, cinder, or paved surface.

The most important aspect of treatment is diagnosis. The extent and depth of damage and the determination of tissue viability (or lack thereof) will dictate surgical treatment. Nonviable skin or damaged skin that will "heal" with excessive scar should be excised. Intravenous fluorescein may be helpful when there is doubt. If tendons or nerves have been severed or avulsed, their repair should await the reestablishment of skin and soft tissue integrity. The case reports that follow illustrate abrasion injuries of various upper limb parts and the factors that determine the choice of skin replacement.

SECTION 1 SKIN PROBLEMS

Case 1

A 4-year old boy was struck by a car, incurring avulsion-abrasion injuries of the face and hand. The facial wounds were repaired by simple closure, and the hand avulsion was covered with split-thickness skin grafts. Two years later the only observable deformity was a hypertrophic scar encircling the skin graft on the hand (Fig. 1-1). Had the deep abrasion surrounding the hand avulsion been excised—as it was in the ankle abrasion shown in Fig. 1-2—this complication could have been avoided.

Deep partial thickness abrasions of the dorsum of the hand should be excised and closed with skin grafts.

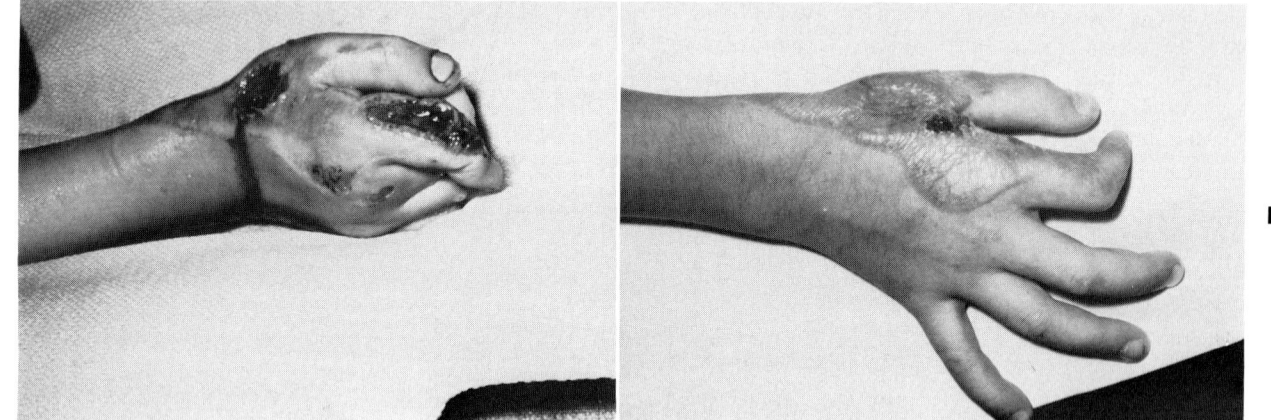

FIG. 1-1. A, Abrasion injury of radial dorsum of hand. Central full-thickness defect at base of thumb was skin grafted, and index finger wound was sutured after reduction of fracture-dislocation. **B,** Wound is virtually healed, but graft is bordered by hypertrophic scar with one area of excoriation.

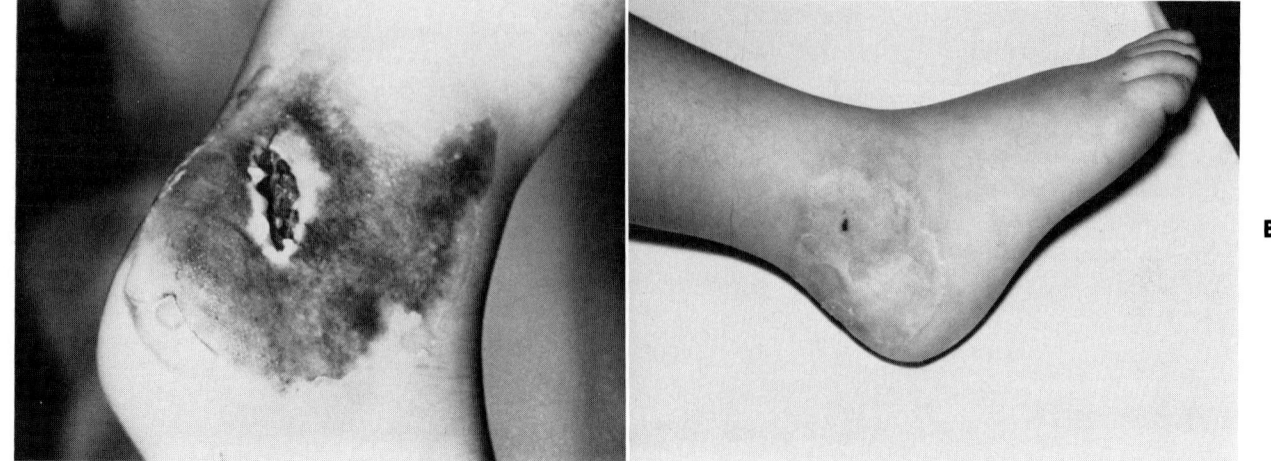

FIG. 1-2. A, Ankle wound comparable to hand injury in Fig. 1-1. Entire area of skin injury was excised and grafted. **B,** Healing without excessive scar.

Case 2

A 31-year-old man injured his hand and wrist by contact with a bench grinder. Friction diced the skin, and although little skin was missing, all shredded tissue was excised. There was a 1-cm exposure of the extensor pollicis brevis and the abductor pollicis longus tendons. Local soft tissue was used to cover the tendons, and the skin defect was closed with a split-thickness skin graft. At 4 months there was good healing and no disability (Fig. 1-3).

Diced or shredded skin should be excised. A split-thickness skin graft should be used for wound closure if the wound is suitable and tendons and nerves are intact and unexposed.

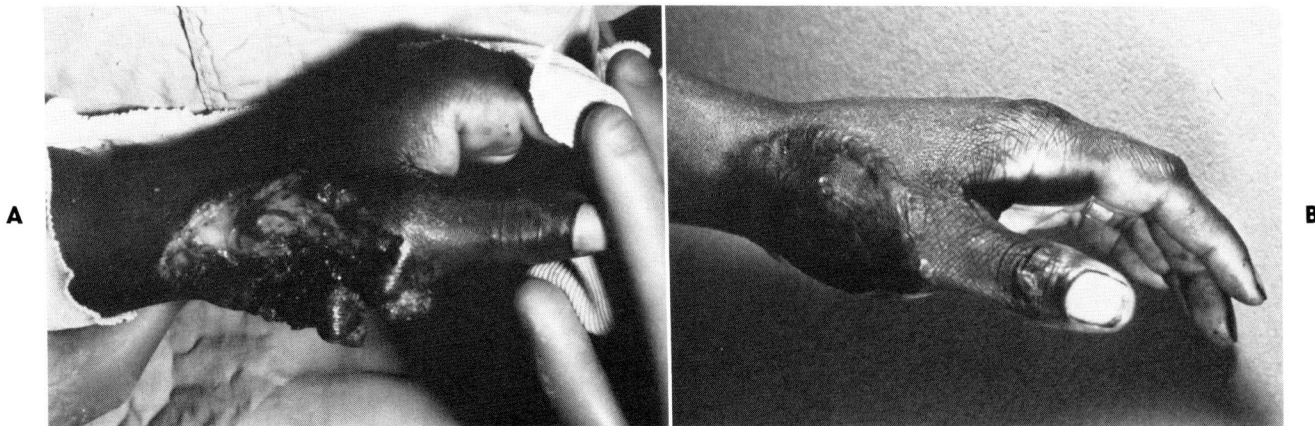

FIG. 1-3. A, Dicing abrasion of hand and wrist. All damaged skin was excised. **B,** Four months after wound closure with split-thickness skin graft.

SECTION 1 SKIN PROBLEMS

Case 3

A 21-year-old man suffered a deep rope-burn abrasion of the medial palm. Flexor tendons to the little finger were severed. The skin wound was debrided and closed with local flaps. Tendon grafting was performed 5 months later (Fig. 1-4).

Restoration of deep structure continuity in abrasion injuries should be deferred until overlying skin integrity has been provided.

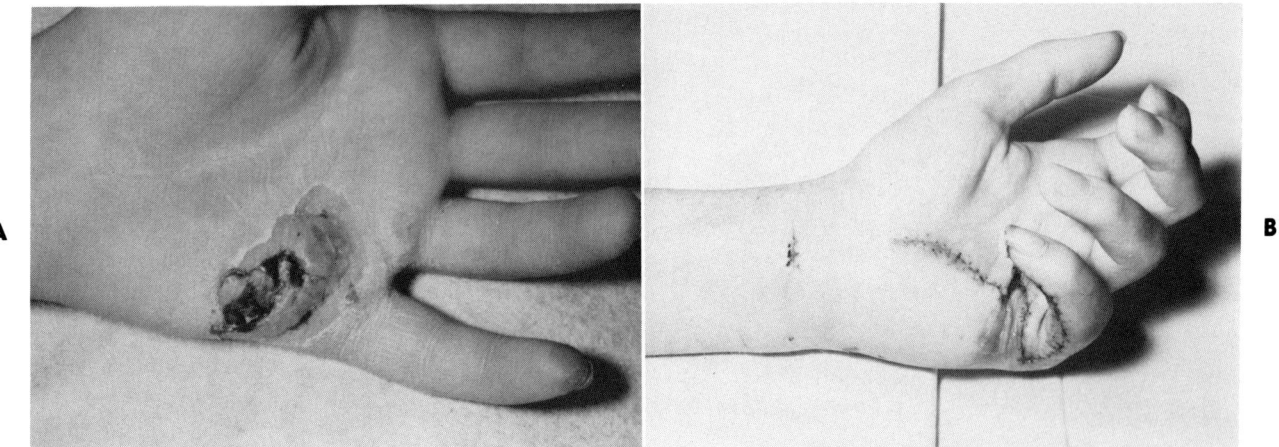

FIG. 1-4. A, Rope-burn abrasion of palm with division of little finger flexor tendons. **B,** Two weeks after placement of flexor tendon graft, 5 months after injury.

Case 4

A 29-year-old man's thumb was caught in a machine, which inflicted multiple parallel oblique lacerations of the flexor surface. The injury extended well into fatty tissue, and each isthmus of skin was of questionable viability. All damaged tissue was excised and the defect closed with a superiorly based anterior chest pedicle flap. Fortunately the slicing injuries of the distal centimeter of the pad were superficial, and this portion of the thumb healed spontaneously. The flap was divided and inset at 3 weeks (Fig. 1-5). When last seen, the patient had normal function and had returned to work. He did not wish to have reduction of the slightly bulky thumb flap.

Use distant coverage only when it is likely to produce the best result.

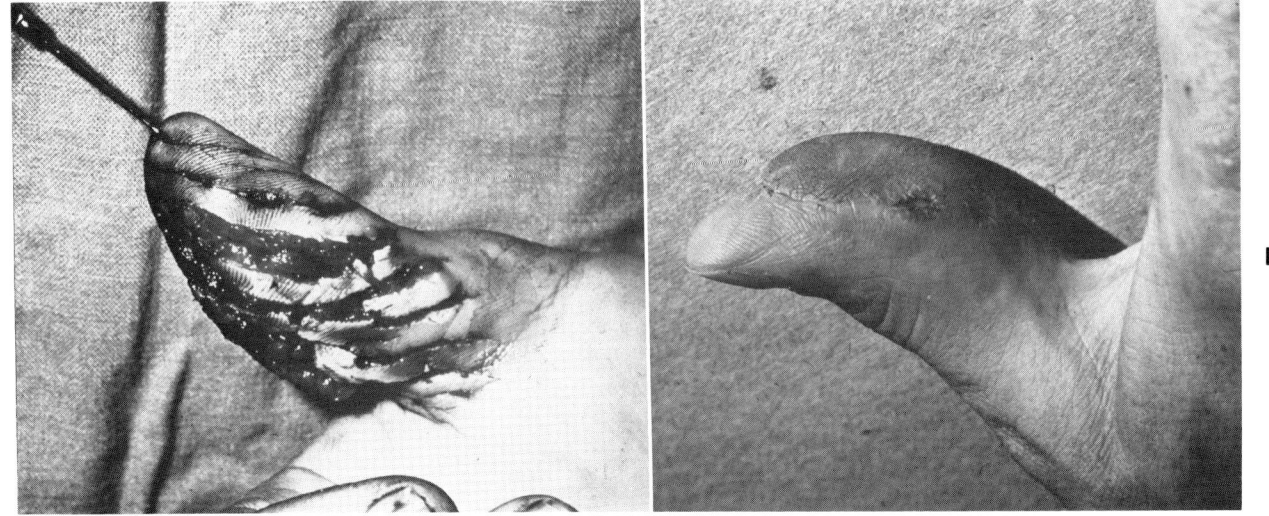

FIG. 1-5. A, Multiple slices of flexor surface of thumb. Area of full-thickness injury excised. **B,** One month after division and inset of chest pedicle to thumb.

SECTION 1 SKIN PROBLEMS

Case 5

The only injury incurred by this 24-year-old man in an automobile accident affected the long, ring, and little fingers of his left hand. The dorsal skin of each was partially scraped away. Skin loss of the fifth digit was least, and the defect was repaired by wound-edge approximation, including that of a divided extensor tendon at the proximal interphalangeal (PIP) joint level. The ring finger defect was closed with a split-thickness skin graft. There was division of the central slip of the extensor tendon of the long finger and disruption of the proximal joint capsule. A chest pedicle flap was used for closure. The flap was divided and inset at 3 weeks. When seen 2 years after injury, his only abnormality was a mallet deformity of the long finger (Fig. 1-6). A letter from the patient 4 years after injury stated that he had no disability and that he used the injured hand for bowling, golfing, writing, and "anything else that is necessary."

The extent and depth of the abrasion wound and the status of deeper structures will often dictate the method of wound repair.

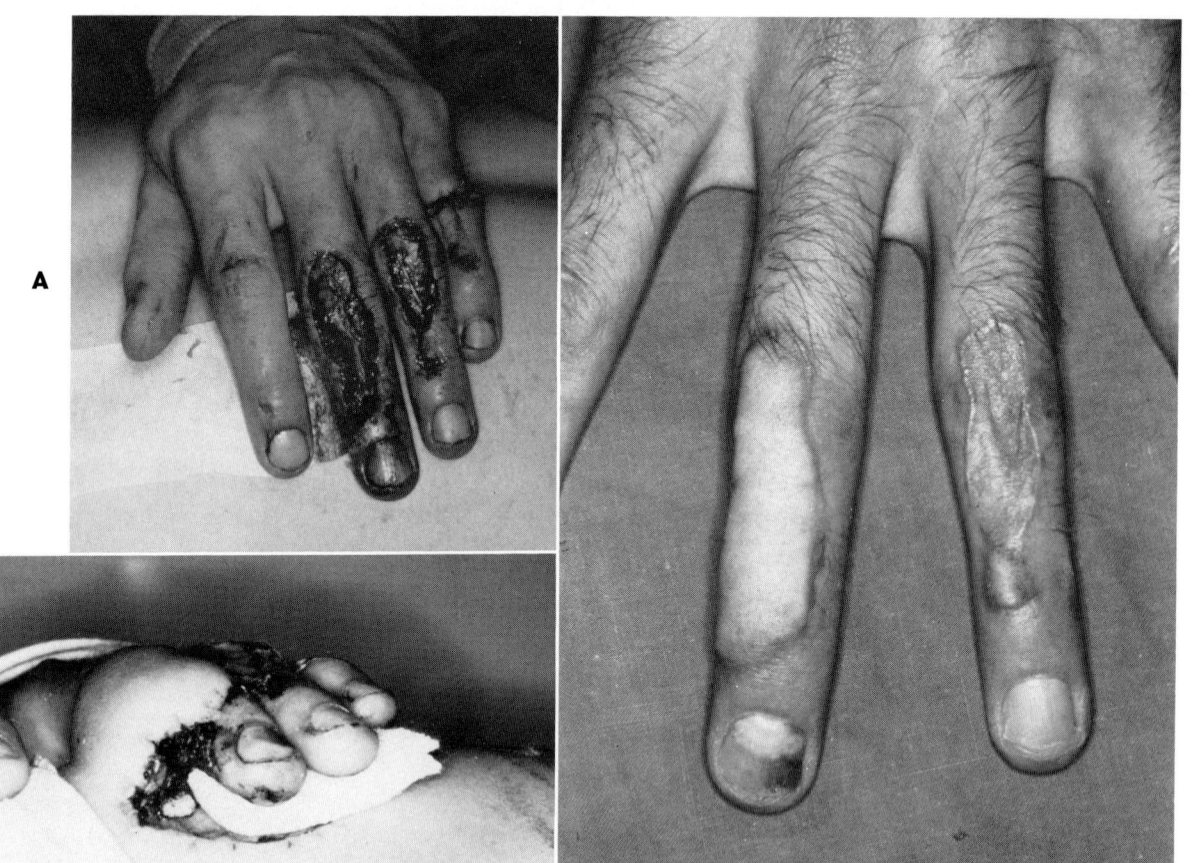

FIG. 1-6. A, Abrasion injury of long, ring, and little fingers. Long-finger wound was deepest, with disruption of PIP joint capsule. **B,** Little finger wound closed by primary suture, ring finger with split-thickness graft, and long finger by chest pedicle flap. **C,** All wounds are healed, and function is normal.

SUMMARY

Management of abrasions of the hand and forearm that will not heal spontaneously without disability or deformity requires an accurate assessment of the extent of injury. Cherry, bronze, or cherry-white skin may actually be full thickness in depth and should be excised at the first treatment. Whether skin replacement is from local tissue, a skin graft, or a distant pedicle flap depends on the nature of the defect, tissue availability, and the integrity of deeper tissues. Repair of tendons and nerves should be deferred until skin and soft tissues have been reconstructed.

Chapter 2   Skin coverage for challenging hand injuries*

Harry J. Buncke

Gerald D. Harris

The basic principles of skin coverage of the injured hand are well established. The skin provided should be supple with adequate sensation and durability. It must not restrict the range of motion of the underlying components of the hand. Skin coverage should be restored in the simplest, fastest, and most reliable manner.

Traditionally, skin coverage has been provided by split-thickness skin grafts, full-thickness skin grafts, local pedicle flaps, distant pedicle flaps, or a combination of these methods. However, the development of microsurgical tissue transplantation and replantation techniques has made possible the transfer in a single operation of large flaps containing full-thickness skin and subcutaneous tissue. These new tissue transfer techniques deserve consideration along with the classic techniques when planning the care of an injured hand. The procedure chosen should best satisfy the aforementioned criteria. The advantages and disadvantages of each method for resurfacing the hand are discussed here.

*Sponsored in part by the Office of Naval Research (Grant no. N00014-76-C-0486).

SPLIT-THICKNESS SKIN GRAFT

The split-thickness skin graft is readily available in large quantities. Split grafts are easily harvested and will survive on most open wounds that are not infected. Exceptions are exposed tendon and bone that lack paratenon or periosteum, respectively. The delicate tissue layers of split grafts provide the vascular support necessary for skin graft survival. If the wound is infected, the graft will not survive but may function as a biologic dressing.

One of the main disadvantages of split-thickness skin grafts is that they are subject to significant contraction as wound healing occurs. This can result in web-space contracture, joint immobility, and limited tendon excursion. In addition, split-thickness skin will ulcerate at points that are subjected to repeated trauma, pressure, or shearing forces, and sensory return is seldom satisfactory except in very small grafts.

FULL-THICKNESS SKIN GRAFTS

Full-thickness skin grafts provide thicker and more durable coverage. They do not contract as do split grafts and consequently are useful in correcting contractures. However, these grafts require excellent uncontaminated vascular beds, which are seldom present except in surgically created wounds. Again, sensory return is poor.

LOCAL FLAPS

Local flaps include cross-finger flaps,[3] palmar flaps,[6] thenar flaps,[5] and neurovascular island flaps.[7] They are used in areas where vascularized skin is needed, i.e., over joints, tendons, and fingertips. They are reliable because they carry their own blood supply. Because they are small and well vascularized, frequently there will be some useful sensory return. The neurovascular island flap, of course, carries its own nerve supply as well as its vascular supply; sensation is usually excellent, although some reeducation must occur to associate the sensory perception of this new location. The disadvantages[11] of these flaps are their limited size and the morbidity associated with the donor sites, which are resurfaced with split-thickness skin grafts.

DISTANT PEDICLE FLAPS

Distant pedicle flaps include the cross-arm flap,[4] the deltopectoral flap,[8] the vertical abdominal flap of Shaw and Payne,[10] and the groin flap recently described by McGregor and Jackson.[8] These flaps offer large amounts of well-vascularized tissue. A disadvantage of distant flaps is the need for multiple-stage procedures for the elevation, delay, division, and transfer of the flap. In addition, the resultant skin coverage is bulky and difficult to tailor because of the thick layer of subcutaneous fat present in these flaps plus the scarring and the contracture that develops during transfer. These flaps are associated with poor sensory return. During the period in which these multiple stages are performed, the recipient hand tends to become swollen and stiff, especially if it is attached to the groin or lower abdomen. The resultant dependent edema plus the stiffness associated with prolonged immobilization may produce irreversible changes.

MICROVASCULAR COMPOSITE TISSUE TRANSPLANTS

Microvascular composite tissue transplants offer many advantages. Large areas of skin can be transferred in a single operation with or without a sensory nerve supply and with or without accompanying bone, tendon, or other specialized structures.[2,12] The principal disadvantages are that the operations are tedious, time consuming, and require special surgical skills and equipment.

GOAL OF SURGEON

The hand surgeon's primary goal in acute hand injuries is to achieve a closed wound to prevent scarring and infection and to protect vital structures. Usually a split-thickness skin graft is preferable to full-thickness grafts or flap coverage. Split-thickness grafts allow the hand to be free and elevated so that associated traumatic edema, stiffness, and scarring are minimized, thus preserving joint motion. Primary flap coverage is provided, if necessary, to protect tendons, bones, joints, and vital structures. Cross-arm, deltopectoral, and submammary flaps permit continuous elevation of the hand, unlike the groin flap or lower abdominal flap. Joint stiffness and immobility following these procedures are not limited to the hand but also include the elbow and shoulder.

The chronic hand injury often requires complex procedures to restore ideal skin coverage. A combination of grafts and flaps may be necessary, but the simplest technique that will satisfy all the needs should be used.

The final objective of all hand operations is to restore sensation, tendon excursion, grip, and pinch. An important by-product of improved hand function is improved appearance of the hand.

CASE HISTORIES

The following case histories illustrate available options for providing ideal skin coverage in acute and chronic hand injuries.

SECTION 1 SKIN PROBLEMS

Case 1

A 17-year-old girl sustained a crushing injury of the left hand with loss of all fingers and the thumb (Fig. 2-1). Three fingers were successfully replanted, and a large dorsal wound proximal to the digits was closed with a split-thickness skin graft. The graft provided coverage for the underlying joint capsules, tendons, and multiple vein grafts inserted across the wound to drain the replants. The replanted thumb was lost and later replaced with a large toe transplant. Again, a split-thickness skin graft was used to cover the base of the toe transplant and the dorsal wound over the area of the first metacarpal. This case illustrates the value of split-thickness skin grafts in primary and secondary reconstructive procedures.

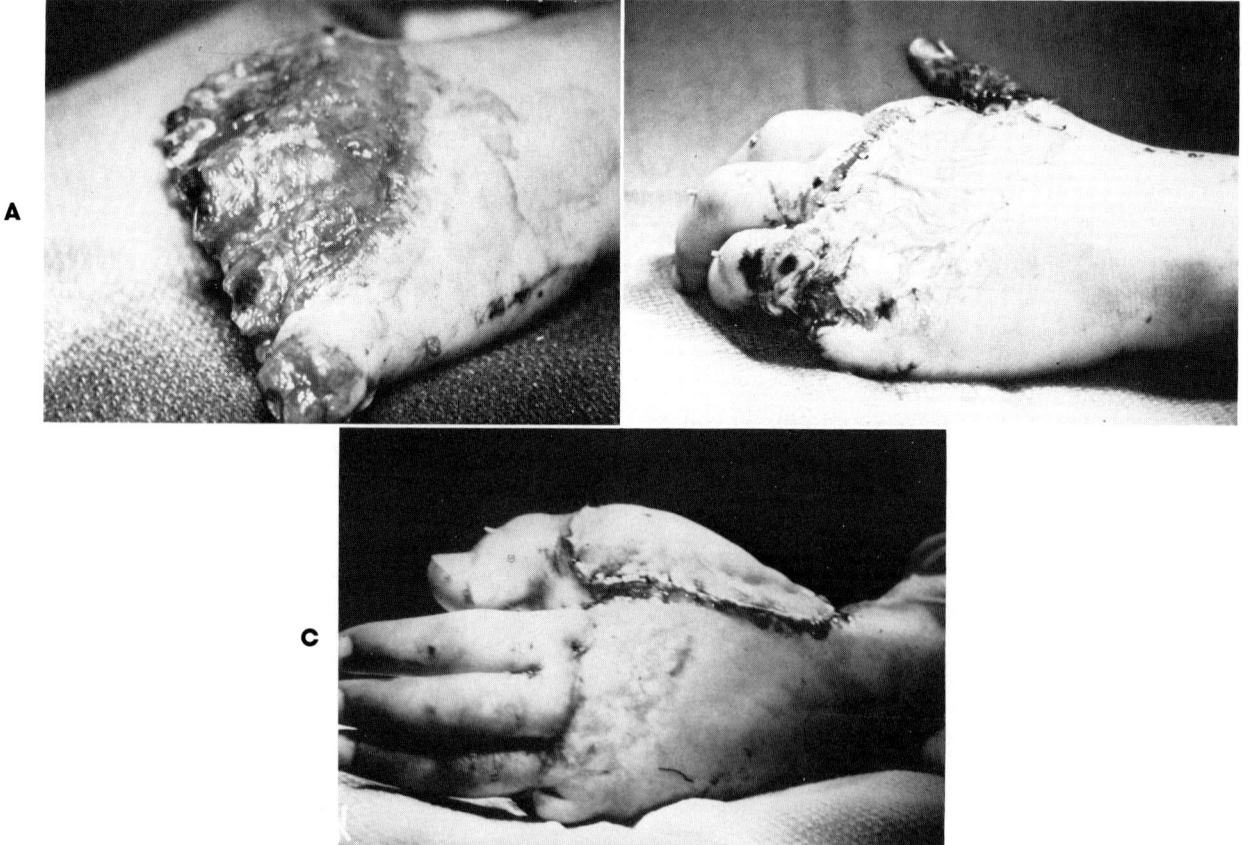

FIG. 2-1. A, Grinding avulsive amputation of all fingers and thumb. **B,** Large split-thickness skin graft used to cover dorsal defect of hand, placing it directly on segmental vein grafts, draining three replanted fingers. Thumb replant failed. **C,** Missing thumb was restored with toe transplant. Again, large split-thickness graft was needed over proximal vascular pedicle.

Case 2

An 18-year-old man sustained an avulsive amputation of his hand. During replantation a volar decompression incision of the forearm was closed with a split-thickness skin graft, which also protected underlying vein grafts in the radial and ulnar arteries (Fig. 2-2). This case also points out the value of split-thickness skin grafts used in cases of acute injury to provide coverage and wound closure without tension.

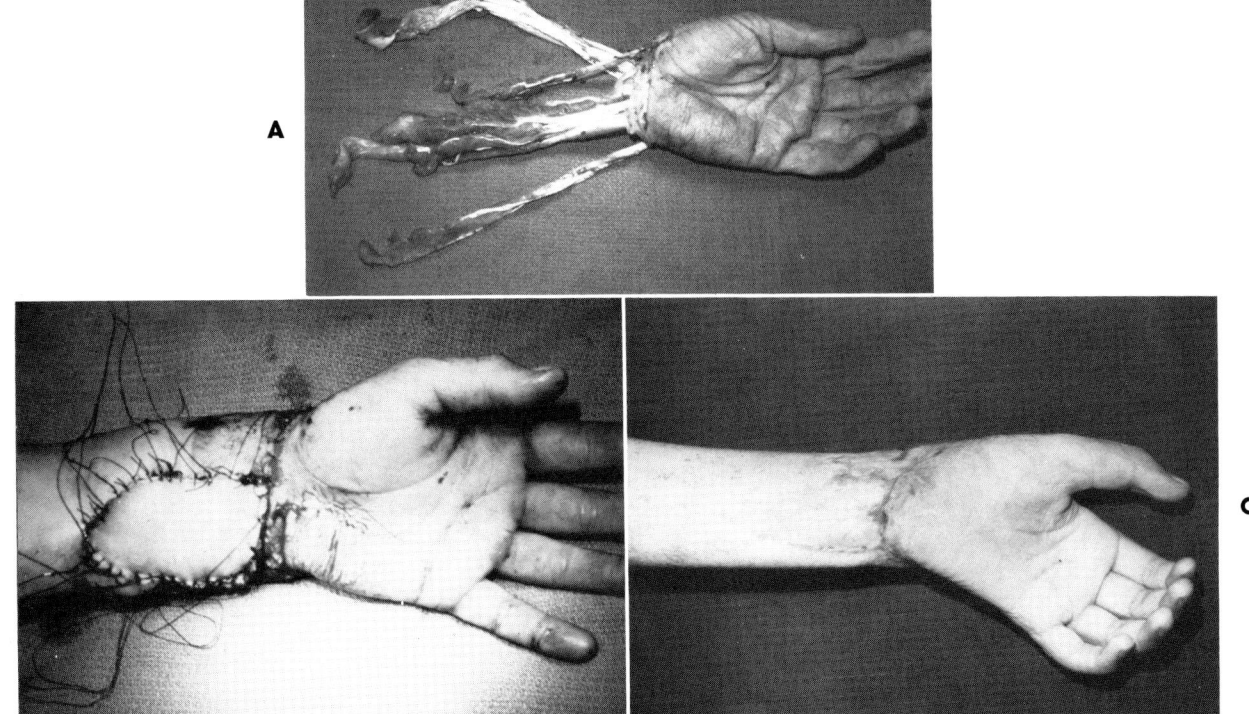

FIG. 2-2. A, Avulsive amputation of hand of 18-year-old man. **B,** Split-thickness skin graft used to cover volar relaxing incision plus underlying long vein grafts in radial and ulnar arteries. **C,** Healed skin graft and viable hand.

SECTION 1 SKIN PROBLEMS

Case 3

A 20-year-old man sustained an extensive injury to the metacarpophalangeal (MCP) joint area on the ulnar side of the left thumb, requiring a bone graft, nerve graft, and tendon repair. A neurovascular island flap was taken from the dorsoradial aspect of the second MCP joint area and was transferred through a skin tunnel to cover the soft tissue loss of the thumb, as well as to the bone graft, nerve graft, and tendon repairs (Fig. 2-3). This case illustrates the early use of a unique local flap in an acute injury.

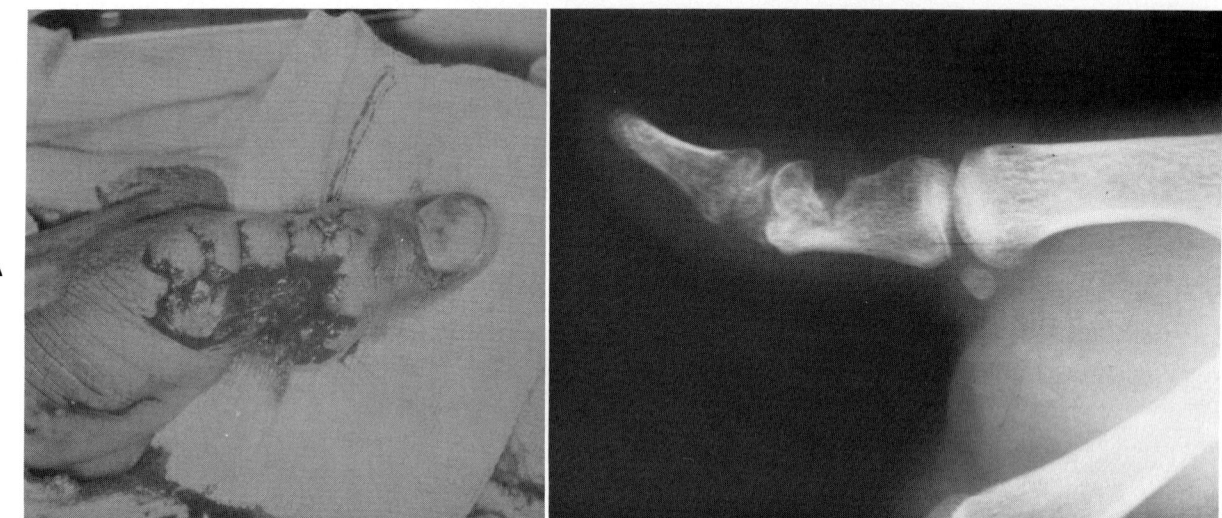

FIG. 2-3. A and **B,** Soft tissue, bone, and nerve defect on radial side of thumb of a 20-year-old man. **C,** Neurovascular island flap from dorsal aspect of second MCP joint area, based on branches of dorsoradial artery and nerve. **D,** Island flap ready to be tunneled across dorsum of thumb to defect on radial side of first MCP joint area. **E,** Healed flap covering bone graft, nerve graft in radial digital nerve, and flexor pollicis longus tendon repair.

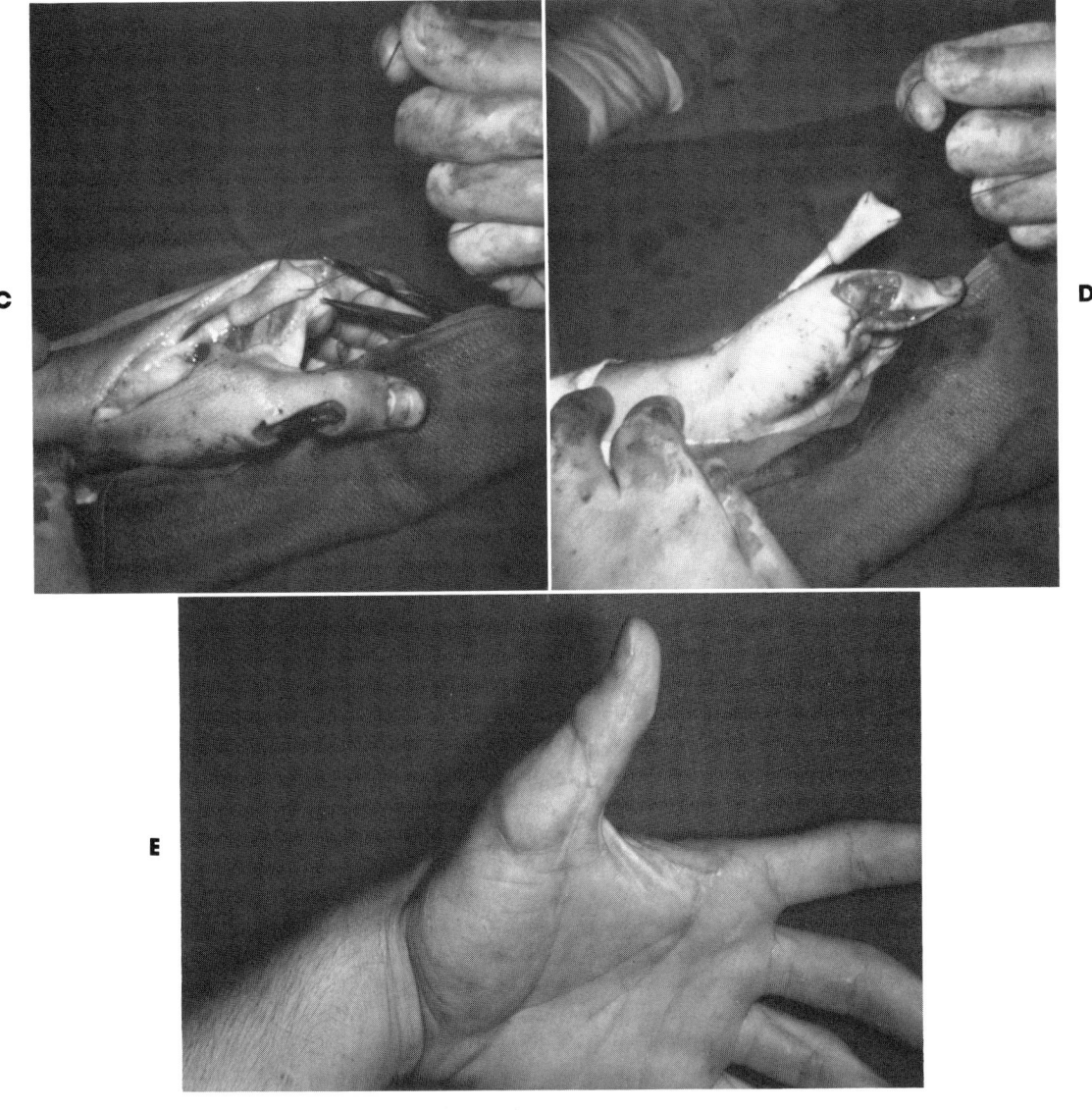

FIG. 2-3, cont'd. For legend see opposite page.

SECTION 1 SKIN PROBLEMS

Case 4

This 32-year-old man had undergone a large toe transplant to reconstruct an amputated thumb. Delayed vascular thrombosis occurred with subsequent loss of the distal phalanx. Subdermal tissues of the proximal phalanx, however, did survive. These viable proximal tissues were salvaged with an immediate deltopectoral flap. A neurovascular island flap from the ulnar side of the ring finger restored sensation to the thumb (Fig. 2-4). This case illustrates the use of a classic distant pedicle flap to provide vascular coverage over exposed bones and joints, plus a local flap to provide critical sensation to the pedicle flap.

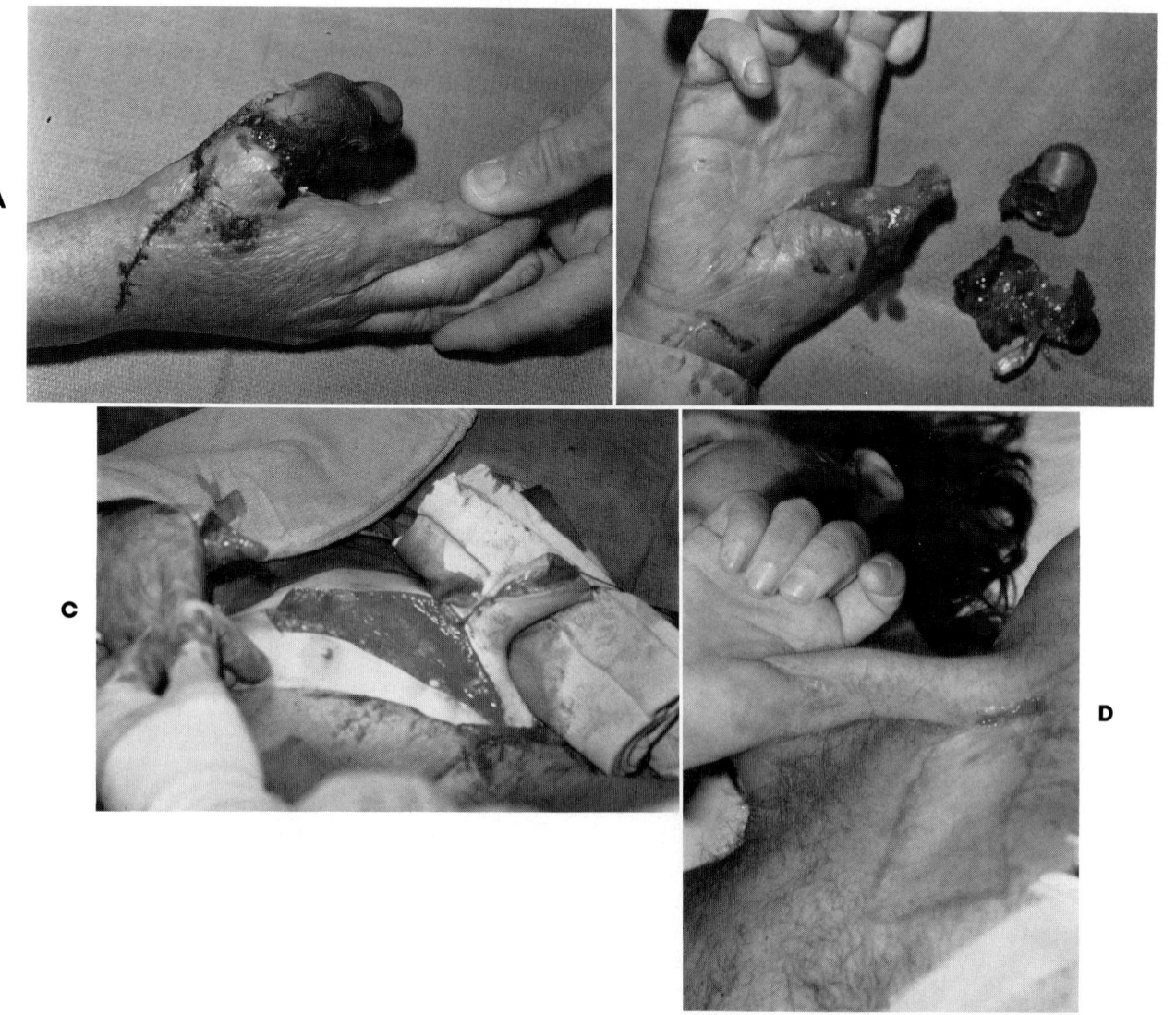

FIG. 2-4. For legend see opposite page.

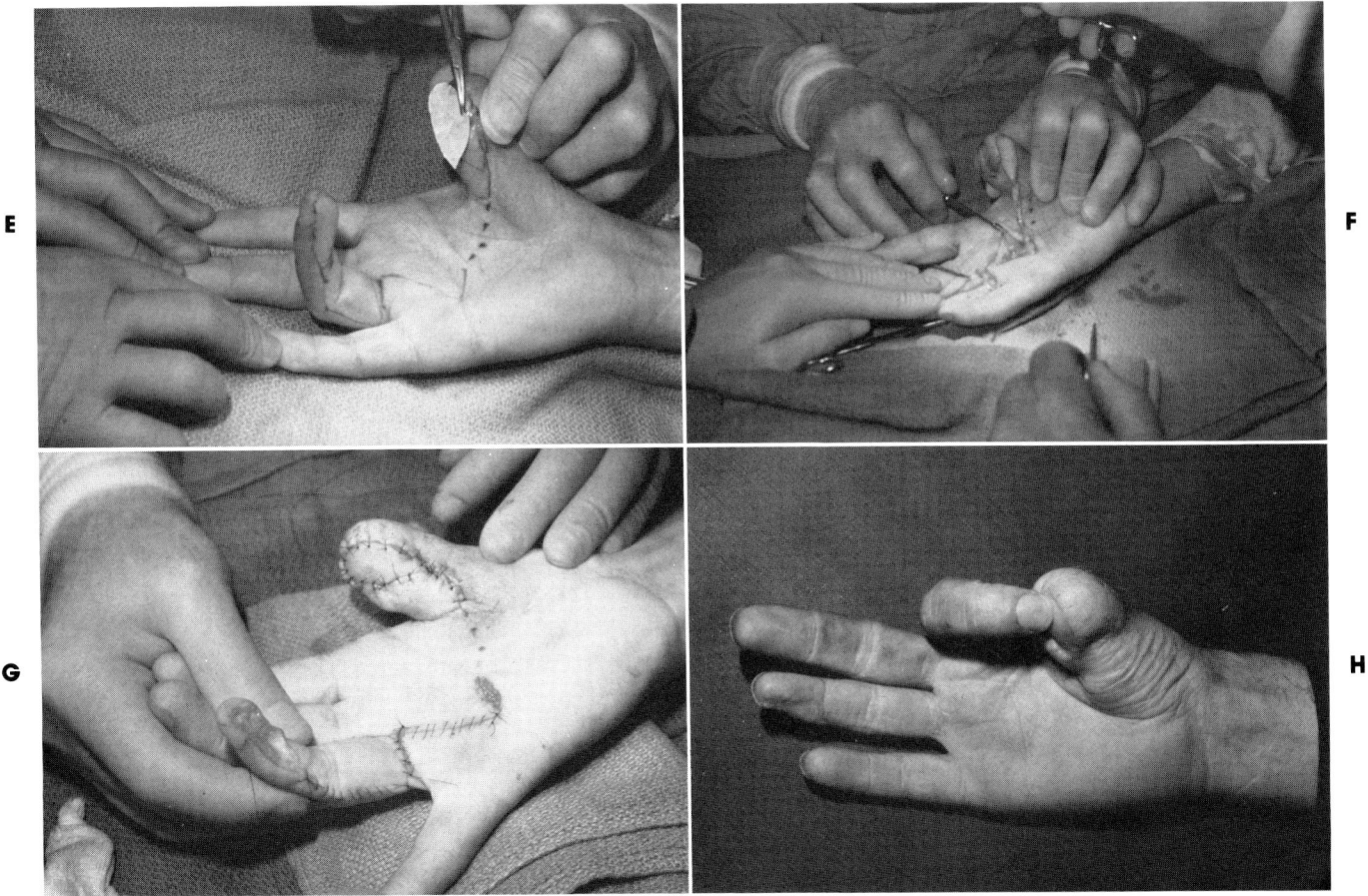

FIG. 2-4. A, Necrotic distal phalanx of large toe transplant. **B,** Viable deeper structures of proximal phalanx of toe transplant. **C,** Contralateral deltopectoral flap based on thoracoacromial vessels laterally being tubed to cover exposed structures on thumb-toe. **D,** Healed tubed flap; minimal swelling in hand because of its elevated position on upper chest. **E,** Neurovascular island flap planned from ulnar side of ring to pinch area on toe–deltopectoral flap–thumb. **F,** Island flap elevated, ready to be tunneled across palm and out on thumb. **G,** Island flap in place. **H,** Healed sensory island on pinch area of shortened toe-pedicle-thumb.

SECTION 1 SKIN PROBLEMS

Case 5

A 62-year-old man had marked flexion contractures of his long, ring, and middle fingers from a childhood burn. The contractures were excised, creating a wound in which the entire distal palm and the proximal phalanges of the fingers were exposed. Tendons, nerves, and blood vessels were bow stringing across the defect. A microvascular groin flap was transplanted to the defect, anastomosing the dorsoradial artery and vena comitans of the first web space to the superficial circumflex iliac vessels of the flap (Fig. 2-5). This case illustrates the use of microvascular transplantation to cover the vital structures in the hands of older persons. Irreversible stiffness of the hand, elbow, and shoulder may result if a conventional distant flap is used in this age group.

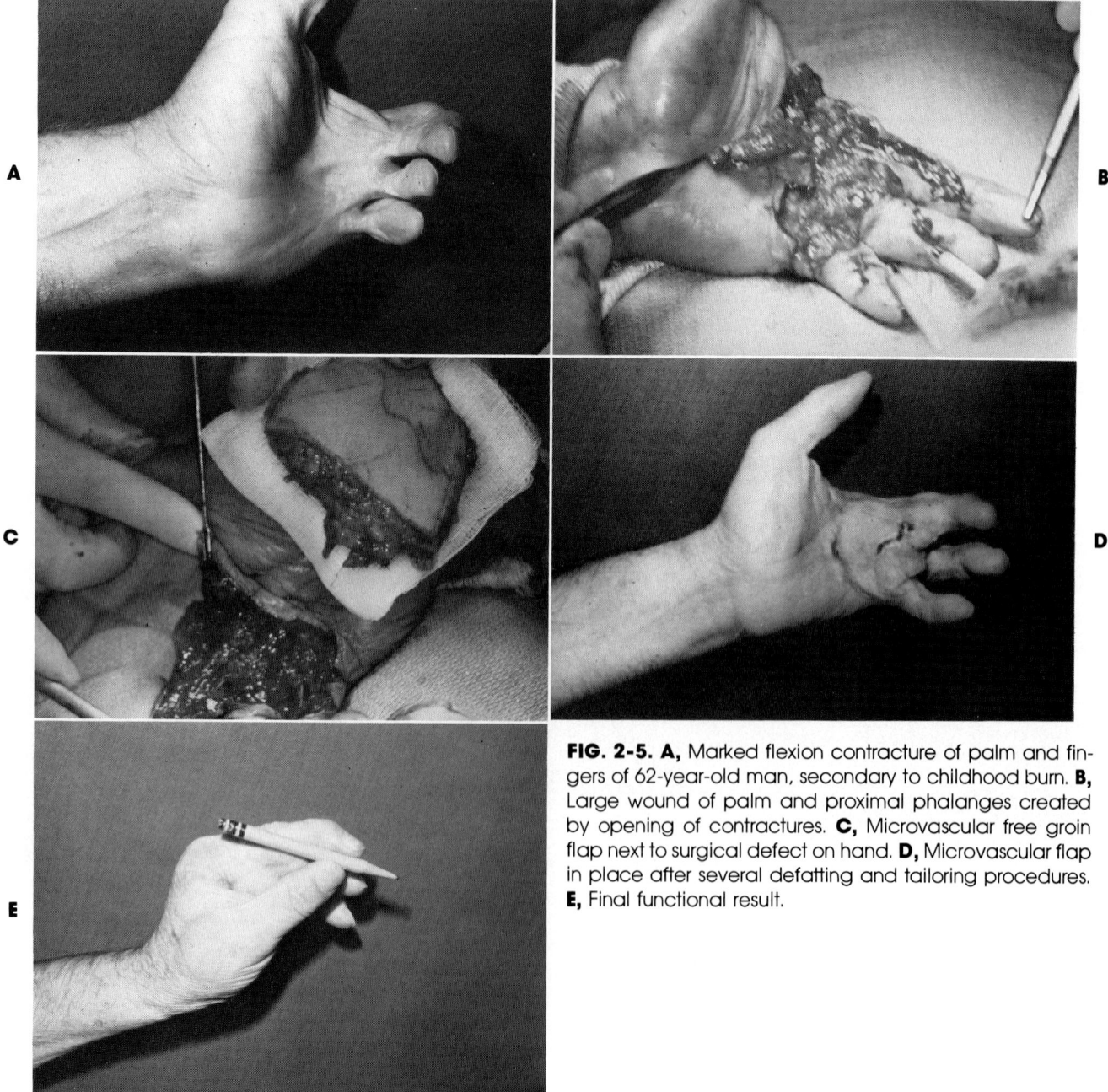

FIG. 2-5. A, Marked flexion contracture of palm and fingers of 62-year-old man, secondary to childhood burn. **B,** Large wound of palm and proximal phalanges created by opening of contractures. **C,** Microvascular free groin flap next to surgical defect on hand. **D,** Microvascular flap in place after several defatting and tailoring procedures. **E,** Final functional result.

CHAPTER 2 SKIN COVERAGE FOR CHALLENGING HAND INJURIES

Case 6

A 12-year-old boy sustained a grinding injury of the dorsoradial surface of his wrist and hand with associated loss of extensor tendons. Primary wound closure was accomplished with a large split-thickness skin graft. A microvascular groin flap then was used to permit the insertion of tendon grafts to the thumb and index and long fingers (Fig. 2-6). This case illustrates the primary use of a split-thickness skin graft to provide wound coverage and prevent infection. A composite vascularized flap was later transferred electively in one stage to replace the skin graft, which provided an ideal recipient site, free from infection and contamination. Recently Taylor and Townsend[12] have described the use of a dorsalis pedis flap with the underlying common extensor tendons carried with the flap as vascularized tendon transplants. Such a procedure would have eliminated secondary tendon grafting as a separate, third stage in this patient.

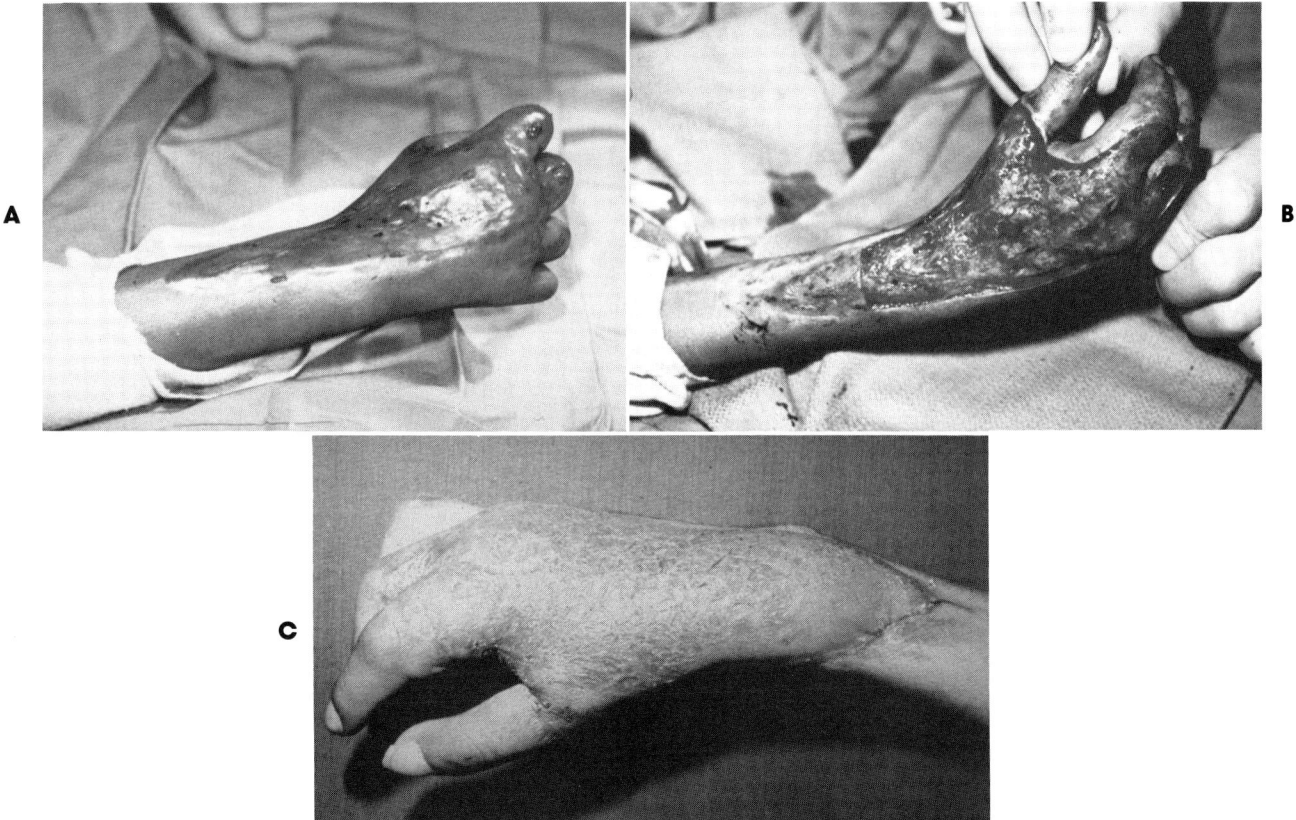

FIG. 2-6. A, Area of split-thickness skin graft on dorsum of wrist, hand, and radial digits. **B,** Graft excised and ready to receive microvascular groin flap cover. **C,** Microvascular flap healed, next to extensor tendons of thumb and index and long fingers.

SECTION 1 SKIN PROBLEMS

Case 7

A 28-year-old man lost all the soft tissue and pulp of the volar distal phalanx of his dominant right index finger after a snakebite. The finger, in essence, was nonfunctional, without sensation, and destined for amputation. To salvage the finger, a neurovascular island flap, consisting of the entire pulp substance of the second toe from the right foot, was transplanted, completely resurfacing and innervating the entire volar surface of the distal phalanx of the finger. The digital nerve of the toe was anastomosed to the radiodigital nerve of the index finger, as was the digital artery of the toe to the radiodigital artery of the index finger. A long venous pedicle was anastomosed to a dorsal vein. The patient now has a useful, pain-free index finger (Fig. 2-7). This case illustrates the use of a specialized free microvascular composite tissue transplant from the foot to restore sensation and function to a fingertip. Such transplants have an advantage over the classic Littler[7] neurovascular island flap in that sensation and coverage are not robbed from another part of an already injured hand.[1] In addition, sensory reeducation is not as essential.

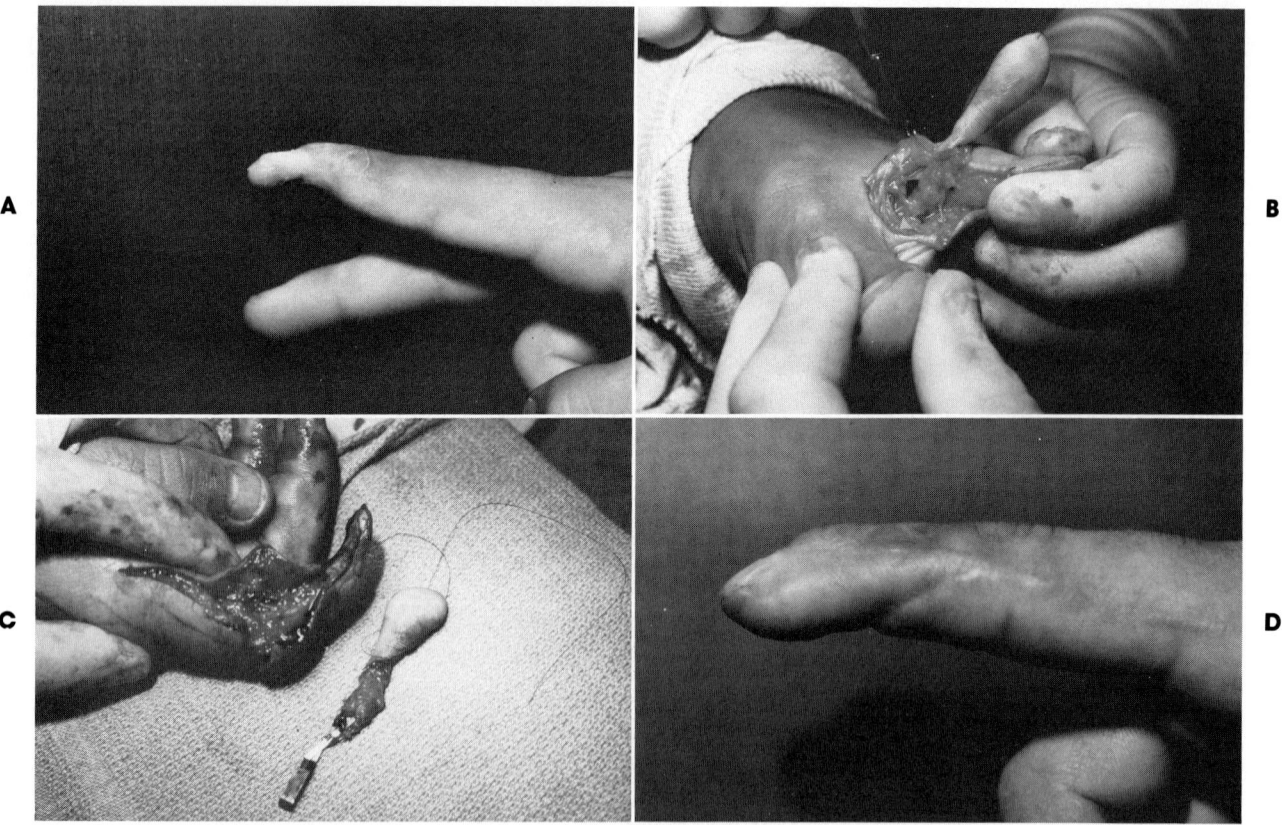

FIG. 2-7. A, Functionless index tip, devoid of pulp, covered with painful, unstable scar. **B,** Neurovascular island flap consisting of entire pulp of second toe. **C,** Microneurovascular transplant next to recipient defect on index finger. **D,** Healed transplant, restoring pulp substance, sensation, and function to index tip.

CONCLUSIONS

These case presentations are intended to illustrate various options for restoring ideal skin coverage to the hand. Other solutions to these same problems are possible; however, the actual techniques used should reflect not only the needs of the patient but also the experience and philosophies of the surgeon.

It is certainly true that new and revolutionary techniques are not necessarily the best, but it is equally true that old and well-established techniques will not always represent the ideal solution to a difficult problem.

REFERENCES

1. Buncke, H.J.: Free toe to hand transplantations by microvascular anastomosis, Trau. Int. Soc. Plast. Surgeons, Sixth Congress, Paris, 1976, Masson.
2. Buncke, H.J., and Rose, E.H.: Free toe to hand neurovascular flaps, Plast. Reconstr. Surg. **63**:607, 1979.
3. Curtis, R.M.: Cross finger pedicle flaps in hand surgery, Ann. Surg. **145**:650, 1957.
4. Delbet, J.P., and Wallich, E.: La plau du cross arm flap dans la chirurgie de la main, Ann. Chir. Plast. **9**:3, 1964.
5. Flatt, A.G.: The thenar flap, J. Bone Joint Surg. **39B**:80, 1957.
6. Fusco, E.M.: Fingertip reconstruction with palmar skin flaps, Am. J. Surg. **87**:608, 1954.
7. Littler, J.W.: Neurovascular stem island transfer in reconstructive hand surgery, Trau. Int. Soc. Plast. Surgeons, Second Congress, London, 1959, E & S Livingstone.
8. McGregor, I.A., and Jackson, I.T.: The extended role of the deltopectoral flap, Br. J. Plast. Surg. **23**:173, 1970.
9. Sharzer, L.A., Barker, D.T., and Adamson, J.E.: Free composite tissue transfer in the upper extremities: a comparison with existing methods. In Serafin, D., and Buncke, H.J., editors: Microsurgical composite tissue transplantation, St. Louis, 1978, The C.V. Mosby Co.
10. Shaw, D.T., and Payne, R.L., Jr.: Repair of surface defects of the upper extremity, Ann. Surg., vol. 123, 1946.
11. Smith, J.R., and Bom, A.F.: An evaluation of fingertip reconstruction by cross finger and palmar pedicle flap, Plast. Reconstr. Surg. **35**:409, 1965.
12. Taylor, G.I., and Townsend, P.: Composite free flap and tendon transfer: an anatomical study and a clinical technique, Br. J. Plast. Surg., **32**:170, 1979.

Chapter 3 Fingernail injuries

Elvin G. Zook

The most common injury to the nail is the subungual hematoma, which is treated by decompression and drainage with infrequent complications. A much less common but more serious injury is the injury to the nail bed and germinal portions of the nail in the nail fold. If the latter is not treated as a serious injury, there is a high incidence of resultant split, rough, and/or nonadherent nail. This deformity can be a real occupational problem for persons who handle cloth or material on which the nail can be caught.

ANATOMY

There is little similarity in the terms used for describing various portions of the nail and surrounding anatomy. Lewis[4] describes a useful map that should enable us to communicate regarding this area (Fig. 3-1). The nail takes its origin from the proximal portion of the floor of the nail fold and one half of the proximal portion of the roof of the fold. The portion of the nail formed by the roof is a minor part of the resultant hard nail.

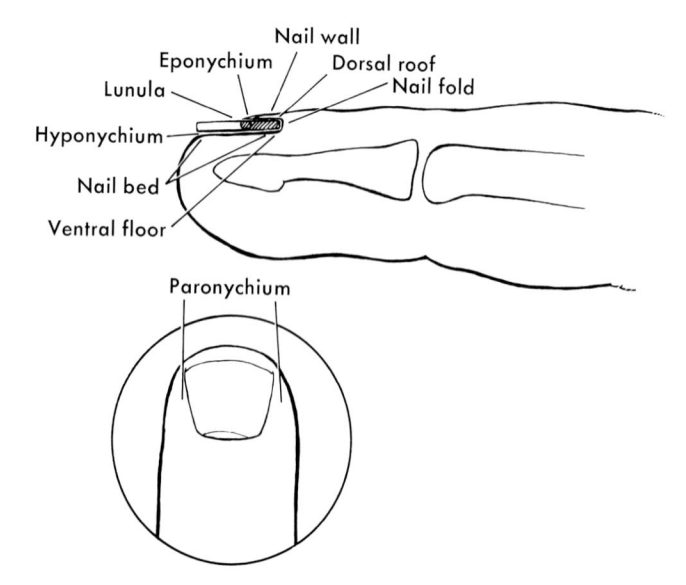

FIG. 3-1. Sagittal and dorsal anatomy of nail. Perionychium is paronychium plus nail bed.

PHYSIOLOGY

After injury to the nail there is a 3-week delay before growth of the nail starts, and then it grows 0.1 mm per day.[1] The portion of the nail proximal to the injury is thicker, since it apparently thickens during the delay but does not move distally. The thickening lasts for 50 days and is followed by 30 days of production of a thinner nail. Therefore at least 100 days pass before a normal nail is produced. The nail does not just adhere to the bed, but the epithelium of the bed actually becomes a part of the nail.[8] Kligman[3] has demonstrated that the dorsal roof of the nail fold and the lateral limits of the cul-de-sac prevent unlimited upward nail growth. This forces it to flatten and grow horizontally in a distal direction. He transplanted segments of the ventral floor of the nail fold of the toe to the forearm, and upward growth rather than lateral growth occurred.

The nails of the longer fingers grow the fastest, and the thumbnail grows the slowest. Although there is no difference between the sexes in the rate of growth, nails grow faster in summer than in winter, and nail biting accelerates growth.[5]

INJURY TO THE MATRIX

When a subungual hematoma involves more than a small portion of the nail or the nail is broken, the tuft fractured, or the nail fold lacerated, the nail should be removed and the injury of the nail bed repaired. This is especially true in females or children where a smooth nail is particularly important functionally as well as cosmetically.

Many times when the nail is removed, a seemingly minor injury is found to involve a severe stellate laceration of the bed (Figs. 3-2 and 3-3). The nail bed should be approximated with fine sutures (7-0 chromic) under loupe magnification (preferably 4×) (Fig. 3-4). The nail is then cleaned and replaced, as advocated by Schiller[6] (Fig. 3-5). He reasons that it maintains a smooth, even surface and positions the matrix edges properly for healing and growth. It is also an excellent splint for the fractured tuft. A few fine drill holes in the nail will allow drainage. If these methods are used, the vast majority of

CHAPTER 3 FINGERNAIL INJURIES

nails should grow out smooth and even (Fig. 3-6). If the nail has been lost, Swanker[7] describes the use of a piece of tantalum as a nail substitute. I prefer to use a nail-shaped piece of 0.020-inch Silastic sheeting held in the nail fold by three horizontal matrix sutures of 5-0 Ethilon. This material is smooth, shapes the nail matrix, and maintains the nail fold accurately.

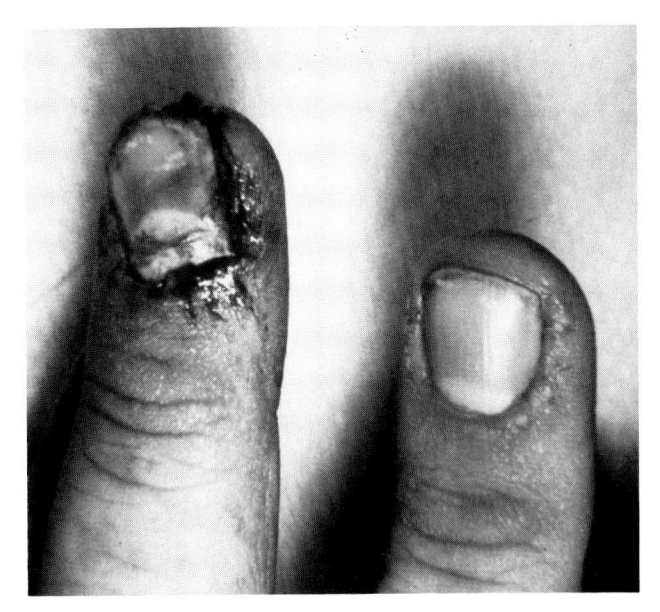

FIG. 3-2. An obvious severe injury of nail bed with nail still partially attached.

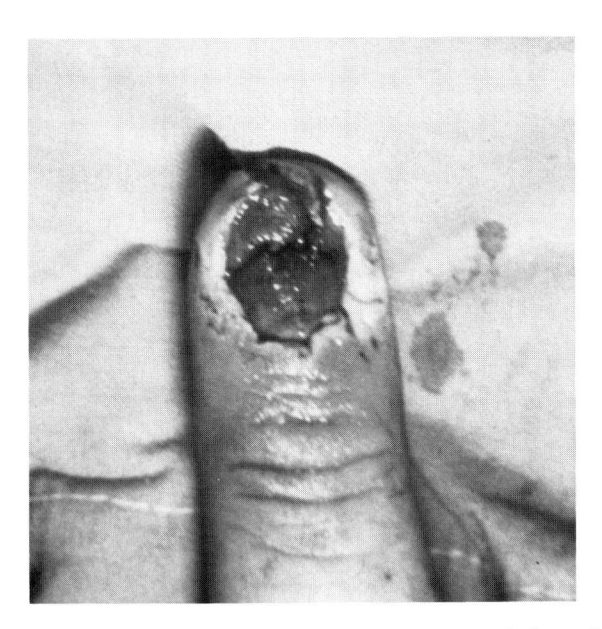

FIG. 3-3. Stellate laceration of nail bed and fingertip found after nail removal.

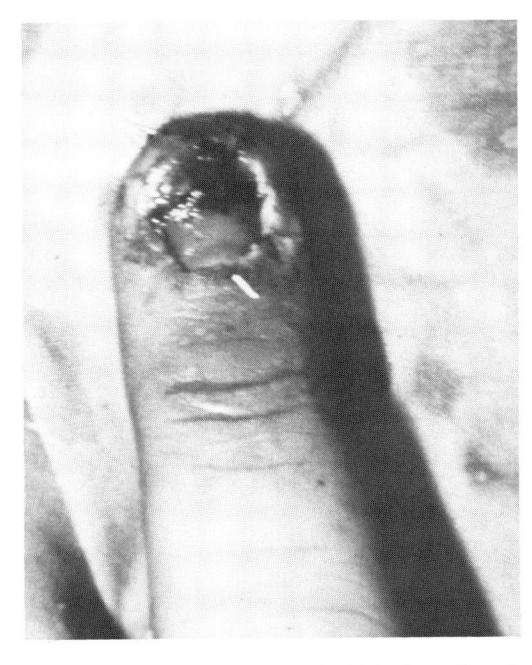

FIG. 3-4. Nail bed repaired with 7-0 chromic suture.

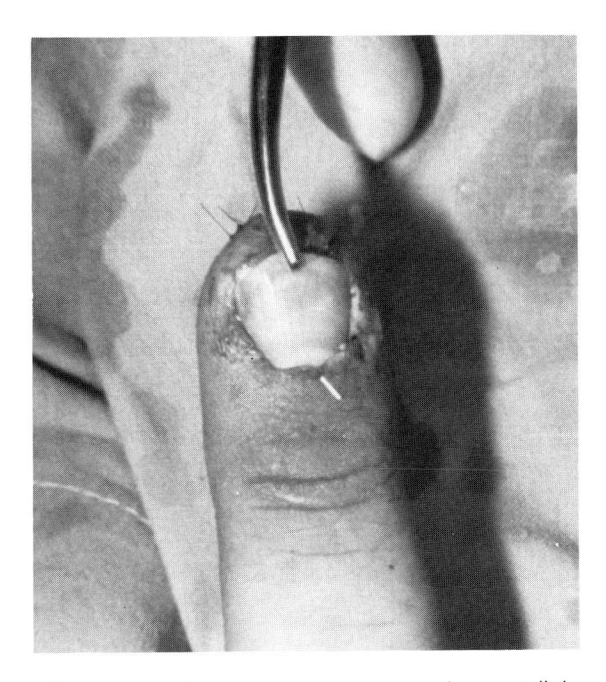

FIG. 3-5. Nail cleaned and replaced as a splint.

SECTION 1 SKIN PROBLEMS

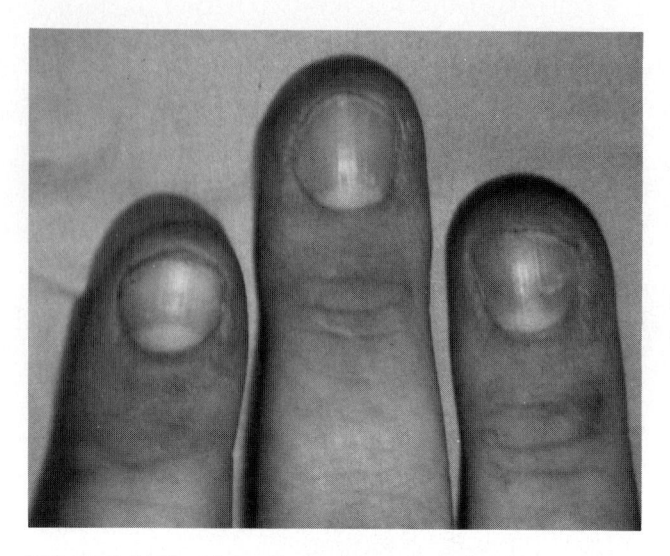

FIG. 3-6. Nail of long finger 8 months after injury without any deformity.

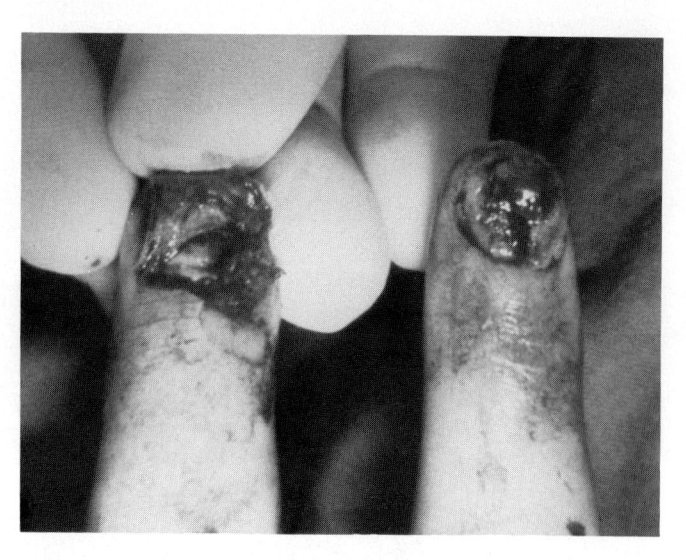

FIG. 3-7. Laceration of roof and floor of nail fold and laceration of nail bed of adjacent finger.

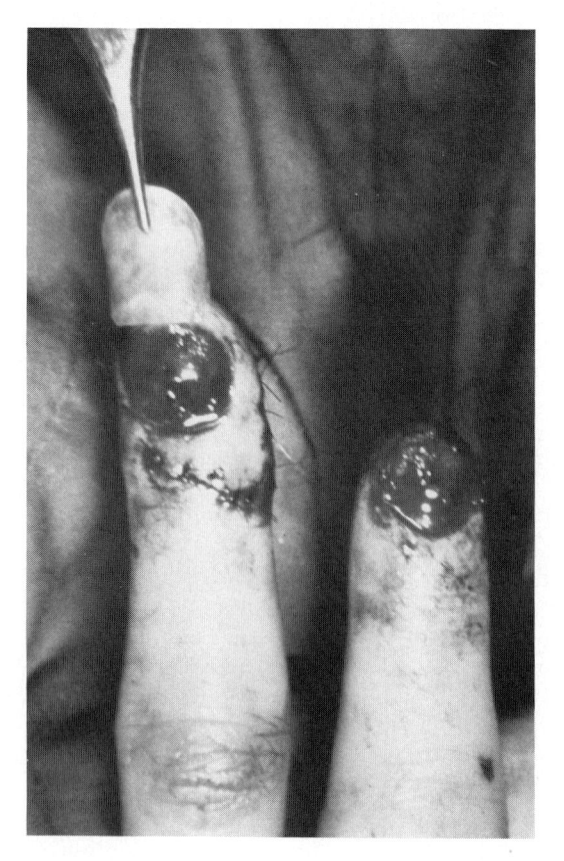

FIG. 3-8. Multilayered closure, with magnification, of nail fold and nail replaced.

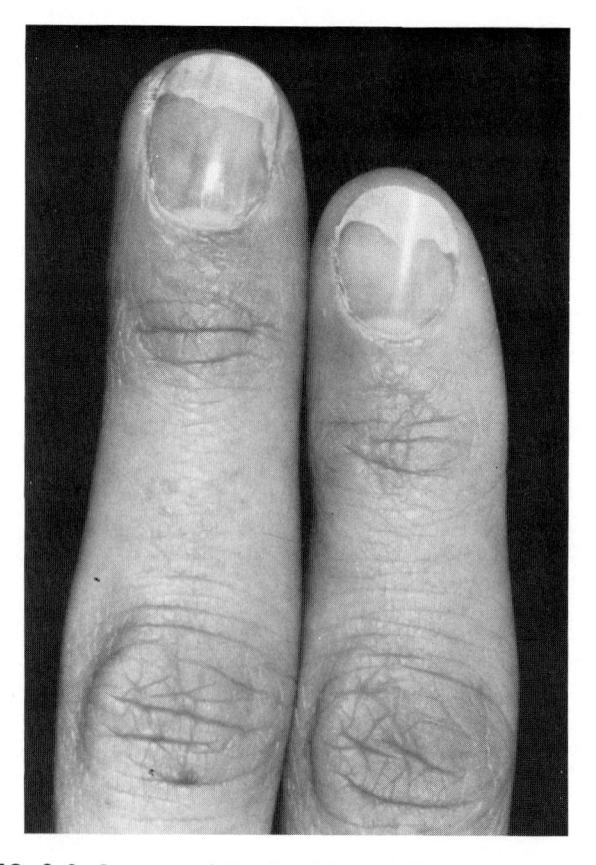

FIG. 3-9. One year following injury. Nails are shown here with only slight deformity.

NAIL FOLD INJURIES

Injuries to the nail fold, where the nail is formed, are even more serious, with good care more critical (Fig. 3-7). The principles of accurate approximation apply here, as in nail bed repairs. Both the dorsal roof and the ventral floor of the nail fold must be approximated with fine absorbable sutures (7-0 chromic). All knots should be placed so that they are in the sulcus of the nail fold and not buried in the soft tissue around it. The skin is sutured with 6-0 monofilament Ethilon. Again, the nail forms a splint to maintain the fold open and in position to form a new smooth nail (Figs. 3-8 and 3-9). Even severe crushing injuries (Fig. 3-10) of the nail bed, nail fold, and dorsal skin of the finger can result in a relatively smooth nail if cleaned, carefully sutured, and splinted with the nail or nail substitute (Figs. 3-11 and 3-12).

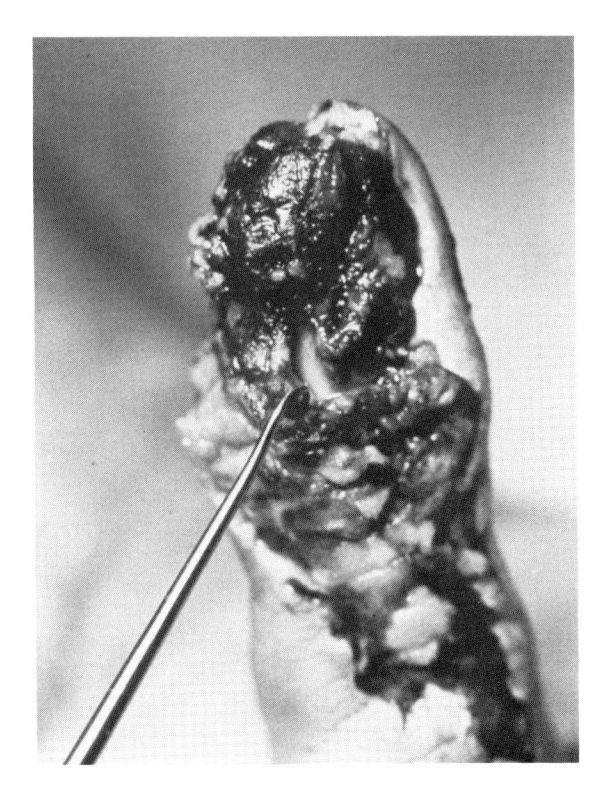

FIG. 3-10. Crushing laceration of the nail bed, nail fold, and dorsum of finger.

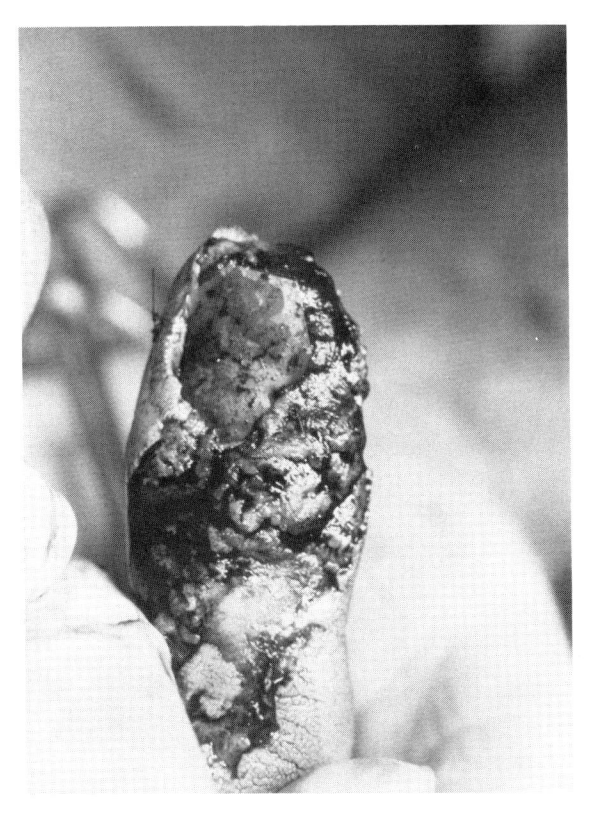

FIG. 3-11. Nail after careful approximation of tissue with magnification, suture with fine chromic suture, and use of Silastic sheeting for nail replacement.

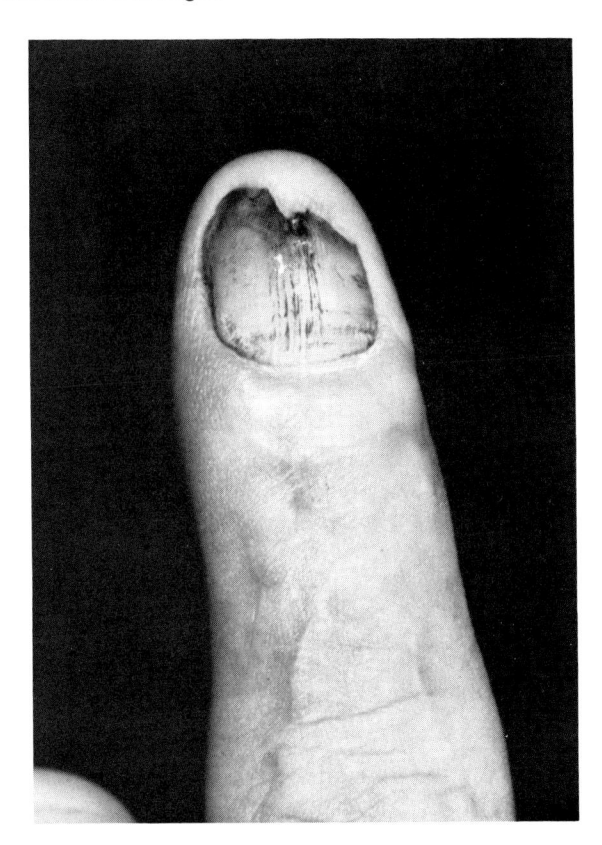

FIG. 3-12. Nine months after injury, nail is not smooth, but result is excellent considering extent of injury.

SECTION 1 SKIN PROBLEMS

FRACTURES OF THE TUFT

In most cases in which the tuft is fractured, reduction, repair of the matrix, and use of the nail as a splint will maintain the bony alignment accurately. In cases of severe fractures or ones that are a few days old, percutaneous longitudinal pinning after reduction may be necessary to maintain position so that accurate matrix repair can be carried out (Figs. 3-13 to 3-15). If the injury shown here had not been accurately repaired, it is my opinion that a severe deformity would have resulted. This encouraged me to repair the injury even though 4 days had passed and infection was a possibility.

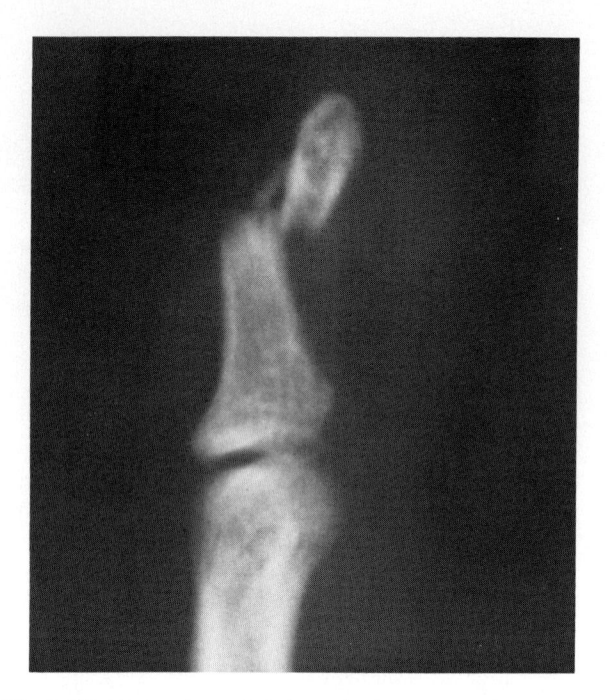

FIG. 3-13. X-ray view of 4-day-old fracture-dislocation of tuft with no approximation of nail bed. Fracture was reduced and pinned and nail bed repaired with fine chromic suture.

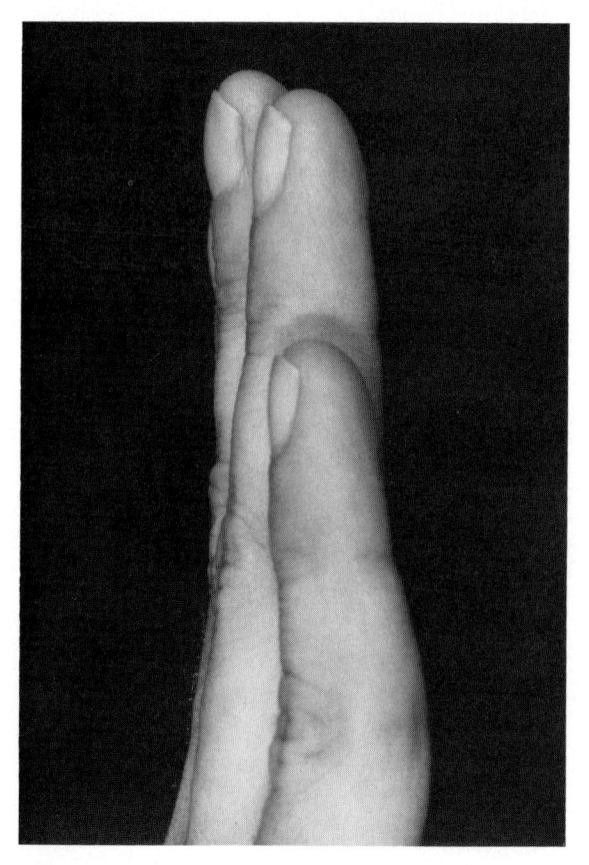

FIG. 3-14. Lateral view showing only slightly more curve of injured nail.

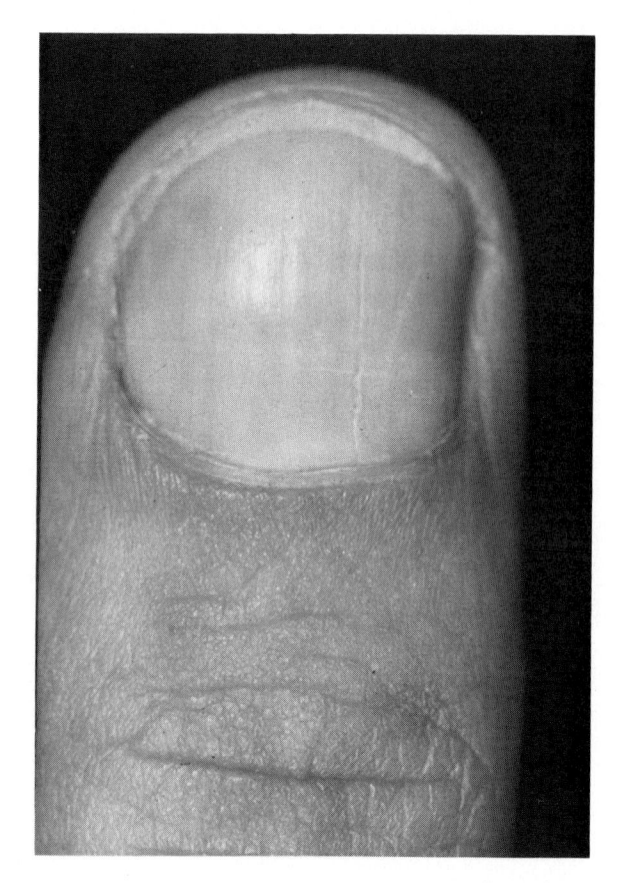

FIG. 3-15. Dorsal view of nail; slight transverse groove can be seen.

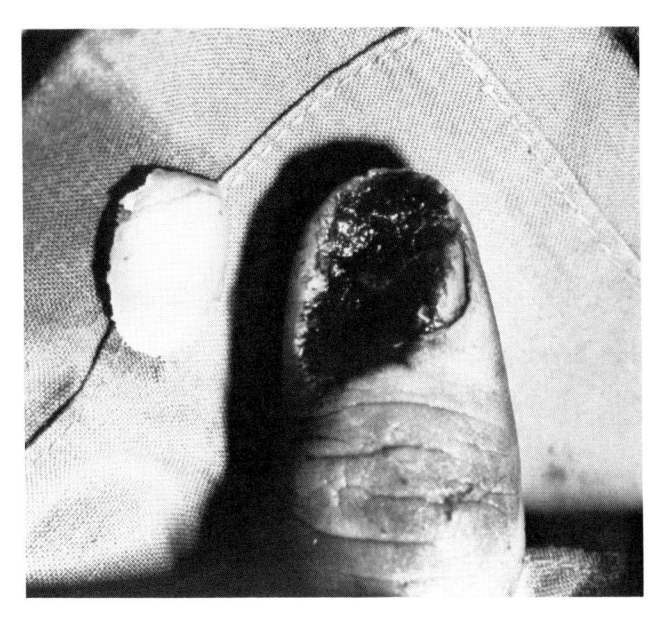

FIG. 3-16. Avulsion of most of nail and nail matrix, including fold of left thumb. It was replaced as a graft and sutured carefully in place.

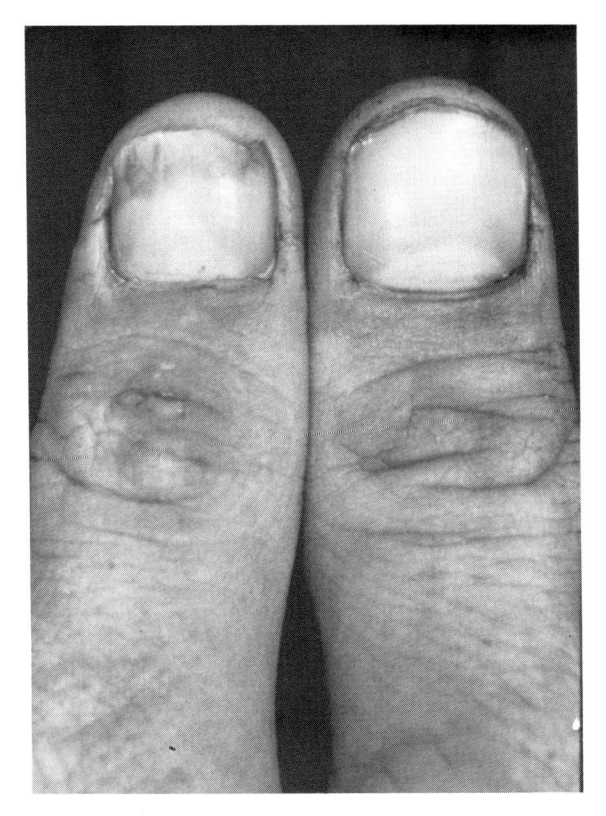

FIG. 3-17. Nine months after injury, patient's left thumb can be seen with only slight deformity.

AVULSION OF MATRIX

If a portion of the matrix is avulsed along with the nail, it should be reapplied without removing it from the nail.[6] The nail then acts as a splint to accurately reposition the matrix to take as a graft (Figs. 3-16 and 3-17). When the avulsed matrix is lost, surgeons have advocated both split-thickness skin grafts[2] and immediate nail matrix grafts from other fingers.[7] I agree with Flatt[2] that a split-thickness skin graft is the safest method of closure. If adherence or splitting of the nail occurs, free nail grafts from other fingers or preferably toes can be used to replace the matrix in a much less traumatized and uncontaminated wound. An as yet unpublished work by Shepard[6a] shows excellent results from the replacement of avulsed segments of the sterile matrix with split-thickness nail bed grafts taken from the remaining nail bed or a toenail. I have used this for several patients and feel it is an excellent technique.

REFERENCES

1. Baden, H.E.: Regeneration of the nail, Arch. Dermatol. **91**:19, 1965.
2. Flatt, A.E.: Nail injuries, Br. J. Plast. Surg. **8**:34, 1955.
3. Kligman, A.M.: Why do nails grow out instead of up? Arch. Dermatol. **84**:181, 1961.
4. Lewis, B.L.: Microscopic studies of fetal and mature nail and surrounding soft tissue, A.M.A. Arch. Dermatol. Syph. **70**:732, 1954.
5. McCash, C.R.: Prenail grafting, Br. J. Plast. Surg. **8**:19, 1955.
6. Schiller, C.: Nail replacement in fingertip injuries, Plast. Reconstr. Surg. **19**:521, 1957.
6a. Shepard, G.: Treatment of nail bed avulsions using split thickness nail bed grafts, Presented at the Annual Meeting of the American Society for Surgery of the Hand, 1980.
7. Swanker, W.A.: Reconstructive surgery of the injured nail, Am. J. Surg. **74**:341, 1947.
8. Tajima, T.: Treatment of open crushing type of industrial injuries of the hand and forearm, J. Trauma **14**:995, 1974.

Chapter 4 Reconstruction of the contracted first web space

James W. Strickland

Injury or disease of the tissues of the first web space often will result in an adduction-flexion deformity that severely restricts the functional capability of the thumb. The deformity may result from injuries to the web space skin, including lacerations, burns, crushing, or poorly planned surgical incisions. More severe first web contractures may result from conditions that cause deep scarring and muscle contracture of the adductor pollicis and first dorsal interosseous muscles. Crushing injuries, especially those which result in a bursting of the musculature through the first web space skin, are particularly likely to result in this type of deformity. Ischemic contracture, median and ulnar nerve paralysis, infection, or even arthritis of the first carpometacarpal (CMC) joint may give rise to this adduction-flexion deformity of the thumb.

It is important for the surgeon to recognize the potential development of an adduction contracture of the first web space immediately after injury and to initiate a prophylactic splinting program, using custom-fitted web space–maintaining splints (Fig. 4-1). The recognition of a developing contracture at an early stage also may allow a reversal of the process by the use of serial web-space splints (Fig. 4-2).

When fixed adduction contractures have developed, splinting programs usually are not effective, and an

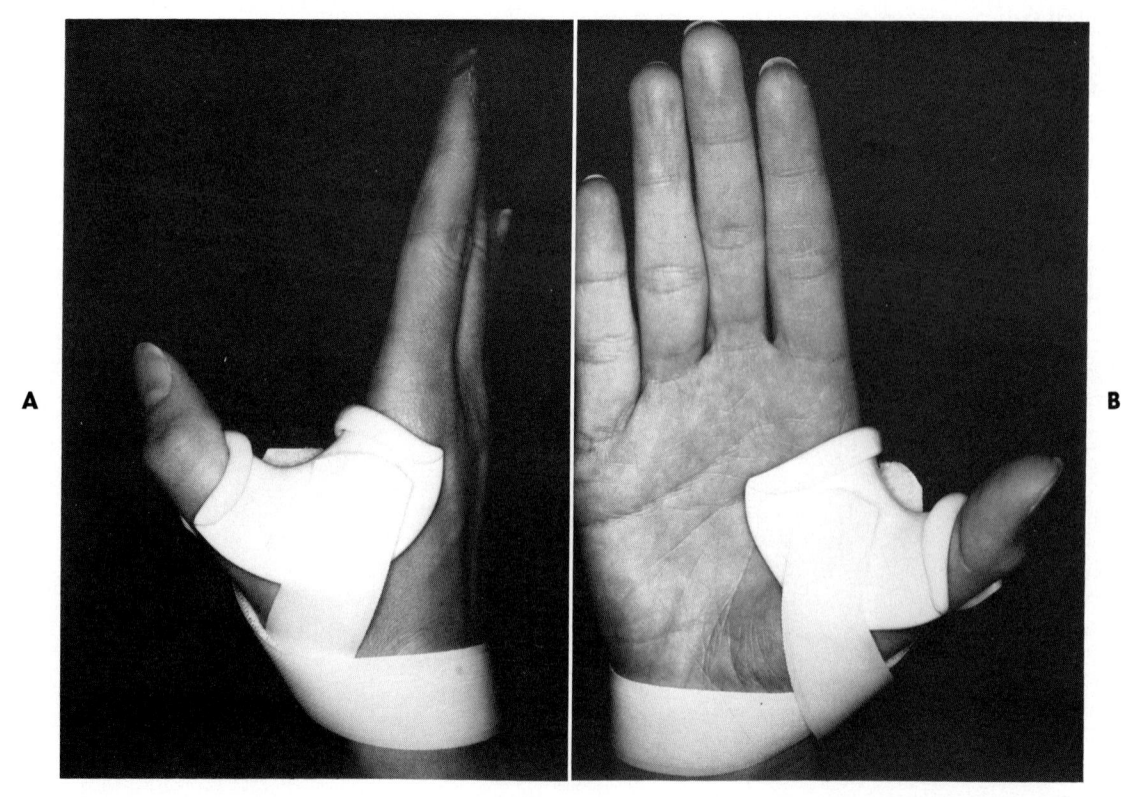

FIG. 4-1. Simple C-shaped Orthoplast splints for maintenance of the first web space. **A,** Dorsal view. **B,** Volar view.

operative deepening of the first web space often may be indicated. Techniques used to mobilize the first metacarpal to an abduction-extension position and to deepen the first web space include the following:

1. Simple Z-plasty
2. Four-flap Z-plasty
3. Free-skin grafting
4. Dorsal rotation flap
5. Cross-arm flap
6. Other remote pedicle flap

Selection of the appropriate surgical technique for a given thumb web contracture will depend on the number and nature of the tisues involved, including the status of the skin, fascia, muscle, and basilar thumb joint, as well as the status of the rest of the hand, including the skin adjacent to the first web. The merits of each of these procedures are discussed in the following sections.

SIMPLE Z-PLASTY

A simple two-flap Z-plasty procedure is probably the simplest technique for opening and deepening a contracted first web space* (Fig. 4-3). The procedure is most applicable when the contracture is not severe, the skin is minimally scarred, and there is a mobile first metacarpal with minimal muscle contracture. The technique is particularly useful when the thumb has been amputated through the proximal phalanx because of the relative thumb lengthening produced by web-space deepening. This method has been called *phalangization*.

Although these procedures are relatively simple, it is important that the surgeon understand the concepts of Z-plasty, including proper flap design, mobilization, and repositioning. The longitudinal axis of the Z-plasty is designed on the distal ridge of the first web space, and oblique proximal palmar and distal dorsal limbs of approximately 60 degrees are then designed. Incisions for the proximal and distal limbs may be reversed if local scar or incisional needs for other reconstructive procedures so mandate. The flaps are dissected back with careful undermining to avoid vascular compromise, and some additional depth can be achieved by partial recession of the distal edge of the web space musculature. The flaps then are reversed and sutured into place. Web-space splinting should be maintained until tissue maturation has occurred.

---

*References 2, 5-7, 9, and 16.

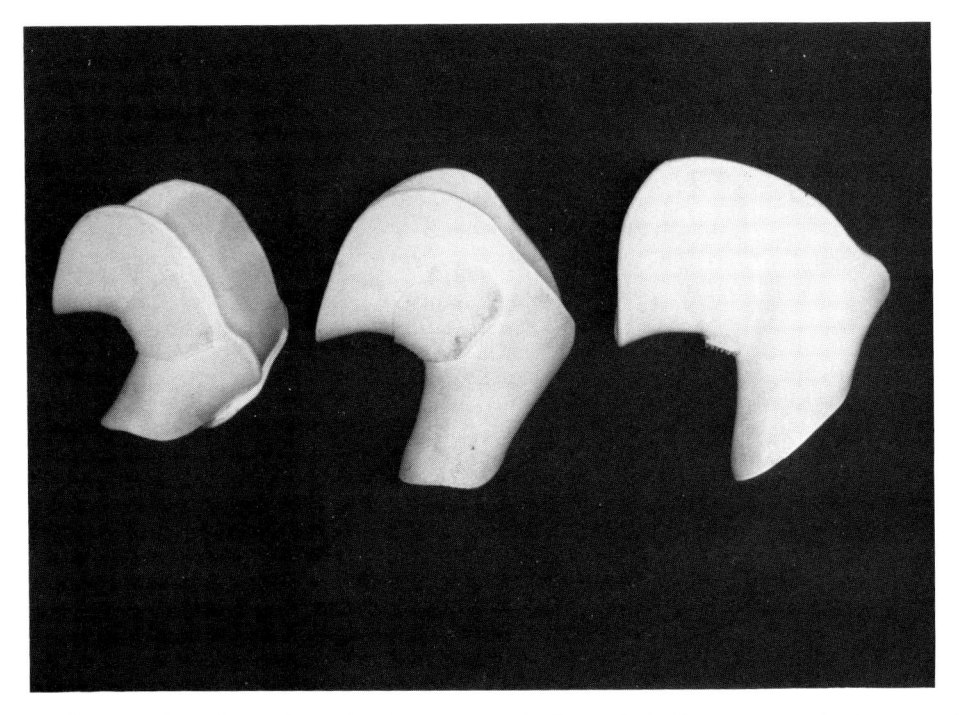

FIG. 4-2. Examples of use of serial web space widening splints. Note progressive increase in width of thumb-index space.

SECTION 1 SKIN PROBLEMS

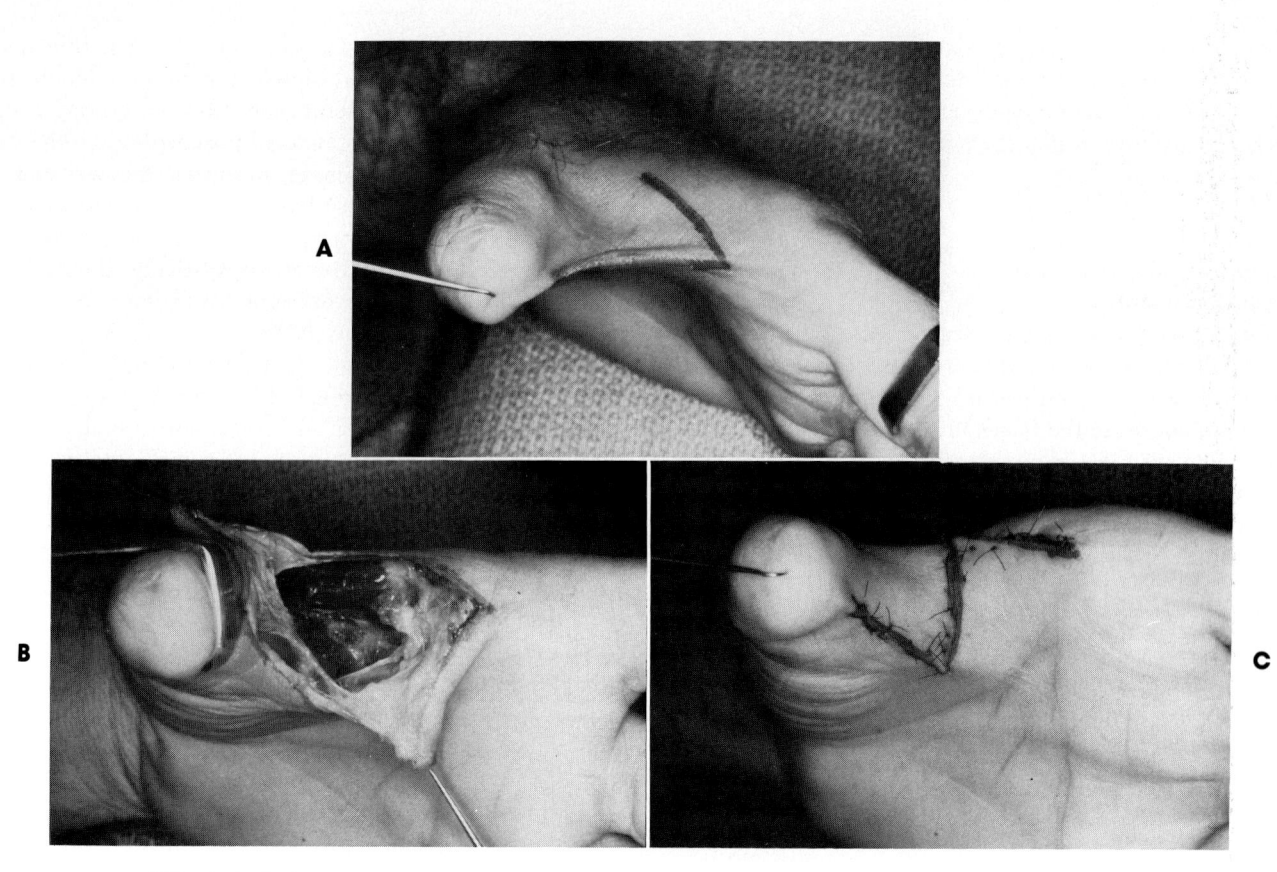

FIG. 4-3. First web space deepening in patient with amputation through distal portion of proximal phalanx of thumb. **A,** Design of Z-plasty. **B,** Mobilization of flaps and recession of first web space musculature. **C,** Appearance of flaps and deepened web after transposition.

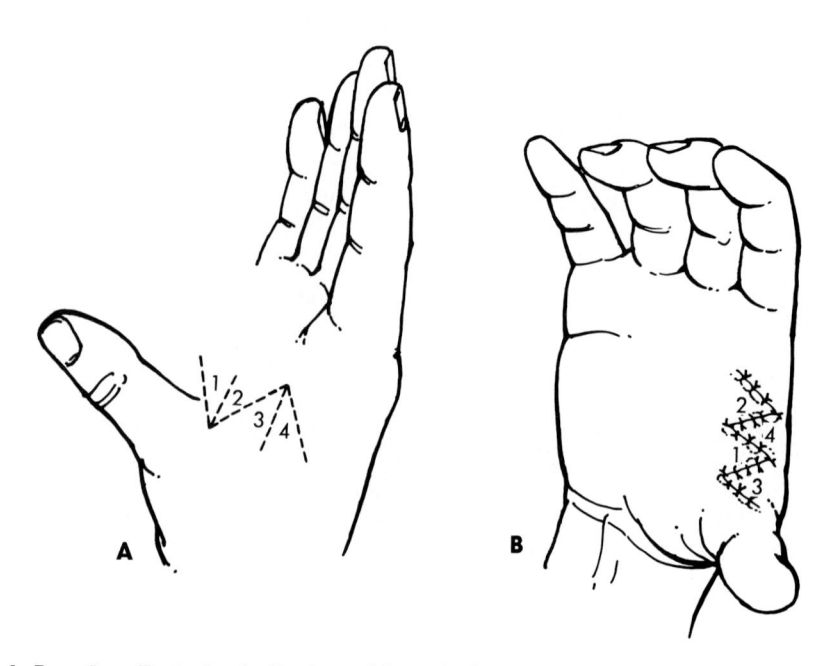

FIG. 4-4. Four-flap Z-plasty. **A,** Design of flaps in first web space. **B,** Appearance of flaps following transposition and suture.

FOUR-FLAP Z-PLASTY

The indications for more elaborate skin mobilization procedures such as the four-flap Z-plasty (Figs. 4-4 and 4-5) are essentially the same as those for a simple Z-plasty, although the former method may permit greater widening of the web space.[18] The technique also requires a mobile first metacarpal with minimal joint or muscle contracture.

Flaps are designed with the longitudinal axis on the distal edge of the thumb web ridge. Proximal volar and distal dorsal incisions varying from 90 to 120 degrees are then made, corresponding in length to that of the longitudinal line. The angles formed by these three lines then are divided equally by oblique incisions extending from their apices, again corresponding in length to that of the other limbs of the double Z-plasty. Incisions are made, and flaps, including skin and a small amount of subcutaneous tissue, are reflected on their bases. A recession of the thumb web musculature may be carried out to provide further depth, and the flaps are then interdigitated so that the common border of the two middle flaps (previously formed by the longitudinal line) comes to lie against the most proximal and distal incision sites. The proximal palmar and distal dorsal flaps are rotated to the midline, and their medial edges (previously formed by the oblique bisecting incisions) are joined. Postoperative web space maintenance splinting may be required.

FREE-SKIN GRAFTING

Free split- or full-thickness skin grafts to cover deficits created by the division of the offending structures at the time of first web space release have a very limited application. On occasion lacerations, burns, or inappropriate incisions will result in contractural scarring of the first web space, which can best be managed by simple skin excision and interpositional skin grafting. Unfortunately, when there has been concomitant involvement of deeper tissues, or when the contracture has been in existence

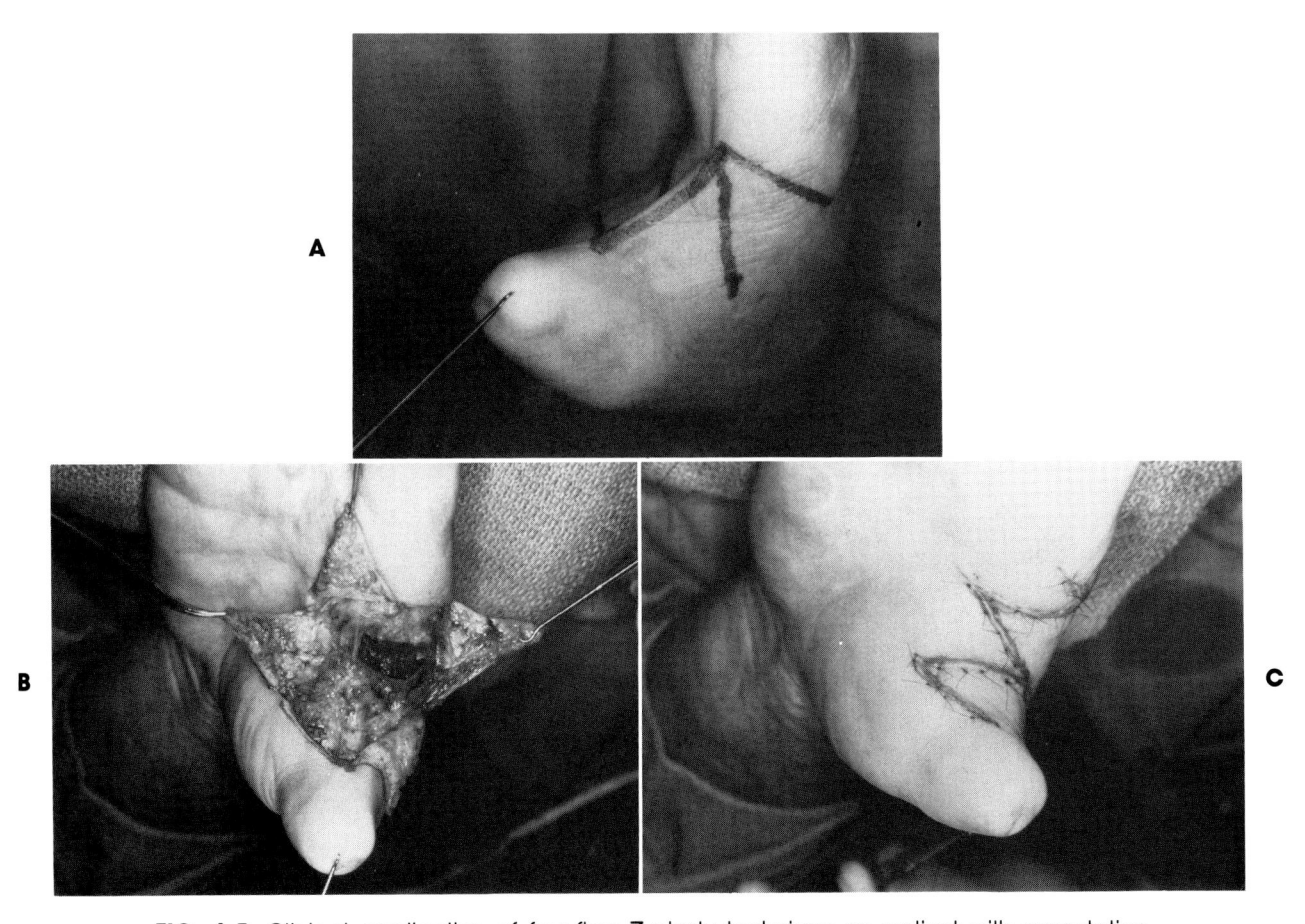

FIG. 4-5. Clinical application of four-flap Z-plasty technique on patient with amputation through distal aspect of proximal phalanx of thumb. **A,** Design of flaps. **B,** Appearance of flaps following mobilization and recession of first web space musculature. **C,** Appearance of deepened thumb web following transposition of flaps.

for a long enough period to allow secondary contracture of the first web space musculature or the basilar thumb joint, simple skin revision will not correct the deformity. Large defects on the opposing sides of the first and second metacarpals, created by wide sequential division of all offending structures, do not lend themselves well to free-graft coverage, particularly when bone and joint surfaces are exposed by the dissection. However, occasionally there will be patients in whom more elaborate procedures, such as rotation flaps or remote pedicle flaps, are contraindicated, and in these instances free grafting, however, inadequate, must be used. The resultant coverage, however, is usually inadequate for the demands of the grasping surfaces of the first web, and loss of correction may result from graft contracture.

DORSAL ROTATION FLAP

Correction of the flexion-adduction contracture of the thumb by the use of dorsal rotation flaps (Figs. 4-6 to 4-8) has been advocated by many.* These techniques are

---

*References 1, 3, 4, 8, 9, and 12-17.

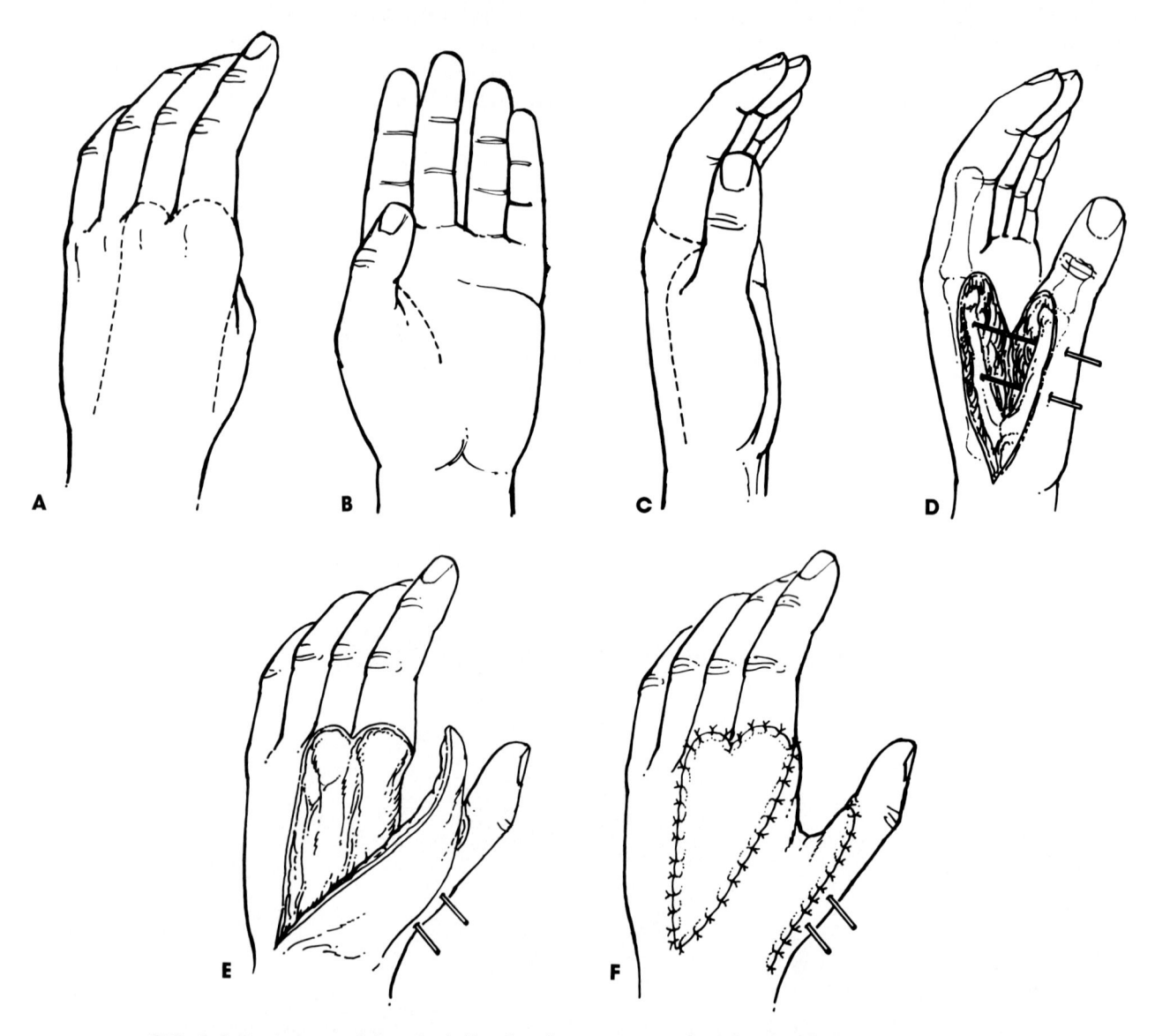

FIG. 4-6. Technique of dorsal rotation flap for coverage of contracted first space. **A,** Design of flap over dorsum of second and third metacarpals and metacarpophalangeal joints. **B,** Linear division of volar web in line with thenar crease. **C,** Dorsal linear division of first web. Incision forms lateral margin of dorsal flap. **D,** Appearance of divided first web space with muscle recession and pin fixation. **E,** Mobilization of dorsal flap. **F,** Appearance of rotated dorsal flap or coverage of first web defect and free-graft coverage of donor site.

CHAPTER 4 RECONSTRUCTION OF THE CONTRACTED FIRST WEB SPACE

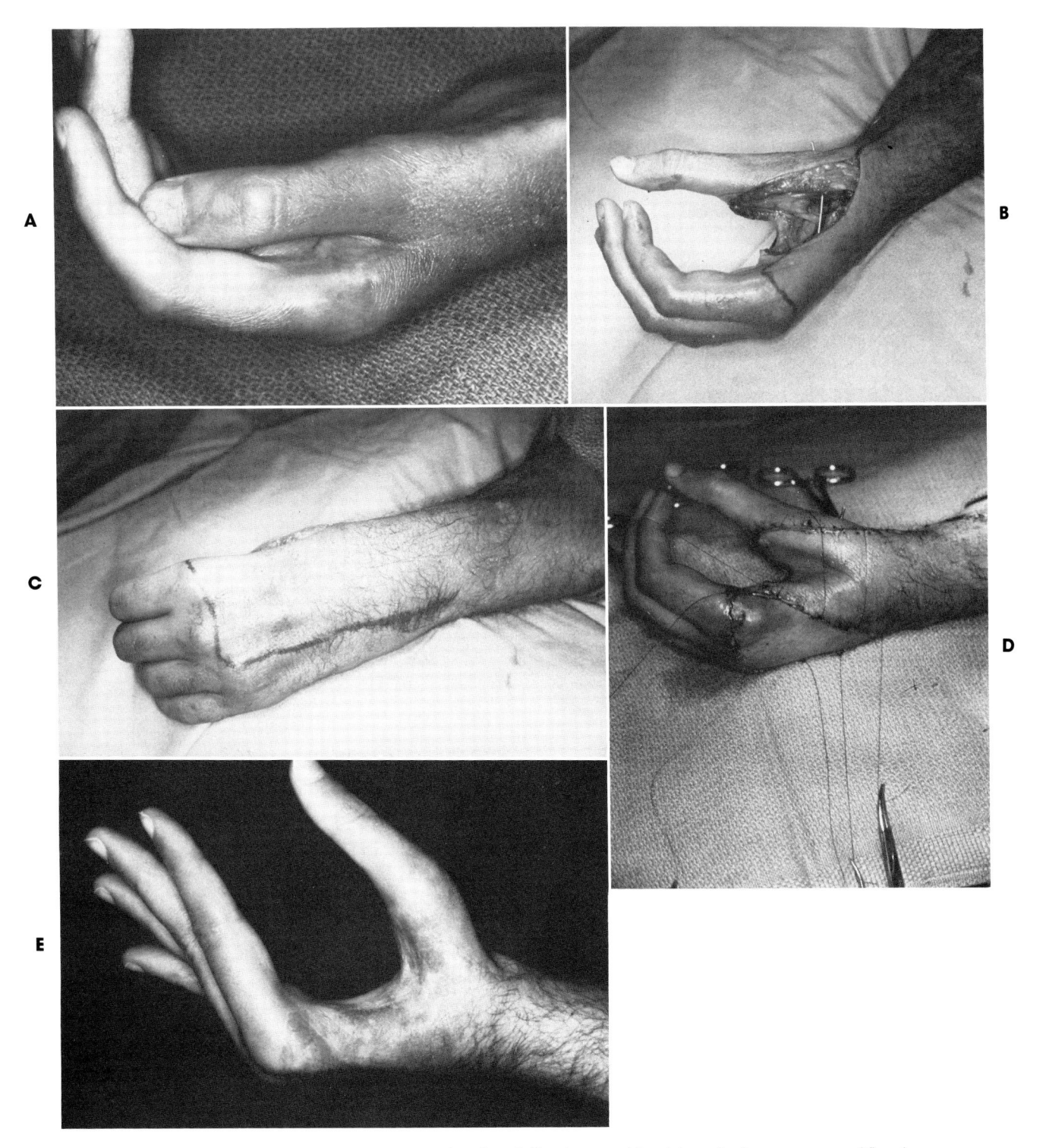

FIG. 4-7. Severe first web-space contracture following crushing injury. **A,** Appearance of fixed first web space contracture at time of surgery. **B,** Appearance of first web space defect following division of skin, scarred muscle, and mobilization of the CMC joint. **C,** Design of dorsal rotation flap over second and third metacarpals. **D,** Appearance of hand following flap transposition and free grafting. **E,** Appearance of widened first web space following rotation flap coverage at 6 months.

SECTION 1 SKIN PROBLEMS

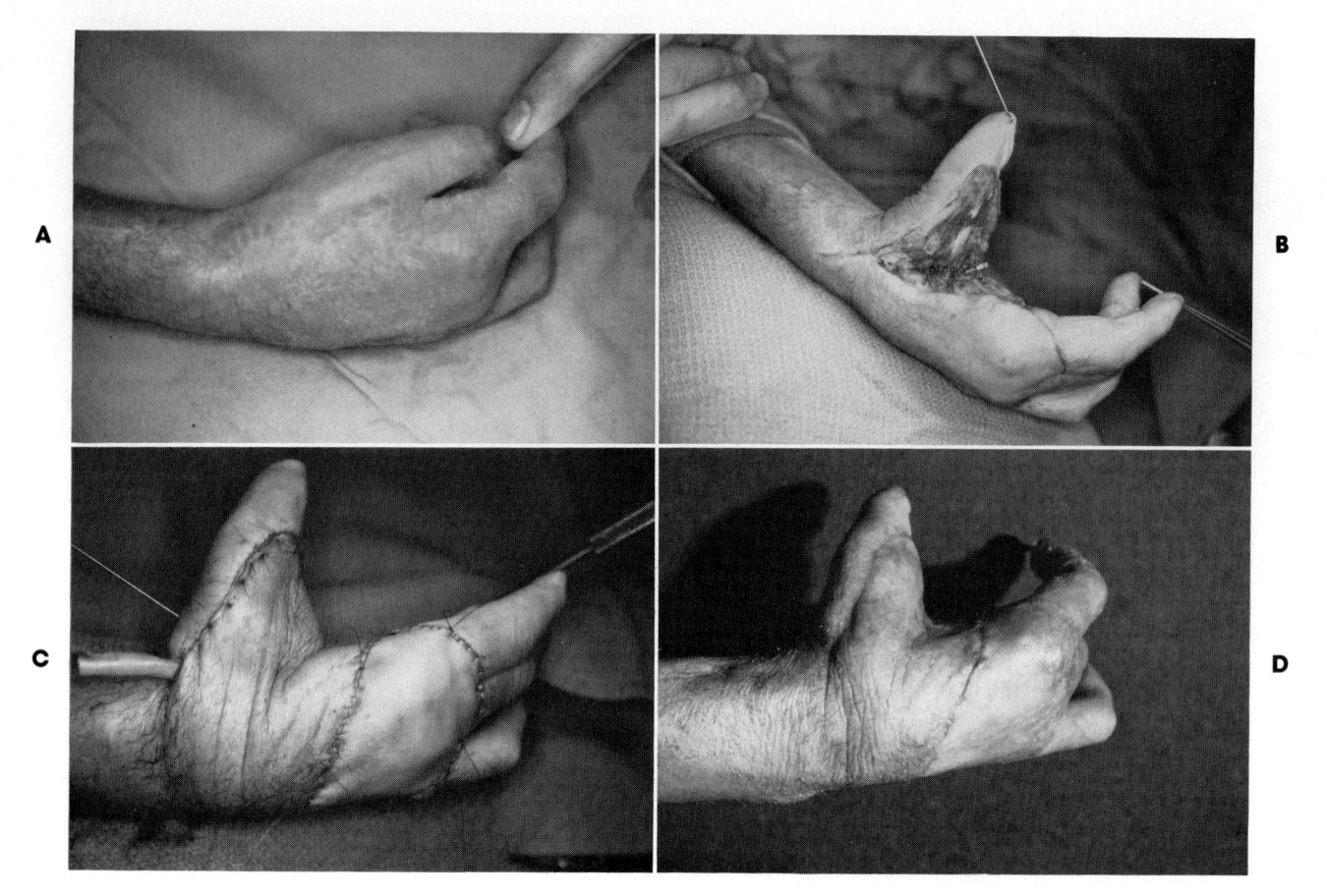

FIG. 4-8. Contracted first web space following mutilating injury to hand with loss of distal aspect of thumb. **A,** Tightly contracted first web space. **B,** Appearance of web space following mobilization and division of all contracting muscle, scar, and joint capsule. **C,** Appearance of reconstructed first web space with rotation flap and free-skin graft coverage of donor site. **D,** Appearance of thumb web and dorsal hand at 3 months.

best used when the injury has resulted in considerable involvement of the first web space musculature and a tight web space deformity has resulted. In these instances procedures more elaborate than simple skin revision will be necessary to mobilize the first metacarpal and restore the web space. Dorsal rotation flap techniques have proved effective in providing deepening, metacarpal mobilization, and partial resurfacing of the metacapal-thumb unit.* The advantage of the dorsal rotation flap is that it provides immediate vascularized coverage with excellent quality skin that retains its sensory innervation. This technique employs a sequential division of all skin, muscle, scar, and capsular adhesions of the first web. It is essential that there be no significant skin or soft tissue damage over the dorsal hand.

A continuous linear dorsovolar incision is carried through the first web, beginning dorsally at the level of the trapeziometacarpal joint and extending along the ulnar border of the first metacarpal. The incision then passes through the thumb web and continues volarly into the palm at the base of the thenar eminence. The origin of the first dorsal interosseous muscle is stripped from the metacarpal, or, if fibrotic, it is divided. The radial artery must be identified and protected, and both the oblique and transverse heads of the adductor are divided. In severe instances mobilization of the first metacarpal by capsular release of the CMC joint or even trapezial excision may be necessary. The thumb is stabilized in the correct position using transfixing Kirschner wires, and a pattern is created over the dorsal hand with its exact configuration being determined by several trial rotations into the thumb web defect. The incision is usually continued from the ulnar web wound dorsally across the radial aspect of the metacarpophalangeal (MCP) joint of the index finger, across the dorsum of the proximal phalanx of that digit, and then proximally and medially over the dorsum of the hand to approximately the base of the fourth metacarpal. The dorsal flap is dis-

---

*References 1, 3, 4, 8, 9, and 12-17.

CHAPTER 4 RECONSTRUCTION OF THE CONTRACTED FIRST WEB SPACE

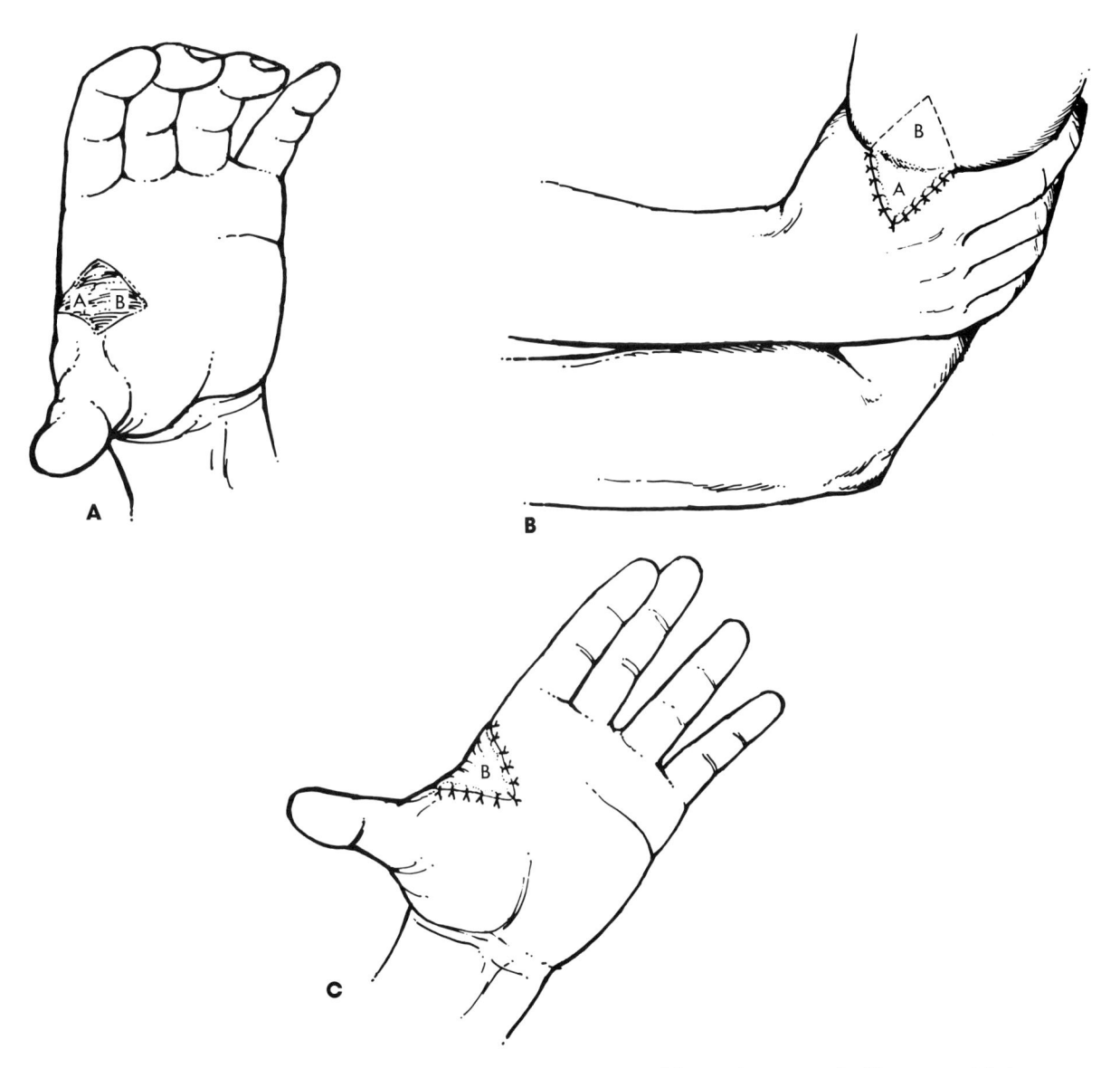

FIG. 4-9. Cross-arm flap technique for reconstruction of first web space. **A,** Diagram of first web space deepening following skin division and muscle recession. **B,** Position of hand with triangular distal flap, *(A)* sutured in dorsal thumb-web defect. Outline of proximal triangular flap *(B)* that will be used for volar web coverage is shown. **C,** Appearance of completed web space reconstruction following transfer of volar flap *(B)*.

sected free from the peritenon and mobilized, and there should be minimal interference with dorsal veins.

In this manner a long, wide, broad-based flap, which may have as much as a 3:1 length to width ratio,[14] is prepared and brings with it excellent skin and soft tissue coverage. The flap is sutured in place, and the resulting triangular defect over the dorso radial aspect of the hand is covered by free-skin grafting. Although pin removal and thumb mobilization are carried out at 4 to 6 weeks postoperatively, a conforming splint is used intermittently in the first web for 3 months.

CROSS-ARM FLAP

When a severe first web space contracture exists with deep muscle and joint contracture and with concomitant compromise of the adjacent dorsal skin, a remote pedicle source must be sought to provide coverage following releasing procedures. The cross-arm technique (Figs. 4-9 and 4-10) can be used occasionally in these circumstances to provide excellent resurfacing of the first web space.[7,11,17] This procedure is excellent both functionally and cosmetically. It provides thin, supple skin, and the contour of the arm is excellent for maintaining the web

SECTION 1 SKIN PROBLEMS

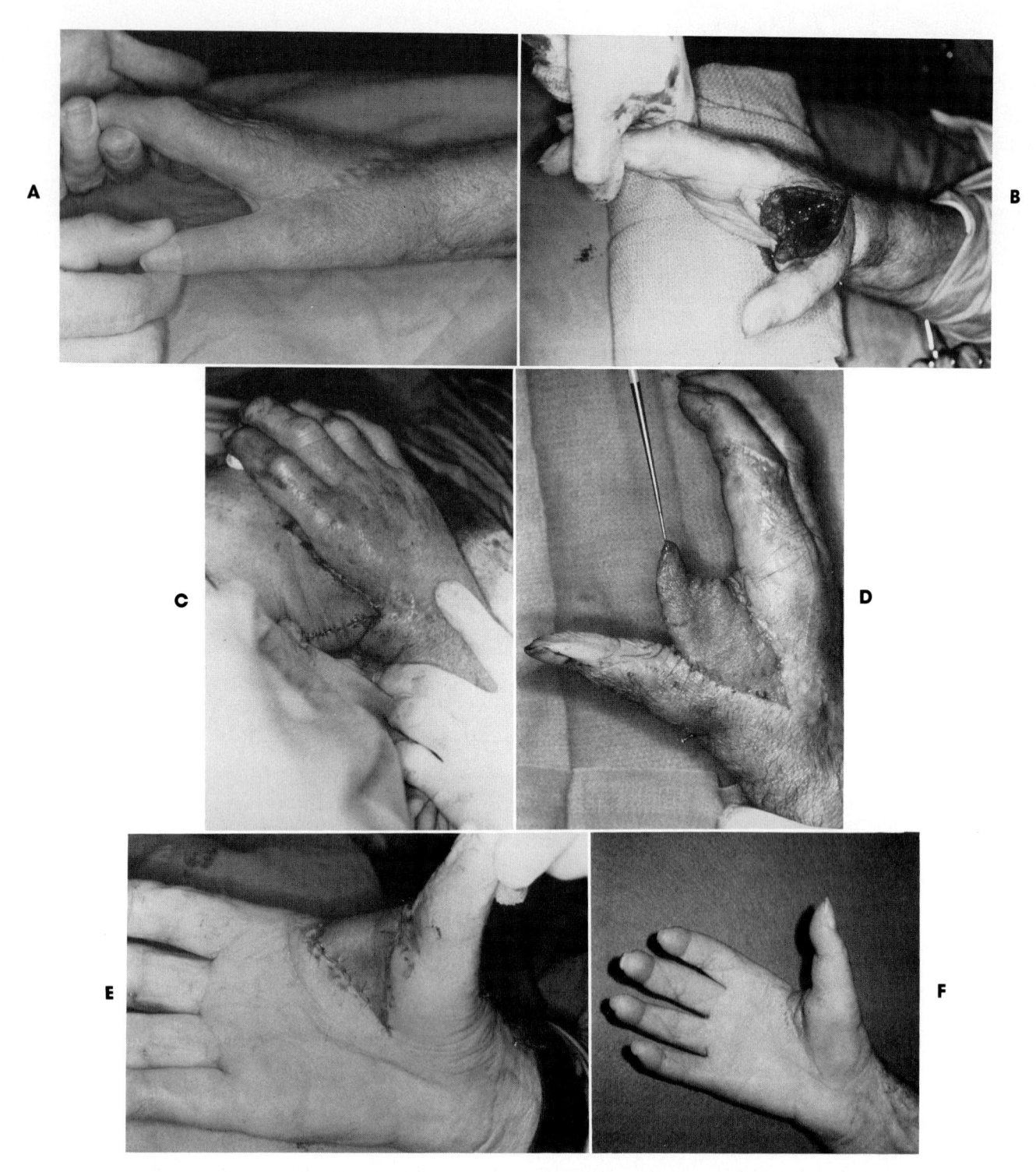

FIG. 4-10. Example of clinical application of cross-arm flap technique. **A,** Tightly contracted first web space with severe injury to dorsal skin. **B,** Appearance of thumb-web defect following skin, muscle, and scar division. **C,** Appearance of dorsal first web space coverage with distal triangular upper arm flap. **D,** At 3 weeks following satisfactory healing of dorsal flap, proximal triangular flap is transposed into volar web defect. **E,** Appearance of volar web coverage at time of insetting. **F,** Appearance of reconstructed first web space using this technique.

space while the pedicle is being vascularized.[11] It has the disadvantage of a resulting defect on the opposite arm as well as the obvious limitation of upper limb function during the period of obligatory immobilization.

The technique again involves a linear dorsal and volar excision through the web space, sequentially dividing all offending structures, including skin, subcutaneous tissue, web space musculature, and on occasion the CMC joint. The hand is then brought into place against the opposite arm in a manner such that the ulnar border of the hand can rest against the anterior surface of the forearm with the thumb comfortably placed around the inner aspect of the upper arm. Patterns are used to design a distal triangular flap that can be used to resurface the dorsal half of the divided web space, and temporary split-thickness skin coverage is placed on the arm and volar hand defects. At 3 weeks a corresponding triangular flap is designed proximally and will be turned into the volar defect after the free graft is excised. Defatting is usually not necessary, although maintenance splinting should be carried out for several months.

OTHER REMOTE PEDICLE FLAPS

On occasion division of a severe adduction-flexion contracture of the first web space may result in a defect in which the use of dorsal rotation or cross-arm flaps is precluded. In these instances other sources such as the abdomen[7,10] or the chest[3] have been advocated. The groin flap, on some occasions has provided an effective source of thumb web coverage, and when the proximal portion of the flap is tubed, some extremity motion can be preserved. Sometimes, however, these flaps will create too much bulk in the thumb web, and defatting procedures may be necessary.

SUMMARY

Long-standing severe adduction contracture of the first metacarpal is a crippling deformity, often totally eliminating prehensile hand function. Surgical release of the deformity is accomplished by a meticulous sequential division of all contracting elements. When the contracture is not great or is of short duration and primarily related to injury of the web space skin, Z-plasty procedures or scar excision and free-skin grafting may be adequate to restore satisfactory thumb abduction-extension. Long-standing contractures, particularly following crushing injuries, will often result in much more severe contractures, and web space restoration in these instances will result in a substantial skin and soft tissue deficit, which may be well covered by the use of a rotation flap from the dorsum of the hand or the use of a cross-arm or other remote pedicle flap. Complications of these procedures incude hematoma formation, flap loss, graft failure, or recurrent adduction contracture. Prolonged splinting is usually necessary to maintain the correction achieved at surgery. If the procedures are carried out with careful attention to technical detail and proper postoperative care, satisfactory restoration of function should be achieved. Additional reconstructive procedures such as tendon transfers may be necessary to further enhance thumb function, although the restoration of the thumb web space and improvement in thumb posture alone will have a profoundly favorable influence on hand performance.

REFERENCES

1. Brown, P.W.: Adduction-flexion contracture of the thumb: correction with dorsal rotation flap and release of contracture, Clin. Orthop. **88**:161, 1972.
2. Bunnell, S.: The management of the nonfunctional hand—reconstruction vs. prosthesis, Artif. Limbs **4**:76, 1957.
3. Chase, R.A.: Atlas of hand surgery, Philadelphia, 1973, W.B. Saunders Co.
4. Flatt, A.E., and Wood, V.E.: Multiple dorsal rotation flaps from the hand for thumb web contractures, Plast. Reconstr. Surg. **45**:258, 1970.
5. Flynn, J.E.: Adduction contracture of the thumb, N. Engl. J. Med. **254**:677, 1956.
6. Howard, L.D.: Contracture of the thumb web, J. Bone Joint Surg. **32A**:267, 1950.
7. Howard, L.D., Jr.: Plastic procedures in hand surgery. In Manual distributed at Instructional Course Lectures, American Academy of Orthopaedic Surgeons, San Francisco, August, 1963.
8. Littler, J.W.: The prevention and correction of adduction contracture of the thumb, Clin. Orthop. **13**:182, 1959.
9. Milford, L.: The hand. In Edmonson, A.S., and Crenshaw, A.H., editors: Campbell's operative orthopaedics, ed. 6., St. Louis, 1980, The C.V. Mosby Co.
10. Miura, T.: Use of paired abdominal flaps for release of adduction contractures of the thumb, Plast. Reconstr. Surg. **63**:242, 1979.
11. Mutz, S.B.: Thumb web contracture, Hand **4**:236, 1972.
12. Peacock, E.E.: Reconstruction of the thumb. In Flynn, J.E., editor: Hand surgery, Baltimore, 1966, Williams & Wilkins Co.
13. Sharpe, C.: Tissue cover for the thumb web, Arch. Surg. **104**:21, 1972.
14. Spinner, M.: Fashioned transpositional flap for soft tissue adduction contracture of the thumb, Plast. Reconstr. Surg. **44**:345, 1969.
15. Strauch, B.: Dorsal thumb flap for release of adduction contracture of the first web space, Bull. Hosp. Joint Dis. **36**:34, 1975.
16. Strickland, J.W.: Restoration of thumb function following partial or total amputation. In Hunter, J.M., Schneider, L.H., Mackin, E.J., et al., editors: Rehabilitation of the hand, St. Louis, 1978, The C.V. Mosby Co.
17. Vilain, R., and Michon, J.: Plastic surgery of the hand and pulp, New York, 1979, Masson Publishing USA, Inc.
18. Woolf, R.M., and Broadbent, T.R.: The four-flap Z-plasty, Plast. Reconstr. Surg. **49**:48, 1972.

Chapter 5 The coverage of difficult digital defects with local rotation flaps

James W. Strickland

The hand surgeon will be confronted occasionally with difficult wound coverage problems following burns, direct trauma, or reconstructive surgery of the fingers. In the acute situation most digital wounds can be at least temporarily covered by the use of free split- or full-thickness skin grafts. More extensive wounds exposing tendon or bone have been traditionally managed by cross-finger flaps, thenar flaps, or pedicle flaps from other remote sources.

Additional coverage problems may be created by the frequent breakdown of skin grafts or by complications after secondary surgical procedures such as tendon reconstruction, capsulectomy, arthroplasty, or arthrodesis in the presence of inadequate or heavily scarred skin. In these instances the need is often created for flap coverage to provide durable resurfacing of the defects. If possible, it is preferable to choose a coverage technique that will provide well-vascularized skin with satisfactory sensory perception and a pleasing cosmetic appearance. It can be seen that neither free-skin grafts nor pedicle flaps can completely satisfy the requirements of these severe coverage problems.

I have found that it is possible in many instances to cover volar or dorsal finger wounds with carefully designed local rotation flaps. The excellent vascularization of the skin of the digits with its rich subdermal plexus permits the rotation of rather large flaps, usually taken from the lateral or dorsal digit, into substantial defects. Full-thickness skin coverage of the donor defect in a less critical anatomic area completes the reconstruction. This technique consistently provides durable, long-lasting coverage with sensate, well-vascularized skin. It has been interesting to note that the cosmetic adaptation of the flap in its new position has been excellent, particularly on the volar digit where skin flexor creases will reappear.

Three examples of the use of local digital rotation flaps are provided here.

CASE 1

A 35-year-old right hand–dominant white man suffered a severe crushing and burn injury of the dorsum of his right hand when it was entrapped by a hot roller. The injury apparently resulted in a total loss of the skin over the dorsum of the index, ring, and small fingers with concomitant underlying tendon injury, particularly to the long and ring fingers. The patient subsequently was managed by local wound care for the first 4 weeks and then underwent Kirschner-wire fixation of the long finger. Ultimately skin grafts were applied on several occasions to the dorsum of the index, long, and ring fingers. Unfortunately the patient continued to have areas of exposed bone and wound breakdown over the dorsum of the long and ring fingers with poor dorsal skin coverage of all digits and fixed flexion deformities of 65 and 75 degrees in the two digits at the proximal interphalangeal (PIP) joint.

At the initial examination, this patient exhibited hypertrophic linear burn scarring of all digits with very thin, poor-quality skin over the dorsum of the PIP joint of the ring finger and exposed bone just proximal to the PIP joint of the long finger (Fig. 5-1, *A*). Fixed flexion deformities in excess of 65 degrees were present in both the long and ring fingers, although the patient had maintained good metacarpophalangeal (MCP) joint motion.

Six months after his initial injury the patient underwent a division of a third web space scar with full-thickness skin graft coverage. Arthrodeses of the PIP joints of the long and ring fingers were carried out with the hope that the additional skin provided by joint extension would allow satisfactory coverage.

At 9 months after injury and 3 months after the arthrodeses the patient had satisfactory bony union but continued to have wound breakdown over the PIP joints of both the long and ring fingers with exposed bone in the long finger (Fig. 5-1, *B*). In addition, there had been a progressive increase in the boutonniere deformity of the small finger. The patient also was concerned about the coverage of the MCP joints of the index, long, and ring fingers and the proximal and middle phalanges of the same digits.

One year after the original injury (6 months after the PIP arthrodeses) excision of the hypertrophic scarring over the dorsum of the index, long, and ring fingers was carried out (Fig. 5-1, *C*). Local rotation flaps were designed over the ulnar lateral aspects of the proximal and middle phalanges of the long and ring fingers to provide full-thickness coverage of the exposed PIP bone (Fig. 5-1, *D*). The flaps were rotated dorsally and sutured in place, and full-thickness coverage of the remaining defects was accomplished, along with repair of the boutonniere deformity and arthrodesis of the distal interphalangeal (DIP) joint of the small finger (Fig. 5-1, *E*). Improved cosmesis of the long, ring, and small fingers was achieved with durable coverage provided to the dorsum of the previously exposed PIP joints (Fig. 5-1, *F*). In 1 year there has been no further wound breakdown, and the patient's hand performance has been markedly improved.

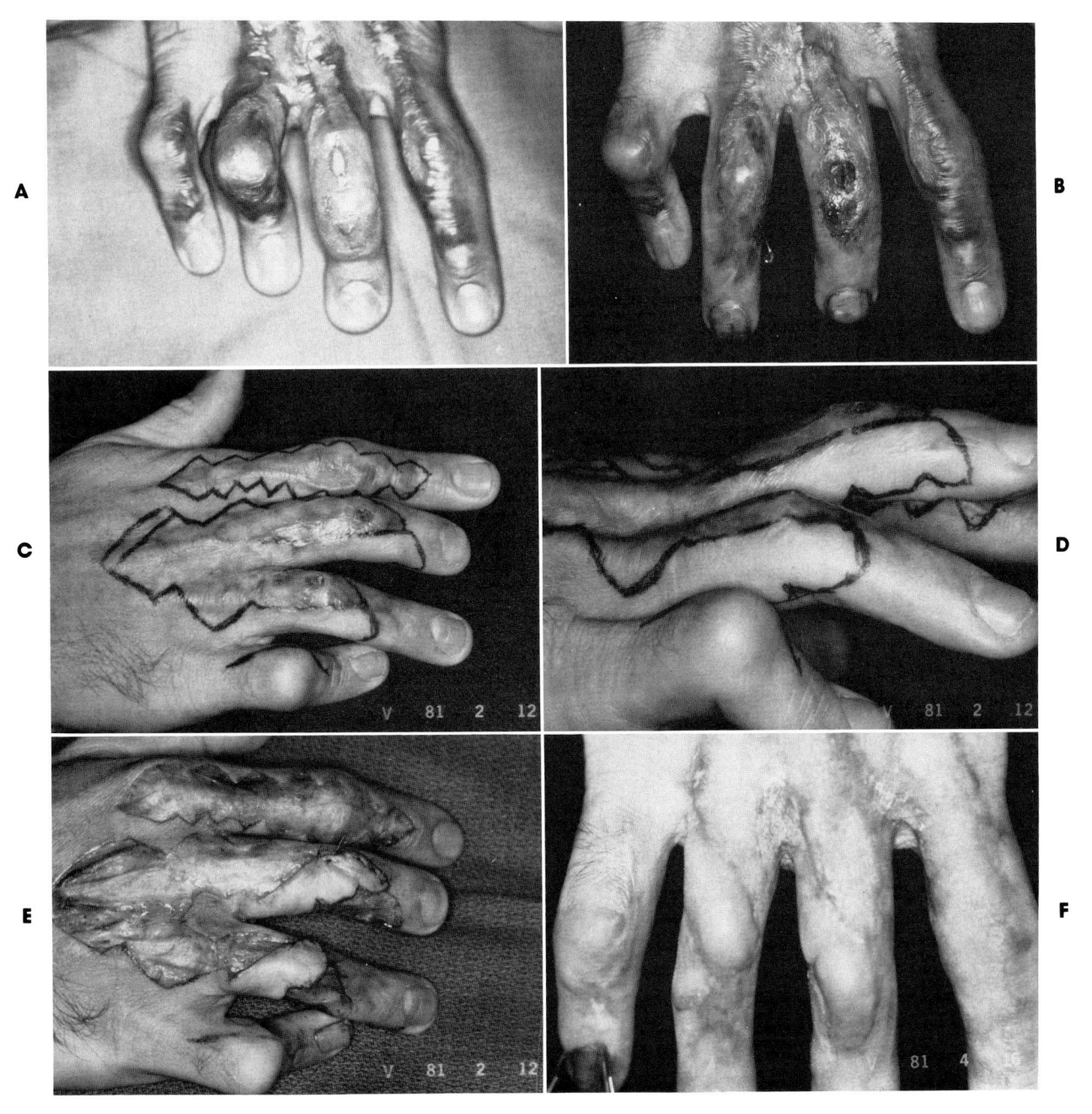

CHAPTER 5 THE COVERAGE OF DIFFICULT DIGITAL DEFECTS WITH LOCAL ROTATION FLAPS

FIG. 5-1

39

SECTION 1 SKIN PROBLEMS

CASE 2

A 51-year-old right hand–dominant man suffered a severe thermal punch injury to his right hand, resulting in traumatic amputation of the index finger and a third-degree burn on the radial side of the long finger (Fig. 5-2, A). Initial debridement was carried out with disarticulation of the index finger at the MCP joint. Subsequent to index ray amputation, full-thickness skin grafting was used to cover a large defect on the proximal and middle phalanges of the long finger.

Unfortunately a complete take of this graft was not achieved, and additional split-thickness skin grafting was necessary in 3 weeks. The patient subsequently experienced chronic fissuring of the graft (Fig. 5-2, B), perhaps resulting from the heavy demand that he placed on his hands in his occupation. Because of this chronic graft breakdown, the patient returned for surgery at 19 months, and approximately 95% of the old graft was excised from the volar radial aspect of the long finger (Fig. 5-2, C and D). A large rotation flap, designed over the entire dorsum of the proximal and middle phalanges of the long finger (Fig. 5-2, E), was

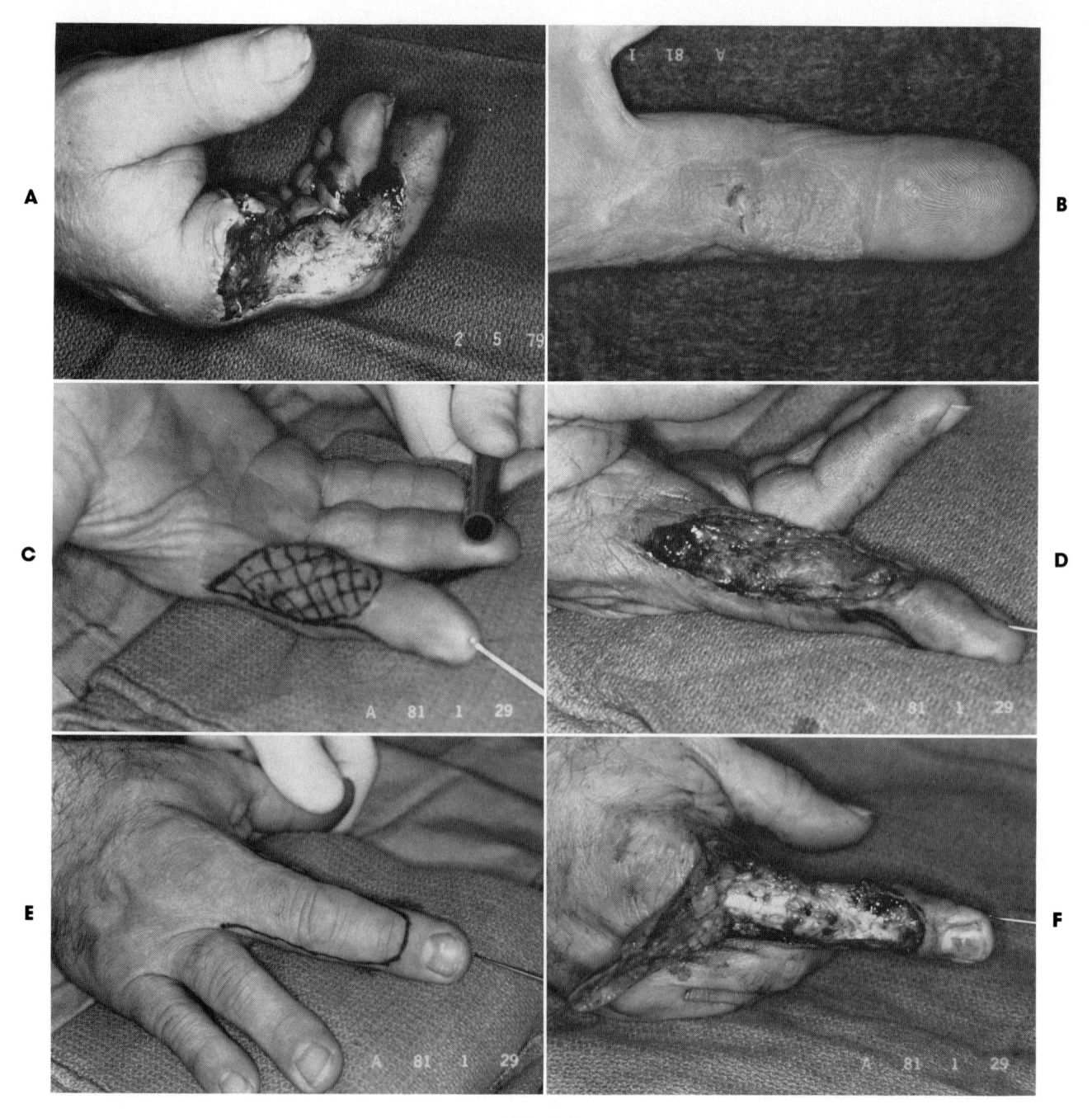

FIG. 5-2

CHAPTER 5 THE COVERAGE OF DIFFICULT DIGITAL DEFECTS WITH LOCAL ROTATION FLAPS

then elevated (Fig. 5-2, *F*) by careful dissection over the epitenon of the extensor mechanism. The flap was then rotated into position (Fig. 5-2, *G*) and sutured in place. The resulting large dorsal defect (Fig. 5-2, *H*) was managed by full-thickness skin grafting (Fig. 5-2, *I*), and a stent dressing was applied (Fig. 5-2, *J*). Satisfactory flap survival was observed at 2 weeks (Fig. 5-2, *K*), and the ultimate performance of the flap on the volar aspect of this digit has been excellent (Fig. 5-2, *L* to *N*). The patient is quite pleased with the flap coverage at 1 year and has satisfactory sensibility and no breakdown problems despite heavy industrial use of the hand.

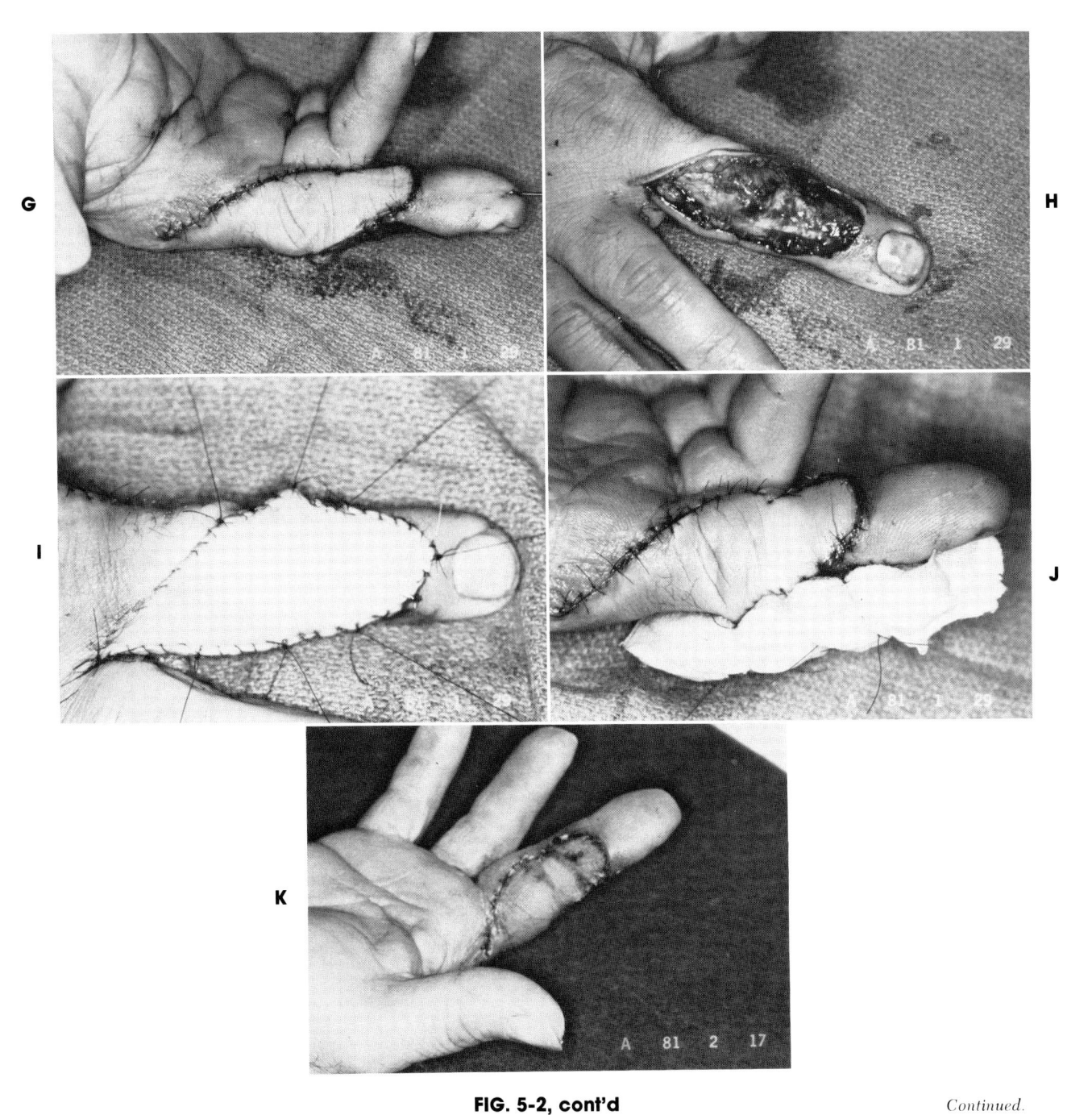

FIG. 5-2, cont'd

Continued.

SECTION 1 SKIN PROBLEMS

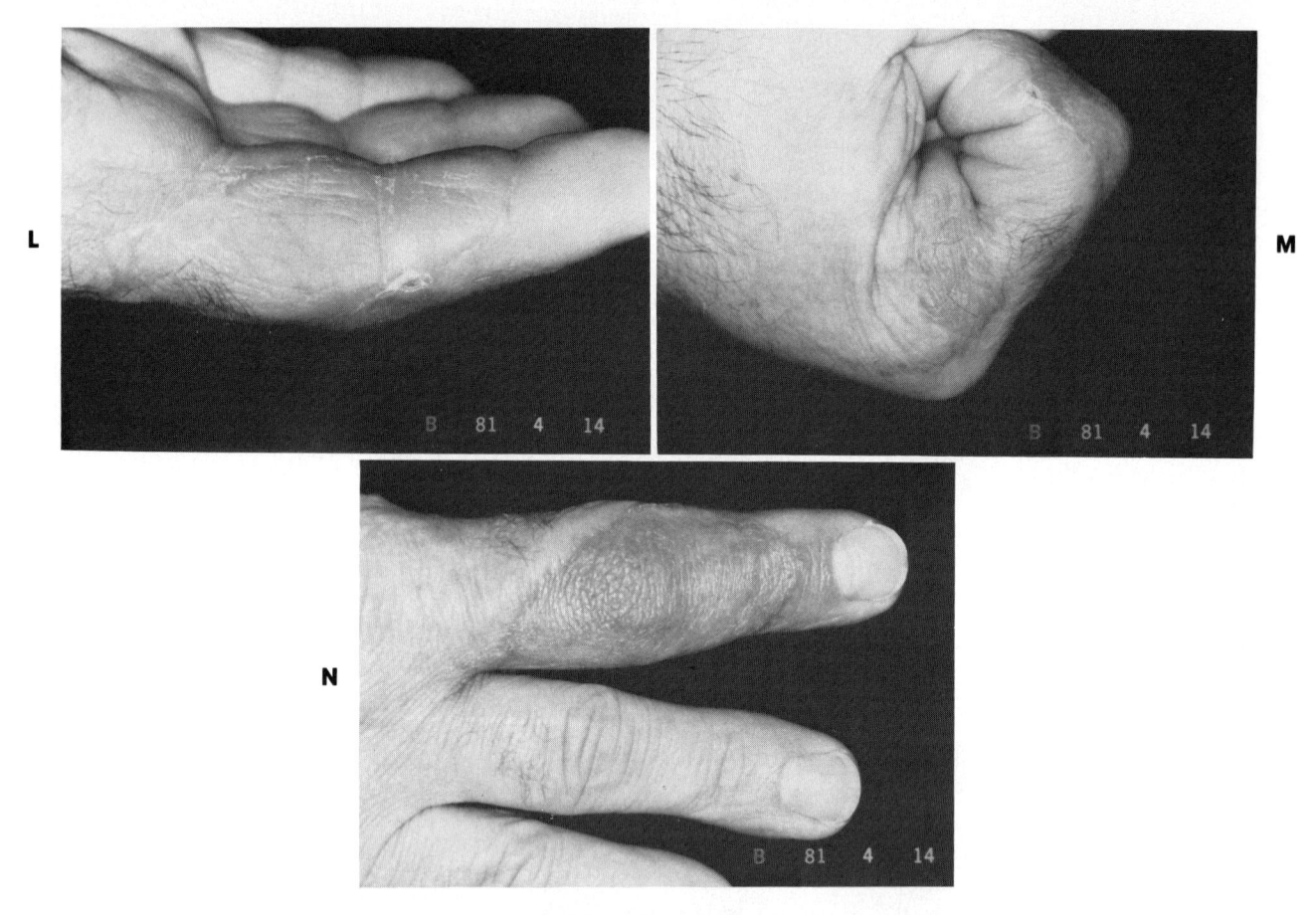

L

M

N

FIG. 5-2, cont'd

42

CHAPTER 5 THE COVERAGE OF DIFFICULT DIGITAL DEFECTS WITH LOCAL ROTATION FLAPS

CASE 3

A 24-year-old man had undergone multiple procedures in an effort to restore flexor tendon function in his right long finger. A dog bite over the middle phalanx had resulted in infection, after which there was a loss of flexor tendon function. A tenolysis of the flexor digitorum superficialis tendon was carried out with excision of the flexor digitorum profundus tendon. After an initial return of good motion, superficialis rupture occurred, and a two-stage tendon reconstruction was initiated with the use of a Hunter rod. Free-tendon grafting ultimately was carried out, but very poor function resulted, and a tenolysis was performed 2 years after the initial injury. Although his initial performance following this procedure was excellent, a dehiscence occurred in the scarred skin at the level of the PIP joint, exposing the tendon graft, and despite conservative efforts, a small, chronically leaking sinus persisted (Fig. 5-3, *A*).

Because of the need to add good-quality skin over the tendon graft and to straighten a progressive flexion deformity of the PIP joint, a volar capsulectomy and dorsal rotation flap were used. A proximal shift of proximal phalangeal skin created a large volar middigital defect with exposed tendon (Fig. 5-3, *B*), and an appropriate dorsoradial rotation flap was designed, mobilized, and sutured in place (Fig. 5-3, *C* and *D*). Excellent, durable volar skin reconstruction has been achieved by this procedure at 14 months (Fig. 5-3, *E* and *F*) with satisfactory cosmetic appearance of the donor site and the return of volar skin creases to the flap. Pulley reconstruction and tenolysis are planned to restore active digital flexion.

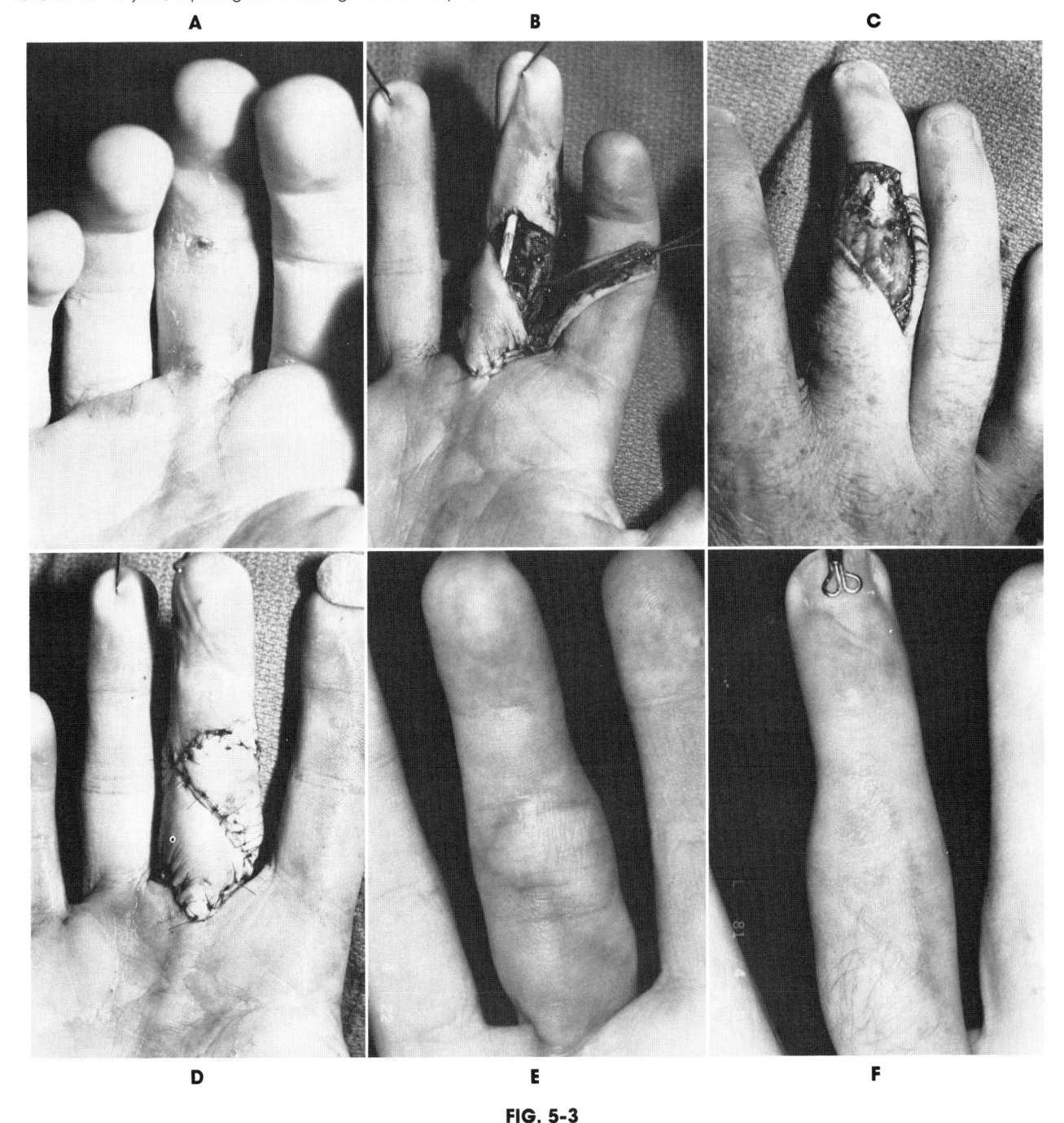

FIG. 5-3

DISCUSSION

Ingenious uses of small digital rotation flaps have been suggested by several authors.[1-4] These techniques have proved useful not only for the coverage of small defects in the digital skin but also for the shifting of sensory perception at the pulp level from the ulnar side of the pad to the radial side, where the sensory demands are greater. Despite the excellent vascularity of the skin of the digit, there has been little mention of the possibility of using large lateral or dorsal flaps to provide coverage of defects on either the dorsal or volar aspects of the proximal or middle phalanges. Provided there is no functional compromise created by the donor defect, the rotation of durable, sensory innervated, well-vascularized skin into areas where coverage of bone, joint, or tendon is required would seem to have considerable and obvious advantages over other methods.

SUMMARY

In this short chapter I have attempted to use three clinical cases to illustrate the efficacy of the local rotation flap technique in providing coverage of problem defects of the digits. I believe that this procedure, although infrequently necessary, is an excellent technique with a high degree of safety and the advantage of providing durable, vascularized, sensate skin without the need to use remote flap sources.

REFERENCES

1. Bunnell, S.: Surgery of the hand, ed. 3., Philadelphia, 1956, J.B. Lippincott Co.
2. Howard, L.D., Jr.: Plastic procedures in hand surgery, San Francisco, 1963, L.D. Howard, Jr.
3. Hueston, J.: The extended neurovascular island flap, Br. J. Plast. Surg. 18:304, 1965.
4. Vilain, R., and Michon, J.: Plastic surgery of the hand and pulp, ed. 2., New York, 1979, Masson Publishing USA, Inc.

SECTION TWO EXTENSOR TENDON PROBLEMS

Chapter 6 Reconstruction in chronic extensor tendon problems

Lawrence H. Schneider

EXTENSORS OF THE WRIST AND FINGERS

The ability to actively extend at the wrist and metacarpophalangeal (MCP) joints of the fingers is the function of the intact long extensor tendon system of the forearm. Disruption of this system, when it results in the loss of wrist extension, greatly handicaps the flexor gripping power of the hand, whereas loss of extension at the MCP joints affects the placement of the fingers in digital function. Adhesions interfering with the gliding function of the distal segments of these disrupted tendons will also effectively produce tenodesis at the wrist and finger joints, further interfering with flexion and grasp activities.[11] It is therefore important to restore an intact, freely gliding system for the extensor mechanism to prevent a great functional loss.

Candidates for reconstruction of the extensor system usually have had failed primary repairs that have either been disrupted or adhered during the healing period. Others have had severe injuries with tendon destruction and original wounds that did not allow primary repair. Another group exists in whom the significance of the original injury was underestimated.

Clinical picture

Functional loss varies greatly in the chronic extensor injury.

Wrist extensors. Loss of the radial wrist extensors, which are rarely injured alone, results in an ulnar deviation deformity when the wrist is extended as a result of the unopposed pull of the extensor carpi ulnaris. Conversely, loss of the continuity of the extensor carpi ulnaris can cause a radial deviation deformity of the wrist in extension. Complete loss of the wrist extensor system may cause the patient to adopt a substitute pattern in which the finger extensors try to take over the lost function. This is not a wholly satisfactory solution.[11] Repair of these wrist extensor injuries should be undertaken only when clinical conditions demand correction and when functional loss justifies the surgery.

Long extensors of the fingers. Individual extensor loss involves a lag or loss of extension at the involved MCP joint. This can be masked by the interconnecting network on the dorsum of the hand (conexus intertendineus) and at times be almost completely compensated for by this system.

Treatment

When confronted with one of these problems, the surgeon has three approaches available. Provided there is good skin and subcutaneous coverage as well as passively mobile joints, the surgeon can perform (1) direct secondary repair, (2) free-tendon graft, or (3) tendon transfer. Each patient's situation has to be individually evaluated. In many cases a final decision as to the technique of reconstruction may not be possible until the actual surgical exploration is undertaken.

One curious phenomenon sometimes occurs in which a patient in whom all the finger extensors had been lost appears to "spontaneously regenerate" the tendons, in this case, while awaiting the maturation of an abdominal pedicle skin graft (Fig. 6-1). No similar events have been found in the literature, although other surgeons have personally reported seeing this phenomenon. Of course, this is not a predictable occurrence and cannot be relied on as a treatment method.

Direct repair. If a great time lapse has not intervened and surgical mobilization of the tendon ends allows approximation without excessive tension, then direct repair is preferable (Fig. 6-2). This gives the best opportunity for the restoration of normal function. If, on direct repair, tension is felt to be excessive, i.e., if 50% of passive flexion is not attainable by the surgeon at the operation, then one of the alternative techniques is considered. Restoration of full extension at the cost of loss of flexion is not often acceptable to the patient.

Tendon graft. In situations where direct repair is not feasible because of excessive tension or where tendon substance is lost, tendon graft may be indicated (Fig. 6-3). Graft material is obtained by the standard techniques and interposed in the defect at the appropriate tension. When determining tension in these extensor tendon problems, the surgeon should put the grafts in

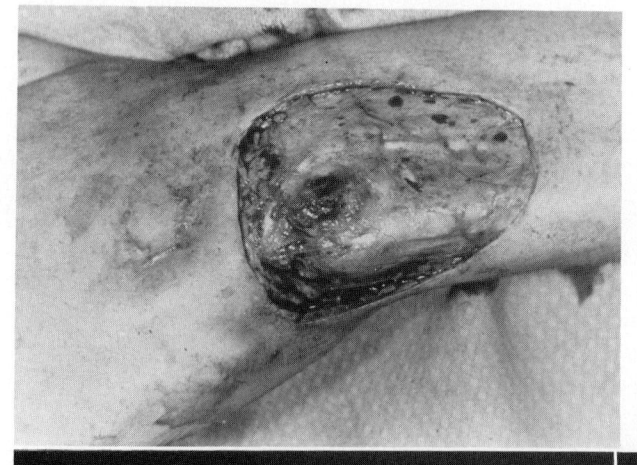

FIG. 6-1. Blast injury in wrist region, with loss of long extensor tendons to the fingers. **A,** Prior to placement of abdominal flap there was no long extensor function, the tendons having been destroyed by injury. **B** and **C,** Three months later active extension and flexion at the MCP joints with no surgery other than application of skin flap.

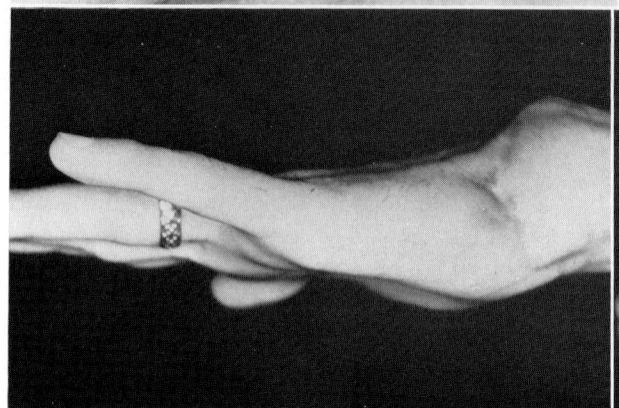

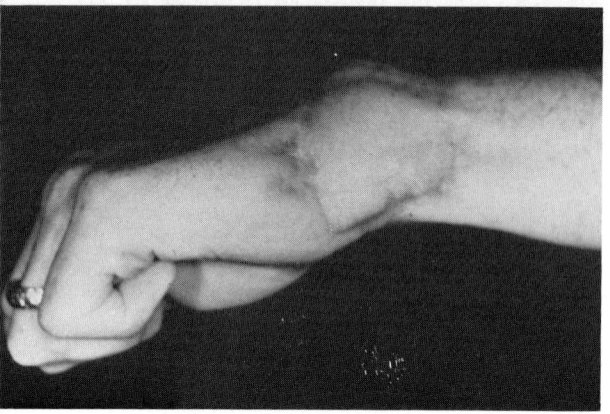

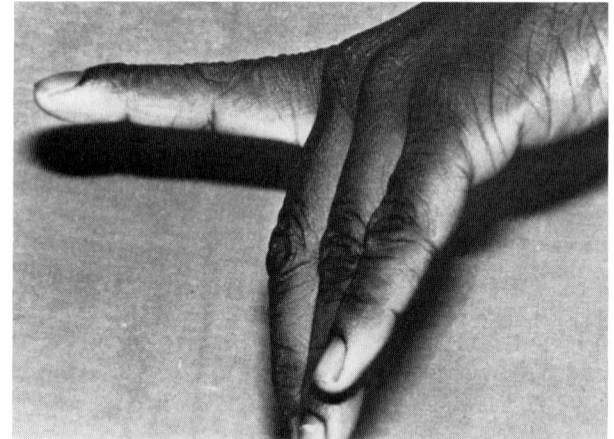

FIG. 6-2. Four-week-old glass laceration of forearm with severance of all long finger extensors except indicis proprius. **A,** Preoperative extensor function. **B,** Extension recovered at 3 months after direct repair. **C,** Full flexion recovered.

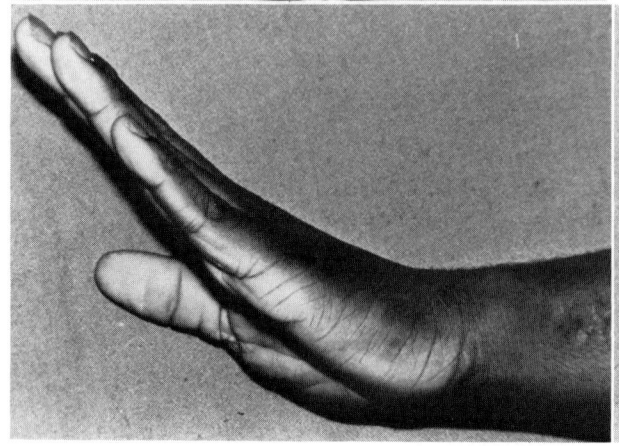

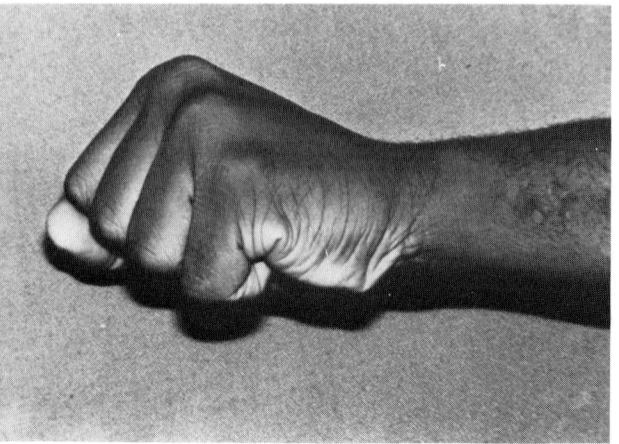

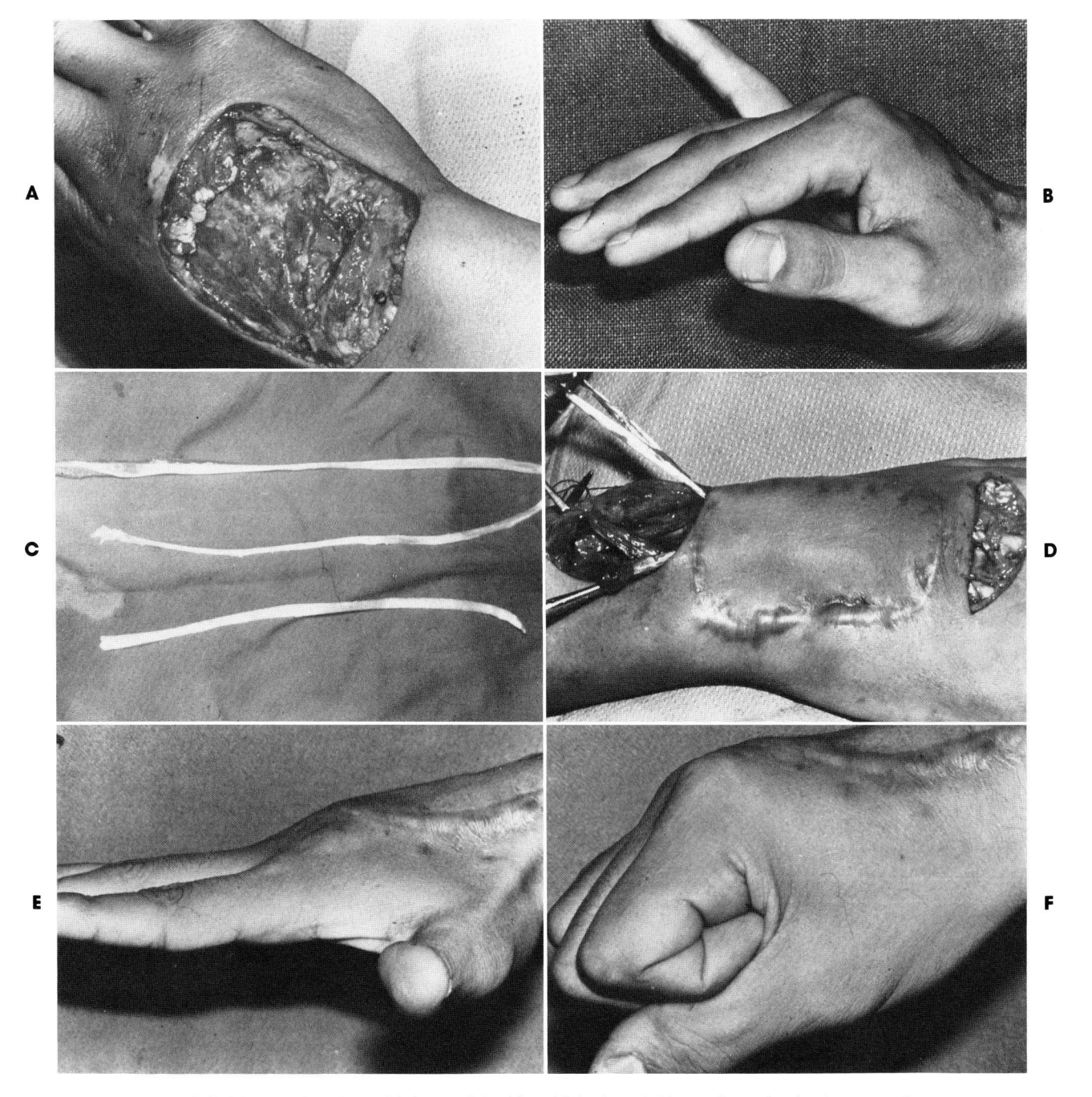

CHAPTER 6 RECONSTRUCTION IN CHRONIC EXTENSOR TENDON PROBLEMS

FIG. 6-3. Victim of motor vehicle accident in which dorsal skin and much of extensor system had been lost. **A,** At time of delayed closure with abdominal flap. **B,** Three months later flap has healed. Attempt at extension shows that extensor digiti minimi has retained function. All other long finger extensors have been lost. **C,** Tendon graft material obtained from plantaris tendon and the palmaris longus. **D,** Grafts are sutured into three extensor hoods distally and interwoven proximally into extensor digitorum communis. **E** and **F,** Extension and flexion obtained at 6 months.

tightly, allowing therapy measures to stretch them free after a 3- to 4-week immobilization period. In cases of loss of all the finger extensor tendons, repair en masse is more practical than attempting individual grafts for each tendon. When the bed is exceedingly poor, the grafting procedure can be staged,[5] placing silicone rubber artificial tendons temporarily in place, to be removed and replaced by a tendon graft at a second stage.

Tendon transfer. In cases where defects cannot be overcome, and especially if the tendon motors are no longer viable, tendon transfer is a good alternative procedure. The well-established rules of tendon transfer[12] must be followed if success is to be forthcoming. The flexor carpi ulnaris as well as the flexor carpi radialis makes an excellent wrist extensor when transferred subcutaneously around the border of the forearm and inserted into the extensor carpi radialis brevis, the more centrally located of the two radial wrist extensors. The pronator teres, as used in radial palsy, is also a good wrist extensor transfer, although its short amplitude limits wrist flexion significantly.

In partial extensor loss the transfer can be as simple as attachment of the distal segment to the adjacent intact extensor tendon or transferring one of the proprius extensors. Having the patient awake and able to cooperate in this aspect of the procedure[6] is very helpful in judging the appropriate tension. In the more massive injuries one of the wrist flexors (Fig. 6-4) elongated by a graft, if needed, is usable, or even use of the flexor digitorum superficialis has been advocated. Since the wrist flexors have a shorter amplitude of action than that needed for full digital extension (3.5 cm compared with 5.0 cm), the interplay of a mobile wrist joint is a helpful adjunct to successful function after this transfer.

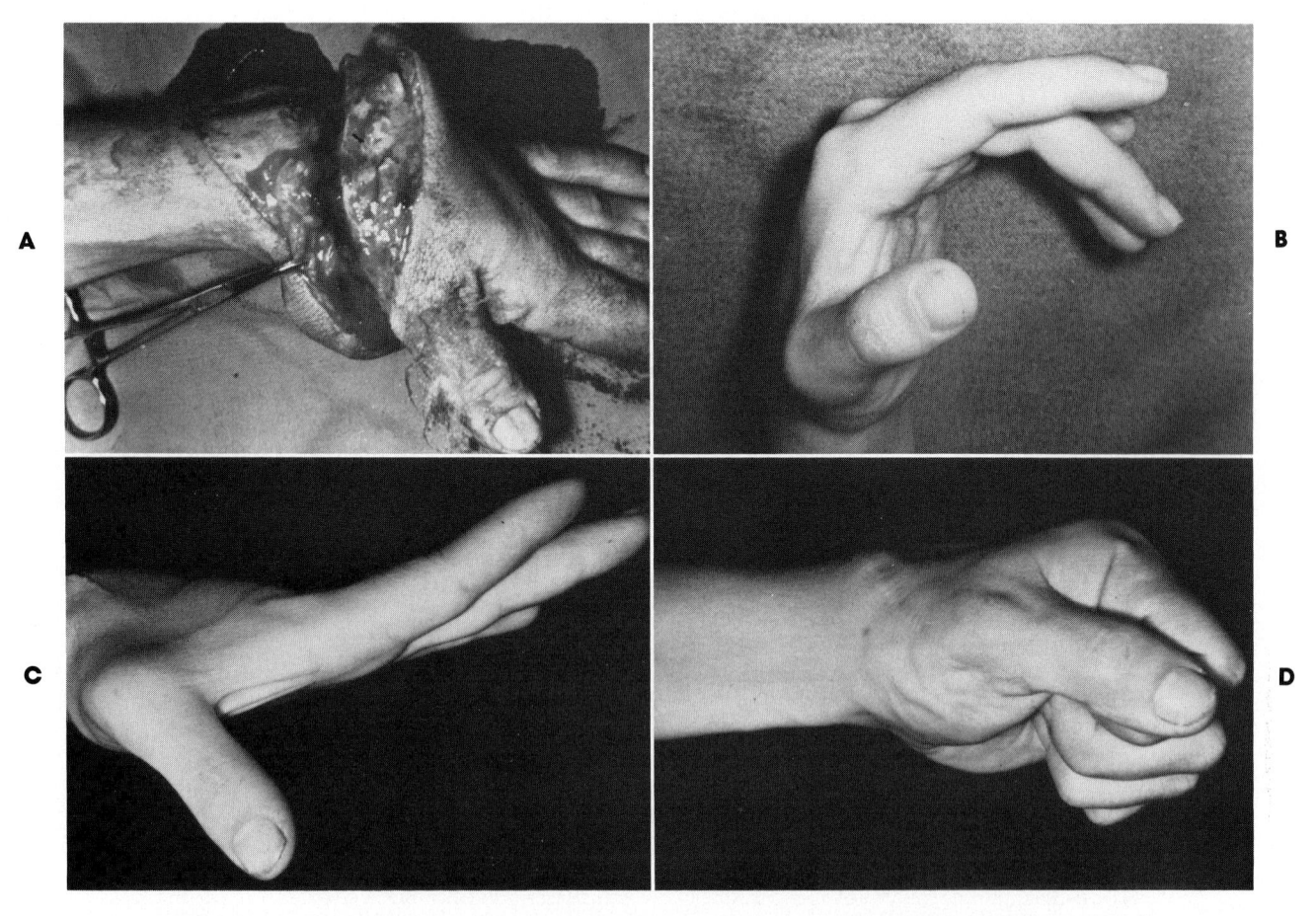

FIG. 6-4. Massive injury to carpal region with transection of all long extensor tendons and carpal bones. **A,** At time of injury the fractures were reduced and pinned. Wound infection precluded early closure and tendon repair. **B,** Wounds healed at 2 months. No active extensor function is present. **C** and **D,** Flexor carpi ulnaris was transferred around ulnar border of forearm into all four long extensor tendons. Flexor superficialis of ring finger was transferred to rerouted extensor pollicis longus. Extension and flexion seen 6 months later.

EXTENSOR POLLICIS LONGUS
Anatomy and function

Loss of extensor pollicis longus tendon function is variable in presentation. The extensor pollicis longus is the primary extensor at the interphalangeal (IP) joint of the thumb, and in many hands it is the most important extensor at the MCP joint as well. It also provides retroposition of the thumb and brings it into the plane of the palm. To test for the integrity of the extensor pollicis longus, the examiner should have the patient strongly extend the thumb in a plane posterior to the plane of the palm. The tendon, if intact, should be visible and palpable (Fig. 6-5). Since, in the absence of extensor pollicis longus function, most patients will still show some degree of active extension at the IP joint by virtue of the insertion of the abductor pollicis brevis, flexor pollicis brevis, as well as extensor pollicis brevis into the extensor aponeurosis, functional loss is greatest where the extensor pollicis longus is the major extensor of the MCP joint (Fig. 6-6). Many patients who have effective extension at the MCP joint through the extensor pollicis brevis will accept the IP weakness and not desire treatment. In the patient with significant functional loss, treatment can restore excellent extensor function to the thumb.

Etiology

Most chronic ruptures of the extensor pollicis longus tendon occur as a rare complication of Colles' fractures (estimated as 1 in 300).[3,14] The tendon rupture usually occurs 6 to 8 weeks after fracture, and there is some disagreement regarding the cause of the tendon injury. There are two general theories as to cause.

Mechanical causes of rupture. Some authors[7,17] believe that the tendon is actually incompletely severed by the bone fragments at the time of injury or reduction. The tendon then completes the rupture at a later date. Others espousing a mechanical cause attribute the problem to attrition of the tendon on a roughened area of the radius near Lister's tubercle.

Vascular theory. Those propounding the vascular theory* think that hemorrhage within the intact tendon sheath sets up a synovial reaction, leading to a decrease in blood supply to the tendon. Recent work[2] has confirmed that the area of the tendon just distal to the dorsal transverse carpal ligament is poorly vascularized, and it is hypothesized that increased pressure within the tendon sheath further reduces the blood flow with resultant degeneration and later rupture. This would explain why

---

*References 1, 2, 10, and 13-16.

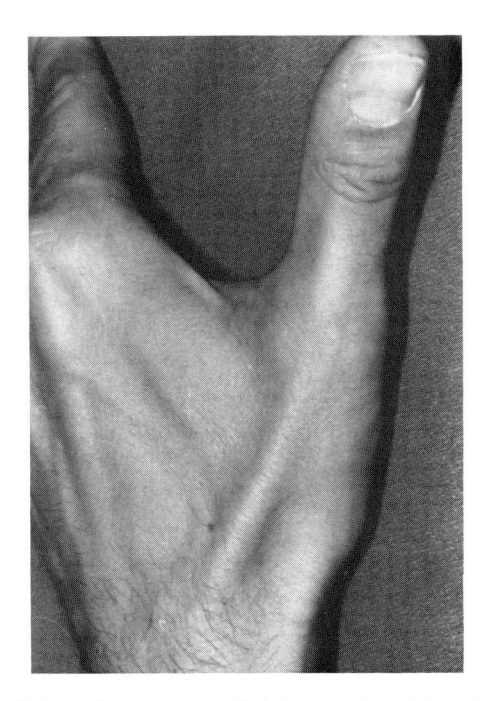

FIG. 6-5. Intact extensor pollicis longus is visible when patient strongly extends the thumb in plane posterior to palm.

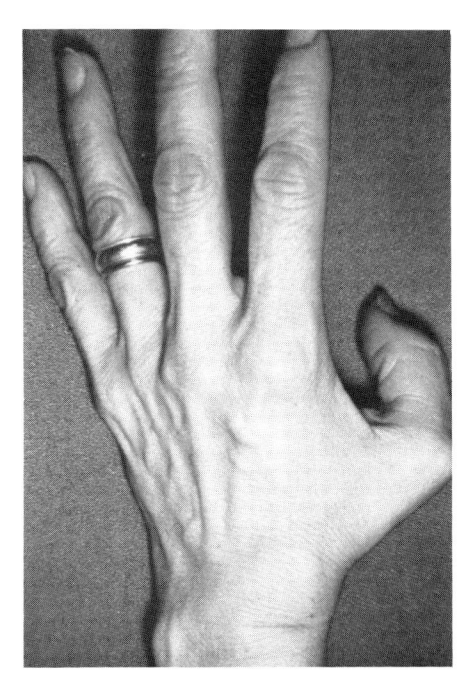

FIG. 6-6. Rupture of extensor pollicis longus with marked loss of thumb function in patient with closed wrist injury and in whom extensor pollicis longus was major extensor of MCP joint.

SECTION 2 EXTENSOR TENDON PROBLEMS

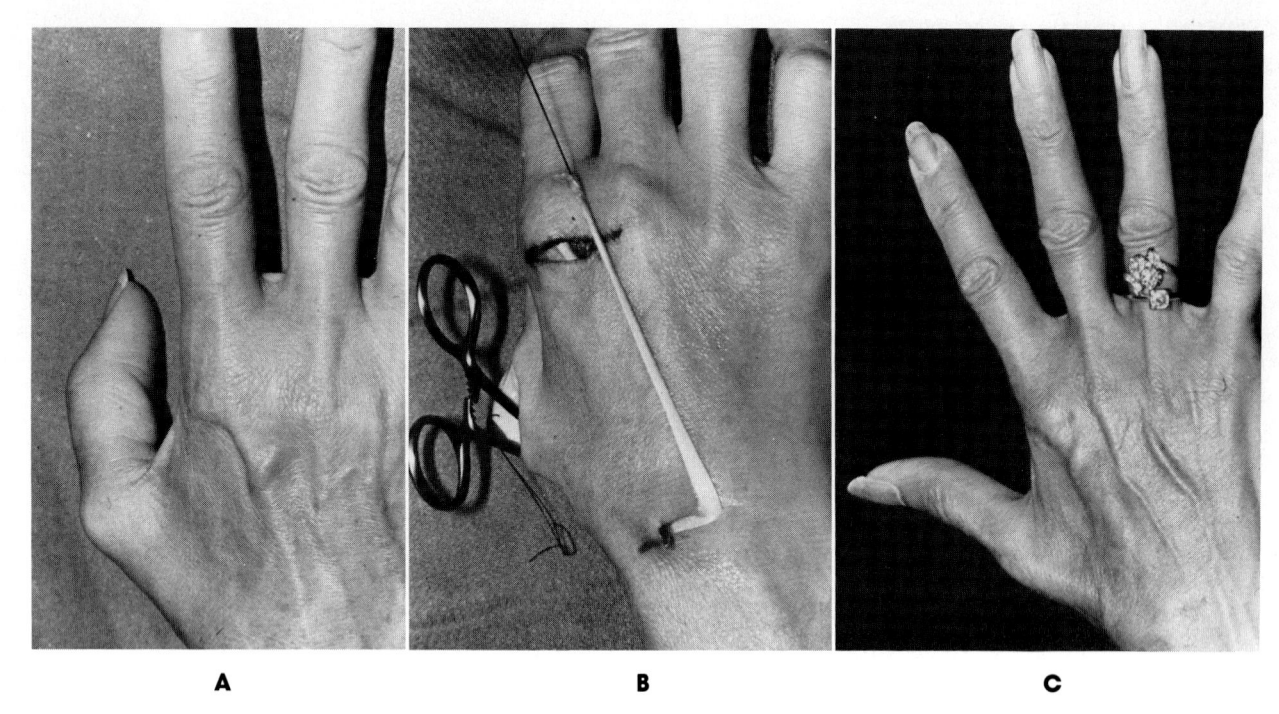

FIG. 6-7. Closed rupture of the extensor pollicis longus tendon after undisplaced Colles fracture. **A,** Preoperative loss of thumb extension. **B,** Extensor indicis proprius transfer; tendon has been mobilized and will be drawn subcutaneously to dorsum of thumb. **C,** Extension recovered 6 months after surgery.

rupture of the extensor pollicis longus tendon is more frequent in undisplaced fractures (not requiring reduction) than in widely displaced injuries in which the tendon sheath is more likely to have been torn. This fact, plus the absence of sharp, bony prominences, in most cases of rupture makes the vascular theory the more reasonable explanation.

Secondary to rheumatoid disease. Another group of patients rupture their extensor pollicis longus tendon secondary to rheumatoid disease where synovial proliferative tissue either invades the tendon directly or competes for the available blood supply, thereby weakening the tendon.

Spontaneous rupture. Spontaneous rupture of the extensor pollicis longus tendon after twisting trauma or wrist sprain without fracture also accounts for a group of patients with this lesion. Repetitive activities resulting in tenosynovitis, most popularly known as *drummer boy's palsy*, were reported with frequency in the German medical literature of the last century.

Treatment of extensor pollicis longus rupture

Direct repair formerly had its proponents,[8,16] but in this chronic condition usually it is not feasible. Tendon grafting[4] can recover function but has the disadvantages of two tendon junctures. A graft cannot be used if the motor capability of the extensor pollicis longus tendon is no longer functional.

Tendon transfer is the most frequent treatment applied to this lesion. Although use of the extensor carpi radialis longus[9] or the extensor pollicis brevis has been advocated, the extensor indicis proprius is the most widely reported in the literature,[1,10,13,16] and results using this transfer have been excellent. This transfer fulfills all the requirements of successful tendon transfer and yields predictable functional results (Fig. 6-7).

In summary, the chronic injury to the long extensor system can yield satisfying functional results through operative procedures that are planned in accord with the basic principles of wound care and tendon surgery.

REFERENCES

1. Christophe, K.: Rupture of the extensor pollicis longus tendon following Colles' fracture, J. Bone Joint Surg. **35A:** 1003, 1953.
2. Engkvist, O., and Lundborg, G.: Rupture of the extensor pollicis longus tendon after fracture of the lower end of the radius, Hand **2:**76, 1979.
3. Frykman, G.: Fracture of the distal radius including sequelae, Acta Orthop. Scand. (Suppl.) **108:**3, 1967.
4. Hamlin, C., and Littler, J.W.: Segmental tendon graft restoration of extensor pollicis longus disruption. In Proceedings of American Society for Surgery of the Hand, J. Bone Joint Surg. **57A:**729, 1975.

5. Hunter, J.M., and Schneider, L.H.: Staged tendon reconstruction. In American Academy of Orthopaedic Surgeons: Instructional Course Lectures 26:134, 1977.
6. Hunter, J.M., Schneider, L.H., Dumont, J., and Erickson, J.C.: A dynamic approach to problems of hand function, Clin. Orthop. 104:112, 1974.
7. Levine, J., and Schneider, M.: Spontaneous rupture of the extensor pollicis longus tendon following the fracture of the carpal navicular bone, J. Bone Joint Surg. 37A:364, 1955.
8. McMaster, P.E.: Late ruptures of the extensor and flexor pollicis longus following Colles' fracture, J. Bone Joint Surg. 14:93, 1932.
9. Pressly, J.A., and Goldner, J.L.: Extensor pollicis longus rupture due to old fracture, collagen degeneration or rheumatoid arthritis: analysis and treatment by transfer of the extensor carpi radialis longus. In Proceedings of American Society for Surgery of the Hand, J. Bone Joint Surg. 56A:1093, 1974.
10. Riddell, D.M.: Spontaneous rupture of the extensor pollicis longus (the results of tendon transfer), J. Bone Joint Surg. 45B:506, 1963.
11. Rosenthal, E.A.: The extensor tendons. In Hunters, J.M., Schneider, L.H., Mackin, E.J., and Bell, J.A., editors: Rehabilitation of the hand, St. Louis, 1978, The C.V. Mosby Co.
12. Schneider, L.H.: Tendon transfers in the upper extremity. In Hunter, J.M., Schneider, L.H., Mackin, E.J., and Bell, J.A., editors: Rehabilitation of the hand, St. Louis, 1978, The C.V. Mosby Co.
13. Simpson, R.G.: Delayed rupture of the extensor pollicis longus tendon following closed injury, Hand 9:160, 1977.
14. Smith, F.M.: Late rupture of the extensor pollicis longus tendon following Colles' fracture, J. Bone Joint Surg. 28:49, 1946.
15. Strandell, G.: Post-traumatic rupture of the extensor pollicis longus tendon: pathogenesis and treatment, Acta Chir. Scand. 109:81, 1955.
16. Trevor, D.: Rupture of the extensor pollicis longus tendon after Colles' fracture, J. Bone Joint Surg. 32B:370, 1950.
17. Vaughn-Jackson, O.J.: Rupture of the extensor tendons by attrition at the inferior radio-ulnar joint, J. Bone Joint Surg. 30B:528, 1948.

Chapter 7 Boutonniere deformity

Julio Taleisnik

Boutonniere deformity of a finger results from a disruption of the integrity of the extensor apparatus at the level of the middle joint. The typical, well-established deformity is characterized by a loss of extension of the proximal interphalangeal (PIP) joint and a secondary hyperextension of the distal joint (Fig. 7-1). The imbalance created by the extensor tendon injury is difficult to correct, particularly in chronic cases, when fixed contractures develop.

ANATOMY

The extensor hood at the base of the finger has been described as "a plexus of tendons within an aponeurotic sheath."[13] Both the extrinsic extensors and the intrinsic tendons contribute to the extensor hood (Fig. 7-2). The extrinsic extensor tendon crosses the metacarpophalangeal (MCP) joint, and proximal to the middle joint it trifurcates into a central slip and two lateral bands. The intrinsic tendons, after contributing to the formation of the extensor hood, bifurcate on each side of the finger. Of the two tendinous slips thus created, the more medial joins the central slip to constitute a common central extensor tendon, which attaches on the proximal dorsal margin of the middle phalanx through a rather thick fibrocartilaginous insertion. The lateral halves of the bifurcating intrinsic tendons are called intrinsic lateral bands. These join the extensor lateral bands to form radial and ulnar common lateral bands, which fuse into a single terminal extensor tendon attaching on the dorsal lip of the distal phalanx through a fibrocartilaginous structure similar to that of the middle joint but not as well developed. This entire tendon complex is intimately related to a retinacular system.[5,19] The transverse retinacular ligament arises from the lateral bands and progresses volarward to a double insertion: superficial, on the overlying dermis dorsal to the neurovascular bundle, and deep, attaching to the flexor tendon tunnel, the volar plate, and the glenoid portion of the collateral ligament.[19] Dorsal and medial to the lateral bands, the transverse retinacular ligament is continuous with a thin retinacular layer that contains the central extensor tendon. Distal to the middle joint, this dorsal retinaculum thickens to bridge the gap between the lateral bands just before they join over the dorsum of the middle phalanx. This is the triangular ligament.

The oblique retinacular ligament[5] is the second major component of the retinacular system. It originates in the distal portion of the volar lateral ridge of the proximal phalanx, from a common attachment with the distal edge of the proximal flexor annular ligament.[11] Earlier descriptions depict this ligament as a cord of variable thick-

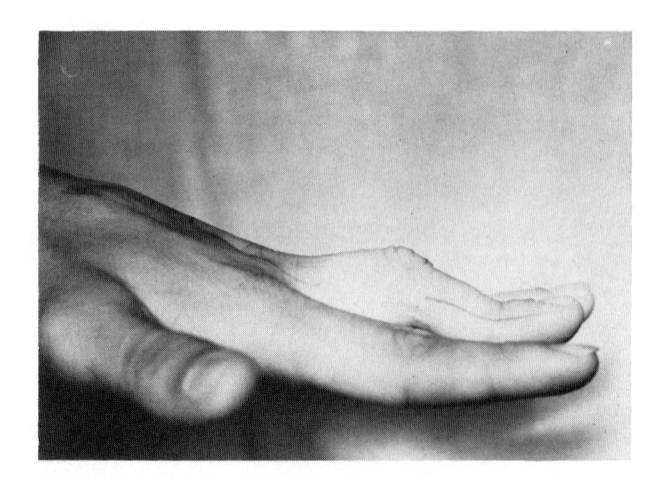

FIG. 7-1. Typical boutonniere deformity: loss of extension of middle joint and hyperextension of distal joint.

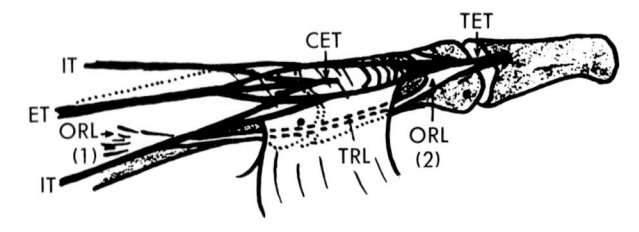

FIG. 7-2. Schematic representation of extensor apparatus of a finger. *IT*, Intrinsic tendons; *ET*, long extensor tendon; *CET*, central extensor tendon; *TET*, terminal extensor tendon; *ORL*, oblique retinacular ligament, origin *(1)* and insertion *(2)*; *TRL*, transverse retinacular ligament.

ness, which progresses distally along the volar margin of the lateral bands and deep to the transverse retinacular ligament,[5,19] volar to the axis of motion of the middle joint, and dorsal to that of the distal joint. Its insertion is mobile, on the edge of the lateral bands at the level of the triangular ligament. More recently Shrewsbury and Johnson[11] found that this ligament was actually complete, as described, in only a small percentage of the fingers they dissected. The ligament varied in completeness and structure among the different fingers of a hand, as well as for both sides of a single digit. Only on the ulnar side of the ring finger did they find an oblique retinacular ligament with any degree of consistency (93% of their specimens). There is also some disagreement as to the functional significance of the transverse and oblique retinacular ligament in the normal digit. It is generally accepted that the transverse retinacular ligament limits the dorsal displacement of the lateral bands during full extension.[5,6,14,19] The role of the oblique retinacular ligament is more controversial. Landsmeer[5] considered it an intercalated factor designed to balance the potentially unstable biarticular digital system. As the distal joint flexes, the oblique retinacular ligament becomes tense, indirectly contributing to the initiation of middle joint flexion. Conversely, initial extension of the distal joint depends largely on the tenodesis effect of the oblique retinacular ligament, whereas the terminal strong extension of the distal joint is directly contributed by the lateral bands.[5,14,19]

A different point of view is offered by Harris and Rutledge,[4] who were unable to observe any change of finger function after severing the oblique retinacular ligament. This ligament was found to be tense only when the middle joint was fully extended while the distal joint was passively flexed beyond 70 degrees, a motion that is not part of normal hand function. Shrewsbury and Johnson[11] found that fingers without an oblique retinacular ligament did not show an alteration of their coordinated motions. Therefore this ligament did not appear to have any dynamic function but rather a static or stabilizing function only. However, although the oblique retinacular ligament may not play a significant role under normal conditions, it can become a deforming factor in some pathologic conditions (particularly Dupuytren's disease, posttraumatic extensor tendon and retinacular imbalance, and burns). An abnormally shortened or contracted oblique retinacular ligament would produce in the *distal* biarticular digital system (middle and distal joints) dynamic changes similar to those found in intrinsic-plus conditions involving the *proximal* biarticular digital system (proximal and middle joints).[5] In the intrinsic-plus deformity, passive hyperextension of the most proximal of the two joints in the *proximal* biarticular system (the MCP joint) results in extension of the middle joint, which is resistant to passive or active flexion attempts. Similarly, in boutonniere deformity any attempt to passively reduce the flexion contracture of the most proximal of the two joints in the *distal* biarticular system (the PIP joint) produces an aggravation of the distal joint hyperextension, which is resistant to passive or active flexion. This has been referred to as a positive intrinsic–intrinsic plus,[1] or retinacular-plus,[19] test (Fig. 7-3).

PATHOGENESIS OF THE DEFORMITY

If the central extensor tendon slip is carefully severed, a boutonniere deformity is not likely to occur. This is part of the rationale of treatment of mallet deformity by central slip tenotomy, as proposed by S.B. Fowler.[8] For a boutonniere deformity to occur a tear of the retinacular component of the dorsal apparatus is required, in addition to the tear of the central tendon. Initially after the injury there is considerable swelling and pain, and a thorough functional examination is rather difficult. The true nature of the injury may be easily missed. The middle joint tends to prolapse dorsally, and the middle phalanx tends to assume a semiflexed position. Normally, in the uninjured digit, gradual flexion of the middle joint progressively increases the load applied to the central extensor tendon slip, while the lateral bands are allowed to migrate in a volar direction. In the boutonniere digit, middle joint flexion tends to keep both ends of the injured central tendon apart. End-to-end healing is not possible as long as the digit is left unprotected. The lateral bands are subluxed. Any attempt by the patient to actively correct the deformity only helps to increase it, since active extension is transmitted to the lateral bands

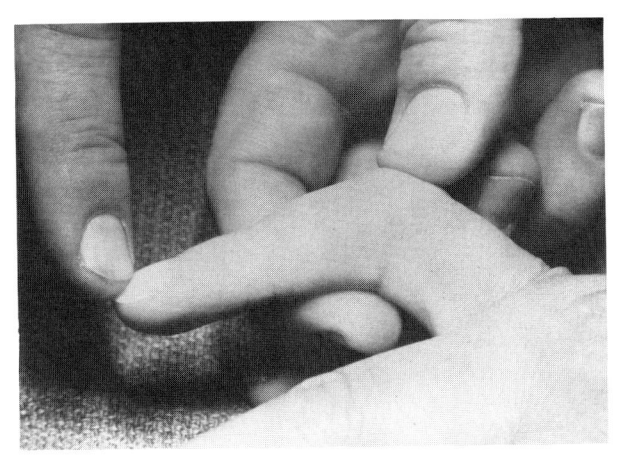

FIG. 7-3. Any passive attempt at reducing middle joint flexion contracture increases distal joint resistance to flexion (positive intrinsic–intrinsic plus, or retinacular-plus, test).

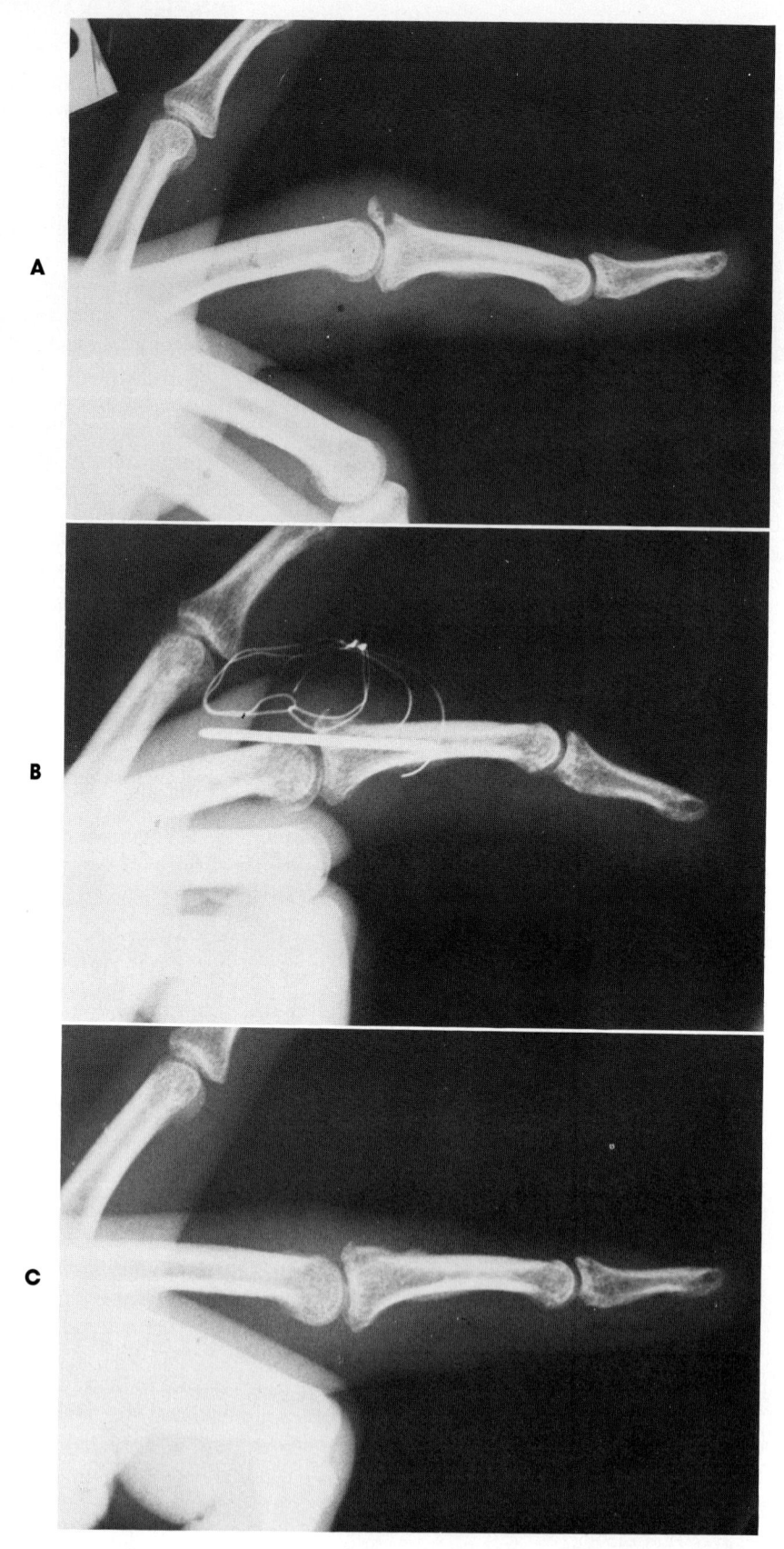

FIG. 7-4. A, Boutonniere deformity secondary to avulsion fracture of central extensor tendon insertion. **B,** Surgical repair. A pullout wire technique was used to reapproximate the avulsed bony fragment, and Kirschner wire to stabilize joint. **C,** Postoperative appearance.

rather than to the injured central tendon; this causes further subluxation of the lateral bands volar to the axis of motion of the middle joint, effectively changing their function to flexion rather than extension of the PIP joint. The more direct line of extensor pull to the distal joint results in secondary hyperextension of the distal interphalangeal (DIP) joint. Initially this typical deformity may be passively corrected. It becomes fixed, however, as soon as the retinacular components of the extensor apparatus shorten to accommodate the new position and length. There are, therefore, several well-defined stages in the progression of the boutonniere deformity. Zancolli[19] recognized an initial stage immediately following the injury, a second period of reducible deformity, a period of retinacular stiffness, and a final stage of fixed deformity.

During the *initial stage* the diagnosis may be easily missed because of swelling, pain, and tenderness. There is voluntary limitation of motion, which makes examination rather unreliable. There is a minimal flexion stance of the middle joint, and motion is present in the distal joint but accompanied by considerable pain and therefore voluntarily restricted. The second stage, *reducible deformity*, is characterized by flexion of the middle joint and hyperextension of the distal joint. Both are passively reducible. The lateral bands are displaced volarly, but there are no retinacular or articular contractures, and both joints can be fully reduced. The intrinsic–intrinsic plus test is therefore negative. When *retinacular contractures* occur, the semiflexed position of the middle joint becomes only partially reducible. As this joint is extended as much as possible, passive flexion of the distal joint becomes severely limited or impossible (Fig. 7-3). The intrinsic–intrinsic plus test is now positive. *Articular contractures*, the fourth stage in the progression of this deformity, occur when there is an actual fixation of the boutonniere deformity stance by periarticular tissue changes.

TREATMENT

Surgical correction of boutonniere deformity is usually limited, in my experience, to the following five categories:

1. Open injuries
2. Boutonniere deformities secondary to intraarticular fractures (Fig. 7-4)
3. Recurrent or chronic deformities that are not responsive to splinting (Fig. 7-5)
4. Boutonniere deformities accompanied by painful posttraumatic degenerative changes of the middle joint
5. The complex deformity seen in collagen diseases, rheumatoid arthritis, and burns (Fig. 7-6)

Overall the boutonniere digit is better managed if treatment is planned according to the stage of development of the deformity. The most important step in the treatment of the initial boutonniere deformity is recognition of the true nature of the injury. Immobilization of the finger with the middle joint semiflexed should be

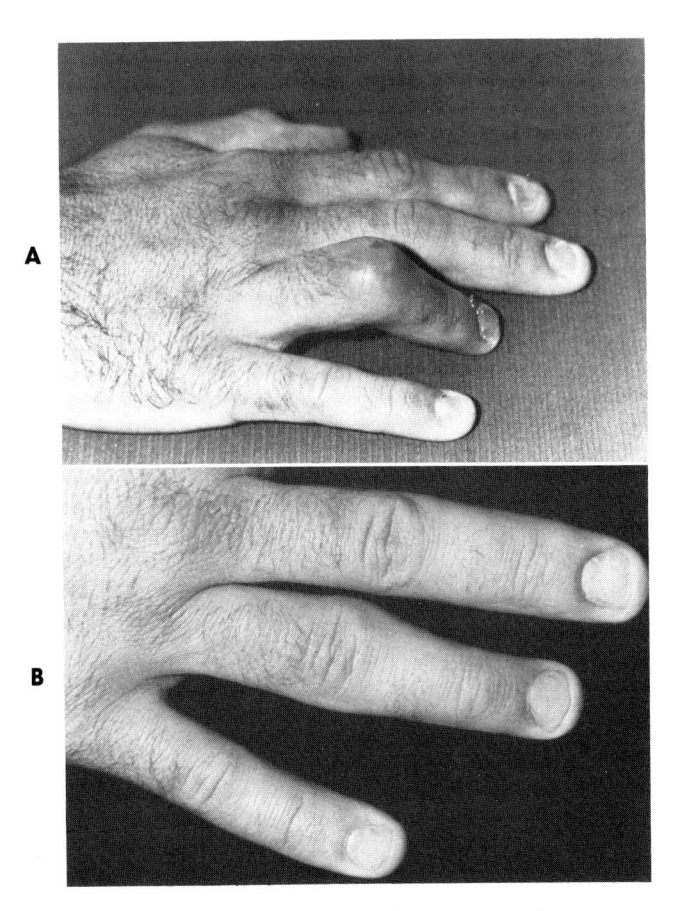

FIG. 7-5. A, Preoperative and, **B,** postoperative appearance of chronic boutonniere deformity.

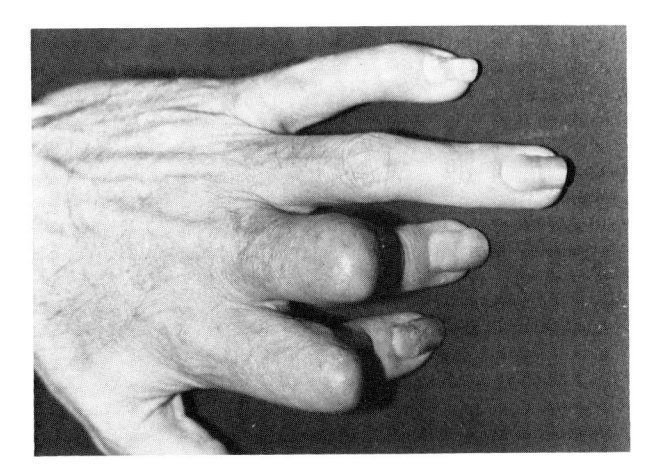

FIG. 7-6. Chronic boutonniere deformity in patient with severe psoriatic arthritis.

SECTION 2 EXTENSOR TENDON PROBLEMS

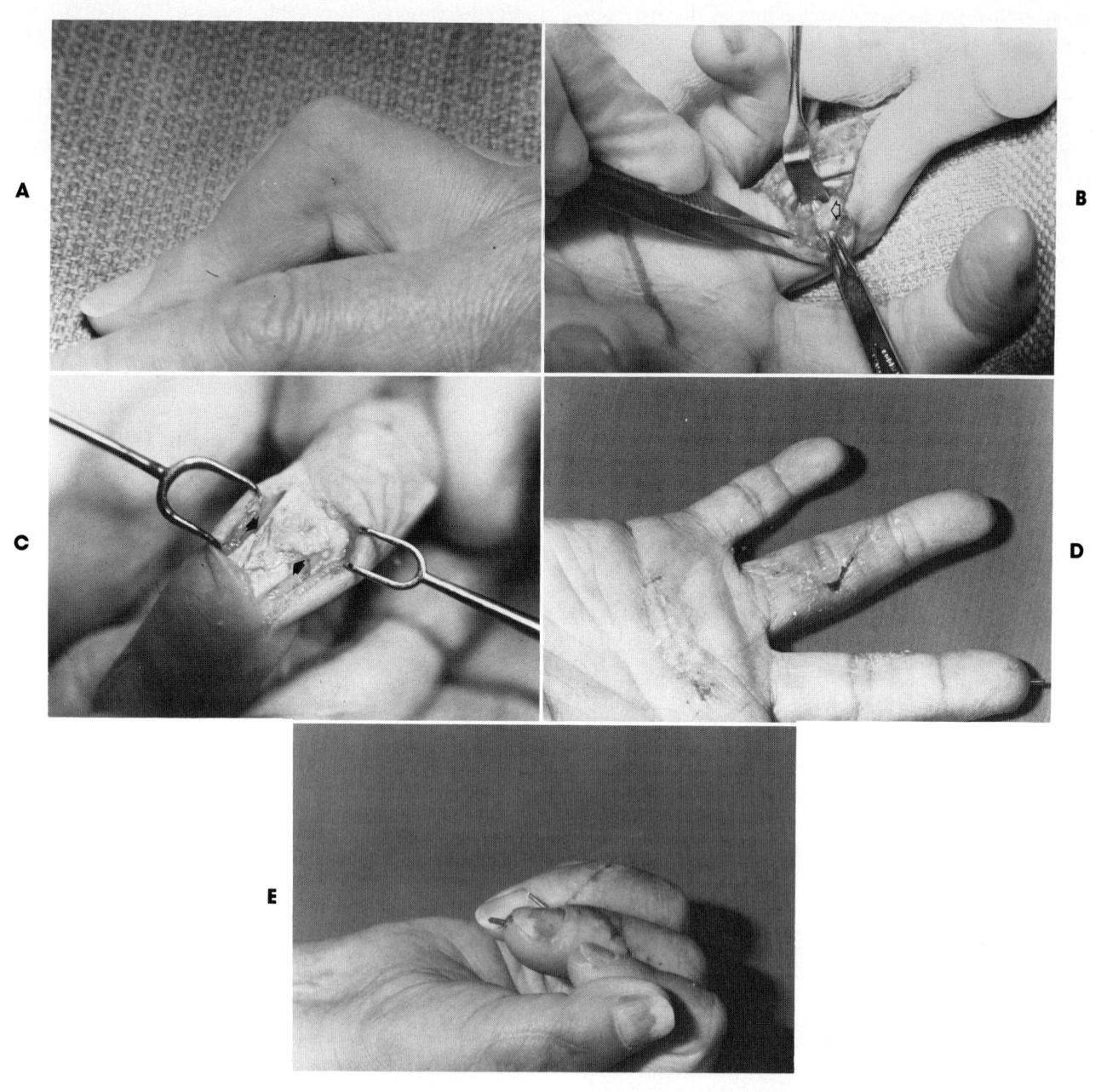

FIG. 7-7. A, Chronic fixed boutonnier deformity of right ring finger. **B,** Check-rein ligament *(arrow).* **C,** Chevron tenotomy of terminal extensor tendon *(arrows).* **D,** Postoperative apearance at 3 weeks following release of middle joint contracture and terminal extensor tendon tenotomy. Palmar incision used to gain control of flexor tendons, to check flexion range after contractures released. **E,** Postoperative range of motion. Long finger shows Kirschner wires used for internal fixation of surgical fusion of its distal joint.

avoided. Stewart[15] proposed that most middle joint injuries be immobilized in extension, provided that the joint surfaces are satisfactory and the flexor tendons are normal. The distal joint is allowed to actively flex and extend during the immobilization of the middle joint, which may assist in the healing of the lacerated or avulsed central tendon and preserve a more normal finger function. Immobilization of the middle joint in extension should be continued for at least 4 weeks and followed by a period of graduated exercises while the finger continues to be protected by removable splints. At the end of a minimum of 6 weeks of treatment the middle joint extension is tested. If it is satisfactory, with minimal or no extension lag, the patient is allowed free use of the digit. A night splint may be of help as long as there is a tendency toward extension lag of the middle joint at the end of a working day. The length of immobilization can be estimated by evaluation of the restoration of full flexion to the distal joint.[1] Immobilization should be continued for a minimum of 4 to 6 weeks or until distal joint flexion is performed fully and freely.

Boutonniere fingers in the second stage, reducible deformity, are similarly treated by splinting of the middle joint in full extension for 4 to 6 weeks or until the distal joint flexes fully. Night splinting may be required for several additional weeks if the finger exhibits a tendency toward a recurrence of deformity during the splint-free period. There may be some degree of flexion contracture, which usually responds to the use of dynamic splints.

When the patient enters the third stage, retinacular contractures interfere with all attempts at permanent restoration of distal joint flexion by nonsurgical means alone. There is a positive intrinsic–intrinsic plus test: the distal joint hyperextension is reducible only when the middle joint is allowed to flex. Active patient cooperation is necessary for the success of treatment, since flexion of the distal joint should be recovered by active motion against the contracted oblique retinacular ligament, while the middle joint is kept in extension. Nighttime splinting for prolonged periods is usually necessary in these patients. When distal joint flexion cannot be obtained or maintained by splinting alone, surgical division of the oblique retinacular ligament should be of help. The terminal extensor tendon is exposed through an oblique incision across the dorsum of the middle segment. The operation is preferably performed with the patient under digital nerve block anesthesia to allow cooperation throughout surgery. Zancolli[19] excises a triangular segment of the lateral margins of the extensor apparatus at the level of the triangular ligament. This excised segment contains the insertion of the oblique retinacular ligament as well as the most lateral fibers of the terminal extensor bands. Dolphin[2] reports improvement in two patients following complete transection of the terminal tendon distal to the triangular ligament. I favor a controlled chevron tenotomy that completely transects both margins of the terminal tendon containing the insertion of the oblique retinacular ligament fibers, distal to the triangular ligament; this is continued centrally by a partial division of the superficial layers of the terminal tendon. The distal joint is then passively flexed, and with the patient awake, the range of active flexion-extension obtained can be evaluated more accurately. At the end of this procedure some tendinous longitudinal fibers can still be seen bridging the gap created by the more superficial chevron tenotomy (Fig. 7-7, C). Active flexion-extension exercises are resumed as soon as postoperative pain and swelling allow, usually at 5 to 7 days postoperative. The digit is protected by intermittent splinting for a minimum of 3 weeks. Tenotomy of the terminal tendon restores balance, or "isometry,"[19] between the central and lateral extensor bands, obviating the need for a direct repair or shortening of the central extensor tendon slip itself.

For a digit in the fourth stage with periarticular and retinacular contractures a 2-week period of progressive plaster splints is first tried (Fig. 7-8). Whether successful or not, it will at least facilitate any operative release that may be undertaken at that point. In the rare case when the contracture is reduced and correction can be maintained, this deformity, in effect, is changed from a stage 4 to a stage 3, becoming amenable to a more permanent correction by terminal extensor tenotomy alone. If, however, surgical correction of the flexion contracture of the middle joint is not possible, or if contracture recurs, then a surgical correction of the joint contracture is indicated. The primary aim of this procedure is the division

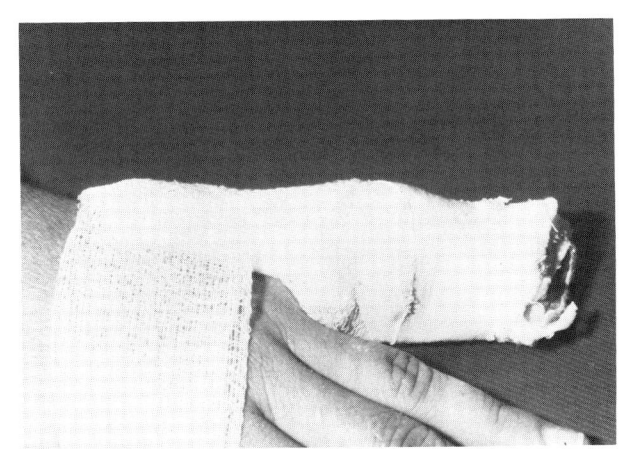

FIG. 7-8. Progressive plaster splints may be used, changed at frequent intervals, in attempt to reduce severe, fixed flexion contracture of middle joint.

of two thick cordlike structures—*check-rein ligaments*[18]—which appear to be responsible for the unyielding contracture. Through an oblique incision across the volar aspect of the proximal digital segment, the flexor sheath is exposed. This incision may be extended into a V for a V-Y–plasty if additional skin length is needed in very severe contractures. In most cases, however, after full extension is obtained, the joint is allowed to flex enough for comfortable skin closure, relying on dynamic splinting to stretch the skin postoperatively and to regain full extension. The flexor sheath over the middle joint is routinely excised. This may provide some release of the flexion contracture. The flexor tendons are then retracted to either side, and the underlying volar plate is identified. The check-rein ligaments "run from thick, broad attachments along the proximal edge of the volar plate, diverge, and insert separately along the volar lateral periosteum of the proximal phalanx"[18] (Fig. 7-7, *B*). After these structures are excised, it is usually possible to manipulate the joint with ease into full extension. A Kirschner wire is used rarely to maintain reduction, but only for the immediate 5 to 7 postoperative days. With the middle joint fully extended the intrinsic–intrinsic plus test becomes clearly positive. The operation should then be completed by a chevron tenotomy of the terminal extensor tendon (Fig. 7-7, *C*).

In this type of boutonniere deformity of very long standing, if the surgical procedure is not performed with the patient awake to cooperate on checking digit motion, it is at times useful to expose the flexor tendons in the palm and check their excursion. Frequently, fine adhesions are felt to tear before the digit can be fully flexed in this manner.

At 5 to 7 days postoperative, external splinting is applied, and an exercise program is instituted, stressing active flexion of the distal joint and active extension and flexion of the middle joint (Fig. 7-7, *D* and *E*), while the digit continues to be protected by intermittent splinting for a minimum of 6 weeks. This is followed by a prolonged period of night splinting and, not infrequently, by part-time day splints as well, as determined by the patient's progress. The patient's cooperation is necessary for this treatment to succeed.

Direct shortening of the central extensor tendon is not necessary, in my experience, for this group of patients. Even in stage 4, balance, or isometry, can be restored to the extensor apparatus in many patients by release of the middle joint contracture, followed by a chevron tenotomy of the terminal tendon and an intensive postoperative rehabilitation program, without directly interfering with the previously damaged central tendon. For those who fail to regain active extension of the middle joint, and for the complex boutonniere deformities, such as those found with burns, rheumatoid arthritis and other collagen diseases, a reconstruction or repair of the attenuated or avulsed central tendon or a fusion may become necessary.

No matter which technique is used of the several described for the restoration of the central tendon function,* it must be kept in mind that the goal of surgery is to rebalance the extensor system. Therefore, after the surgical repair is completed and prior to the insertion of any internal fixation, the finger should show a change from its boutonniere stance to a position of near extension of the middle joint and semiflexion of the distal joint—in effect a reversal of the boutonniere deformity. A good range of passive flexion of the middle joint without disruption of the central tendon repair or reconstruction should also be possible. Only then may a Kirschner wire be inserted to protect the repair for at least the immediate postoperative period. This is replaced by external splinting at 5 to 7 days postoperatively. Full-time immobilization is continued for a minimum of 4 weeks, after which a graduated program of exercises is prescribed while intermittent protective splinting is continued until a satisfactory tissue balance is obtained. For the complex boutonniere deformity with painful middle joint changes, a salvage procedure (fusion, arthroplasty) is indicated.

SUMMARY

Treatment of the initial stage of the boutonniere deformity is directed at protecting the middle joint in full extension while encouraging active flexion of the distal joint; the treatment of the second stage of reducible deformity is similar, except that some degree of dynamic splinting may be required to correct early middle joint contractures, and prolonged night splinting may be required as well. When retinacular contractions are present, some form of terminal extensor tendon tenotomy is indicated to restore extensor tendon balance. The fourth stage of chronic boutonniere deformity is treated by surgical release of the middle joint contracture, accompanied by a terminal extensor tendon tenotomy. It is rarely necessary to directly visualize or treat the actual central tendon deficit, except for those patients who fail to gain active middle joint extension and for the more complex boutonniere deformities.

---

*References 3, 6, 7, 9, 10, 12, 16, 17, and 19.

REFERENCES

1. Boyes, J.H.: Bunnell's surgery of the hand, ed. 5, Philadelphia, 1970, J.B. Lippincott Co.
2. Dolphin, J.A.: Extensor tenotomy for chronic boutonniere deformity of the finger, J. Bone Joint Surg. **47A**:161, 1965.
3. Elliott, R.A., Jr.: Injuries to the extensor mechanisms of the hand, Clin. Orthop. North Am. **1**:335, 1970.

4. Harris, C., Jr., and Rutledge, G.L.: The functional anatomy of the extensor mechanism of the finger, J. Bone Joint Surg. **54A:**713, 1972.
5. Landsmeer, J.M.F.: The coordination of finger-joint motions, J. Bone Joint Surg. **45A:**1654, 1963.
6. Littler, J.W., and Eaton, R.G.: Redistribution of forces in the correction of the boutonniere deformity, J. Bone Joint Surg. **49A:**1267, 1967.
7. Matev, I.: Transposition of the lateral slips of the aponeurosis in treatment of longstanding "boutonniere deformity" of the fingers, Br. J. Plast. Surg. **17:**281, 1964.
8. Milford, L.: Mallet finger. In Crenshaw, A.H., editor: Campbell's operative orthopedics, ed. 6, St. Louis, 1971, The C.V. Mosby Co.
9. Planas, J.: Buttonhole deformity of the fingers. In Stack, H.G., and Bolton, H., editors: The proceedings of the Second Hand Club, Thirteenth meeting, Paris, 1962, British Society for Surgery of the Hand.
10. Rothwell, A.G.: Repair of the established post traumatic boutonniere, Hand **10:**241, 1978.
11. Shrewsbury, M.M., and Johnson, R.K.: A systematic study of the oblique retinacular ligament of the human finger: its structure and function, J. Hand Surg. **2:**194, 1977.
12. Souter, W.A.: The problem of boutonniere deformity, Clin. Orthop. **104:**116, 1974.
13. Stack, H.G.: Muscle function in the fingers, J. Bone Joint Surg. **44B:**899, 1962.
14. Stack, H.G.: Mallet finger, Hand **1:**83, 1969.
15. Stewart, I.M.: Boutonniere finger, Clin. Orthop. **23:**220, 1962.
16. Suzuki, K.: Reconstruction of post-traumatic boutonniere deformity, Hand **5:**145, 1973.
17. Tubiana, R.: Surgical repair of the extensor apparatus of the fingers, Surg. Clin. North Am. **48:**1015, 1968.
18. Watson, H.K., Light, T.R., and Johnson, T.R.: Checkrein resection for flexion contracture of the middle joint, J. Hand Surg. **4:**67, 1979.
19. Zancolli, E.: Structural and dynamic bases of hand surgery, Philadelphia, 1968, J.B. Lippincott Co.

Chapter 8 Results of surgical treatment of chronic boutonniere deformity: an analysis of prognostic factors

James B. Steichen

James W. Strickland

William H. Call

Stephen G. Powell

The anatomy of the extensor mechanism as it affects the function of the proximal interphalangeal (PIP) joint of a digit has been a subject of great interest for many hand surgeons.* A complete knowledge of the normal anatomy is essential to completely understand the pathology of abnormal conditions about the PIP joint. Treatment of the posttraumatic boutonniere deformity has stimulated many surgeons to formulate many methods of treatment,† both operative and nonoperative, in the hope that better results would follow each suggested idea for this very difficult problem.

It has been our experience that, if the diagnosis is correctly made within the first 6 to 8 weeks of injury, there are then many choices of treatment that will give good to excellent results.[32,36] If it has been over 8 weeks since the injury, however, and the patient presents with the characteristic posture of metacarpophalangeal (MCP) joint hyperextension, PIP joint flexion, and distal interphalangeal (DIP) joint hyperextension, then the results of treatment of this lesion are very unpredictable and influenced by many important variables.

Although many authors have stressed the good results obtained with their techniques, detailed analysis of the factors involved in treating the *chronic* deformity are difficult to find. Souter[33,34] has reported on a series of 106 central slip lesions from Pulvertaft's clinic with excellent follow-up analysis of these injuries. However, the majority of these patients were treated within 6 weeks of injury, and an analysis of chronic lesions over 8 weeks old or lesions with fixed flexion contracture of the PIP joint is not available. Rothwell[28,29] reported on 12 patients with established boutonniere deformities but did not include an analysis of the many factors involved. We feel that many factors determine the final result achieved in patients with established chronic boutonniere deformities, and these are important in determining the eventual treatment as well as the degree of improvement that may be obtained. Although boutonniere injuries also may be caused by burns,[17,20] rheumatoid arthritis, and other indirect injuries to the dorsum of the PIP joint, the posttraumatic lesion caused by direct or indirect trauma to the central slip has been isolated for the purpose of analysis.

ANATOMY OF BOUTONNIERE DEFORMITY

We define boutonniere deformity as an interruption of the central slip of the extensor mechanism with loss of the ability to extend actively the PIP joint or flex actively the DIP joint. To create this deformity, the central slip of the extrinsic extensor mechanism has been separated traumatically at or near its insertion into the middle phalanx with a tear of the triangular ligament fibers. As the flexor digitorum superficialis tendon pulls the digit into flexion at the PIP joint, and the extrinsic extensor tendon now exerts its pull on the proximal phalanx, the MCP joint is pulled into extension or hyperextension, and the intrinsic lateral bands fall volar to the axis of rotation of the PIP joint. The head of the proximal phalanx may buttonhole through the volarly subluxed lateral bands as the triangular ligamentous fibers separate. The pull of the lateral bands now flexes the PIP joint as they extend or hyperextend the DIP joint. The transverse retinacular ligaments may contract with time, thus holding the lateral bands anteriorly. The oblique retinacular ligaments of Landsmeer or Weitbrecht, which are initially relaxed with the PIP joint in flexion, may then tighten and contract as the deformity becomes chronic and thereby cause greater tension in the extended DIP joint. If the PIP joint is not kept passively extended or the DIP joint is not kept passively flexed, then fixed contractures will develop in these joints with time and complicate the treatment of these chronic lesions.

---

*References 2, 4, 11-14, 24, 31, and 38-40.

†References 1, 3, 9, 10, 13, 15, 16, 19, 21-23, 25, 30, and 35.

CHAPTER 8 RESULTS OF SURGICAL TREATMENT OF CHRONIC BOUTONNIERE DEFORMITY

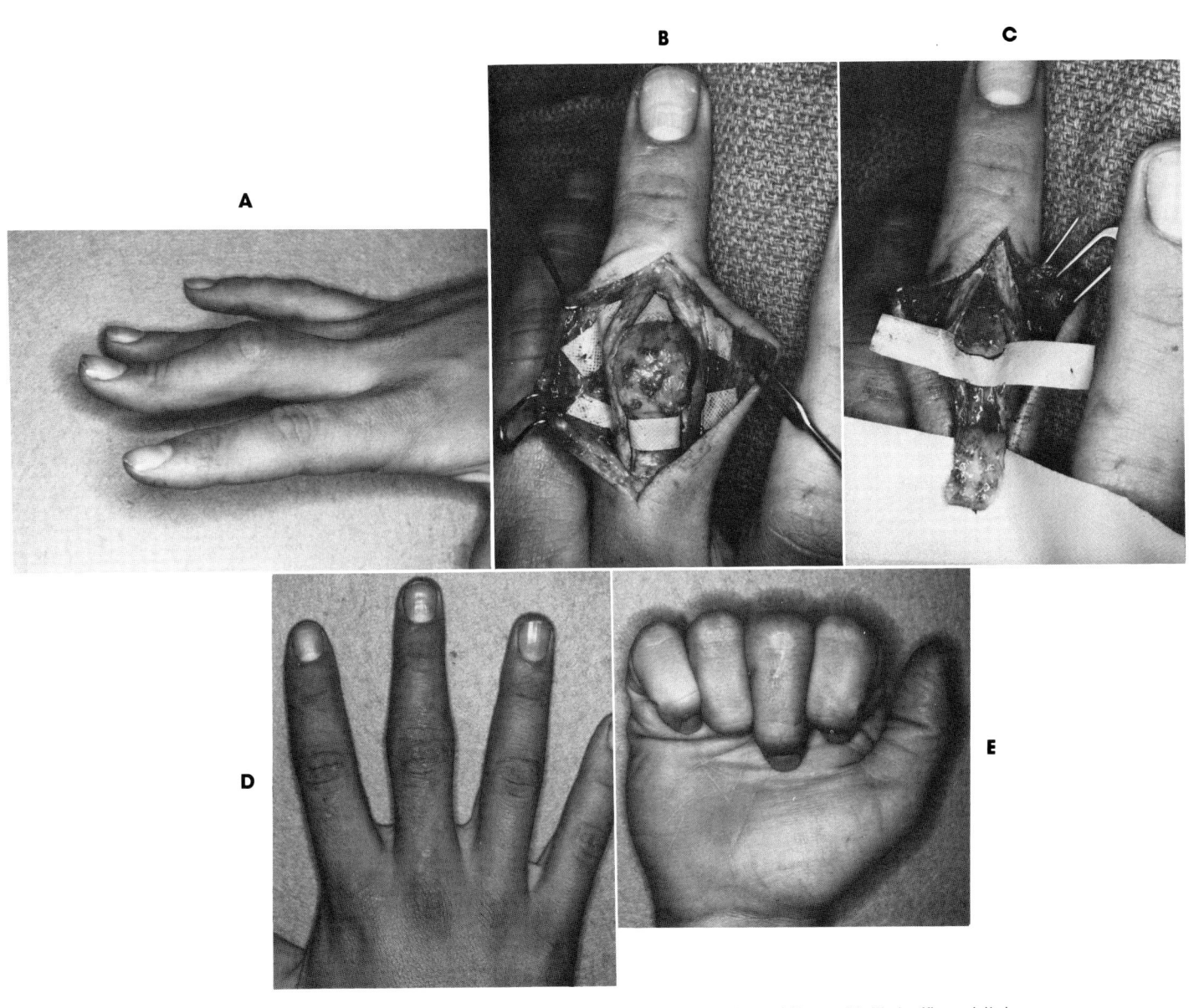

FIG. 8-1. A, Chronic boutonniere deformity of 4 months' duration at time of initial office visit, in 21-year-old man after open laceration over PIP joint. Typical presentation with MCP joint hyperextension, PIP joint flexion, and DIP joint hyperextension is illustrated, as patient attempts to maximally extend PIP joint. Full passive extension to neutral was present at initial office visit. **B,** Surgical reconstruction of chronic boutonniere deformity with Elliott[6-8] anatomic repair. Lateral bands have been freed and mobilized and brought dorsal, and central slip has been tenolysed. Redundant scar of central slip is apparent. **C,** PIP joint has been transfixed in full extension with oblique Kirschner wire. Scar of redundant central slip has been incised proximal to its insertion into middle phalanx, and redundant proximal central slip is reflected proximally. Procedure is completed by excision of redundant excess scar, as described by Elliott, with end-to-end repair of central slip scar and repair of triangular ligament. **D,** Full active extension achieved 4 months postoperatively. **E,** Full active flexion of PIP joint 4 months postoperatively with almost full flexion at DIP joint.

TREATMENT

For many years our approach to the patient with a chronic posttraumatic boutonniere deformity of 8 weeks' or greater duration has been initially conservative. An intensive therapy program is instituted consisting of dynamic splinting of the PIP joint to achieve full extension; then extension of the PIP joint is maintained for an additional 6 weeks while active DIP joint motion is encouraged. Any patient who could not maintain active extension at the PIP joint after a prolonged splinting program was then considered for surgical correction.

Procedure

Over a 10-year period a single surgical procedure for "anatomic reconstruction of the extensor mechanism," as suggested by Elliott,[6-8] has been used for these chronic deformities (Fig. 8-1, A). The repair consists of dorsal mobilization of the displaced lateral bands after division of the deforming transverse retinacular fibers (Fig. 8-1, B). The PIP joint is brought to its maximal and, it is hoped, full degree of extension and then held there with a transarticular Kirschner wire. An extensor tenolysis of the lengthened central slip is carefully performed, and then the scar over the joint is transected proximal to the joint, leaving a cuff of tendon attached to the middle phalanx (Fig. 8-1, C). Next the mobilized central slip is overlapped and the excess scar resected. The tendon or scar ends are sewn end to end with 4-0 nonabsorbable suture, and very carefully the lateral bands are brought dorsal only at the triangular ligament area and only to their original position. If the DIP joint is then resistive to passive flexion and this is not a result of joint arthrofibrosis, then a decision is made about a terminal tendon release, as advocated by S.B. Fowler[18] or Dolphin,[5] or a release of the oblique retinacular ligaments. Elliott,[8] however, feels that a terminal tenotomy is never indicated. Postoperatively the Kirschner wire is left in place for 6 to 8 weeks, and active flexion of the DIP joint begins immediately. After the pin has been removed, active flexion is started at the PIP joint with use of a resting splint in full PIP extension between exercise periods. Dynamic traction is added later, if needed, to increase PIP and DIP motion (Fig. 8-1, D and E).

MATERIAL

In an attempt to isolate the many variables that may contribute to the long-term results of this condition, we analyzed a retrospective series of 36 digits in 35 patients with boutonniere deformities present for 8 weeks or more after trauma. All were unresponsive to conservative treatment and were treated with this single surgical procedure for late boutonniere reconstruction.

The average postoperative follow-up analysis was 6½ months with a range of 3 to 24 months. The majority of these injuries (69%) occurred in young adults 33 years old or younger, with the average age being 29.5 years. Males (69%) were more frequently involved than females. The incidence of the injury in the dominant hand and the presence of an open or closed wound were equally distributed. The index finger was least often injured, but the three ulnar fingers were equally involved. The predominant mechanisms of injury were sharp lacerations and "jamming" incidents. Work, home, and sports settings were essentially equally common in the production of these lesions. Thirty-four digits had the boutonniere deformity as a single abnormality. Two digits had the boutonniere deformity as part of a larger hand injury. Two lesions occurred after infection developed following satisfactory repair of an open laceration.

Indications for surgical repair

Although the exact criteria for boutonniere reconstruction were somewhat variable among the senior surgeons, no patient was considered for operative treatment who could extend the PIP joint actively to within 30 degrees of neutral. It was also considered optimal that full passive extension be achieved by the time of surgery. This principle was compromised when patients presented at surgery with small increments of flexion deformity at the PIP joint that had developed subsequent to their last office visit. When the anatomic repair was done in this circumstance, the compromise proved to be almost uniformly disastrous. Elliott's admonition[8] that "the final result will seldom exceed the pre-operative passive range of motion" proved to be true.

All digits in this study were monitored for at least 3 months after initiation of postoperative mobilization, unless an obvious failure resulted in early reoperation.

RESULTS

The surgical results in these patients were evaluated and graded based on the *active* range of motion of the PIP joint.

An excellent result required active PIP flexion of 90 degrees or more, with an active PIP extension lag of 20 degrees or less. A good result achieved PIP flexion of 80 degrees or more, with a PIP extension lag of 30 degrees or less. A fair result achieved PIP flexion of 70 degrees or more, with a PIP extension lag of 40 degrees or less. A poor result achieved less than 70 degrees of PIP flexion, with a PIP extension lag of greater than 40 degrees. Inability to flex the DIP joint greater than 30 degrees resulted in a one-grade decrease in the final assessment classification.

Multiple variables then were studied to determine their effects on the final results. Since no patient could actively extend the PIP joint to within 30 degrees of neutral preoperatively, the established *passive* flexion contracture was used for analysis.

CHAPTER 8 RESULTS OF SURGICAL TREATMENT OF CHRONIC BOUTONNIERE DEFORMITY

The passive motion status of the PIP joint at the initial examination proved to be a sensitive indicator of final postoperative joint performance. PIP flexion contractures of 0 to 30 degrees at initial examination were demonstrated in 17 patients. Sixty-five percent of these were graded excellent or good at final evaluation, whereas 35% were graded fair or poor. PIP flexion contractures of 31 to 60 degrees at initial examination were seen in 11 patients. Only 27% were graded excellent or good, and 73% were graded fair or poor. PIP flexion contractures of greater than 60 degrees at initial examination were seen in seven patients. None of these digits was graded excellent or good; all were graded fair or poor (Table 8-1).

We had felt that the ability to attain full passive PIP joint extension prior to surgery, whether present at initial examination or obtained through dynamic splinting, also would be an important prognostic factor and would certainly contribute to an excellent result. There were 22 patients who demonstrated full passive PIP extension before surgery, however, and only 59% of these were graded excellent or good at final evaluation, whereas 41% were graded fair or poor. Thirteen patients, despite a dynamic splinting program, never attained full passive PIP extension before surgical repair. Only *one* patient was graded excellent or good at final evaluation; 92% were graded fair or poor (Table 8-2).

The ages of the patients selected for surgical treatment of this lesion were helpful in predicting the results. There were 12 patients in this study group under 21 years of age at the time of surgery. Fifty-nine percent of these were graded excellent or good at final evaluation; 41% were graded fair or poor. In the group between 21 and 45 years of age at the time of surgery there were 18 patients. Thirty-three percent were graded excellent or good, whereas 67% were graded fair or poor. In the group older than 45 years of age at the time of surgery there were five patients. One patient, or 20%, was graded good; 80% were graded fair or poor (Table 8-3).

Table 8-1. PIP flexion contracture at initial evaluation

Results	0 to 30 degrees: number of patients (%)	31 to 60 degrees: number of patients (%)	Greater than 60 degrees: number of patients (%)
Excellent	9 (53)	1 (9)	0 (0)
Good	2 (12)	2 (18)	0 (0)
Fair	2 (12)	3 (28)	1 (14)
Poor	4 (23)	5 (45)	6 (86)
TOTAL	17	11	7

Table 8-2. Full passive PIP extension

Results	Attained before surgery: number of patients (%)	Not attained before surgery: number of patients (%)
Excellent	9 (41)	1 (8)
Good	4 (18)	0 (0)
Fair	3 (14)	3 (23)
Poor	6 (27)	9 (69)
TOTAL	22	13

Table 8-3. Results of surgical treatment of chronic boutonniere deformity according to patient age

Results	Under 21 years old: number of patients (%)	Age 21 to 45: number of patients (%)	Over 45 years old: number of patients (%)
Excellent	6 (50)	4 (22)	0 (0)
Good	1 (9)	2 (11)	1 (20)
Fair	1 (9)	4 (22)	1 (20)
Poor	4 (32)	8 (45)	3 (60)
TOTAL	12	18	5

If, however, we analyzed the results relative to patient age based on a sole division at 33 years of age, then we find that 88% of all excellent or good results occurred in patients 33 years of age or younger. However, even in their group only 56% of the digits achieved good or excellent results. We must keep in mind that, by contrast, 82% of the digits in patients over the age of 33 achieved only fair or poor results.

The presence of a significant fracture about the PIP joint at the time of original injury, excluding small avulsion fragments, adversely affected long-term performance of boutonniere repair. A significant fracture about the PIP joint was demonstrated in six patients at initial injury. Thirty-four percent were graded excellent or good at final evaluation; 66% were graded fair or poor. No significant fracture about the PIP joint was demonstrated at the time of original injury in 29 patients. Forty-two percent of these were graded excellent or good, and 58% were graded fair or poor (Table 8-4).

The nature of the original injury had some bearing on the results of treatment of these lesions. Injuries that were originally open fared better than closed ones. Eighteen patients originally had open central slip injuries. Fifty percent of these were graded excellent or good at final evaluation; 50% were graded fair or poor.

Seventeen patients originally had closed central slip injuries. Only 30% were graded excellent or good, whereas 70% were graded fair or poor, which we felt was usually a result of initial misdiagnosis and lack of proper initial treatment, resulting in more severe flexion contracture at the time of our original evaluation.

Previous local surgery was demonstrated to have a strong negative correlation with final function after surgical repair of chronic boutonniere deformity. Ten patients had had prior surgery about the PIP joint at the time of definitive reconstruction. Only 20% of these were graded excellent or good at final evaluation; 80% were graded fair or poor.

Twenty-five patients had had no prior surgery about the PIP joint before definitive reconstruction was undertaken. Forty-eight percent were graded excellent or good, and 52% were graded fair or poor.

SUMMARY

Although the literature on multiple techniques for the repair of the boutonniere deformity is plentiful, information on important variables relating to the outcome of the chronic boutonniere deformity has been scarce. Surgeons involved in the management of these long-standing deformities are well aware that results are often disappointing despite careful efforts to reproduce described techniques that are reported to restore excellent function.

From our data we conclude that the final result after surgical repair of *chronic* boutonniere deformity present for more than 8 *weeks* at initial examination is disappointing. It is apparent that the ultimate performance of a digit after late central slip reconstruction is strongly prejudiced by a fixed PIP joint flexion contracture greater than 30 degrees at the time of initial evaluation or an inability to achieve full PIP joint extension preoperatively. The tendency to accept *almost* complete PIP joint extension prior to surgery, with full extension attempted at the time of surgical correction, proved to be disastrous. Age greater than 45 years, significant associated fracture, an initial closed injury with probable misdiagnosis, or a history of prior surgery also militated against a good result.

CONCLUSIONS

Despite the numerous surgical procedures recommended in the literature that allegedly correct chronic boutonniere deformity,* the failure to provide statistical evidence in their support is not helpful in planning a treatment program. It would appear from this study that patients with chronic boutonniere deformities who exhibit those prognostic factors which adversely affect the final result should be considered for alternative procedures.

There can be no question that we have markedly altered our position on the management of this lesion as a result of these findings. The disappointing results following our use of the well-accepted Elliott[8] technique of central slip reconstruction has led us to pursue a much more conservative approach, consisting of prolonged splinting, often initiated many months after the original injury.

Our present approach to this difficult problem has evolved from our experience and also from the ability of our hand therapists to deal successfully with patients

Table 8-4. Results of surgical treatment of chronic boutonniere deformity according to fracture involvement at initial injury

Results	Significant fracture present: number of patients (%)	No significant fracture present: number of patients (%)
Excellent	1 (17)	9 (31)
Good	1 (17)	3 (11)
Fair	1 (17)	5 (17)
Poor	3 (49)	12 (41)
TOTAL	6	29

*References 19, 21, 26, 27, and 41.

who have difficult contractures of the digital joints. We now start all patients with boutonniere deformities with associated active or passive extension lag on a program of dynamic splinting. Depending on the degree of the fixed flexion contracture, we may start with a short dorsal outrigger splint and then, as the deformity decreases, substitute that with a Joint Jack or a Bunnell safety-pin splint. As the flexion deformity becomes even less but also more resistant to passive correction, we have had excellent results with gentle manipulation and cylinder casting. This requires changing the cast frequently, however, which is a problem for patients who live a great distance from the treatment center.

Once we achieve full passive extension at the PIP joint, we then maintain this full passive extension of only the PIP joint for a minimum of 8 weeks before any flexion is allowed at the PIP joint. During this time the DIP joint is left free, and active and passive motion is possible and encouraged to help rebalance the dorsal apparatus. At the 8-week examination, if active extension is possible, progressive exercise is allowed and encouraged at the PIP joint. This program of prolonged splinting to allow the central slip scar to mature and contract without surgical excision and repair has given encouraging results.

If, while the patient is on this program of prolonged splinting for chronic deformities, the passive flexion contracture cannot be extended, we may do a volar capsulotomy of the PIP joint to achieve full passive extension and then resume the splinting program as outlined previously.

Many patients with chronic boutonniere deformity, after a thorough evaluation and analysis, are not troubled by the flexion contracture of the PIP joint as much as

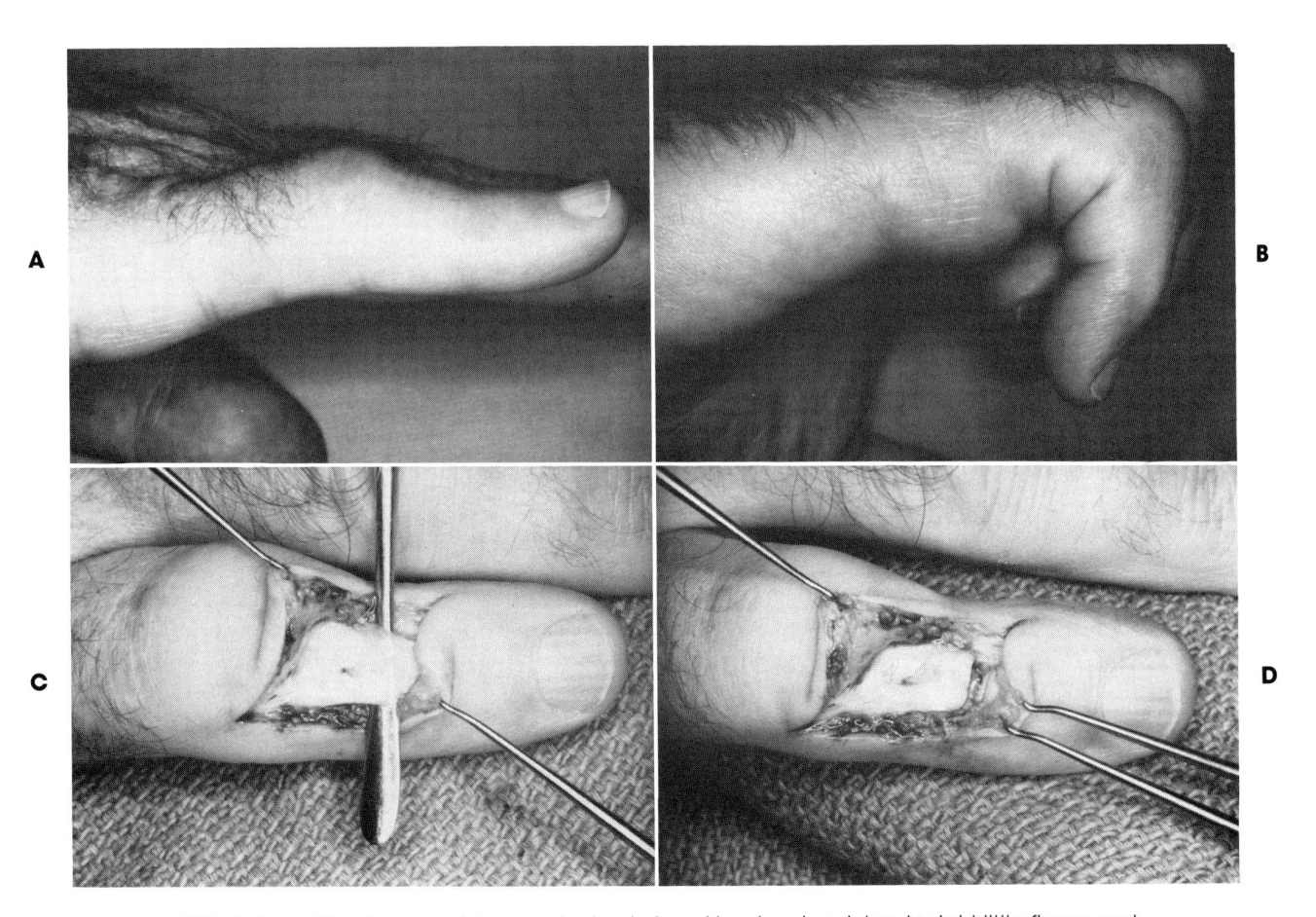

FIG. 8-2. A, Fifty-six–year-old man who had closed boutonniere injury to right little finger and presented 2 months after injury, with a 55-degree fixed flexion contracture of PIP joint. After 2 months of dynamic splinting he had 25-degree flexion contracture of PIP joint, as shown here. **B,** His only remaining functional problem was lack of active flexion of DIP joint. **C,** Under local digital block anesthesia, Dolphin[5] (Fowler)[18] procedure is performed by mobilization of terminal extensor tendon over middle phalanx. **D,** Terminal tendon is now transected distal to triangular ligament and proximal to insertion of oblique retinacular ligaments.

Continued.

SECTION 2 EXTENSOR TENDON PROBLEMS

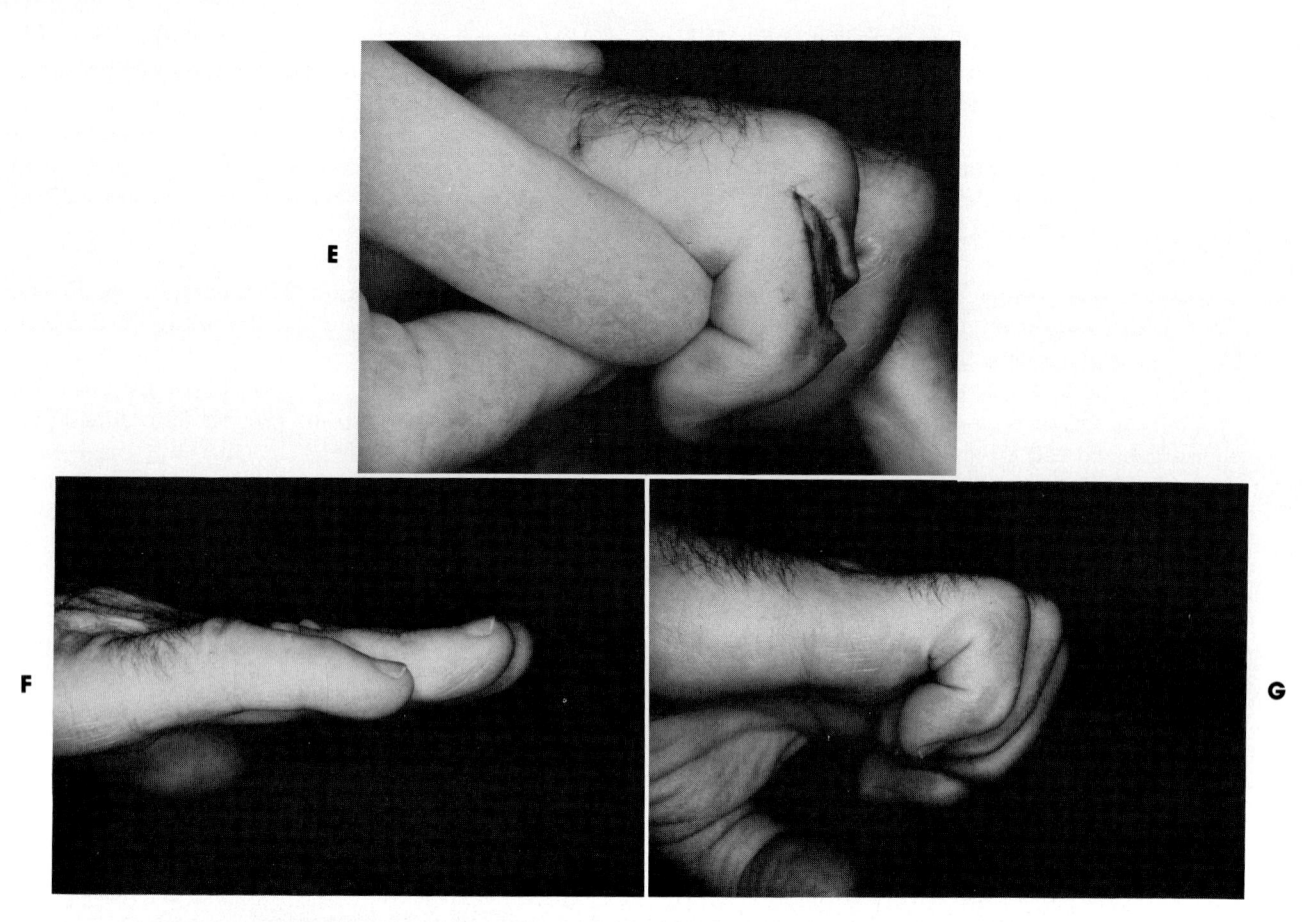

FIG. 8-2, cont'd. E, Patient now can actively flex DIP joint freely after surgical release. **F,** Six months postoperatively there is only 10-degree active extension lag at DIP joint, and PIP joint has only 15-degree extension lag. **G,** Active flexion at 6 months postoperatively is to 90 degrees at PIP joint and 60 degrees at DIP joint with good patient satisfaction.

they are by the loss of active flexion of the DIP joint. This is a functional loss of grasp and grip strength. For these patients we now use the simple distal extensor releases, done with the patient under local anesthesia, as advocated by Fowler[18] and modified by Dolphin[5] (Fig. 8-2).

If formal procedures are needed, however, for the PIP joint fixed contracture, then consideration is given to the predictable reconstruction afforded by interpositional arthroplasty[37] or arthrodesis.

REFERENCES

1. Bingham, D.L.C., and Jack, E.A.: "Buttonholed" extensor expansion, Br. Med. J. **2:**701, 1937.
2. Bunnell, S.: Bunnell's surgery of the hand, ed. 4, Philadelphia, 1964, J.B. Lippincott Co.
3. Burton, R.J., and Eaton, R.G.: Common hand injuries in the athlete, Orthop. Clin. North Am. **4:**809, 1973.
4. Chan, G.E., Zuska, A.J., and McNeill, T.W.: Boutonniere deformity, Ill. Med. J. **146:**532, 1974.
5. Dolphin, J.A.: Extensor tenotomy for chronic boutonniere deformity of the finger: report of two cases, J. Bone Joint Surg. **47A:**161, 1965.
6. Elliott, R.A., Jr.: Extensor-tendon injuries at the interphalangeal joint levels, J. Bone Joint Surg. **47A:**633, 1965.
7. Elliott, R.A., Jr.: Injuries to the extensor mechanism of the hand, Orthop. Clin. North Am. **1:**335, 1970.
8. Elliott, R.A., Jr.: Boutonniere deformity. In Cramer, L.M., and Chase, R.A., editors: Symposium on the hand, St. Louis, 1971, The C.V. Mosby Co.
9. Entin, M.A.: Repair of extensor mechanism of the hand, Surg. Clin. North Am. **40:**275, 1960.
10. Goldner, J.L.: Deformities of the hand incidental to pathological changes of the extensor and intrinsic muscle mechanisms, J. Bone Joint Surg. **35A:**115, 1953.
11. Grant, J.C.: Grant's atlas of anatomy, ed. 6, Baltimore, 1972, Williams & Wilkins Co.
12. Harris, C., Jr., and Rutledge, G.L.: The functional anatomy of the extensor mechanism of the finger, J. Bone Joint Surg. **54A:**713, 1972.
13. Kaplan, E.B.: Anatomy, injuries and treatment of the ex-

tensor apparatus of the hand and digits, Clin. Orthop. **13:** 24, 1959.
14. Kaplan, E.B.: Functional and surgical anatomy of the hand, ed. 2, Philadelphia, 1965, J.B. Lippincott Co.
15. Kilgore, E.S., Jr., and Graham, W.P., III: Operative treatment of boutonniere deformity, Surgery **64:**999, 1968.
16. King, T.: Treatment of boutonniere deformity, J. Bone Joint Surg. **52B:**800, 1970.
17. Larson, D.L., Wofford, B.H., Evans, E.B., et al.: Repair of the boutonniere deformity of the burned hand, J. Trauma **10:**481, 1970.
18. Littler, J.W.: Principles of reconstructive surgery of the hand. In Converse, J.M., editor: Reconstructive plastic surgery, vol. 4, Philadelphia, 1964, W.B. Saunders Co.
19. Littler, J.W., and Eaton, R.G.: Redistribution of forces in the correction of the boutonniere deformity, J. Bone Joint Surg. **49A:**1267, 1967.
20. Maisels, D.O.: The middle slip or boutonniere deformity in burned hands, Br. J. Plast. Surg. **18:**117, 1965.
21. Matev, I.: Transposition of the lateral slips of the aponeurosis in treatment of long-standing "boutonniere deformity" of the fingers, Br. J. Plast. Surg. **17:**281, 1964.
22. McCue, F.C., and Abbott, J.L.: The treatment of mallet finger and boutonniere deformities, Va. Med. Mo. **94:**623, 1967.
23. McCue, F.C., Honner, R., Johnson, M.C., Jr., et al.: Athletic injuries of the proximal interphalangeal joint requiring surgical treatment, J. Bone Joint Surg. **52A:**937, 1970.
24. Micks, J.E., and Hager, D.: Role of the controversial parts of the extensor of the finger, J. Bone Joint Surg. **55A:**884, 1973.
25. Milch, H.: Button-hole rupture of the extensor tendon of the finger, Am. J. Surg. **13:**244, 1951.
26. Nichols, H.M.: Repair of the extensor-tendon insertions in the fingers, J. Bone Joint Surg. **33A:**836, 1951.
27. Planas, J.: Buttonhole deformity of the fingers, J. Bone Joint Surg. **45B:**424, 1963.
28. Rothwell, A.G.: The repair of established boutonniere and mallet finger deformities, J. Bone Joint Surg. **58B:**384, 1976.
29. Rothwell, A.G.: Repair of the established post traumatic boutonniere deformity, Hand **10:**241, 1978.
30. Selig, S., and Schein, A.: Irreducible buttonhole dislocations of the fingers, J. Bone Joint Surg. **22:**436, 1940.
31. Smith, R.J.: Boutonniere deformity of the fingers, Bull. Hosp. Joint Dis. **27:**27, 1966.
32. Souter, W.A.: Division of the central slip of the extensor expansion of the fingers, J. Bone Joint Surg. **48B:**587, 1966.
33. Souter, W.A.: The boutonniere deformity: a review of 101 patients with division of the central slip of the extensor expansion of the fingers, J. Bone Joint Surg. **49B:**710, 1967.
34. Souter, W.A.: The problem of boutonniere deformity, Clin. Orthop. **104:**116, 1974.
35. Spinner, M., and Choi, B.Y.: Anterior dislocation of the proximal interphalangeal joint: a cause of rupture of the central slip of the extensor mechanism, J. Bone Joint Surg. **52A:**1329, 1970.
36. Stewart, I.M.: Boutonniere finger, Clin. Orthop. **23:**220, 1962.
37. Swanson, A.B.: Implant resection arthroplasty of the proximal interphalangeal joint, Orthop. Clin. North Am. **4:**1007, 1973.
38. Tubiana, R.: Surgical repair of the extensor apparatus of the fingers, Surg. Clin. North Am. **48:**1015, 1968.
39. Tubiana, R., and Valentin, P.: The physiology of the extension of the fingers, Surg. Clin. North Am. **44:**907, 1964.
40. Wallace, A.F.: An early boutonniere deformity, Br. J. Plast. Surg. **19:**251, 1966.
41. Weeks, P.M.: The chronic boutonniere deformity: a method of repair, Plast. Reconstr. Surg. **40:**248, 1967.

SECTION THREE FLEXOR TENDON PROBLEMS

Chapter 9 Functional recovery after flexor tendon severance in the finger: the state of the art

James W. Strickland

Regaining digital function after tendon interruption within the flexor sheath has long been one of the most difficult problems in hand surgery. In recent years there have been substantial advances in our understanding of tendon anatomy, nourishment, and healing, accompanied by the development of improved techniques for tendon repair and the postoperative restoration of tendon excursion. The ability to reconstruct a gliding flexor tendon system in the presence of severe tissue scarring also has been a significant improvement in tendon surgery in this difficult area. This chapter only briefly summarizes meaningful contributions to our understanding of the performance of severed and repaired digital flexor tendons, tying these contributions to preexisting concepts and experience to create a logical clinical approach to the management of these injuries.

FLEXOR TENDON HEALING

In an excellent review of the many concepts proposed for healing of the flexor tendons following severance within the digits, Ketchum[23] documents what has been a continuing controversy among the students of this process. Until recent years it was fairly well accepted that a flexor tendon lacked the intrinsic capability to heal itself but rather relied on the activity of cells emanating from adjacent tissues.[52-56,58,59] Later evidence, however, gives strong support to the concept that there is, at least in ideal situations, an intrinsic capability of flexor tendons to heal themselves.* Interestingly, the observation of Mason and Allen[41] that a flexor tendon repair has no tensile strength until it is stressed has remained relatively unchallenged.

TENDON NUTRITION

Important studies have been carried out recently to identify patterns of vascularity of flexor tendons within the digital sheath system.† Although the patterns within a given digit are somewhat variable,[6,7] it has been well demonstrated that the vascular distribution to flexor tendons is supplied through the short and long vincular systems, is segmental in nature, is richer on the dorsal surface of the tendons than on the volar side, and results in several reasonably avascular tendon segments[6,7,46] (Fig. 9-1). The clinical importance of these findings is obvious when one considers the well-known adhesion-provoking tendency of avascular tissues in other areas of the body such as the bowel.

There is an increasing awareness of the prejudicial effect on tendon amplitude that may result from interference with the vincular blood supply either by injury or surgical dissection. Additional work to define the restoration of blood supply to tendon grafts after conventional techniques[29] or after the two-stage silicone-rod method[68] has also provided important information.

A second valuable source of flexor tendon nutrition has been demonstrated to be the synovial fluid within the digital sheath.* The work of Manske and his associates[36-40] in particular strongly suggests that this system may provide nutrition comparable with or superior to that of the vincular vessels. The evidence now appears irrefutable that tendons can heal in an isolated synovial environment, leading to renewed emphasis on sheath repair following tendon suture.[32,34]

THE PULLEY SYSTEM

Detailed descriptions by Doyle and Blythe of the flexor pulley system in the digits[8] and thumb[9] probably have been the most important anatomic contributions in this area (Figs. 9-2 and 9-3). Clinical discussions of the condition of the four annular and three cruciate digital pulleys after flexor tendon injury and surgery have become commonplace and emphasize the growing awareness of the value of these restraining cylinders in ensuring tendon efficiency. Clinical studies[8] have indicated that at least A_2 and A_4 pulleys are necessary to attain full digital flexion. However, the biomechanical impact of the loss of the A_3 and to a lesser extent the A_1 pulleys, in allowing the flexor tendon to move away from the proximal interpha-

---

*References 12, 14, 28, 30, 32-34, 43, and 44.
†References 2, 6, 7, 33, and 46.

*References 32, 34, 36-40, and 42.

SECTION 3 FLEXOR TENDON PROBLEMS

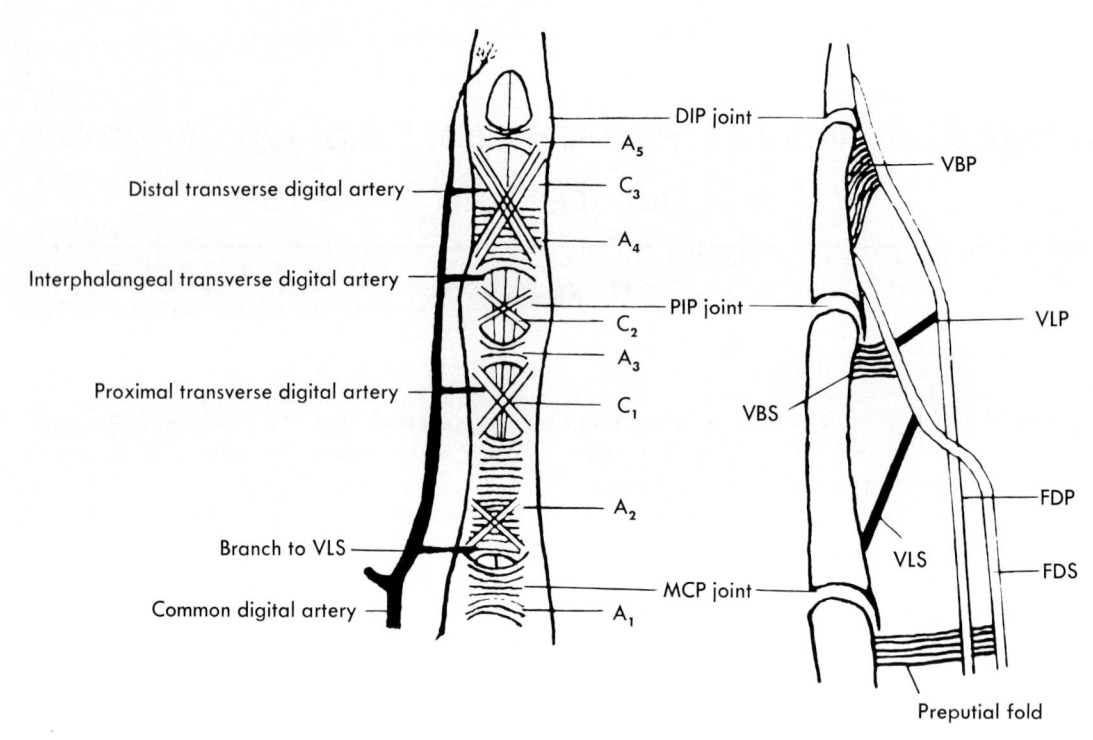

FIG. 9-1. Scheme of fibrous pulley system, vincular system, and four transverse communicating branches of the common digital artery. *VLS,* Vinculum longum superficialis; *VBS,* vinculum breve superficialis; *VBP,* vinculum breve profundus; *VLP,* vinculum longum profundus; *FDP,* flexor digitorum profundus; *FDS,* flexor digitorum superficialis. (From Ochiai, N., et al.: J. Hand Surg. **4:**322, 1979.)

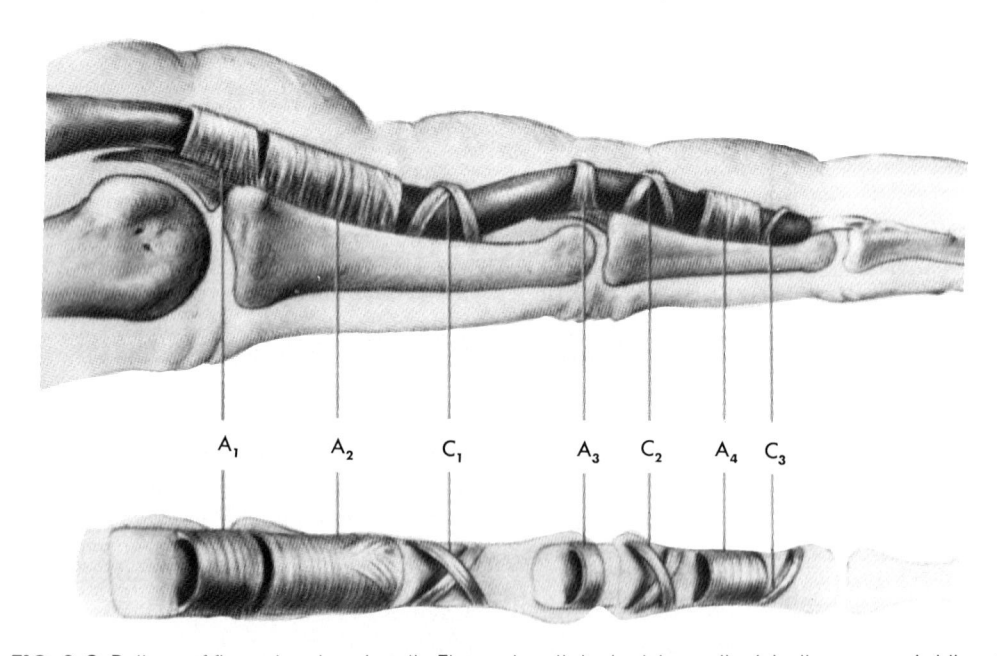

FIG. 9-2. Pulleys of flexor tendon sheath. Flexor sheath is double-walled, hollow, synovial-lined connective tissue tube that encloses flexor tendons. Four annular and three cruciform pulleys are noted in their relative locations. Annular pulleys are thick, rather rigid fibrous tissue structures in contrast to cruciform bands, which are thin and pliable. Second and fourth annular pulleys are the most important functionally. (From Doyle, J.R., and Blythe, W.F.: The finger flexion tendon sheath and pulleys: anatomy and reconstruction. In American Academy of Orthopaedic Surgeons: Symposium on Tendon Surgery in the Hand, St. Louis, 1975, The C.V. Mosby Co.)

CHAPTER 9 FUNCTIONAL RECOVERY AFTER FLEXOR TENDON SEVERANCE IN THE FINGER: THE STATE OF THE ART

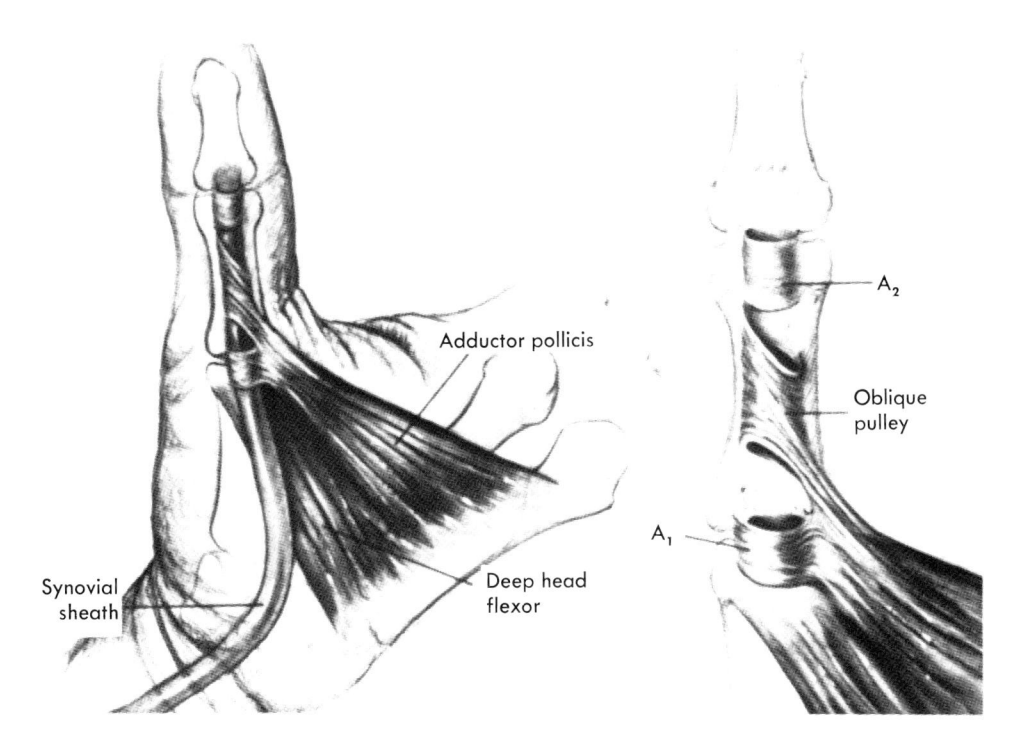

FIG. 9-3. Thumb flexor pulley system. Thumb flexor synovial sheath is double-walled, hollow tube sealed at both ends. Sheath begins 2.0 cm proximal to radial styloid and ends just distal to interphalangeal (IP) joint. On top of sheath and closely applied to it are three constant pulleys — two annular and one oblique. First annular, located at MCP joint, is 7 to 9 mm wide and 0.5 mm thick. Oblique pulley courses from ulnar-proximal to radial-distal and is 9 to 11 mm wide at its midaspect. Second annular pulley is near site of insertion of flexor pollicis longus and is 8 to 10 mm wide but quite thin. (From Doyle, J.R., and Blythe W.F.: J. Hand Surg. **2:**150, 1977.)

langeal (PIP) and metacarpophalangeal (MCP) joints, respectively, has taken on considerable clinical significance. Efforts to salvage and reconstruct these pulleys have become an extremely important part of flexor tendon surgery (Figs. 9-4 and 9-5).

TENDON REPAIR

Pioneered by the work of Verdan and associates[70-74] and Kleinert and Bennett,[25] "no man's land" has largely been dropped from the vocabulary of the hand surgeon, and primary flexor tendon repair within the digital sheath has become routine, under favorable circumstances[34] (Fig. 9-6). The concept that tendons could be repaired in this area with the expectation of returning to a favorable amount of amplitude and digital motion has advanced from being regarded with suspicion and doubt to general acceptance. Results that originally were thought to be no better than those obtained with flexor grafting now have been shown to be superior in almost all studies.* Furthermore, the consideration of flexor tendon repairs as an absolute surgical emergency has been effectively overcome, and several studies indicating equal or better results from delayed primary flexor tendon suture have made surgical procrastination a credible alternative to late-night repair.[35,64] In addition, it has been effectively demonstrated that in most instances it is preferable to repair both the flexor digitorum profundus and superficialis tendons rather than the profundus alone, as was thought to be the wiser option in previous years.[25,28,70-72]

Although the specific techniques for tendon suture have not changed greatly since the original emphasis by Bunnell[3] on atraumatic methods, the classic Bunnell pullout or crisscross sutures have lost popularity when compared with other simpler or stronger repairs.[22,25,31] Urbaniak,[69] in an excellent study of the tensile strength of eight different tendon junctures, indicated the superiority of the Kessler-type repair[68] for the type of end-to-end juncture that is required for the severed flexor tendon. Other more ingenious techniques of tendon reconstruction have been received with less enthusiasm.[47]

*References 26, 28, 45, 68, 70, and 74.

SECTION 3 FLEXOR TENDON PROBLEMS

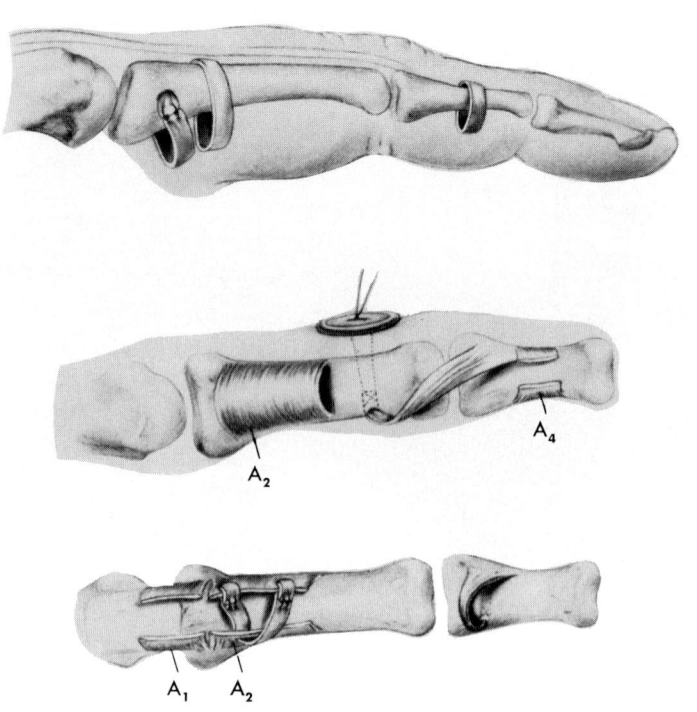

FIG. 9-4. Techniques of pulley reconstruction. Pulleys may be reconstructed by using free-tendon grafts or by using slip of superficialis tendon near its insertion. In proximal phalanx, grafts may be placed through bone or around or underneath extensor tendon. Remnants of annular bands may be used as anchors for free graft, which can be woven into and sutured to band. Attachments of reconstructed pulleys must be strong and preferably attached to bone. Reconstructed pulley should hold flexor tendon as close as possible to bone without loss of free tendon motion. (From Doyle, J.R., and Blythe, W.F.: The finger flexion tendon sheath and pulleys: anatomy and reconstruction. In American Academy of Orthopaedic Surgeons: Symposium on Tendon Surgery in the Hand, St. Louis, 1975, The C.V. Mosby Co.)

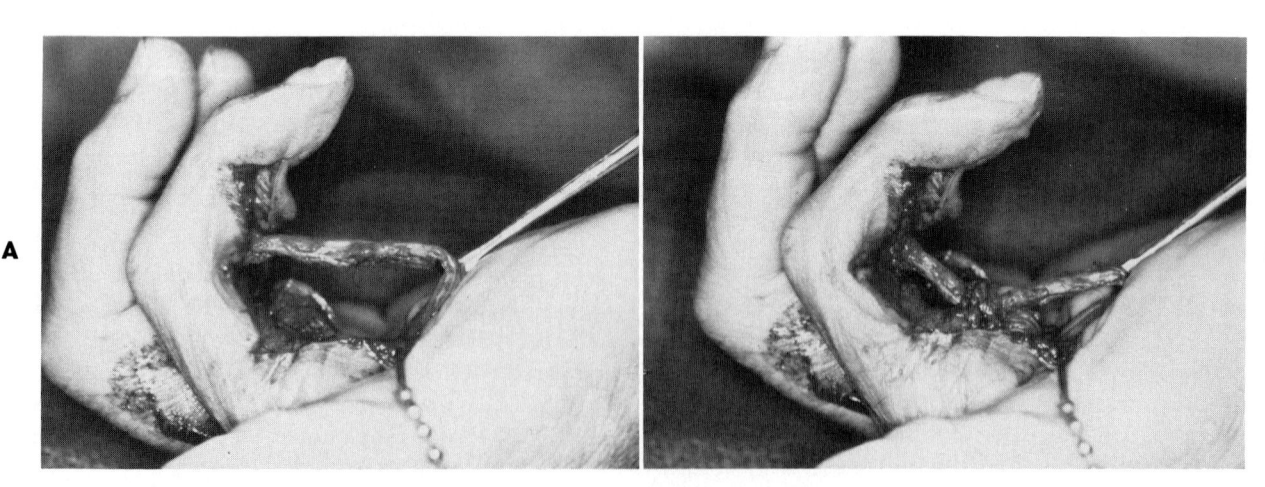

FIG. 9-5. Importance of digital pulley system. **A,** Severe bowstringing of lysed flexor profundus tendon in the absence of the A_1, A_2, and A_3 pulleys. **B,** Improved tendon restraint following reconstruction of A_2 pulley.

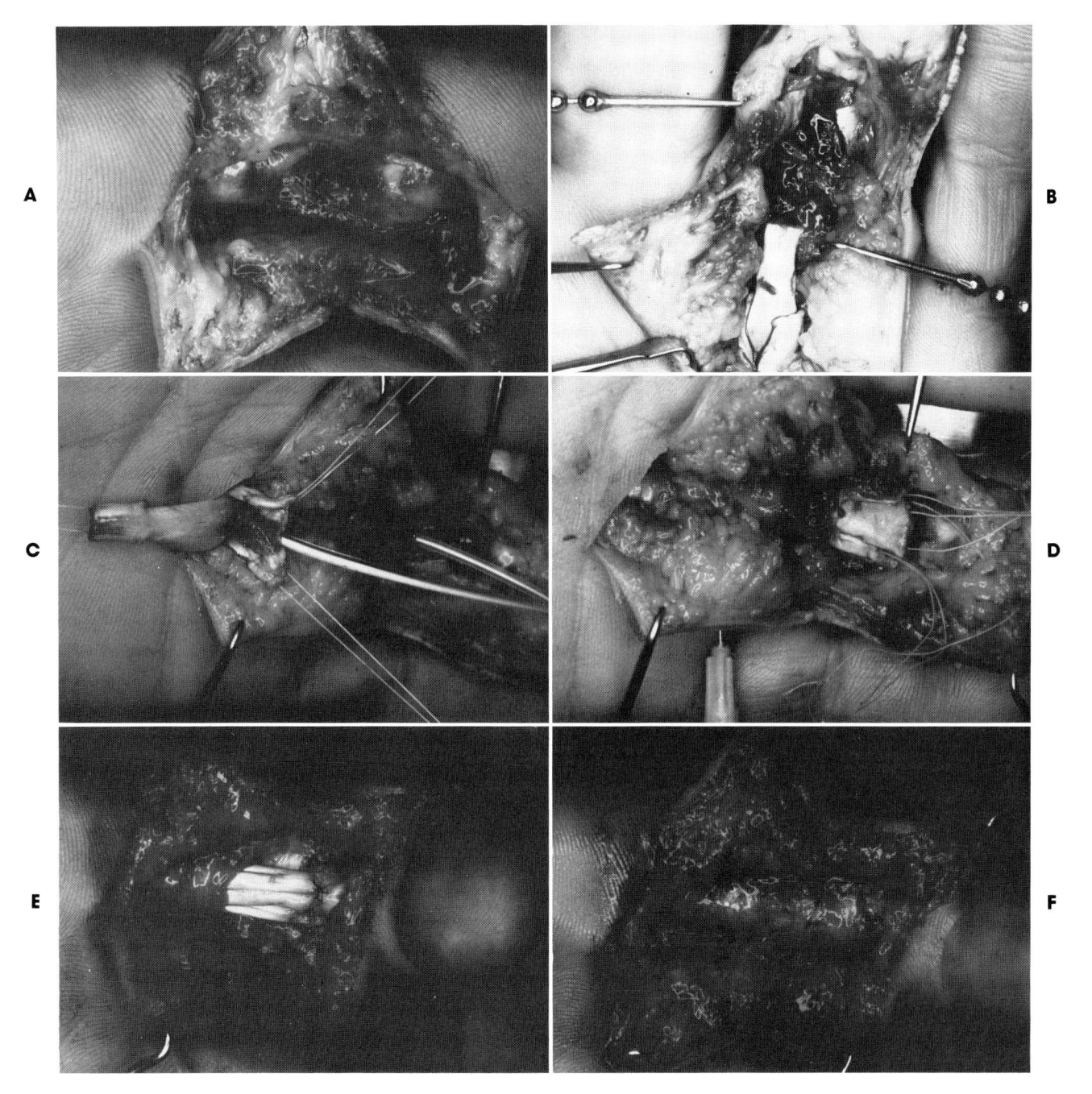

CHAPTER 9 FUNCTIONAL RECOVERY AFTER FLEXOR TENDON SEVERANCE IN THE FINGER: THE STATE OF THE ART

FIG. 9-6. Repair of severed flexor digitorum profundus and superficialis in digit. **A,** Appearance of empty flexor sheath between A_2 and A_3 pulleys after severance in distal aspect of proximal phalanx. **B,** Appearance of retracted flexor tendon stumps proximal to A_1 pulleys in palm and distal tendon stumps over proximal aspect of middle phalanx with preservation of intervening pulley systems. **C,** Placement of proximal modified Kessler sutures in preparation for delivery of tendons into distal aspect of finger using infant-feeding tube. **D,** Appearance of proximal tendon stumps after passage into distal digit, maintained by use of small 25-gauge transversely placed hypodermic needle. **E,** Completion of tendon repair by joining proximally and distally placed Kessler sutures with knots in juncture site. Additional 6-0 peripheral running sutures are used to tidy repair site. **F,** Repair of overlying flexor tendon sheath using fine nonabsorbable sutures.

SECTION 3 FLEXOR TENDON PROBLEMS

PHARMACOLOGIC ADHESION CONTROL

Research continues in the development of methods of tendon-adhesion modification[51] or prevention[54,57] by the use of local or systemic medications. Although no drug has yet been identified that can produce consistently good results without delaying wound or tendon healing or producing systemic reactions, it would not be surprising if an effective drug were to be found within the next decade.

POSTOPERATIVE MANAGEMENT

Despite the historical reluctance to stress a repaired flexor tendon by means of early active or passive mobilization and the advice of Peacock and associates,[52] who emphasized the biologic contradiction of such techniques, evidence is building that early motion in fact *can* produce better results. The proponents* of early active motion emphasize that little tension is actually placed on the site of tendon juncture, the rupture rate is low, and functional results are substantially better. Other studies have indicated that at least comparable results can be achieved by passive mobilization methods as described by Harmer[15-18] and Young and Harmon[78] and recently popularized by Duran and associates.[10,11] A recent study[67] comparing the results of immobilization versus early passive motion in zone II flexor tendon injuries indicates the superiority of a modification of Duran's technique (Fig. 9-7).

TENDON GRAFTS

The techniques and results of conventional free-tendon grafting, so beautifully demonstrated by Boyes and Stark[1] and Pulvertaft,[62,63] remain unchallenged today, although the indications have varied. Far more emphasis is placed on primary repair than on secondary grafting, and the badly injured digit is more likely to undergo a

*References 13, 19, 22, 27, and 31.

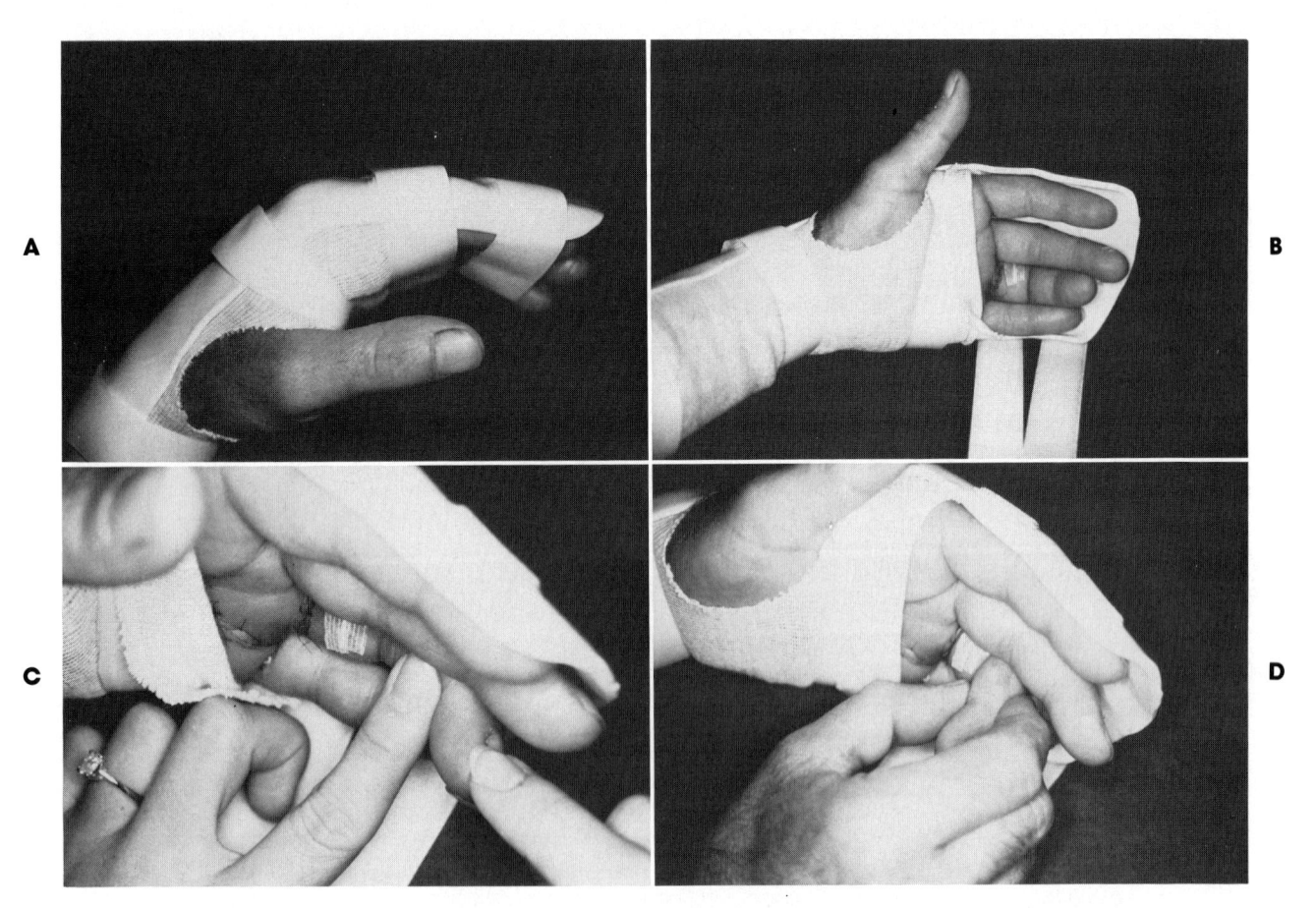

FIG. 9-7. Method of early passive tendon immobilization. **A,** Use of molded orthoplast splint maintaining wrist and MCP joint flexion and relatively extended position of digits. **B,** Velcro straps removed in preparation for passive motion exercises. **C,** Blocking exercises of DIP joint to isolate profundus excursion. **D,** Gentle flexion and extension of PIP, moving both tendons.

two-stage salvage effort than a seemingly ill-fated one-stage tendon graft. Nonetheless, in those digits with flexor tendon division and minimal tissue reaction and scarring, a properly conceived and carried out conventional free-tendon graft remains the procedure of choice and can be expected to frequently return satisfactory digital performance. The predicted rate of functional recovery following tendon grafting has been reported by Weeks, Wray, and Stromberg.[76]

Considerable controversy still exists with regard to the advisability of carrying out free-tendon grafting in the presence of an intact flexor digitorum superficialis tendon. Most experienced authors temper their advice on this subject with a great deal of caution.[62,63,66] Pulvertaft[62,63] stated that "tendon grafting through an intact superficialis should not be advised unless the patient is determined to seek perfection and the surgeon is confident of his ability to offer a reasonable expectation of success without undue risk of doing harm." He recommended a less involved procedure such as arthrodesis or tenodesis for most patients. Stark and associates[66] felt that the prerequisites for grafting with an intact superficialis tendon included a superficialis that was normal, full passive motion, minimal soft tissue scarring, and patient age between 10 and 21.

Tendon homografts and allografts have been used with varying degrees of clinical success,* although a small number of composite sheath-tendon allografts were shown to provide an astonishingly good return.[49,50] Logistic difficulties with regard to securing, preserving, and implanting these grafts remain as obstacles to their widespread use, although future improvements are a possibility.

The development of the two-stage reconstruction of the digital flexor tendon system as popularized by Hunter and associates[20,21] has provided an extremely important addition to the armamentarium of the hand surgeon (Fig. 9-8). The procedure involves the implantation of a silicone or silicone-Dacron–reinforced gliding prosthesis into a scarred flexor tendon bed, resulting in the formation of a mesothelium-lined pseudosheath about the rod. Following maturation of the pseudosheath, a tendon graft is inserted to replace the prosthesis with the expectation of minimal adhesion formation about the graft (Fig. 9-9). Particularly in those instances where there is a scarred flexor tendon bed, good passive motion, and a well-motivated patient, the technique has proved valuable in allowing the restoration of tendon gliding when the situation otherwise might have been unsalvageable. It is recognized that one must carefully follow the technical advice provided by the developers of the technique[20,21] and that complications such as joint contracture and infection may be somewhat more frequent than from other digital tendon procedures. Nonetheless, when considering the severity of the condition of the tissues in the digits selected for this restorative effort and the unlikelihood of restoring satisfactory function by any other means, the procedure is an excellent one. Functional recovery after this technique has been compared with that of other grafts and is surprisingly favorable.[75] It is perhaps not unreasonable to assume that, with the advance in the development of biologically compatible materials, a true functioning tendon prosthesis with

*References 4, 5, 48, 54, 60, and 61.

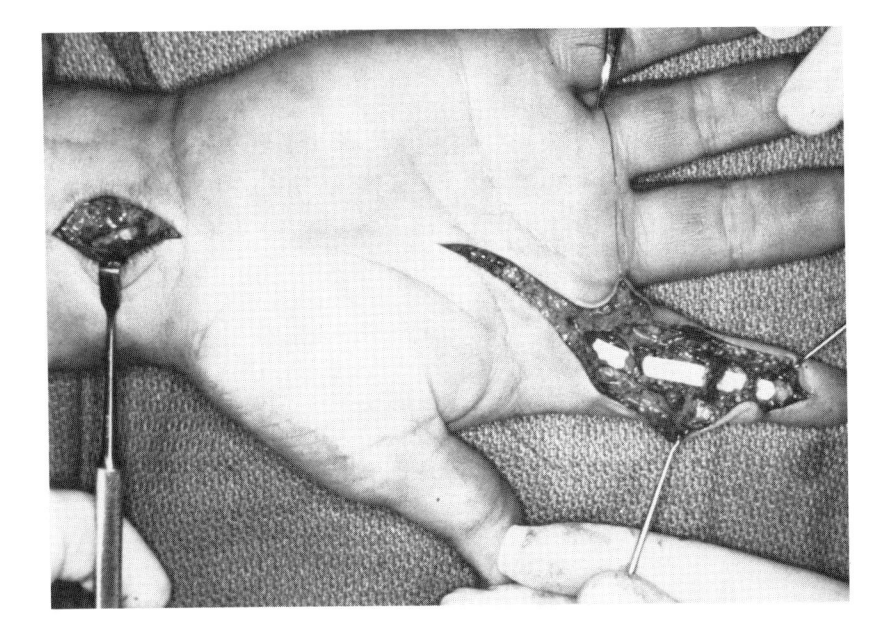

FIG. 9-8. Implantation of silicone-Dacron gliding tendon prosthesis into badly scarred bed of index finger in this 32-year-old man. Note preservation or reconstruction of pulleys.

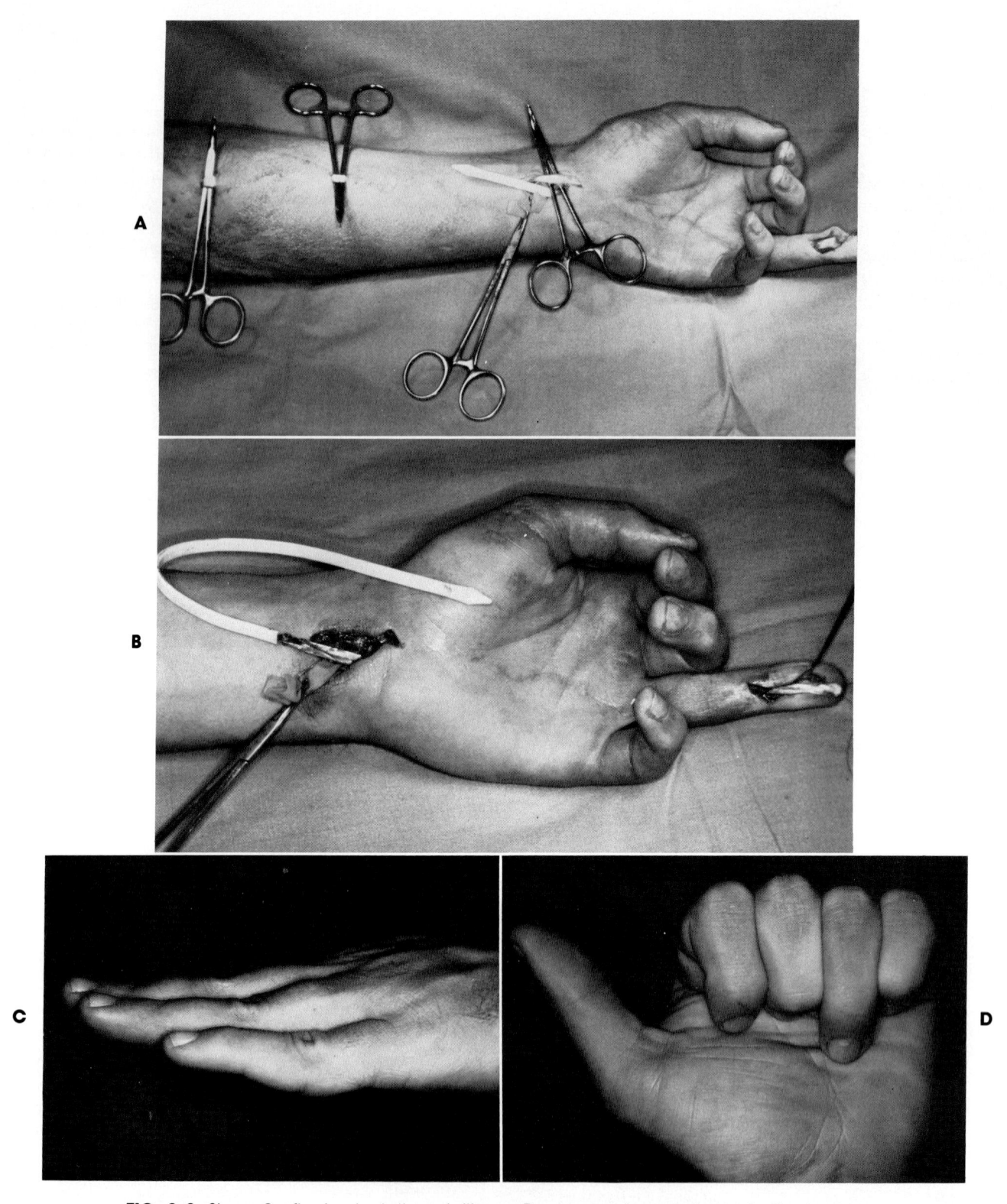

FIG. 9-9. Stage 2 after implantation of silicone-Dacron tendon prosthesis. **A,** Proximal and distal identification of silicone rod in wrist and over distal phalanx. In addition, palmaris longus has been readied for extraction for use as free-tendon graft. **B,** Passage of free-tendon graft into pseudosheath at time of rod extraction. **C,** Excellent extension after two-stage reconstruction of profundus tendon to right finger. **D,** Nearly full flexion of right finger at 20 weeks. (Courtesy James B. Steichen, M.D.)

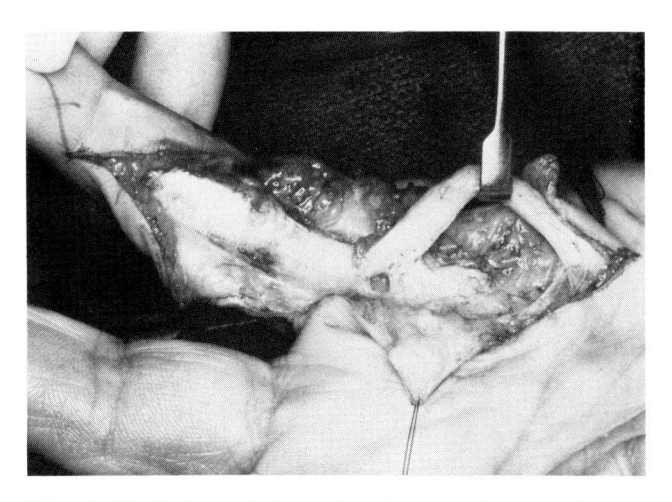

CHAPTER 9 FUNCTIONAL RECOVERY AFTER FLEXOR TENDON SEVERANCE IN THE FINGER: THE STATE OF THE ART

FIG. 9-10. Failure of flexor tendon repair secondary to severe amplitude-restricting adhesions in digit.

adequate proximal motor and distal bone junctures will be developed in the not too distant future.

TENOLYSIS

The surgical mobilization of adherent flexor tendons in the digital canal has historically been a controversial procedure (Fig. 9-10). Much of the criticism of this procedure was a result of the unpredictability of results because of either the recurrence of adhesions or tendon rupture. However, recent reviews of large numbers of flexor tenolyses in the palm and digits have indicated that, when thoroughly carried out and confirmed by either a "flexor check" at the wrist (Fig. 9-11) or by active motion in the locally anesthetized patient (Fig. 9-12), the procedure can be quite gratifying with consistent improvement in digital flexion and a low incidence of tendon rupture.[65,77] Particularly when the qual-

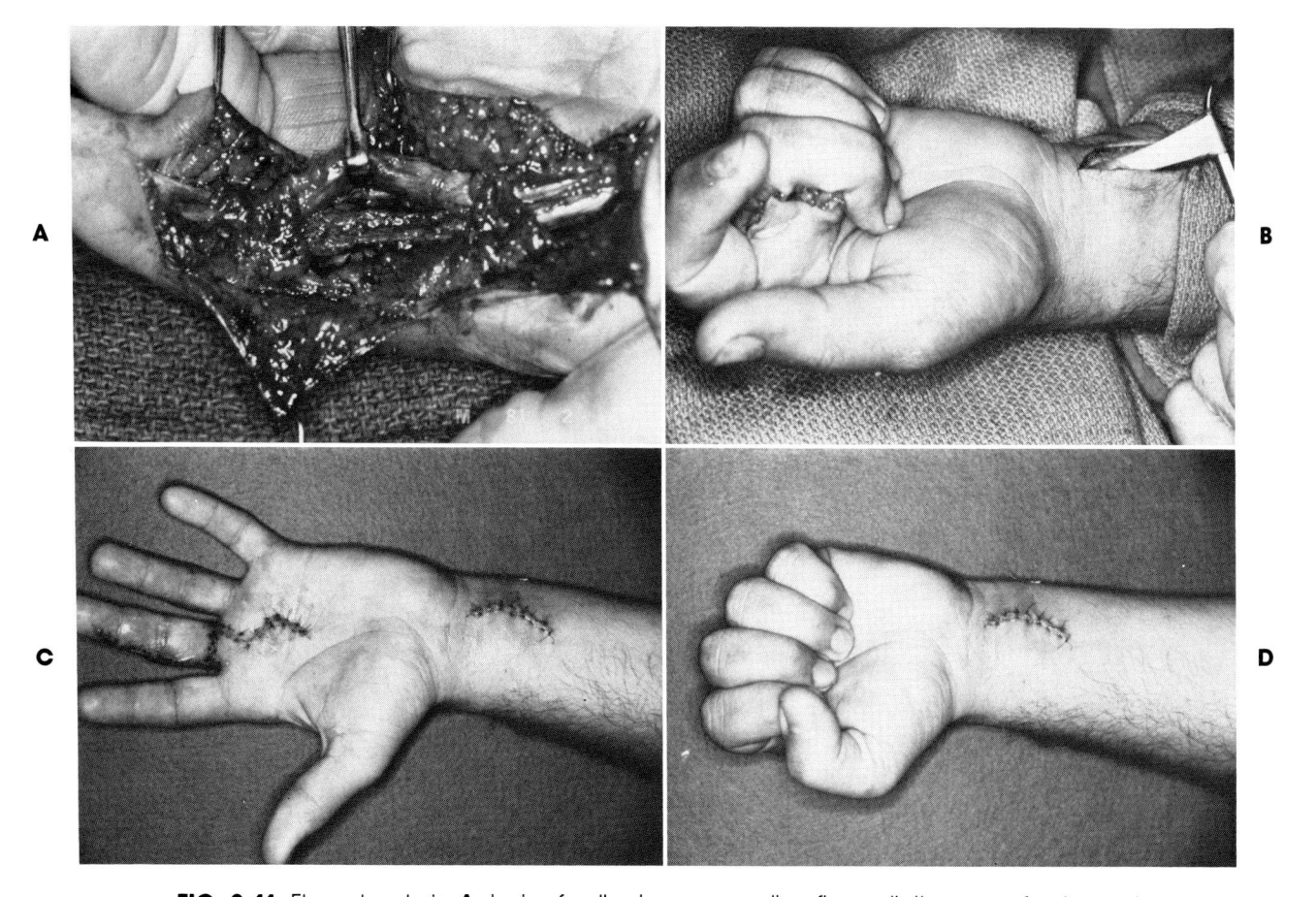

FIG. 9-11. Flexor tenolysis. **A,** Lysis of adhesions surrounding flexor digitorum profundus and supeficialis in finger, maintaining A_2 and A_4 pulleys. **B,** "Flexor check" at wrist, establishing proximal amplitude of lysed tendon. **C,** Appearance of hand at 2 days with full extension and, **D,** full flexion.

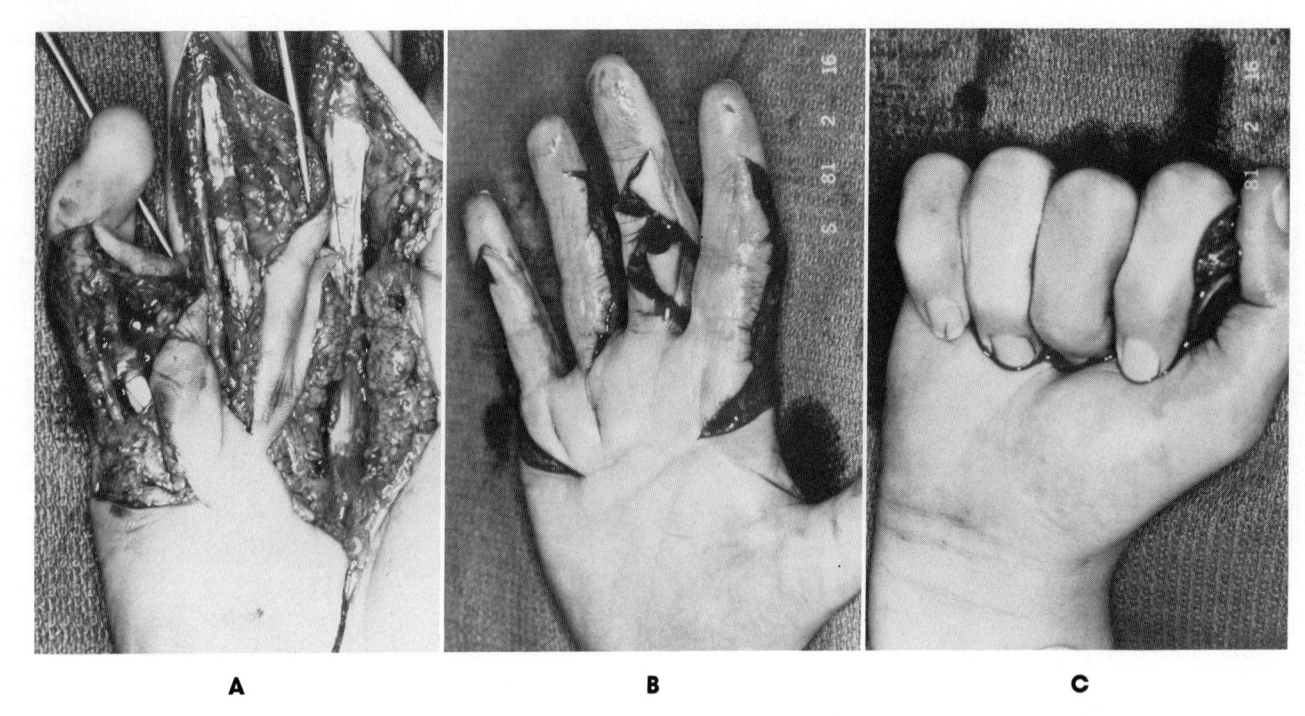

FIG. 9-12. Simultaneous lysis of flexor tendons in all four digits under local (wrist block) anesthesia. **A,** Appearance of previously repaired flexor tendons following lysis. **B,** Nearly full digital extension following tourniquet release. Note use of both midlateral and zigzag incisions, depending on factors unique to digits involved. **C,** Nearly full digital flexion demonstrated by patient at time of anesthesia confirms success of procedure.

ity of the lysed tendons is good, one can proceed almost immediately with vigorous active and passive exercise programs, and with the proper guidance and patient cooperation, satisfactory motion can be regained and maintained.

Tenolysis always must be considered as the potential final procedure following tendon repair, conventional grafting, or two-stage grafting, and patients should be forewarned that a definite percentage of each of these procedures will result in tendon adherence sufficient to require lysis. It also should be emphasized to these patients that a good range of passive motion is an absolute prerequisite to attempts at surgical mobilization of flexor tendons.

PULLEY REPAIR

Recent emphasis on the value of the digital pulleys has led to the recognition that inadequate pulley systems must be reconstructed. The techniques for pulley reconstruction vary somewhat according to the preference of the surgeons. Passing tendons over the flexors and either through phalangeal bone or around the phalanx have been perhaps the most popular procedures,[8] although recent techniques[24] using the fibrous rim forming the lateral walls of the flexor sheath also have been popularized (Fig. 9-13). These procedures can be carried out at the time of tendon grafting, silicone-rod insertion, or tenolysis, although in the latter procedure they must be carefully protected postoperatively, usually by small circumferential adhesive-tape rings.

SUMMARY

Recent advances in the understanding of tendon healing and nourishment, the pulley system, and the techniques of repair, pulley preservation, and adhesion modification have provided us with a current "state of the art" that allows a rational systematic approach to flexor tendon surgery.

Primary or delayed primary flexor tendon repair of both the profundus and superficialis should be carried out following interruption of the digital flexor tendons. The use of nonabsorbable sutures with a Kessler or modified Kessler technique would seem appropriate with careful preservation of the vincular system and, whenever possible, repair of the flexor tendon sheath. A well-supervised program of early motion using either active or passive techniques currently would seem to be appropriate.

The use of conventional free-tendon grafts should be reserved for those cases seen late where the tissue bed is

CHAPTER 9 FUNCTIONAL RECOVERY AFTER FLEXOR TENDON SEVERANCE IN THE FINGER: THE STATE OF THE ART

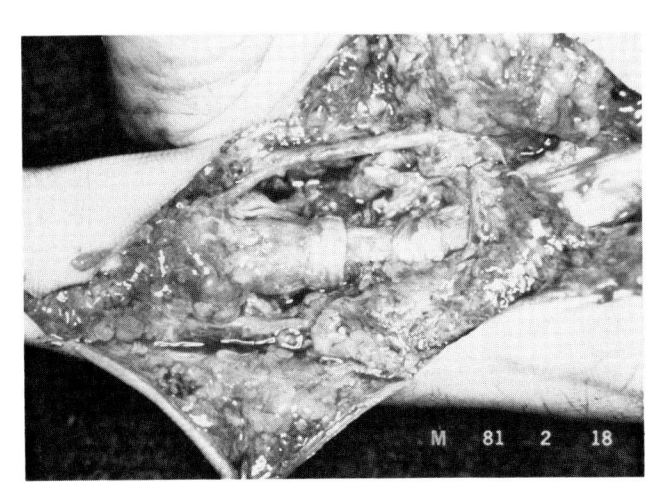

FIG. 9-13. Repair of A_3 (tendon graft around phalanx) and A_3 (tendon graft to lateral fibrous rims) pulleys to enhance flexor tendon efficiency and minimize volar displacement away from PIP joint.

ideal and passive motion complete. Two-stage reconstruction consisting of the implantation of a silicone rod followed by free-tendon grafting is reserved for those severe salvage situations in which flexor grafting must await the preparation of a smooth gliding bed. Tenolysis remains a reliable final mobilizing procedure following either repair or graft techniques and is best carried out with the patient under local anesthesia and analgesia. Attention to pulley salvage and reconstruction is important in all these procedures.

It is obvious that the restoration of function to a digit following flexor tendon interruption may be a long and tedious procedure, requiring the development of a strong rapport between surgeon and patient. When initiating the care of a patient with such an injury, the surgeon should spend considerable time explaining the problems related to the particular tendon injury, the likelihood of achieving success, and the number of procedures that may be required. A high degree of patient motivation must be established to ensure the proper participation in the demanding preoperative and postoperative regimen associated with these procedures.

With the important advances occurring in many areas of flexor tendon surgery, it is realistic to believe that in the near future the techniques described in this chapter will be substantially altered and modified. Results should continue to improve until the patient and surgeon can realistically expect to return all digits to nearly full function after flexor tendon interruption.

REFERENCES

1. Boyes, J.H., and Stark, H.H.: Flexor-tendon grafts in the fingers and thumb: a study of factors influencing results in 1000 cases, J. Bone Joint Surg. **53A**:1332, 1971.
2. Brokis, J.G.: The blood supply of the flexor and extensor tendons of the fingers in man, J. Bone Joint Surg. **35B**:131, 1953.
3. Bunnell, S.: Repair of tendons in the fingers and description of two new instruments, Surg. Gynecol. Obstet. **26**: 103, 1918.
4. Cameron, R.R., Conrad, R.N., Sell, K.W., et al.: Freeze-dried composite tendon allografts: an experimental study, Plast. Reconstr. Surg. **47**:39, 1971.
5. Cameron, R.R., Sell, K., and Latham, W.D.: The experimental transplantation of freeze-dried composite flexor tendon allografts, J. Bone Joint Surg. **52A**:1065, 1970.
6. Caplan, H.S., Hunter, J.M., and Merklin, R.J.: Intrinsic vascularization of flexor tendons. In American Academy of Orthopaedic Surgeons: Symposium on Tendon Surgery in the Hand, St. Louis, 1975, The C.V. Mosby Co.
7. Caplan, H.S., Hunter, J.M., and Merklin, R.J.: The intrinsic vascularization of flexor tendons in the human, J. Bone Joint Surg. **57A**:726, 1975.
8. Doyle, J.R., and Blythe, W.F.: The finger flexion tendon sheath and pulleys: anatomy and reconstruction, In American Academy of Orthopaedic Surgeons: Symposium on Tendon Surgery in the Hand, St. Louis, 1975, The C.V. Mosby Co.
9. Doyle, J.R., and Blythe, W.F.: Anatomy of the flexor tendon sheath and pulleys of the thumb, J. Hand Surg. **2**:149, 1977.
10. Duran, R.J., and Houser, R.G.: Controlled passive motion following flexor tendon repair in zones 2 and 3. In American Academy of Orthopaedic Surgeons: Symposium on Tendon Surgery in the Hand, St. Louis, 1975, The C.V. Mosby Co.
11. Duran, R.J., Houser, R.G., Coleman, C.R., et al.: A preliminary report in the use of controlled passive motion following flexor tendon repair in zones II and III, J. Hand Surg. **1**:79, 1976.
12. Flynn, J.E., and Graham, J.H.: Healing with tendon suture and tendon transplants. In Flynn, J.E., editor: Hand surgery, Baltimore, 1966, Williams & Wilkins Co.
13. Furlow, L.T.: Early active motion in flexor tendon healing, J. Bone Joint Surg. **54A**:911, 1972.
14. Furlow, L.T.: The role of tendon tissues in tendon healing, Plast. Reconstr. Surg. **57**:39, 1976.
15. Harmer, T.W.: Tendon suture, Bost. Med. Surg. J. **176**: 808, 1917.
16. Harmer, T.W.: Cases of tendon and nerve repair, Bost. Med. Surg. J. **194**:739, 1926.
17. Harmer, T.W.: Certain aspects of hand surgery, N. Engl. J. Med. **214**:613, 1936.
18. Harmer, T.W.: Injuries to the hand, Am. J. Surg. **42**:638, 1938.
19. Hernandez, A., Velasco, F., Rivas, A., et al.: Preliminary report on early mobilization for the rehabilitation of flexor tendons, Plast. Reconstr. Surg. **40**:354, 1967.
20. Hunter, J.M., and Salisbury, R.E.: Flexor-tendon reconstruction in severely damaged hands: a two-stage procedure using a silicone-Dacron reinforced gliding prosthesis prior to tendon grafting, J. Bone Joint Surg. **53A**:829, 1971.
21. Hunter, J.M., Schneider, L.H., and Fietti, V.G., Jr.: Re-

construction of the sublimis finger, J. Hand Surg. **4**:282, 1979.
22. Kessler, I., and Nissim, F.: Primary repair without immobilization of flexor tendon division within the digital flexor sheath, Acta Orthop. Scand. **40**:587, 1969.
23. Ketchum, L.D.: Primary tendon healing: a review, J. Hand Surg. **2**:428, 1977.
24. Kleinert, H.E., and Bennett, J.B.: Digital pulley reconstruction employing the always present rim of the previous pulley, J. Hand Surg. **3**:297, 1978.
25. Kleinert, H.E., Kutz, J.E., Ashbell, T.S., et al.: Primary repair of lacerated flexor tendons in "no man's land," J. Bone Joint Surg. **49A**:577, 1967.
26. Kyle, J.B., and Eyre-Brook, A.L.: The surgical treatment of flexor tendon injuries in the hand, results obtained in a consecutive series of 57 cases, Br. J. Surg. **41**:502, 1954.
27. Lahey, F.H.: A tendon suture which permits immediate motion, Bost. Med. Surg. J. **188**:851, 1923.
28. Lindsay, W.K.: The fibroblast in flexor tendon healing, J. Bone Joint Surg. **46A**:909, 1964.
29. Lindsay, W.K., and McDougall, E.P.: Digital flexor tendons: an experimental study. III. The fate of autogenous digital flexor tendon grafts, Br. J. Plast. Surg. **13**:293, 1961.
30. Lindsay, W.K., and Thomson, H.G.: Digital flexor tendons: an experimental study. I. The significance of each component of the flexor mechanism in tendon healing, Br. J. Plast. Surg. **12**:289, 1960.
31. Lister, G.D., Kleinert, H.E., Kutz, J.E., et al.: Primary flexor tendon repair followed by immediate controlled mobilization, J. Hand Surg. **2**:441, 1977.
32. Lundborg, G.: Experimental flexor tendon healing without adhesion formation—a new concept of tendon nutrition and intrinsic healing mechanisms: a preliminary report, Hand **8**:235, 1976.
33. Lundborg, G., Myrhage, R., and Rydevik, B.: The vascularization of human flexor tendons within the digital synovial sheath region—structure and functional aspects, J. Hand Surg. **2**:417, 1977.
34. Lundborg, G., and Rank, F.: Experimental intrinsic healing of flexor tendons based upon synovial fluid nutrition: a new aspect of the biology of tendon repair, J. Hand Surg. **2**:231, 1977.
35. Madsen, E.: Delayed primary suture of flexor tendons cut in the digital sheath, J. Bone Joint Surg. **52B**:264, 1970.
36. Manske, P.R., Bridwell, K., and Lesker, P.A.: Nutrient pathways to flexor tendon of chickens using tritiated proline, J. Hand Surg. **3**:352, 1978.
37. Manske, P.R., Lesker, P.A., and Bridwell, K.: Experimental studies in chickens on the initial nutrition of tendon grafts, J. Hand Surg. **4**:565, 1979.
38. Manske, P.R., Lesker, P.A., and Bridwell, K.: Experimental studies on the initial nutrition of flexor tendon grafts, J. Hand Surg. **4**:282, 1979.
39. Manske, P.R., Lesker, P.A., Bridwell, K., et al.: Nutrient pathways to flexor tendons within the flexor sheath, J. Hand Surg. **3**:287, 1978.
40. Manske, P.R., Whiteside, L.A., and Lesker, P.A.: Nutrient pathways to flexor tendons using hydrogen washout technique, J. Hand Surg. **3**:32, 1978.
41. Mason, M.L., and Allen, H.S.: The rate of healing of tendons: an experimental study of tensile strength, Ann. Surg. **113**:424, 1941.
42. Matthews, P.: The fate of isolated segments of flexor tendons within the digital sheath: a study in synovial nutrition, Br. J. Plast. Surg. **29**:216, 1976.
43. Matthews, P., and Richards, H.: The repair potential of digital flexor tendons: an experimental study, J. Bone Joint Surg. **56B**:618, 1974.
44. Matthews, P., and Richards, H.: The repair reaction of flexor tendon within the digital sheath, Hand **7**:27, 1975.
45. Miller, H.: Repair of severed tendons of the hand and wrist: statistical analysis of 300 cases, Surg. Gynecol. Obstet. **75**:693, 1942.
46. Ochiai, N., Matsui, T., Miyaji, N., et al.: Vascular anatomy of flexor tendons. I. Vincular systems and blood supply of the profundus tendon in the digital sheath, J. Hand Surg. **4**:321, 1979.
47. Paneva-Holevich, E.: Two-stage tenoplasty in injury of the flexor tendons of the hand, J. Bone Joint Surg. **51A**:21, 1969.
48. Peacock, E.E.: Morphology of homologous and heterologous tendon grafts, Surg. Gynecol. Obstet. **109**:735, 1959.
49. Peacock, E.E.: Restoration of finger flexion with homologous composite tissue tendon grafts, Am. J. Surg. **26**:564, 1969.
50. Peacock, E.E., and Madden, J.W.: Human composite flexor tendon allografts, Ann. Surg. **166**:624, 1967.
51. Peacock, E.E., and Madden, J.W.: Some studies on the effects of B-aminoprorionitrile in patients with injured flexor tendons, Surgery **66**:215, 1969.
52. Peacock, E.E., et al.: Postoperative recovery of flexor tendon function, Am. J. Surg. **122**:686, 1971.
53. Potenza, A.D.: Tendon healing within the flexor digital sheath in the dog: an experimental study, J. Bone Joint Surg. **44A**:49, 1962.
54. Potenza, A.D.: Critical evaluation of flexor-tendon healing and adhesion formation within artificial digital sheaths, J. Bone Joint Surg. **45A**:1217, 1963.
55. Potenza, A.D.: Healing and fate of lyophilized homologous flexor-tendon grafts within the flexor digital sheath, J. Bone Joint Surg. **46A**:908, 1964.
56. Potenza, A.D.: The healing of autogenous tendon grafts within the flexor digital sheath in dogs, J. Bone Joint Surg. **46A**:1462, 1964.
57. Potenza, A.D.: Prevention of adhesions to healing digital flexor tendons, J.A.M.A. **187**:187, 1964.
58. Potenza, A.D.: The mechanism of healing of digital flexor tendons, Hand **1**:40, 1969.
59. Potenza, A.D.: The healing process in wounds of the digital flexor tendons and tendon grafts: an experimental study. In Verdan, C., editor: Tendon surgery of the hand, Edinburgh, Scotland, 1979, Churchill Livingstone.
60. Potenza, A.D., and Melone, C.W.: Functional evaluation of freeze-dried flexor tendon grafts in the dog, J. Hand Surg. **2**:233, 1977.
61. Potenza, A.D., and Melone, C.W.: Evaluation of freeze-dried flexor tendon grafts in the dog, J. Hand Surg. **3**:157, 1978.

62. Pulvertaft, R.G.: Experiences in flexor tendon grafting in the hand, J. Bone Joint Surg. **41B:**629, 1959.
63. Pulvertaft, R.G.: Tendon grafts for flexor tendon injuries in the fingers and thumb: a study of technique and results, J. Bone Joint Surg. **38B:**175, 1971.
64. Salvi, V.: Delayed primary suture in flexor tendon division, Hand **3:**181, 1971.
65. Schneider, L.H., and Hunter, J.M.: Flexor tenolysis. In American Academy of Orthopaedic Surgeons: Symposium on Tendon Surgery in the Hand, St. Louis, 1975, The C.V. Mosby Co.
66. Stark, H.H., Zemel, N.P., Boyes, J.H., et al.: Flexor tendon graft through intact superficialis tendon, J. Hand Surg. **2:**456, 1977.
67. Strickland, J.W., and Glogovac, S.V.: Digital function following flexor tendon repair in zone II: a comparison of immobilization and controlled passive motion techniques, J. Hand Surg. **5:**537, 1980.
68. Urbaniak, J.R., Bright, D.S., Gill, L.H., et al.: Vascularization and the gliding mechanism of free flexor-tendon grafts inserted by the silicone-rod method, J. Bone Joint Surg. **56A:**473, 1974.
69. Urbaniak, J.R., Cahill, J.D., Jr., and Mortensen, R.A.: Tendon suturing methods: analysis of tensile strengths. In American Academy of Orthopaedic Surgeons: Symposium on Tendon Surgery in the Hand, St. Louis, 1975, The C.V. Mosby Co.
70. Verdan, C.: Primary repair of flexor tendons, J. Bone Joint Surg. **42A:**647, 1960.
71. Verdan, C.: Practical considerations for primary and secondary repair in flexor tendon injuries, Surg. Clin. North Am. **44:**951, 1964.
72. Verdan, C.: Primary and secondary repair of flexor and extensor tendon injuries. In Flynn, J.E., editor: Hand surgery, Baltimore, 1966, Williams & Wilkins Co.
73. Verdan, C.: Half a century of flexor tendon repair: current status and changing philosophies, J. Bone Joint Surg. **54A:**472, 1972.
74. Verdan, C., and Michon, J.: Le traitement des plaies des tendons fleschisseurs des doigts, Rev. Chir. Orthop. **47:**285, 1961.
75. Weeks, P.M., and Wray, R.C.: Rate and extent of functional recovery after flexor tendon grafting with and without silicone rod preparation, J. Hand Surg. **1:**174, 1976.
76. Weeks, P.M., Wray, R.C., and Stromberg, B.V.: The rate of functional recovery after flexor tendon grafting, J. Hand Surg. **1:**75, 1976.
77. Whitaker, J.H., Strickland, J.W., and Ellis, R.K.: The role of flexor tenolysis in the palm and digits, J. Hand Surg. **2:**231, 462, 1977.
78. Young, R.E.S., and Harmon, J.M.: Repair of tendon injuries of the hand, Ann. Surg. **151:**562, 1960.

Chapter 10 Problems in the management of flexor tendon injuries in zones I and II

Robert J. Duran

Robert G. Houser

This chapter presents some of the problems encountered in the management of flexor tendon injuries in zones I and II (Fig. 10-1). It is important to remember that the zones represent the location of tendon injury and not the cutaneous injury. Cases are presented along with analyses of specific problems and the choices considered for their correction.

ZONE I

Zone I is the area distal to the proximal interphalangeal (PIP) joint. The following injury represents a zone I problem.

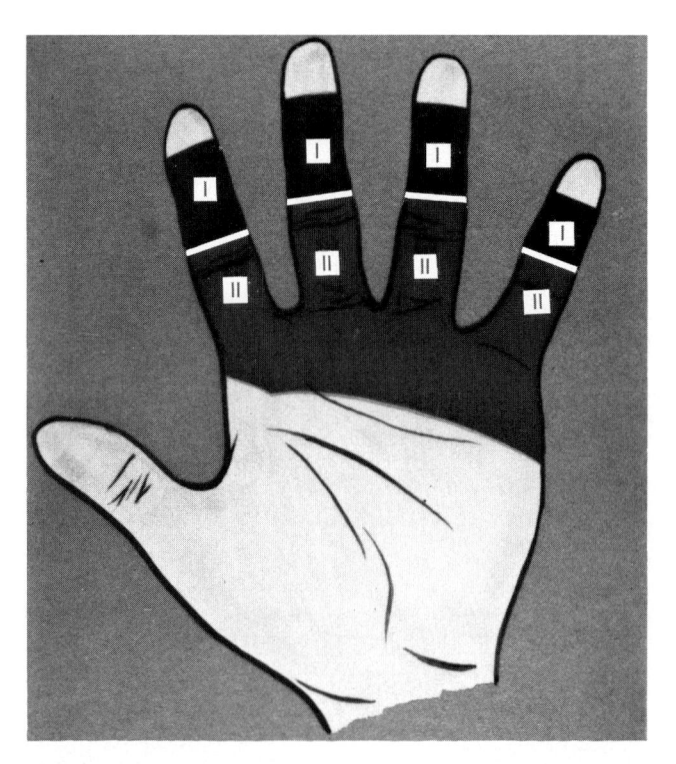

FIG. 10-1 Surgical zones I and II of flexor tendons of fingers.

CHAPTER 10 PROBLEMS IN THE MANAGEMENT OF FLEXOR TENDON INJURIES IN ZONES I AND II

Case 1

A 26-year-old factory worker lacerated his left long finger just proximal to the distal finger crease. The skin laceration was sutured, and the patient returned to work, which required the lifting of heavy boxes. Weakness of grip, loss of tip strength, and tenderness in the distal palm of the hand made it increasingly difficult for the patient to perform his duties. He was examined approximately 9 weeks after the original injury, and a diagnosis of lacerated flexor digitorum profundus tendon was made (Fig. 10-2). Sensation, range of joint motion, and flexor digitorum superficialis function were normal.

The choices considered for treatment of this injury were the following:
1. Stabilizing procedures of the distal interphalangeal (DIP) joint
    a. Tenodesis
    b. Capsulodesis
    c. Arthrodesis
2. Tendon advancement procedure
3. Secondary tenorrhaphy
4. Tendon graft through flexor digitorum superficialis decussation
    a. One stage
    b. Two stage

Considerable controversy continues to exist as to the management of the flexor digitorum profundus injury when seen late. We are referring only to those patients with normal flexor digitorum superficialis function. Age, occupation, and the finger involved, as well as the condition of the finger, are important factors to consider in planning the treatment. It is our opinion that primarily this requires a decision based on the particular needs of the patient. In this patient it was determined that his particular needs would be tip strength and motion; therefore stabilizing procedures were not considered. The procedures discussed were tendon advancement or secondary tenorrhaphy. If these procedures were not possible, then primary or staged tendon grafting through the intact flexor digitorum superficialis tendon would be considered. The decision therefore would have to be made by the surgeon when conditions were visualized at the time of surgery. This was acceptable to the patient.

At operation, the proximal end of the flexor digitorum profundus was firmly fixed in the midportion of annulus two (A_2). Degeneration and swelling of the tendon were present in the palm. The distal end of the flexor digitorum profundus tendon was firmly adherent to A_4. Secondary tendon repair was obviously impossible. Repair was undertaken with resection of the distal tendon and dilatation of all five annular pulleys as well as decussation of the flexor digitorum superficialis. Approximately 20% of the distal portion of A_4 had to be sacrificed. Because of scarring in the bed and collapse of portions of the annular system, a staged procedure was considered advisable. The proximal portion of the flexor digitorum profundus tendon was beveled and secured to the external surface of A_1 to maintain the balance of the profundus and lumbrical systems. A silicone rod was threaded through the pulley system and attached distally to the flexor digitorum profundus stump. Proximally, the rod was allowed to remain free at the level of the lumbrical muscle with the finger extended.

After 4 months a palmaris longus tendon graft was placed through the flexor digitorum superficialis decussation with distal attachment into the distal phalanx, using a pullout technique. Proximally, the graft was imbricated through the flexor digitorum profundus tendon.

Approximately 4 months after removal of the intratendinous wire the final range of motion had been achieved. A total active motion of 275 degrees was gained with a permanent 5-degree deficit in extension at the DIP joint (Figs. 10-3 to 10-5). The patient returned to his original job.

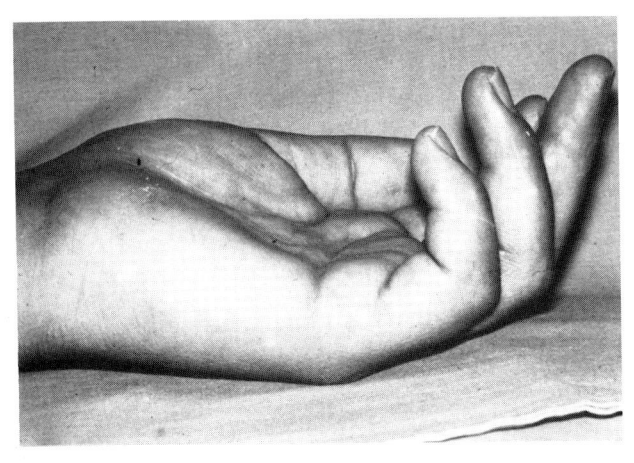

FIG. 10-2. Loss of DIP-joint flexion in long finger with normal function of flexor digitorum superficialis (case 1).

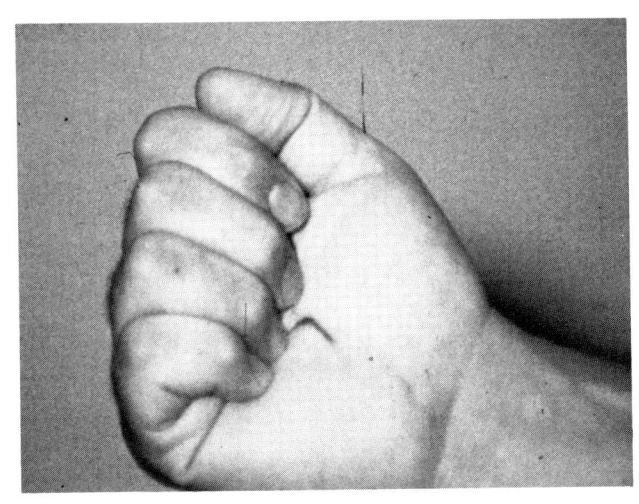

FIG. 10-3. Flexion gained in long finger after tendon graft through intact flexor digitorum superficialis tendon (case 1).

SECTION 3   FLEXOR TENDON PROBLEMS

Discussion

It is generally agreed that a flexor digitorum profundus tendon advancement should be avoided if the tendon has been lacerated more than 1 cm from the point of insertion. Advancing the tendon a greater distance could result in flexion contracture (Fig. 10-6) or tendon imbalance, interfering with normal flexion of neighboring fingers. This is particularly true in the long, ring, and little fingers. Verdan[3] describes this imbalance as the syndrome of the Quadriga. When the laceration is more than 1 cm from the insertion, we advocate that primary repair of the flexor digitorum profundus tendon be followed by controlled passive motion exercises postoperatively[1] (Figs. 10-7 to 10-10).

Stabilizing procedures are reserved for patients not requiring tip strength or motion who have excellent flexor digitorum superficialis function or those in whom the risk of a pull-through graft would not be justified because of other injuries, such as DIP joint injury with minimal motion.

The decision to employ the two-stage tendon reconstruction in this patient was based on the collapse of the superficialis decussation and the pulley system, as well as the scarring present. The choice of this method is in accord with the indications of Wilson and associates[4] for flexor profundus reconstruction.

ZONE II

Zone II extends from the first annular ligament to the proximal PIP.

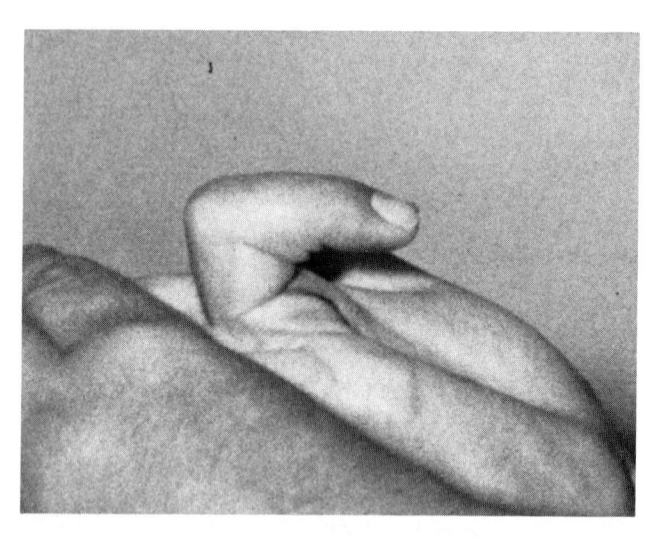

FIG. 10-4. Maintenance of flexor digitorum superficialis function following tendon graft (case 1).

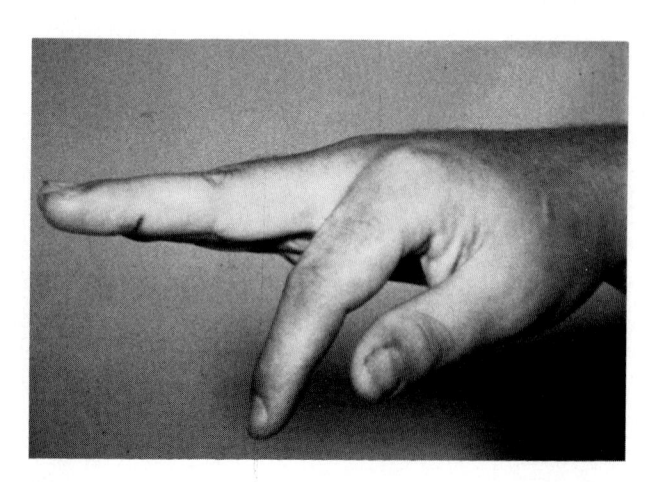

FIG. 10-5. Extension achieved after flexor digitorum profundus tendon graft through decussation of flexor digitorum superficialis (case 1).

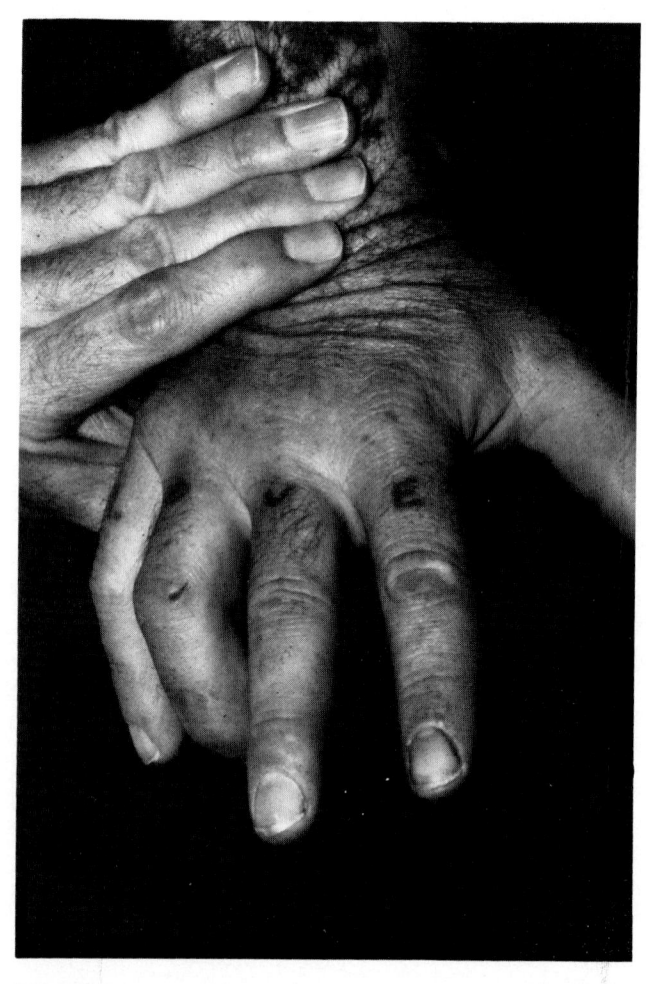

FIG. 10-6. Postoperative flexion contracture of ring finger in 42-year-old laborer after excessive advancement of flexor digitorum profundus tendon in zone I.

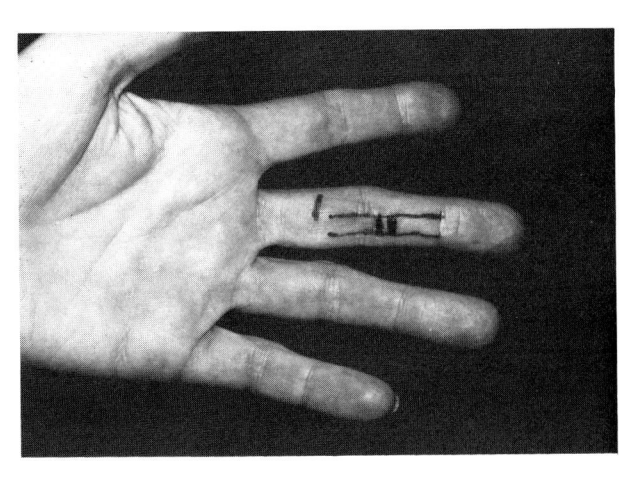

CHAPTER 10 PROBLEMS IN THE MANAGEMENT OF FLEXOR TENDON INJURIES IN ZONES I AND II

FIG. 10-7. Zone I laceration of flexor digitorum profundus in 45-year-old physician; stab wound with finger flexed. Cutaneous wound is marked proximally.

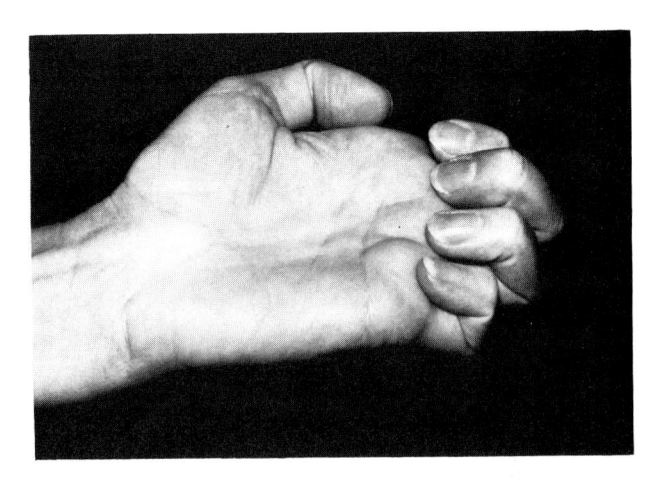

FIG. 10-8. Postoperative flexion gained after primary repair of flexor digitorum profundus and use of controlled passive motion postoperatively.

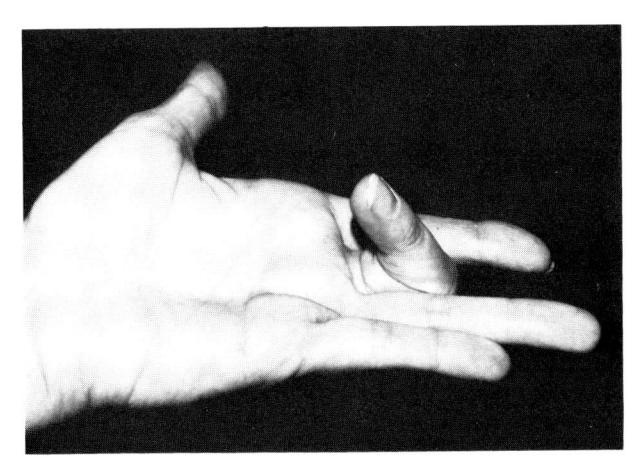

FIG. 10-9. Postoperative flexion of flexor digitorum superficialis after primary repair of flexor digitorum profundus and use of controlled passive motion postoperatively.

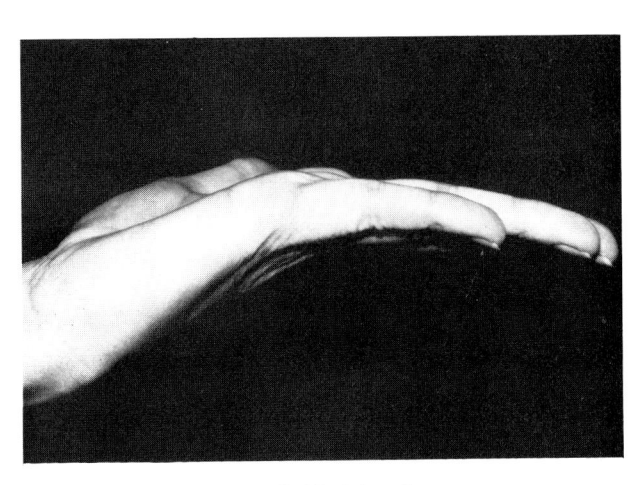

FIG. 10-10. Extension.

Case 2

A 34-year-old farmer injured his left hand in a combine accident. His left index finger was partially amputated, and he sustained a deep laceration at the base of the long finger. The flexor digitorum profundus and flexor digitorum superficialis were severed, along with the volar digital nerve on the radial side.

Treatment consisted of neurorrhaphy of the volar digital nerve on the radial side and tenorrhaphy of the flexor digitorum profundus. A splint was applied with the wrist acutely flexed and rubber-band finger traction holding the finger in flexion. He was instructed to follow a postoperative motion program, but he failed to cooperate and later admitted that he had not moved the finger. The splint was removed at 4 weeks, and the patient was unable to actively flex or extend the long finger at the PIP or DIP joint. Consultation was sought 10 months after primary treatment (Fig. 10-11). A flexion contracture of 54 degrees was present at the PIP joint. The patient was unable to fully flex the DIP joint of the uninjured ring finger and noticed weakness in little finger flexion (Fig. 10-12). The index finger stump was not tender and was used for lateral pinch. Two-point discrimination in the volar aspect of the finger on the radial side was 9 mm.

Immobilization in this case resulted in loss of gliding of the repaired flexor digitorum profundus tendon of the long finger. Since the patient did not follow instructions for postoperative exercise, it can be assumed that the anastomosis became adherent distal to the level of injury as a result of severe flexion of the wrist. It can be assumed also that the flexed position of the finger did not permit proximal migration of the tendon, possibly because of swelling of the anastomosis and inability to negotiate the annulus. When use of the splint was discontinued and the wrist returned to normal position, an imbalance existed in the ring finger and to a lesser extent in the little finger.

At operation, using a sensory nerve block, a tenolysis of the flexor digitorum profundus was performed from midpalm to the distal phalanx, improving flexion of the long finger as well as restoring flexion to the ring and little fingers. Extension was improved by resecting the distal portion of the flexor digitorum superficialis tendon as it crossed the PIP joint as well as resecting the check-rein ligaments of the PIP joint. A final TAM (total active motion) of 240 degrees, including a 20-degree extension deficit of the PIP joint, was attained (Figs. 10-13 and 10-14).

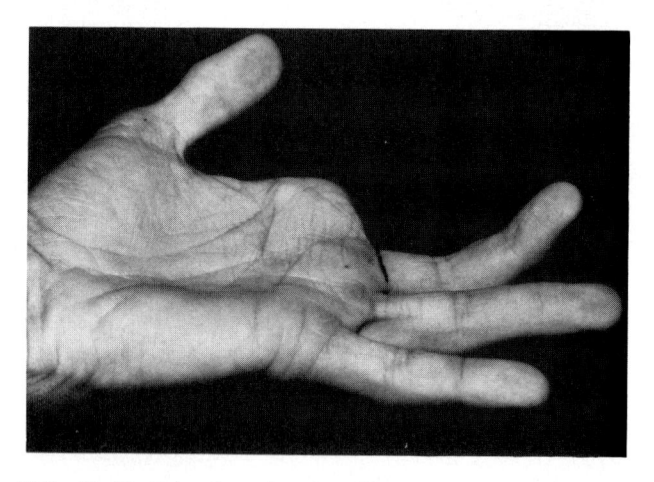

FIG. 10-11. Extension showing flexion contracture of PIP joint (case 2).

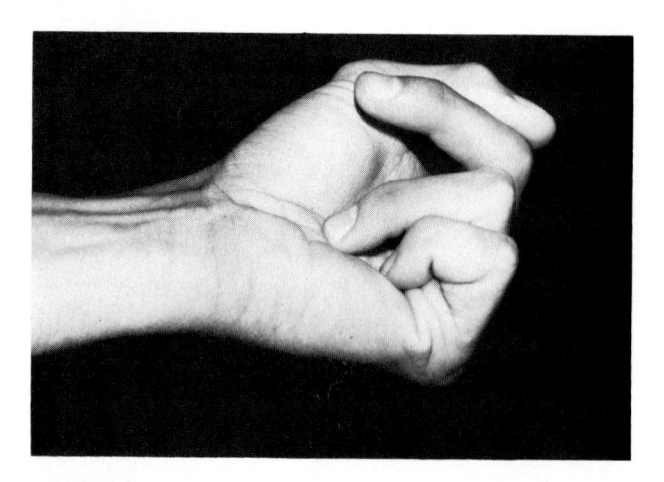

FIG. 10-12. Patient attempting to flex injured long finger. Note inability to fully flex distal joint of uninjured ring finger (case 2).

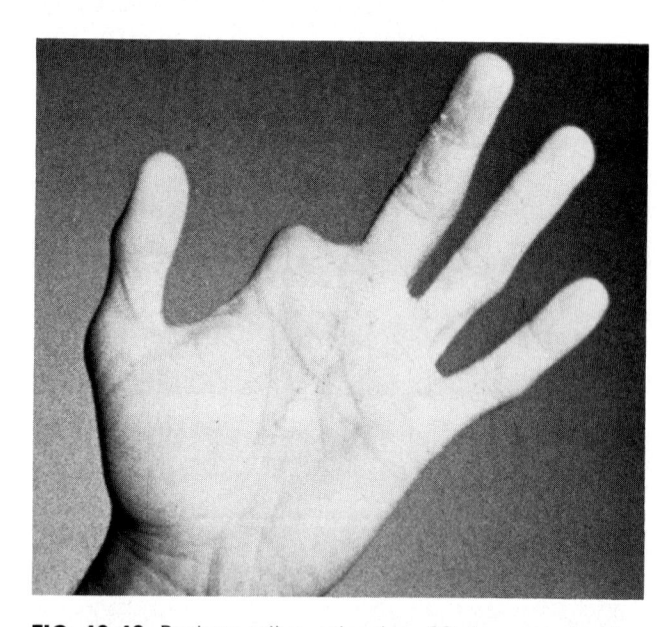

FIG. 10-13. Postoperative extension: 20-degree extension deficit is present at PIP joint (case 2).

Discussion. In this patient adhesion-imbalance affected not only the injured long finger but also the uninjured ring and little fingers. Flexion contracture of the PIP joint resulted from the flexed position of the PIP joint held in rubber-band traction. Flexion contracture was fixed by flexor digitorum profundus tendon adhesion and by the distal portion of the flexor digitorum superficialis, which crossed the PIP joint.

This patient was a candidate for primary repair of the flexor digitorum superficialis and flexor digitorum profundus tendons, followed by a postoperative motion program. The surgeon who first treated the patient intended that motion be used postoperatively, but the patient failed to cooperate.

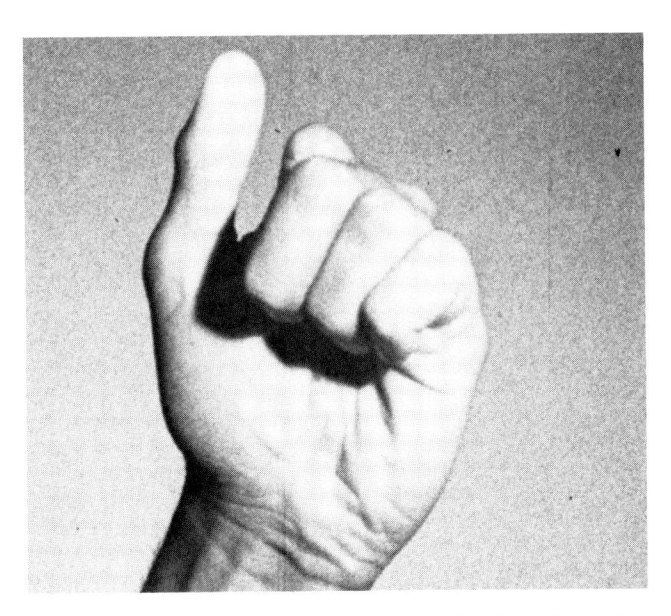

FIG. 10-14. Postoperative flexion gained in long finger following tenolysis of flexor digitorum profundus. Note increased flexion of uninjured ring finger (case 2).

SECTION 3 FLEXOR TENDON PROBLEMS

Case 3

A 29-year-old housewife lacerated the left little finger in proximal zone II, severing the flexor digitorum profundus and flexor digitorum superficialis tendons. Primary tenorrhaphy of only the flexor digitorum profundus tendon was performed, and the wrist and finger were immobilized. One week later the tendon ruptured, and a second tenorrhaphy was performed. Six months later the patient was unable to fully extend the finger and lacked active flexion, so a third procedure, a tenolysis of the flexor digitorum profundus tendon, was carried out. Postoperatively the finger progressively flexed, and the patient was unable to extend it (Fig. 10-15).

Examination 2 years after the original injury disclosed PIP joint flexion contracture of 80 degrees in the little finger. Passive extension of the distal phalanx made active flexion at the DIP joint possible, but bowing of the flexor digitorum profundus tendon across the PIP joint indicated that the pulley mechanism was absent in this area.

Multiple problems were present in this zone II injury. On the basis of three previous operations and such a severe PIP joint flexion contracture, it seemed highly probable that a two-staged flexor tendon reconstruction would be necessary. This was acceptable to the patient.

At surgery the previous lateral incision in the finger was used and extended into the palm in a zigzag manner. The annular system was absent from mid-A_2 to A_4. PIP joint contracture was the result of a shortened flexor digitorum profundus tendon bowing across the PIP joint. In addition, there was a retrotendinous band and secondary PIP joint contracture. Excision of the flexor digitorum profundus tendon, the retrotendinous band, and the checkrein ligaments of PIP joint resulted in a PIP joint extension deficit of

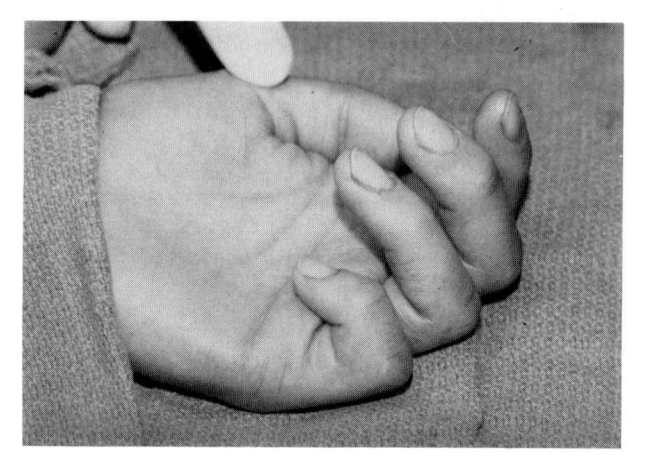

FIG. 10-15. Fixed PIP joint contracture of 80 degrees following zone II flexor digitorum profundus repair, secondary repair after tendon rupture, and tenolysis as third procedure (case 3).

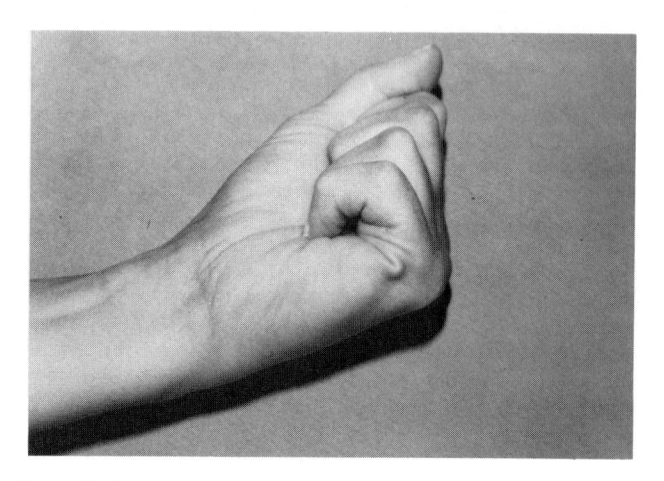

FIG. 10-16. Flexion after two-stage flexor tendon reconstruction (case 3).

only 10 degrees. A silicone rod was placed, sutured distally to the residual flexor digitorum profundus stump, and allowed to remain in a pocket posterior to the flexor digitorum profundus at the lumbrical muscle level. A reconstruction of distal A_2 and A_3 using the Weilby technique[2] completed the procedure.

Four months later a second stage tendon graft procedure was performed. The wrist was placed in moderate flexion to maintain the extended position of the PIP joint to avoid recurrence of the flexion contracture.

Three months after stage 2 an extension deficit of 9 degrees at the PIP joint and 15 degrees at the DIP joint was present. TAM was 211 degrees at that time (235 degrees minus extension loss of 24 degrees) (Figs. 10-16 and 10-17).

Discussion. This particular problem is being seen more often as a complication of primary flexor tendon repair in zone II. The importance of stage 1 in flexor tendon reconstruction is well illustrated in this case. The opportunity to correct the flexion contracture, reconstruct the pulley mechanism, and place a silicone rod to improve the scarred bed in stage 1 had produced a satisfactory result for this patient after tendon grafting in stage 2.

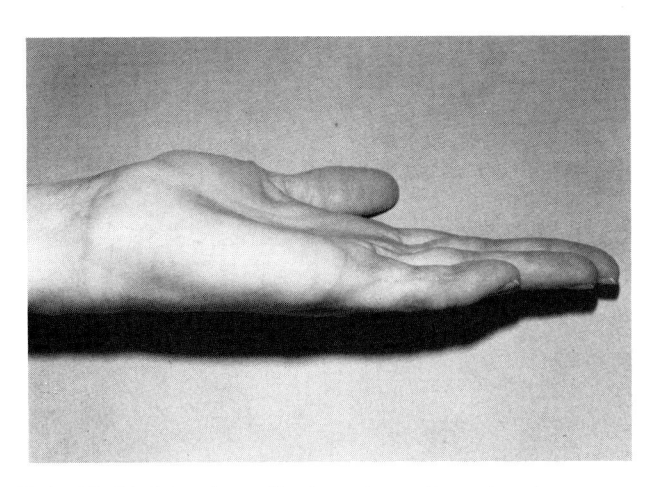

FIG. 10-17. Extension after two-stage flexor tendon reconstruction (case 3).

REFERENCES

1. Duran, R.J., Houser, R.G., and Stover, M.G.: Management of flexor tendon lacerations in zone 2 using controlled passive motion postoperatively. In Hunter, J.M., Schneider, L.H., Mackin, E.J., and Bell, J.A., editors: Rehabilitation of the hand, St. Louis, 1978, The C.V. Mosby Co.
2. Kleinert, H.E., and Bennett, J.B.: Digital pulley reconstruction employing the always present rim of the previous pulley, J. Hand Surg. **3**:297, 1978.
3. Verdan, C.E.: Primary and secondary repair of flexor and extensor tendon injuries. In Flynn, J.E., editor: Hand surgery, Baltimore, 1966, Williams & Wilkins Co.
4. Wilson, R.L., Carter, M.S., Holdeman, V.A., and Lovett, W.L.: Flexor profundus injuries treated with delayed two-stage tendon grafting, J. Hand Surg. **5**:74, 1980.

Chapter 11 The pulley system: rationale for reconstruction

James M. Hunter

John F. Cook, Jr.

Crucial to any successful exploration or reconstruction of a finger flexor tendon system is a thorough knowledge of the supporting framework about the tendon. This framework provides for optimal efficiency of the tendon system. The difference between a mediocre and an excellent result in flexor tendon surgery is determined not solely by the treatment of the tendon itself but also by consideration of important structural aspects of the pulley system and the vincular blood supply.

Flexor tendon surgery in the finger is complex and difficult. We propose that adherence to the strict anatomic and surgical principles here can significantly alter the surgeon's results and the patient's satisfaction.

Fig. 11-1 illustrates the difference between a result that was previously considered good to excellent and a much better one in which silicone, passive tendon implant replaces the flexor tendons in the long finger of a Burmese monkey.[11] This laboratory experiment dramatically emphasizes the need to critically study the pulley systems that will produce optimal function following flexor tendon reconstruction.

ANATOMY

The normal anatomic pulley system is a continuum of reinforcing fibers, interlacing to provide a supporting framework about the tendons for optimal flexor efficiency. There are five annular pulleys: A_2 and A_4, long, rigid retinaculum arising exclusively from bone, and A_1, A_3, and A_5, arising from bone and volar plate. The three cruciate pulleys serve as reinforcing extensions of the annular pulleys, along with an area of variable fiber between A_1 and A_2[9,10] (Fig. 11-2). In addition, the superficialis tendon reinforces the profundus tendon proximal to the chiasm of Camper.

The proper digital arteries give four transverse tributaries that enter the flexor retinaculum at the cruciate pulley areas and feed the vincular system, which in turn nourishes the flexor tendons (Fig. 11-3).

CHAPTER 11 THE PULLEY SYSTEM: RATIONALE FOR RECONSTRUCTION

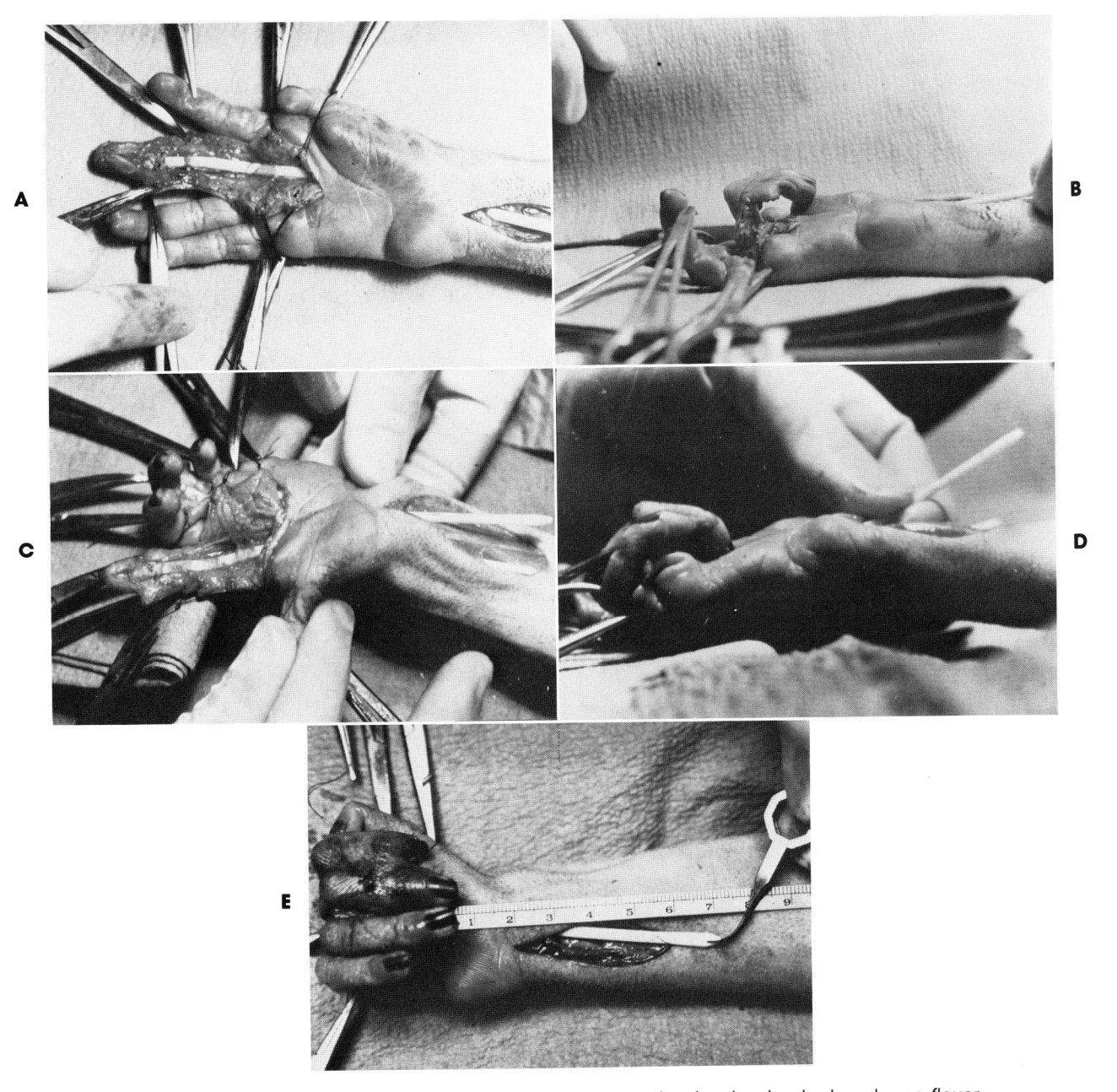

FIG. 11-1. Evaluation of pulley system. **A,** Silicone passive tendon implant replaces flexor tendons in long finger of Burmese monkey. A_2 and A_4 pulleys remain in place. **B,** As implant is pulled proximally, finger pulp–to–distal palmar crease measurement is 1 inch. **C,** Four annular pulleys in place. **D,** Finger pulp–to–distal palmar crease distance is obliterated. **E,** Same gliding excursion was applied to implant in both instances. Four-pulley system is most efficient.

SECTION 3 FLEXOR TENDON PROBLEMS

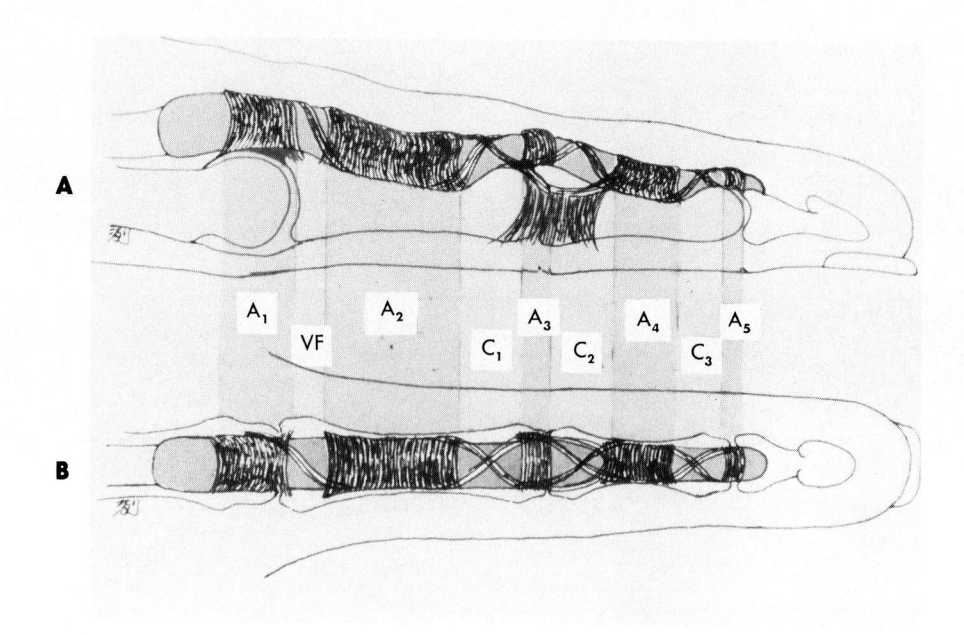

FIG. 11-2. A, Lateral and, **B,** anteroposterior finger flexor retinaculum. Note five annular pulleys (A_1 to A_5). A_2 and A_4 are anchored to bone. A_1, A_3, and A_5, arising from bone and volar plate, are adjusting pulleys. Note three cruciform pulleys (C_1 to C_3) and one variable fiber *(VF)* area between A_1 and A_2. These pulleys interlace with and arise from annulars in a continuum. With finger flexion, these pulleys fold up in accordion-like fashion.

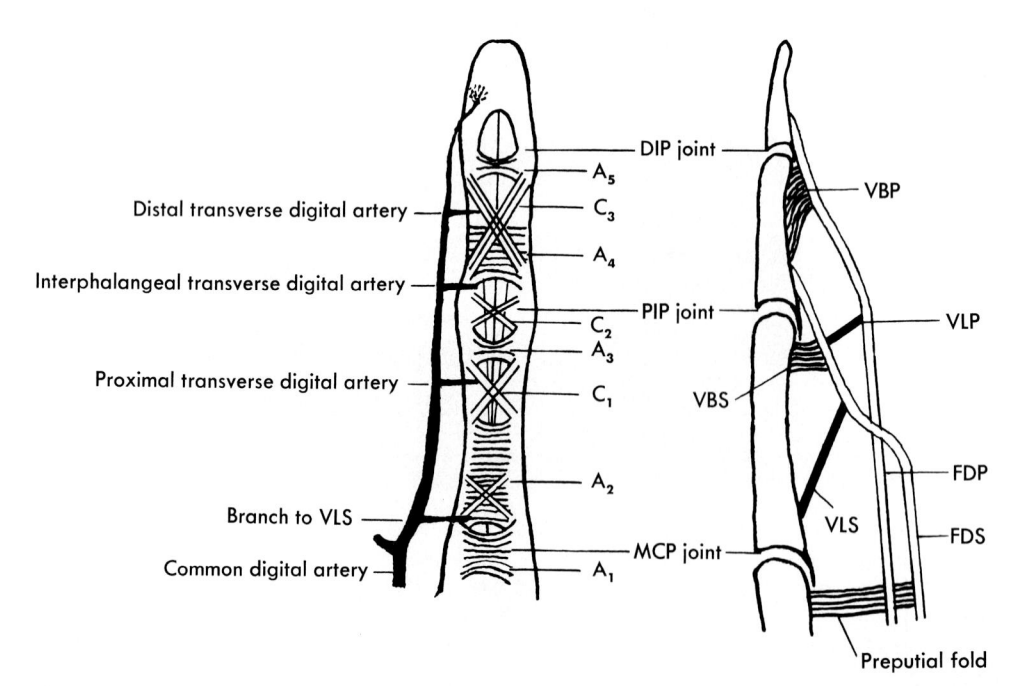

FIG. 11-3. Diagram of blood supply flexor tendon via proper digital artery to four transverse communicating branches, which penetrate retinaculum at cruciate and variable fiber areas and feed vincula.[19] *VLS,* Vinculum longum superficialis; *VBS,* vinculum brevem superficialis; *VBP,* vinculum breve profundus; *VLP,* vinculum longum profundus; *FDP,* flexor digitorum profundus; *FDS,* flexor digitorum superficialis. (From Ochiai, N., et al.: J. Hand Surg. **4:**322, 1979.)

CHAPTER 11 THE PULLEY SYSTEM: RATIONALE FOR RECONSTRUCTION

EXPLORATION OF THE FLEXOR RETINACULUM

Based on previous studies,[10] it appears acceptable to surgically enter the tendon sheath at the cruciate pulley areas, bearing in mind that the blood supply to the vincula enters at these areas as well. Resecting cruciate pulleys and A_5 while leaving the other annular pulleys intact in the two tendon flexor systems results in no change from the normal flexion ability. Therefore in surgical exploration of a flexor system the major pulleys to be left intact are A_1, A_2, A_3, and A_4.

The surgeon may be required to adapt to certain less than optimal situations. Tendon rupture may require resection of key pulleys for tendon repair. Trauma may damage part of or all the retinaculum, requiring pulley reconstruction. Tendons themselves may require grafting or complete sacrifice in favor of a silicone implant for staged reconstruction.[11]

Principles

As pulleys are resected, the efficiency of the flexor system is reduced. As suggested by Bunnell,[6] loss of pulleys results in the flexor tendons bowstringing, or moving away from their normal proximity to bones and joints, while taking the shortest distance between two adjacent pulleys. This gives the muscle-tendon unit increased mechanical advantage in flexing the bowstrung joint but results in a distinct loss of motion of the joint at a constant tendon excursion. Loss of flexion power of the finger ensues because bowstringing at one joint weakens flexion of the remaining joints.[2,5,14] As the tendon bows away from its bed, subtendinous scarring occurs, resulting in decreased tendon gliding, tendon adhesions, and flexion contractures of the joint. Tendon forces concentrate on the few remaining pulleys, increasing their susceptibility to rupture (Fig. 11-4).

Problems associated with a bowed tendon include the following:

1. Decreased range of joint motion
2. Decreased flexion power
3. Flexion contracture of the joint
4. Tendon adhesions
5. Increased risk of pulley rupture

Key pulleys, then, are those which diminish bowing by binding the tendon close to the concavities of the phalanges and close to the center of rotation of the joints.

Clinical application of principles

The proximal interphalangeal (PIP) joint is the most important joint in moving the finger tip to the distal palmar crease. It has the largest arc of motion of the three finger joints. The PIP joint moves the fingertip in a vertical direction toward the palm, thus gaining the most fingertip-to–distal palmar crease distance per degree of arc. Therefore the pulleys surrounding the PIP joint should be preserved, if at all possible. These include the distal portion of A_2 (A_{2b}), all of C_1, A_3, and C_2, and the proximal portion of A_4 (A_{4a}). (We now divide the large annular pulleys—A_2 and A_4—into two parts, a and b.) The same logic applies to the metacarpophalangeal (MCP) and distal interphalangeal (DIP) joints.

As previously mentioned, resecting cruciate pulleys from an intact system results in no change from normal. However, as annular pulleys are resected, the cruciates assume an increasingly larger role in preventing bowstringing.[10] It must be emphasized that, in a compromised system, effort must be made to avoid iatrogenic damage to *any* pulleys, including cruciates.

Should tendon repair require further pulley sacrifice for adequate exposure, transverse incisions into annular pulleys may be made or flaps created and resutured later. Intermediate portions of large annular pulleys may be incised with less penalty than if done to end sections. A_5 is the least important of the annulars. A_3 would be next sacrificed (not without penalty), provided that A_{2b} and A_{4a} were intact. If A_{2b} or A_{4a} need to be incised, care

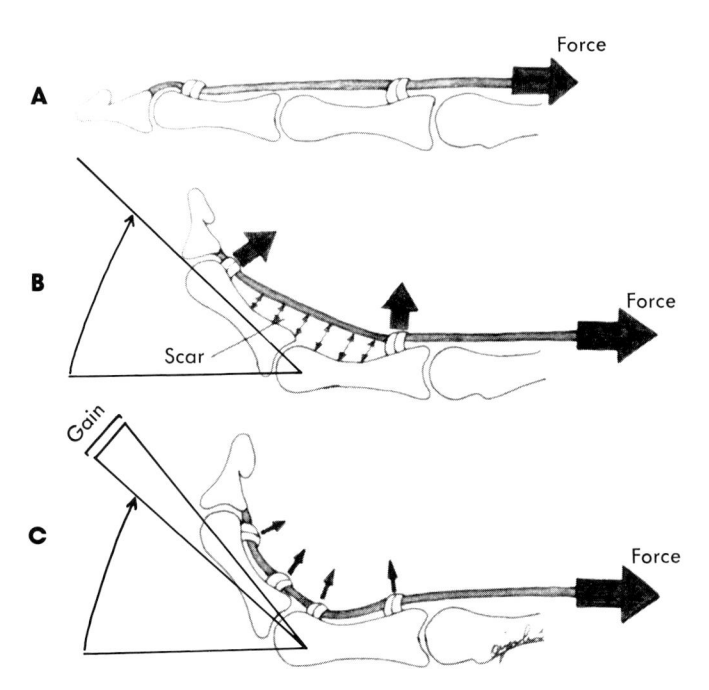

FIG. 11-4. Forcing pulley system. **A,** Two-pulley, one-tendon simplified system. **B,** As tendon is pulled proximally, tendon bows away from PIP joint, allowing subtendinous scar buildup, resulting in flexion contracture of joint. Decreased tendon gliding then results in tendon adhesions. Tendon forces concentrate on two remaining pulleys, increasing their susceptibility to rupture. **C,** More normal, four-pulley system eliminates tendon bowing and scar, joint contractures, and tendon adhesions. Tendon forces are better distributed along this pulley system, and range of flexion is improved.

must be taken to retain C_1 and C_2. It must be reiterated that key pulleys are those which bind the tendons close to the center of rotation of the joints. A_1, A_2, and A_4 remain necessities.

After tendon exploration or repair, active finger motion should be observed intraoperatively. We recommend the use of neuroleptanalgesia with fentanyl citrate (Innovar), in association with local lidocaine infiltration, to allow active finger motion by the patient during tenolysis procedures.[12] (See Chapter 35.) Should the choice of anesthesia preclude the patient's active participation, active motion should be simulated by passively pulling the tendon proximally and measuring the fingertip-to–distal palmar crease distance. If motion is not full, an instrument may be used to simulate a pulley in the appropriate location, and motion again is measured. Should there be a significant difference, we recommend pulley reconstruction.

Reconstruction of pulleys

Construction of pulleys in the clinical situation requires consideration of other factors that influence results:

1. The quality and size of pulley material
2. The size of the tendon, tendon graft, or tendon implant around which pulleys are to be built
3. The number of pulleys
4. The location of pulleys

Doyle and Blythe's basic tenets[9] of pulley construction require pulleys to be of strong material, broad and tight fitting, and with firm anchorage. Of the various methods of pulley reconstruction,* we prefer using tendon graft material placed through drill holes in bone or around the phalanx beneath the extensor tendon (Figs. 11-5 to 11-7).

A fact not generally considered in tendon grafting is that when a small diameter graft replaces two normal tendons, an element of bowing within the system occurs, resulting in decreased efficiency (Fig. 11-8). This suggests that, when possible, larger donor grafts should be used.

The same problem arises when pulleys are reconstructed around tendons. It is difficult to construct a pulley tight enough around the tendon to avoid bowing within the system yet loose enough to allow smooth gliding of the tendon and strong enough to withstand the forces applied to it in postoperative finger flexion. Also, a very carefully supervised postoperative regimen of initial passive motion followed by gradual gentle active motion must be instituted. Use of a tendon implant as the first stage in tendon reconstruction allows construction of properly snug pulleys with little risk of rupture. The pulley should be built as tightly as possible, since the final product is generally looser than it was thought to be

---

*References 1, 3, 7, 10, 13, 15, 19, 21, and 22.

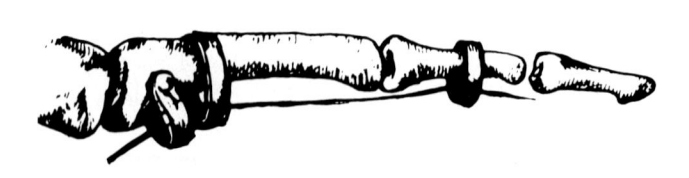

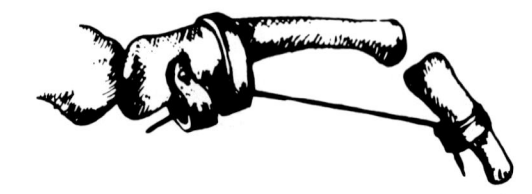

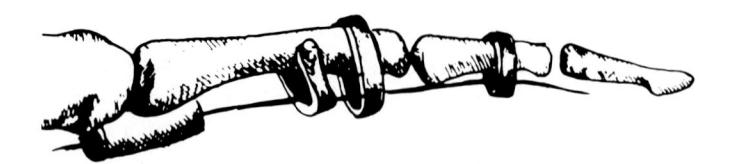

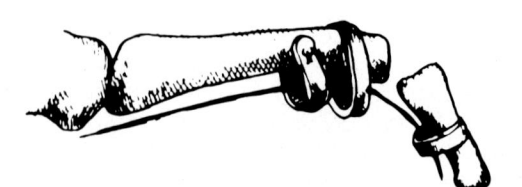

FIG. 11-5. Tendon bowing caused by absent pulley, corrected by placement of new pulley close to joint axis.

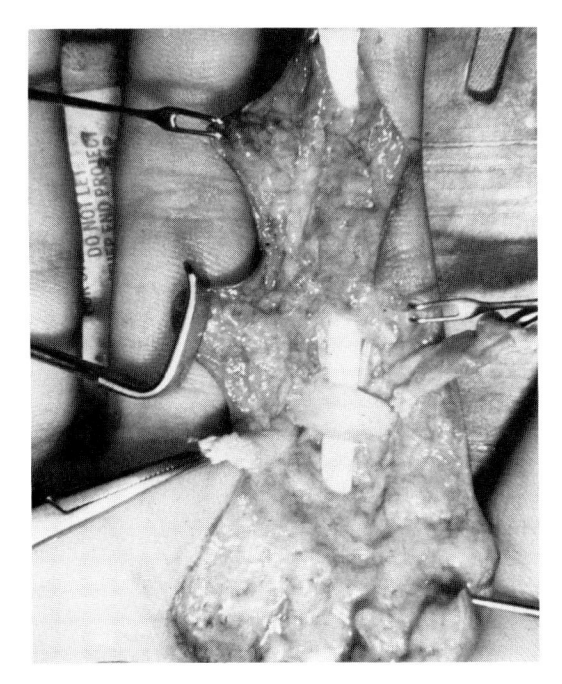

FIG. 11-6. Pulley reconstruction: tendon graft is passed dorsal to proximal phalanx under extensor tendon. Neurovascular bundle is pulled lateral and protected.

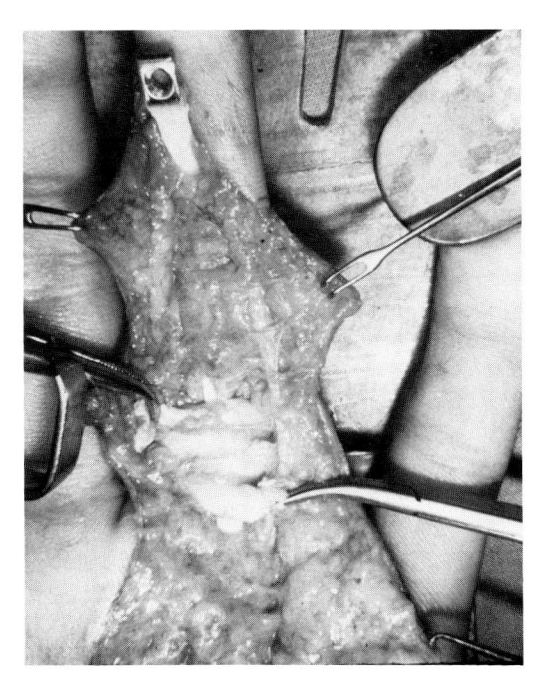

FIG. 11-7. Pulley reconstruction: A_{2a+b} level is made longer and more efficient by wrapping graft wound bone second time.

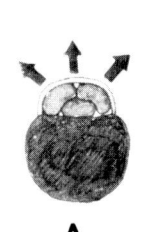

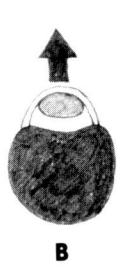

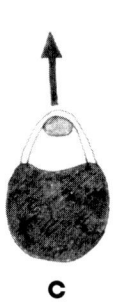

FIG. 11-8. Bowstringing within system. **A,** Two-tendon system with two slips of flexor superficialis and one of flexor profundus. Tendon forces are symmetrically distributed along all sides of pulley. **B,** One-tendon system: with loss of flexor superficialis, profundus bows away from bone in flexion, while tendon force is concentrated at smaller pulley area. **C,** Use of small tendon graft such as plantaris or toe extensor results in further bowing, with deformation of pulley and forces concentrated solely at one point. Attenuation of pulley may result. (See section on problems associated with bowed tendon.)

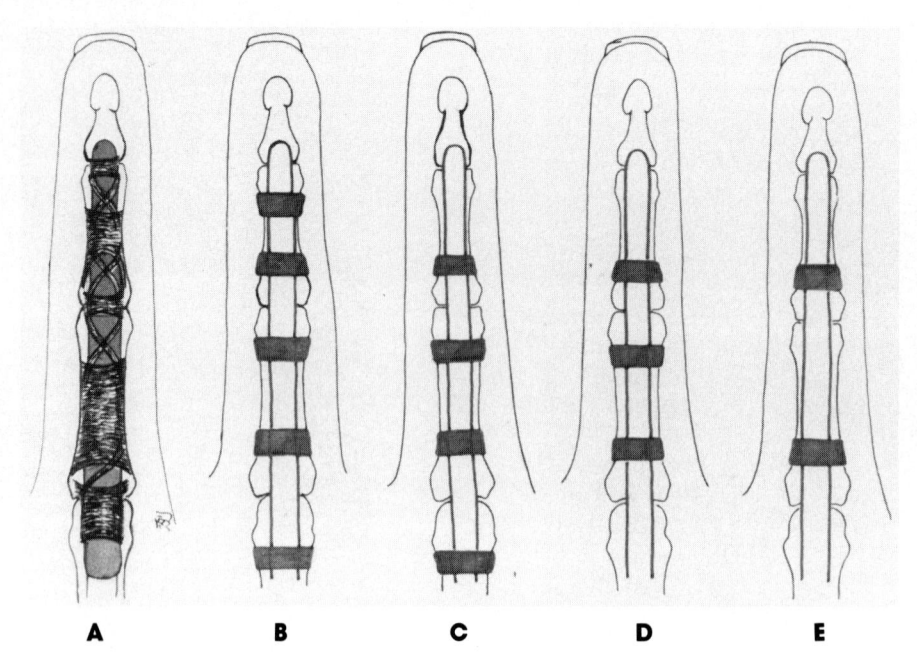

FIG. 11-9. Pulley reconstruction. **A,** Anatomic flexor retinaculum. **B,** Five-pulley reconstructed system, which best approaches ideal. **C** and **D,** Efficient three- and four-pulley systems. **E,** Least efficient two-pulley system. Note key pulleys located at bases of proximal and middle phalanges. Four- and five-pulley systems should be strived for in pulley reconstruction.

at the time of surgery. With general use of relatively small plantar tendons or toe extensors as second-stage grafts, we now use a smaller size stage 1 implant (size 4) when possible to more accurately approximate the size of the future graft.

The number and location of reconstructed pulleys to achieve optimal flexor efficiency have been a matter of controversy.* Based on cadaveric anatomic investigations, we propose that the five-pulley reconstructed system, with proper location of well-built pulleys, best approaches the ideal.[10] As already mentioned, key pulleys are those which diminish bowing and its accompanying hazards by binding the tendon close to the centers of rotation of the joints. Ideally, the pulleys should be placed as close to the distal edge of the joints as possible, i.e., at the bases of the proximal and middle phalanges. However, placement of pulleys close to the proximal aspect of the joints (e.g., closer to the PIP joint than is C_1) results in impingement of the volar plate and collateral ligaments on the pulley and limits motion. Key pulley locations, then, would be A_1, A_{2a}, C_1, A_3, C_2, A_{4b}, and A_5. Reconstruction of tight, broad, strong pulleys at the A_3 and A_5 locations, which would move with the volar plates, is not possible in our hands. We then are left with locations A_1, A_{2a}, C_1, and A_{4b}, which essentially are the pulleys on either side of the three joints, except for distal to the DIP joint. Our five-pulley reconstructed system places one pulley at each of these locations (Fig. 11-9).

In the clinical situation, construction of five pulleys can be difficult and tedious. We would only attempt this sort of reconstruction about a stage 1 tendon implant. When dealing with severely damaged flexor systems, a compromise sometimes is reached. Often a four-pulley system can provide nearly the same results if done properly, and the distal pulley might be eliminated. We would hesitate to use less than four properly placed pulleys.

A distinct improvement was noted at the beginning of this chapter between the two-pulley system and the four-pulley system in the Burmese monkey. Fig. 11-10 shows clinical examples of results achievable in severely damaged flexor systems by adherence to the principles outlined.

SUMMARY

Tendon and pulley problems in the area of the finger flexor retinacular pulley system pose a tremendous chal-

---

*References 2, 4, 7, 11, 16, 17, 20, and 22.

CHAPTER 11 THE PULLEY SYSTEM: RATIONALE FOR RECONSTRUCTION

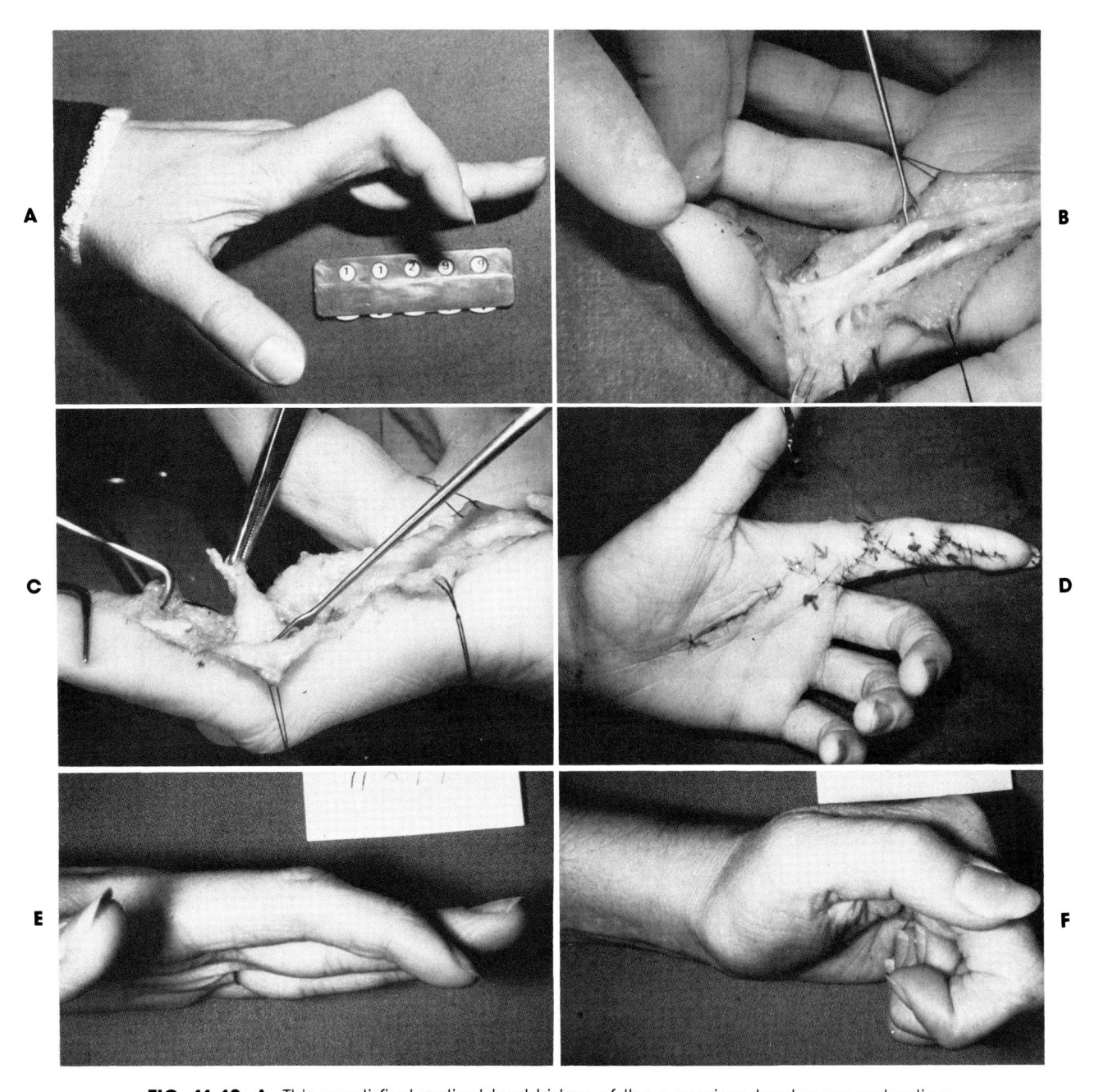

FIG. 11-10. A, This unsatisfied patient had history of three previous tendon reconstructions, resulting in this joint contracture and tendon bowing. **B,** At surgery, expected scarring anterior to PIP joint was noted. **C,** Hypertrophied scar is resected as contracture is released. Proper pulley placement might have prevented this problem. **D,** Skin closure stage 1 flexor tendon reconstruction contracture released, PIP joint pinned, pulleys reconstructed, and multiple V-Y skin shifts made. **E,** Ten months postoperatively, finger is soft, extension lag represents firm soft tissue envelope, and actual joint contracture is 10 degrees. **F,** Ten months postoperatively, final result after pulley reconstruction. Patient has reached her functional potential.

lenge to any surgeon's ability. In striving to achieve optimal results, tendon bowstringing must be minimized. To this end, we conclude that:
1. The major pulleys to be left intact for optimal function are A_1, A_2, A_3, and A_4 in their entirety.
2. In surgical reconstruction the five-pulley system best approaches the ideal, with key pulley placement focused at the bases of the proximal and middle phalanges.

REFERENCES

1. Bader, K.F., Sethi, G., and Curtin, J.W.: Silicone pulleys and underlays in tendon surgery, Plast. Reconstr. Surg. **41**:157, 1968.
2. Barton, N.J.: Experimental study of optimal location of flexor tendon pulleys, Plast. Surg. **43**:125, 1969.
3. Boyes, J.H.: Bunnell's surgery of the hand, ed. 5, Philadelphia, 1970, J.B. Lippincott Co.
4. Boyes, J.H., and Stark, H.H.: Flexor tendon grafts in the fingers and thumb, J. Bone Joint Surg. **53A**:1332, 1971.
5. Brand, P.W., Cranor, K.C., and Ellis, J.C.: Tendon and pulleys at the metacarpophalangeal joint of a finger, J. Bone Joint Surg. **53A**:779, 1975.
6. Bunnell, S.: Repair of tendons in the fingers and description of two new instruments, Surg. Gynecol. Obstet. **26**:103, 1918.
7. Cleveland, M.: Restoration of the digital portion of a flexor tendon and sheath in the hand, J. Joint Surg. **15**:762, 1933.
8. Cook, J.F., and Hunter, J.M.: Unpublished data.
9. Doyle, J.R., and Blythe, W.: The finger flexor tendon sheath and pulleys: anatomy and reconstruction. In American Academy of Orthopaedic Surgeons: Symposium on Tendon Surgery in the Hand, St. Louis, 1975, The C.V. Mosby Co.
10. Hunter, J.M., Cook, J.F., Ochiai, N., Konikoff, J., Merlin, R., and Mackin, G.: The pulley system, J. Hand Surg. **5**:283, 1980.
11. Hunter, J.M., and Salisbury, R.E.: Flexor tendon reconstruction in severely damaged hands, J. Bone Joint Surg. **53A**:829, 1971.
12. Hunter, J.M., Schneider, L.H., Dumont, J., and Erickson, J.C.: A dynamic approach to problems of hand function, Clin. Orthop. **104**:112, 1974.
13. Kleinert, H.E., and Bennett, J.B.: Digital pulley reconstruction employing the always present rim of the previous pulley, J. Hand Surg. **3**:297, 1978.
14. Landsmeer, J.M.F.: Studies in the anatomy of articulation. I. The equilibrium of the intercalated bone, Acta Morphol. Neerl. Scand. **3**:287, 1961.
15. Lister, G.D.: Reconstruction of pulleys employing extensor retinaculum, J. Hand Surg. **4**:461, 1979.
16. Littler, J.W.: Free tendon grafts in secondary flexor tendon repair, Am. J. Surg. **74**:315, 1947.
17. Manske, P.R., and Lesker, P.A.: Strength of human pulleys, Hand **9**:147, 1977.
18. Ochiai, N., Matsui, T., Miyaji, N., et al.: Vascular anatomy of flexor tendons. I. Vincular system and blood supply of the profundus tendon in the digital sheath, J. Hand Surg. **4**:321, 1979.
19. Posch, J.L.: Primary tenorrhaphies and tendon grafting procedures in hand injuries, Arch. Surg. **73**:609, 1956.
20. Rank, B.K., Wakefield, A.R., and Hueston, J.T.: Surgery of repair of applied to hand injuries, ed. 4, Baltimore, 1973, Williams & Wilkins Co.
21. Weckesser, E.: Technique of tendon repair. In Flynn, J.E., editor: Hand surgery, ed. 2, Baltimore, 1975, Williams & Wilkins Co.
22. Wray, R.C., and Weeks, P.M.: Reconstruction of digital pulleys, Plast. Reconstr. Surg. **53**:534, 1974.

SECTION FOUR BONE PROBLEMS

Chapter 12 Scaphoid fractures

Donald C. Ferlic

Much as been written about fractures of the scaphoid, and in reviewing the literature a great number of opinions can be found with regard to etiology, treatment, and results. Russe[4] has pointed out that fractures of the distal third occur in 10% of the cases, the middle third in 70%, and the proximal third in 20%. He has listed the approximate times of union as 6 to 8 weeks in the distal third and middle third and 10 to 12 weeks in the proximal third. He also has related the obliquity of the fracture in the middle third to the healing time, with horizontal oblique and transverse fractures being healed in a shorter period. The vertical oblique fracture has a shearing force that accounts for the delayed healing time of 10 to 12 weeks. Other authors, as well as my experience, have indicated healing times (or at least what is accepted as healing according to x-ray examinations) to be considerably longer than did Russe.

Weber and Chao[8] have demonstrated the mechanism of injury for fractures through the midportion of the scaphoid. They have shown that for the fracture to occur the wrist must be in a position of dorsiflexion from 95 to 100 degrees and that the radial portion of the palm receives the major part of the load. With these forces applied, the scaphoid lies between the radial lip dorsally and the palmar radiocarpal ligament.

BLOOD SUPPLY OF THE SCAPHOID

The blood supply of the scaphoid has been described in the past, but Taleisnik and Kelly,[6] using perfusion techniques, showed three principal vessels supplying the scaphoid. These generally come from the radial artery but occasionally from the superficial volar arch. The principal blood supply was from a lateral volar artery, which was supplemented with a small distal and a small dorsal branch. Their investigation of the intraosseous anatomy confirms the often mentioned fact of distal penetration of the bone by these nutrient arteries, which may result in avascular necrosis of the proximal segment after a fracture of the middle or proximal third of the scaphoid.

DIAGNOSIS

To make the diagnosis of a scaphoid fracture, one must be constantly aware of the possibility of an occult fracture whenever there is tenderness in the anatomic snuff box. Routine x-ray views are taken that consist of an anteroposterior, posteroanterior, lateral, oblique, posteroanterior with the wrist in marked ulnar deviation (which can be seen to open up a fractured scaphoid in many cases), and also a special view (the Stecher view) with the wrist in ulnar deviation, which angles the x-ray tube down the shaft of the first metacarpal. If the x-ray examination does not demonstrate a fracture of the scaphoid, although one is suspicious of this, the wrist is immobilized, and it is radiographically examined again in 10 to 14 days.

MANAGEMENT OF SCAPHOID FRACTURES

In the closed treatment of scaphoid fractures numerous types of immobilization and positions of the wrist are listed in the literature. After a thorough search one can find support for any position, ranging from radial deviation in dorsiflexion to ulnar deviation in palmar flexion. In addition, one can find support for a long-arm cast, a short-arm cast, with the thumb in, or with the thumb out. All the fingers have been left in plaster, and three-finger casts have been used. All authors give support to their findings, and generally their results will be satisfactory in about 90% of the cases. They compare their results with other series that have had fewer good results, but variables exist in each series that cannot be reconciled. The cast that I use has been described by Vichick[7] and is a short-arm cast with the wrist in a neutral position and the thumb abducted. He has shown that the distracting forces are eliminated with the neutral wrist. The palmar abduction of the thumb locks the scaphoid in place, eliminates transmitted motion to the scaphoid from finger motion, and provides compression of the fracture by aligning the long axis of the scaphoid with the shaft of the thumb metacarpal. He has found in 125 consecutive cases that clinical union was achieved in each case at an average of 8.5 weeks of immobilization.

The problem therefore exists of what to do with the displaced fracture, the one with delayed union, the one with established nonunion, or the one with aseptic necrosis. In the old or unrecognized fracture, simple immobilization may be all that is necessary to heal the fracture. Mazet and Hohl[3] have listed criteria that may be used if one contemplates only plaster immobilization in these old ununited fractures. These are (1) absence of arthritis, (2) no sclerosis of the proximal fragment, (3) reasonable approximation of fragments, (4) no avascular changes, and (5) willingness of the patient to wear a cast for an indefinite period. Many authors have demonstrated the healing of fractures with plaster even though the fractures were unrecognized for a number of months. For the accepted nonunion, again one can find many different surgical procedures in the literature with good to satisfactory results reported for each procedure. These include simply drilling the fracture fragments, interpositional arthroplasty, and excision of the radial styloid, proximal fragment, entire scaphoid, or the proximal row. Arthrodesis of either the wrist or an intercarpal arthrodesis, compression screw fixation, implant arthroplasty, and bone grafting are additional alternatives. In my series of scaphoid fractures I have performed most of these procedures for specific indications.

My standard operation for delayed union is bone graft using the volar Russe[4] approach. This has been advocated to best preserve the blood supply of the fracture; also, through the volar approach one is better able to restore the normal contour of the bone, since the fractured scaphoid tends to collapse volarward. In my series and in others this type of bone grafting procedure has resulted in a high rate of union. Although I feel that the radial styloid gives some stability to the scaphoid after bone graft, I will excise it if there are arthritic changes between it and the scaphoid.

Another point of disagreement in bone grafting the scaphoid is the location from which the donor bone should be taken. I have taken local bone from the radius and from the proximal ulna but generally have not been satisfied with this, since it is desirable to have one large segment of bone, and there is difficulty taking this large piece locally. I therefore routinely take the bone graft from the iliac crest. If the fracture is not seen to be stable at the time of surgery, Kirschner wires are used for immobilization, since the postoperative dressing is bulky and gives little support to the fragments.

In the case of nonunion with significant degenerative changes or aseptic necrosis a simple styloidectomy alone has proved to be satisfactory in a few very select cases. Proximal row carpectomy also usually gives a satisfactory but not a normal wrist. Wrist fusion is reserved for an occasional patient with marked arthritic changes or one for whom other methods have failed.

Replacement arthroplasty is rapidly gaining popularity, and Swanson[5] has reported satisfactory use of this procedure. Although good results have been obtained, a number of potential problems exist, and many questions are left unanswered: how long will this procedure give a satisfactory result? What is to be done in case of failure? Another problem is dislocation of the prosthesis, which is the greatest cause of failure of this procedure. One must pay careful attention to the operative technique outlined by Swanson, using pin fixation and ligamentous reconstruction by tendon transfer where necessary. The prosthesis is particularly unstable when a styloidectomy has been done previously. In these cases in which the bony buttress that gives lateral support is missing, replacement arthroplasty should not be done.

The last issue in dealing with a fractured scaphoid is the congenital bipartite scaphoid. Does this exist or not? Numerous reports have appeared in the literature, raising this question. Boyes[1] has enumerated five criteria that give support to the diagnosis of congenital bipartite scaphoid: (1) the absence of a history of trauma, (2) the presence of bilateral scaphoid bipartition, (3) equal size and density of both ossicles, (4) the absence of degenerative changes in the radial scaphoid–carpal articulation, and (5) a clear space between the components with smooth edges at the joint surfaces.

Lewis and associates[2] presented five cases that suggested the presence of a congenital bipartite scaphoid, but after doing microscopic sections of numerous embryologic specimens, they concluded that the bipartite scaphoid is of traumatic origin, and they failed to find evidence to substantiate the possibility of the entity called *congenital bipartite scaphoid.*

REFERENCES

1. Boyes, J.H.: Bunnell's surgery of the hand, ed. 5, Philadelphia, 1970, J.B. Lippincott Co.
2. Lewis, D.S., Calhoun, T.P., Garn, S.M., Carroll, R.E., and Burdi, A.R.: Congenital bipartite scaphoid—fact or fiction? J. Bone Joint Surg. **58A:**1108, 1976.
3. Mazet, R., and Hohl, M.: Fracture of the carpal navicular, J. Bone Joint Surg. **45A:**82, 1963.
4. Russe, O.: Fracture of the carpal navicular, J. Bone Joint Surg. **42A:**759, 1960.
5. Swanson, A.B.: Silicone rubber implants for the replacement of the carpal scaphoid and lunate bones, Orthop. Clin. North Am. **1:**299, 1970.
6. Taleisnik, J., and Kelly, P.J.: The extraosseous and intraosseous blood supply of the scaphoid bone, J. Bone Joint Surg. **48A:**1125, 1966.
7. Vichick, D.A.: Fractures of the carpal scaphoid, Presented at the Annual Meeting of the Western Orthopedic Association, Colorado Springs, Oct. 1977.
8. Weber, E.R., and Chao, E.Y.: An experimental approach to the mechanism of scaphoid waist fractures, J. Hand Surg. **3:**142, 1978.

Chapter 13 Articular fractures: beware of the "unseen" forces

James H. House

This chapter emphasizes the importance of considering the functional anatomy of the joint and the influence of the soft tissues when treating patients with articular fractures. Rational treatment of articular fractures requires an understanding of the dynamic and stabilizing forces acting on each fragment. Radiographs show only the bony elements of these injuries; however, the points of attachment of the important supportive ligaments and the muscle and tendon relationships that significantly contribute to the resulting deformity must be understood when evaluating these injuries. Bennett's fracture is a relatively frequent injury of the thumb, and the importance of accurate anatomic reduction of this fracture-dislocation of the first metacarpal on the trapezium is well known. Isolated fracture-dislocation of the fifth metacarpal–hamate joint is less frequent but an injury that can be easily missed on initial radiographs and, if inadequately treated, may lead to chronic pain and weakness of grasp. Articular fractures of the proximal interphalangeal (PIP) joint are likewise potentially disabling injuries and deserve discussion.

A review of the anatomy of the carpometacarpal (CMC) joints of the first and fifth metacarpals and a comparison of Bennett's fracture of the thumb and fracture-dislocation of the fifth metacarpal–hamate joint emphasize the similarity of these injuries and call attention to the importance of considering the "unseen" soft tissue structures when treating articular fractures.

BENNETT'S FRACTURE: ANATOMY OF INJURY

The CMC joint of the thumb is a saddle joint in which the flexion-extension axis is rotated approximately 90 degrees from the plane of the palm. The base of the first metacarpal is concave in relation to this axis and convex in relation to its lateral plane. The corresponding articular surface of the trapezium is essentially opposite that of the metacarpal with slightly different radii of the "saddle" permitting flexion-extension, adduction-abduction, and limited rotation of the metacarpal at this joint. Rotation about the longitudinal axis of the first metacarpal (15 to 20 degrees) occurs primarily in flexion because of the relative laxity of the capsule in this position. This very mobile joint is dynamically stabilized volarly by the thenar intrinsic muscle group and dorsally by the extrinsic thumb extensors. The thenar muscles provide volar support across the CMC joint because of their origins at the scaphoid, flexor retinaculum, and trapezium with insertion into the thumb and the radial border of the first metacarpal. The *adductor pollicis* muscle, with its oblique head arising from the carpal bones and the transverse head from the shaft of the third metacarpal, inserts on the volar ulnar aspect of the proximal phalanx and into the extensor aponeurosis of the thumb. The *abductor pollicis longus* tendon, which arises from the middle third of the dorsal surface of the ulna, radius, and interosseous membrane and inserts at the radial side of the first metacarpal, is the most important extrinsic tendon influencing the stability of this joint. The most important ligamentous support at the first metacarpal trapezial joint is the *anterior oblique*, or *deep ulnar*, ligament, which extends from the proximal volar aspect of the first metacarpal to the tubercle of the trapezium.

Bennett's fracture occurs when an axial blow is directed against the partially flexed thumb metacarpal, creating a shearing force that results in an articular fracture of the base of the metacarpal (Fig. 13-1). This volar ulnar fragment of the metacarpal remains in place on the trapezium because of the strong anterior oblique ligament. The metacarpal shaft component is pulled dorsally and radially by the abductor pollicis longus, and the adduction force of the adductor pollicis at the ulnar side of the distal metacarpal angulates the metacarpal on the trapezium. The deforming forces of the unopposed abductor pollicis longus and the adductor pollicis, as well as the axial tension of the thenar muscles, make accurate reduction and immobilization of this articular fracture-dislocation very difficult. Reduction can be obtained by axial traction on the thumb with application of direct pressure over the dorsum of the thumb metacarpal while adducting the thumb to relax the tension of the adductor pollicis. Maintenance of the reduction by cast treatment alone is often unsuccessful, and internal fixation is usually indicated to provide stability through fixation of the CMC joint in anatomic alignment. After closed reduc-

SECTION 4 BONE PROBLEMS

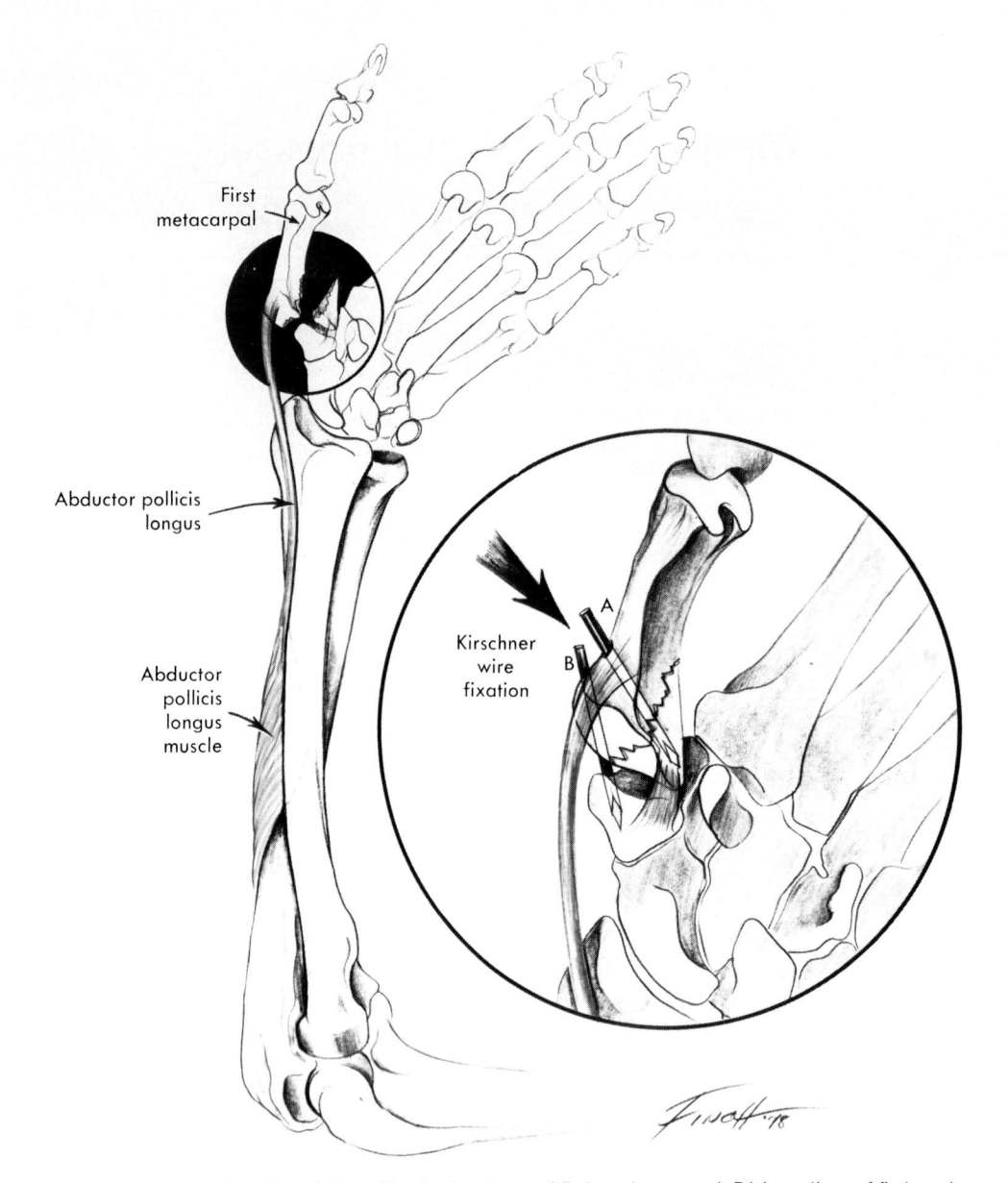

FIG. 13-1. Bennett's fracture: intraarticular fracture of first metacarpal. Dislocation of first metacarpal from trapezium results from unopposed force of abductor pollicis longus tendon. After reduction, a Kirschner wire *(B)* is used to prevent recurrent dislocation. An additional Kirschner wire *(A)* may be used to internally fix articular fracture of base of first metacarpal.

tion, percutaneous fixation of the fracture and/or the CMC joint is usually possible; however, if the reduction is unacceptable, open reduction with direct visualization of the fracture should be performed through a volar radial incision. Continuous traction methods employing a pin through the thumb connected to an outrigger on a cast cause unnecessary stiffness of the metacarpophalangeal (MCP) joint of the thumb. Immobilization should be continued in the cast for 4 to 6 weeks, followed by gentle active range of motion exercises.

FIFTH METACARPAL—HAMATE JOINT FRACTURE: ANATOMY OF INJURY

The hamate–fifth metacarpal joint is also a modified saddle joint, but the base of the fifth metacarpal is *convex* in a volar dorsal plane and slightly concave in a radioulnar plane. It articulates with the ulnar facet of the hamate, which is concave in a dorsal volar plane, allowing flexion and extension through approximately a 30-degree arc of motion. The ulnar facet of the hamate is convex in the radioulnar plane, but fifth metacarpal ab-

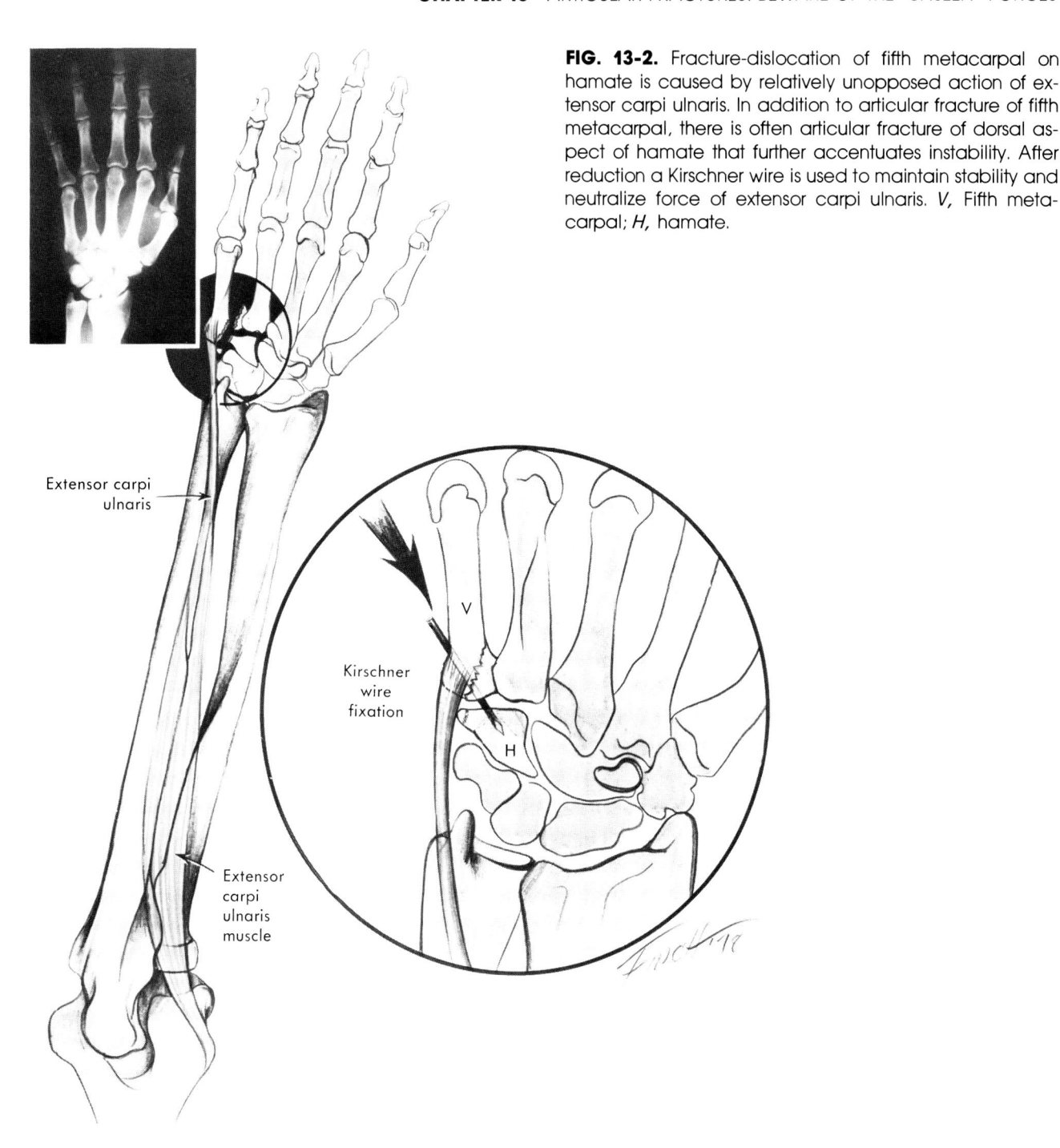

CHAPTER 13 ARTICULAR FRACTURES: BEWARE OF THE "UNSEEN" FORCES

FIG. 13-2. Fracture-dislocation of fifth metacarpal on hamate is caused by relatively unopposed action of extensor carpi ulnaris. In addition to articular fracture of fifth metacarpal, there is often articular fracture of dorsal aspect of hamate that further accentuates instability. After reduction a Kirschner wire is used to maintain stability and neutralize force of extensor carpi ulnaris. *V*, Fifth metacarpal; *H*, hamate.

duction does not occur because of fixation to the fourth metacarpal proximally and the deep transverse metacarpal ligament distally. The radial facet of the hamate articulates with the fourth metacarpal base, which is more limited in flexion-extension because of smaller articular surface contact and ligamentous attachments to the more stable third metacarpal. The radial side of the fifth metacarpal base articulates with the fourth metacarpal, the ulnar aspect serves as the origin of the opponens digiti minimi muscle, and the dorsal ulnar base is the insertion of the extensor carpi ulnaris tendon. Slight rotation about the longitudinal axis of the fifth metacarpal is permitted at the CMC joint, and gliding motion occurs between the fourth and fifth metacarpal bases. These motions allow normal cupping of the palm while grasping and are produced by the hypothenar muscles, which insert on the fifth ray. Further stability of the fifth metacarpal bone in the hand is established by volar and dorsal hamate-metacarpal ligaments, which reinforce the joint capsule, and volarly by the strong pisometacarpal ligament, which is continuous with the insertion of the flexor carpi ulnaris tendon. The intermetacarpal ligaments provide stability between the bases of the fourth and fifth metacarpals adjacent to the articulation.

When the fifth metacarpal–hamate joint is injured by an axial force, an articular fracture may occur, and a volar and radial intraarticular metacarpal fragment often remains articulating with the fourth metacarpal and hamate because of the intermetacarpal and volar ligaments (Fig. 13-2). A dorsal fragment of the hamate also may be sheared off and remain attached to the metacarpal shaft component. The hypothenar muscles and the extensor carpi ulnaris tendon produce deforming forces, resulting in instability. The extensor carpi ulnaris pulls directly at the fifth metacarpal base in a proximal ulnar direction, and the flexion-adduction force of the hypothenar muscles at the distal metacarpal (producing a dorsal ulnar lever at the base) usually prevents stable reduction. Internal fixation of the fifth metacarpal–hamate joint will neutralize the effects of these deforming forces and facilitate treatment.

Proper radiographs require precise positioning so that the articular contours can be visualized. It is particularly difficult to accurately evaluate the articular surfaces of the fifth metacarpal–hamate joint. The usual antero-

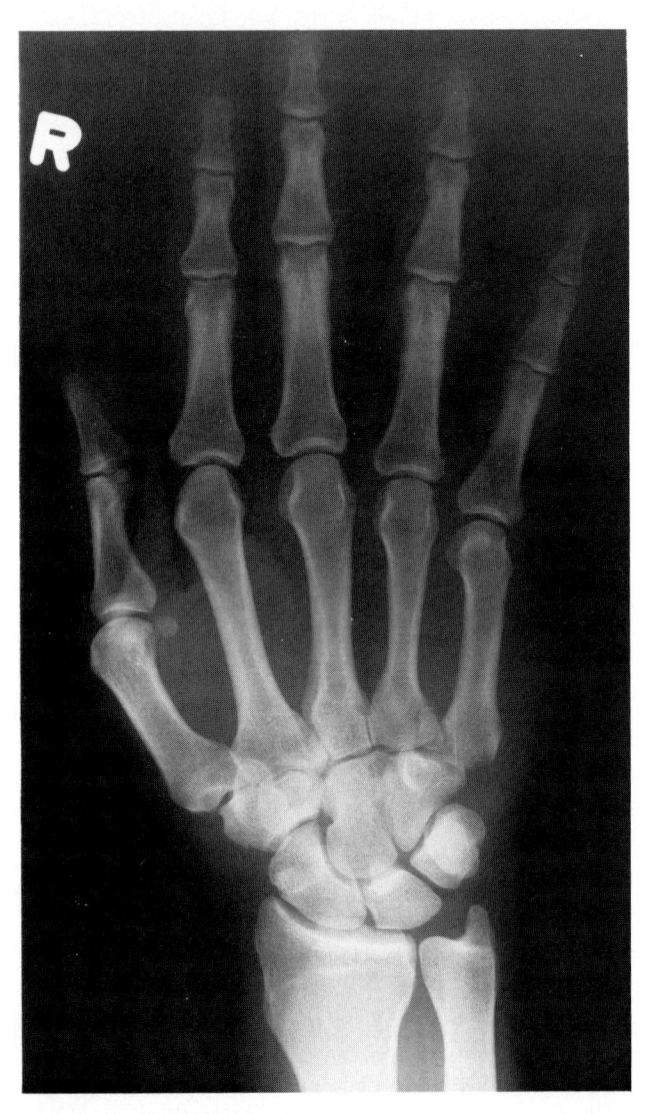

FIG. 13-3. Articular fracture of base of fifth metacarpal is partially concealed by base of fourth metacarpal. Note that there is persistent subluxation of fifth metacarpal on hamate in a dorsal and ulnar direction.

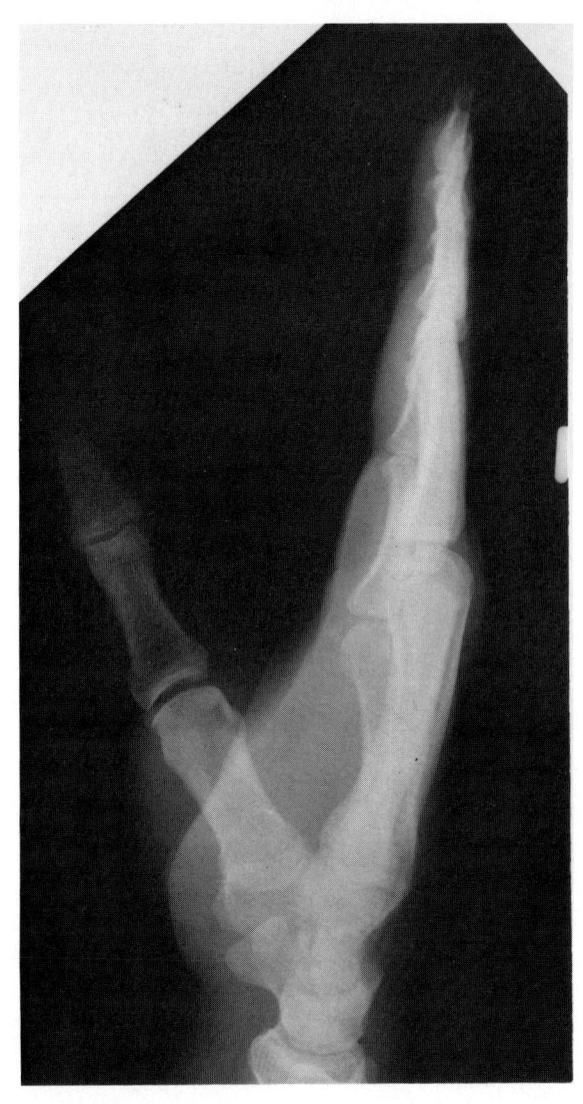

FIG. 13-4. Superimposition of bases of metacarpal prevents direct visualization of fifth metacarpal–hamate joint on lateral view; however, palmar angulation of distal portion of fifth metacaral is important radiographic clue to this injury.

CHAPTER 13 ARTICULAR FRACTURES: BEWARE OF THE "UNSEEN" FORCES

posterior and lateral x-ray views are inadequate because of superimposition of the other metacarpals on the lateral view and some normal apparent overlap of the hamate and fifth metacarpal on most anteroposterior views. If the hand is pronated approximately 30 degrees more than in the usual palm-down anteroposterior x-ray position, and if the beam is directed perpendicular to the joint, the surfaces usually can be well visualized[1] (Fig. 13-3).

Observe the position of the fifth metacarpal shaft relative to the other metacarpals on a true lateral view when this injury is suspected (Fig. 13-4). Apparent flexion of the fifth metacarpal may be caused by the dorsal ulnar dislocation of the base with resulting angulation of the shaft by the pull of the hypothenar intrinsic muscles. Tomograms may be taken to further clarify the nature of the articular fracture and to confirm adequate reduction.

DISCUSSION

Proper treatment of all articular fractures requires a careful assessment of the structural injury to the joint as well as a consideration of the dynamic and stabilizing forces of the muscles, tendons, and ligaments related to that joint.

Since many articular fractures occur in association with dislocation at the time of injury, the radiograph may not indicate the degree of displacement that occurred. The dislocation often reduces spontaneously or is reduced by the patient, a coach, or a bystander before the radiograph is taken. These factors have been presented in considerable detail with respect to Bennett's fracture and fifth metacarpal–hamate joint injuries.

Similar consideration must be given to the relatively common fracture of the PIP joint of the finger (Fig. 13-5), an injury that is often improperly treated, resulting in

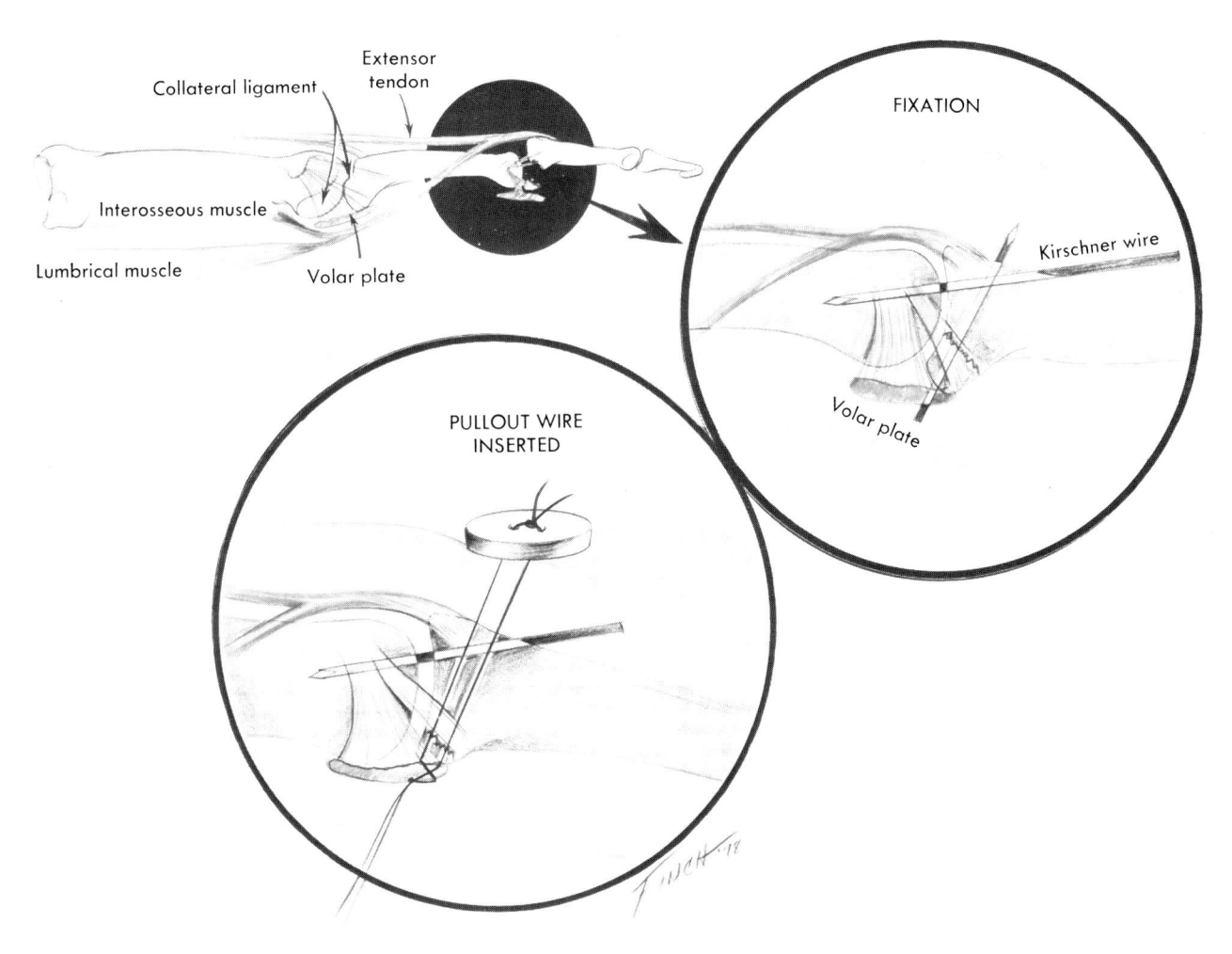

FIG. 13-5. Articular fracture involving volar aspect of base of middle phalanx often renders PIP joint unstable because majority of collateral ligament and volar plate attaches to this small fragment. In extension, pull of central slip of extensor mechanism causes dorsal dislocation of middle phalanx. It is often necessary to use Kirschner wire to prevent dislocation and either pullout suture or Kirschner wire to internally fix articular fragment.

SECTION 4 BONE PROBLEMS

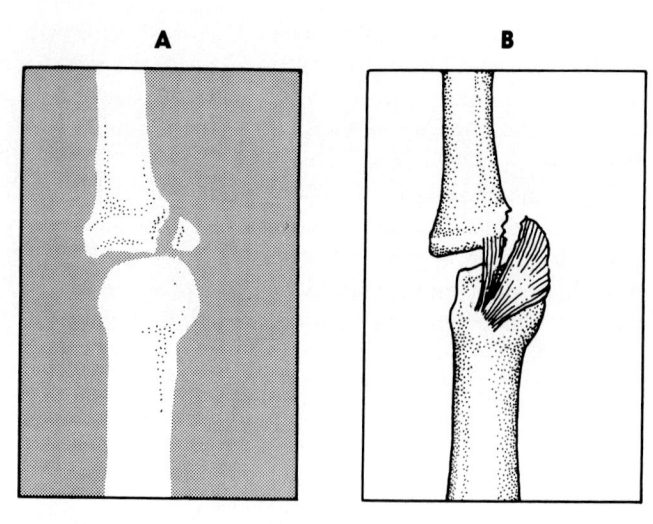

FIG. 13-6. Sketch emphasizes that relatively small bone fragment seen on radiograph is actually primary attachment of collateral ligaments and volar plate. **A,** X-ray appearance. **B,** Ligament attachments.

chronic dorsal subluxation, limited range of motion, and painful posttraumatic arthritis. The anteroposterior radiograph may appear to be normal, and the lateral radiograph may suggest that a very simple fracture has occurred when only a relatively small fragment of bone is observed to have been fractured from the volar aspect of the base of the middle phalanx (Fig. 13-6). This fragment, however, is the major attachment of the collateral ligaments and the volar plate and may render the joint grossly or potentially unstable, depending on the size of the fragment. When this fragment involves more than 30% of the articular surface, the dorsal articular component, along with the remainder of the middle phalanx, is likely to sublux dorsally because of the pull of the central slip of the extensor mechanism as the middle phalanx goes into extension. For fragments that are up to 30% of the articular surface, extension-block splinting (Fig. 13-7) is usually successful; when larger articular fractures are present, open reduction and internal fixation with precise restoration of the articular surface are indicated. Supplemental pin fixation of the PIP joint to

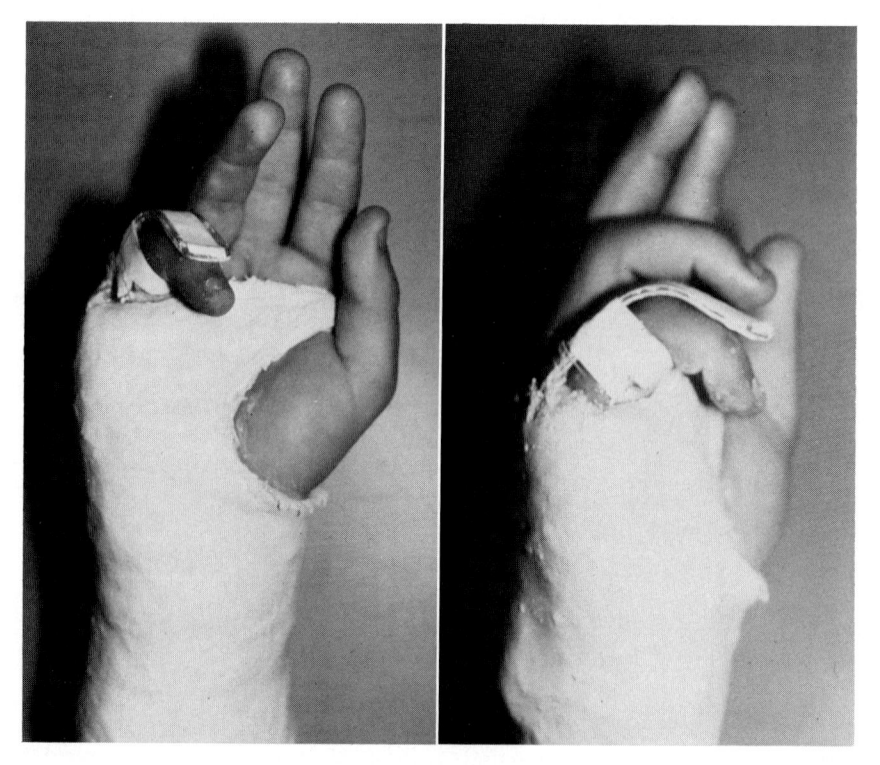

FIG. 13-7. Extension-block splint: double thickness aluminum splint, incorporated into short-arm cast, is used to prevent dislocation. This technique also allows relatively early active flexion, minimizing problems of joint stiffness.

prevent dorsal dislocation may be temporarily employed if significant dorsal subluxation instability exists. Internal fixation may be supplemented by extension-block splinting to allow early motion and prevent subluxation as the joint is extended.

It is not the purpose of this chapter to discuss all articular fractures or to present all treatment modalities for those fractures discussed but rather to reiterate the importance of considering the "unseen" soft tissues when evaluating all fractures and dislocations, particularly those involving the articular surface.

SUMMARY

Articular fractures often are associated with dislocation of the joint at the time of injury. Awareness of this fact and careful consideration of the soft tissue structures contributing to the dynamic and structural stability of each joint are essential. There is a striking similarity between the well-known Bennett fracture and the often undiagnosed fifth metacarpal–hamate joint fracture, which emphasizes these points. Even slightly displaced fifth metacarpal fractures may produce an articular incongruity that predisposes the patient to chronic pain with traumatic arthritis, loss of motion, and weakness of grip. Precise anatomic reduction with internal fixation either percutaneously or by surgical exposure gives the best prognosis in these potentially disabling injuries. Careful consideration of the functional anatomy as it relates to the x-ray projection of the skeleton is essential to understanding these injuries and allows a rational and flexible concept for the treatment of these common problems.

REFERENCE

1. Bora, W.F., and Didizian, N.H.: The treatment of injuries to the carpometacarpal joint of the little finger, J. Bone Joint Surg. **56A**:1459, 1974.

SELECTED READINGS

Agee, J.M.: Unstable fracture dislocations of the proximal interphalangeal joint of the fingers: a preliminary report of a new treatment technique, J. Hand Surg. **3**:386, 1978.

Boyes, J.H.: Bunnell's surgery of the hand, ed. 5, Philadelphia, 1970, J.B. Lippincott Co.

Eaton, R.G.: Joint injuries of the hand, Springfield, Ill., 1971, Charles C Thomas, Publisher.

Hsu, J.D., and Curtiss, R.M.: Carpometacarpal dislocations on the ulnar side of the hand, J. Bone Joint Surg. **52A**:927, 1970.

Ker, H.R.: Dislocation of the fifth carpometacarpal joint, J. Bone Joint Surg. **37B**:254, 1955.

McElfresh, E.C., Dobyns, J.H., and O'Brien, E.T.: Management of fracture-dislocation of the proximal interphalangeal joints by extension-block splinting, J. Bone Joint Surg. **54A**:1705, 1972.

Robertson, R.C., Cowley, J.J., and Faris, A.M.: Treatment of fracture-dislocation of the interphalangeal joints of the hand, J. Bone Joint Surg. **28**:68, 1946.

Waugh, R.L., and Yancey, A.G.: Carpometacarpal dislocations, J. Bone Joint Surg. **30A**:397, 1978.

Wilson, J.N., and Rowland, S.A.: Fracture-dislocations of the proximal interphalangeal joint of the finger, J. Bone Joint Surg. **48A**:293, 1966.

Chapter 14 Complex fractures of the finger metacarpals

James L. Becton

The metacarpal bones, which are the proximal portion of the digital ray, are arranged in a configuration such that they form arches in both longitudinal and transverse directions. The marginal metacarpal bones of the thumb and little finger are quite mobile, with 90 degrees of motion for the thumb and 40 degrees of motion for the little finger at their respective carpometacarpal (CMC) joints. However, the index and long finger metacarpals are stable at their CMC joints. Injuries to the hand that result in fractures of the metacarpals often involve the mobile metacarpals of the thumb and little finger.

It is the purpose of this chapter to present cases of fractures of the finger metacarpals, which are less common but often complex. A method of treatment for each is suggested.

CHAPTER 14 COMPLEX FRACTURES OF THE FINGER METACARPALS

FRACTURE-DISLOCATION OF INDEX METACARPOPHALANGEAL (MCP) JOINT
Case 1

A 10-year-old boy was playing football and sustained an injury to his hand. A roentgenogram of the hand showed a dislocation of the index MCP joint with a fracture of the metacarpal head. The suggested treatment was open reduction of the dislocation by a dorsal approach and Kirschner wire fixation of the fracture of the metacarpal head (Fig. 14-1).

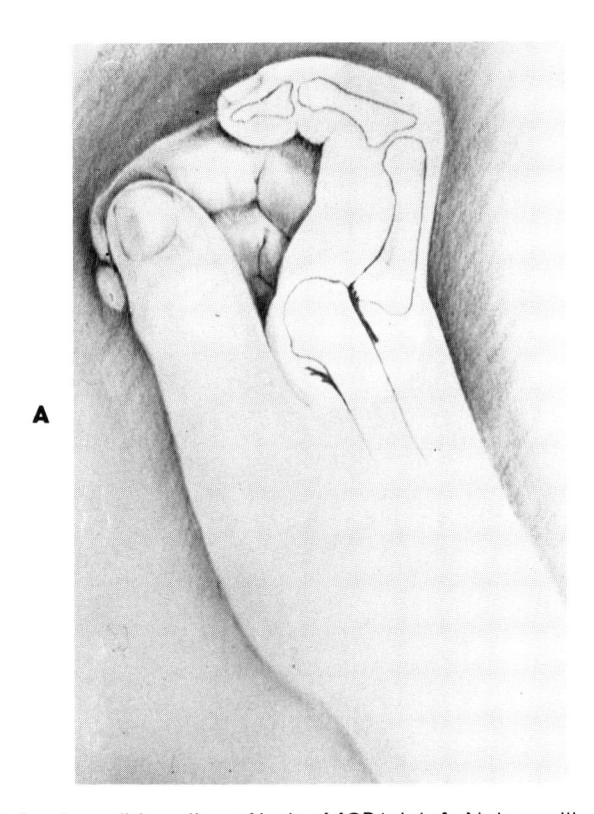

FIG. 14-1. Case 1: fracture-dislocation of index MCP joint. **A,** Note position of finger in hyperextension at MCP joint. Volar plate is trapped behind metacarpal head.

Continued.

B

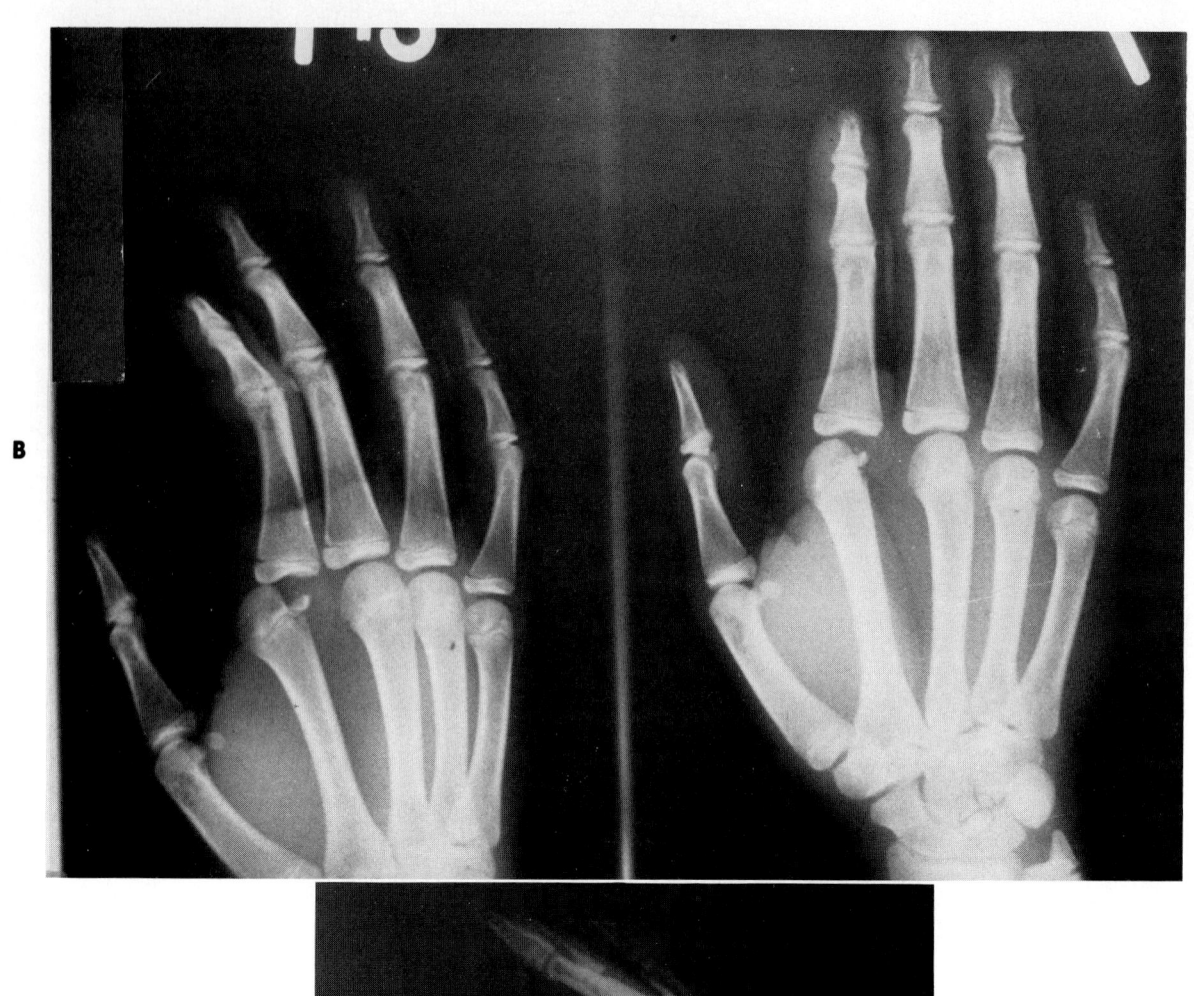

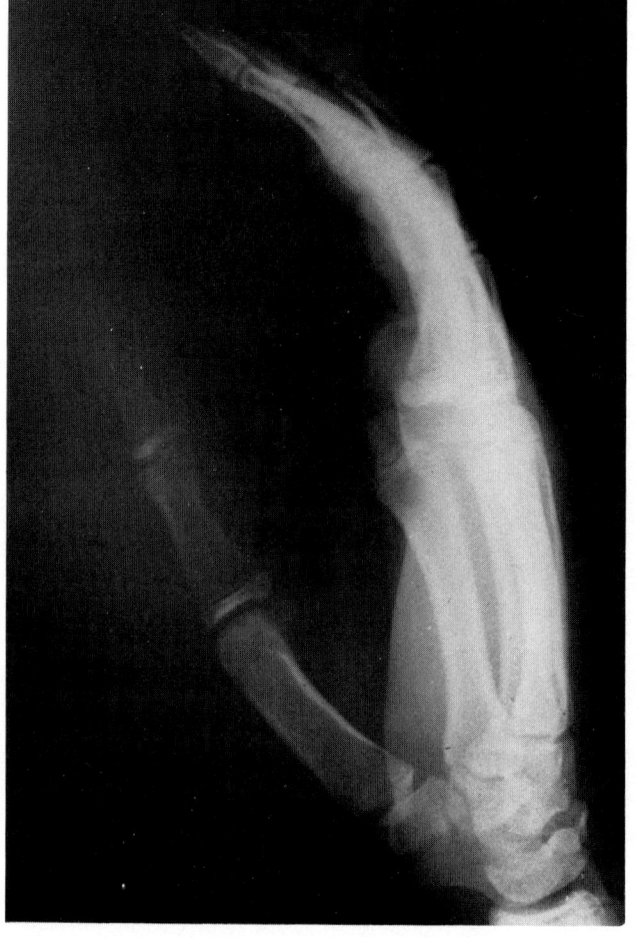

C

FIG. 14-1, cont'd. For legend see opposite page.

CHAPTER 14 COMPLEX FRACTURES OF THE FINGER METACARPALS

Discussion

At the time of this dislocation the volar plate becomes trapped dorsal to the metacarpal head and is the main structure blocking reduction. At the same time the lumbrical muscle comes to lie on the radial side of the metacarpal neck, and the profundus and sublimis tendons lie on the ulnar side of the metacarpal neck. The transverse fibers of the parlmar fascia form a sling around the volar side of the metacarpal neck. However, the volar plate is the primary structure blocking reduction, and once this is released and brought over the metacarpal head, the other structures easily clear the metacarpal head.

Closed reduction is usually unsuccessful, and open reduction is required. The dislocated joint can be approached by either a volar or dorsal approach. The advantages of using a dorsal longitudinal approach for exposure is that the volar plate can be visualized and incised and the entrapped metacarpal head reduced. The fracture of the metacarpal head is in full view and can be reduced and fixed with a Kirschner wire. The digital nerve from the radial side of the index finger is stretched over the volar surface of the metacarpal head and lies just beneath the skin. It can be lacerated easily when making a volar incision. A volar approach alone does not allow visualization of the metacarpal head once the joint is reduced, and the fracture cannot be reduced and fixed. Therefore I would suggest using a dorsal approach for open reduction of the fracture-dislocation of the index metacarpal head.

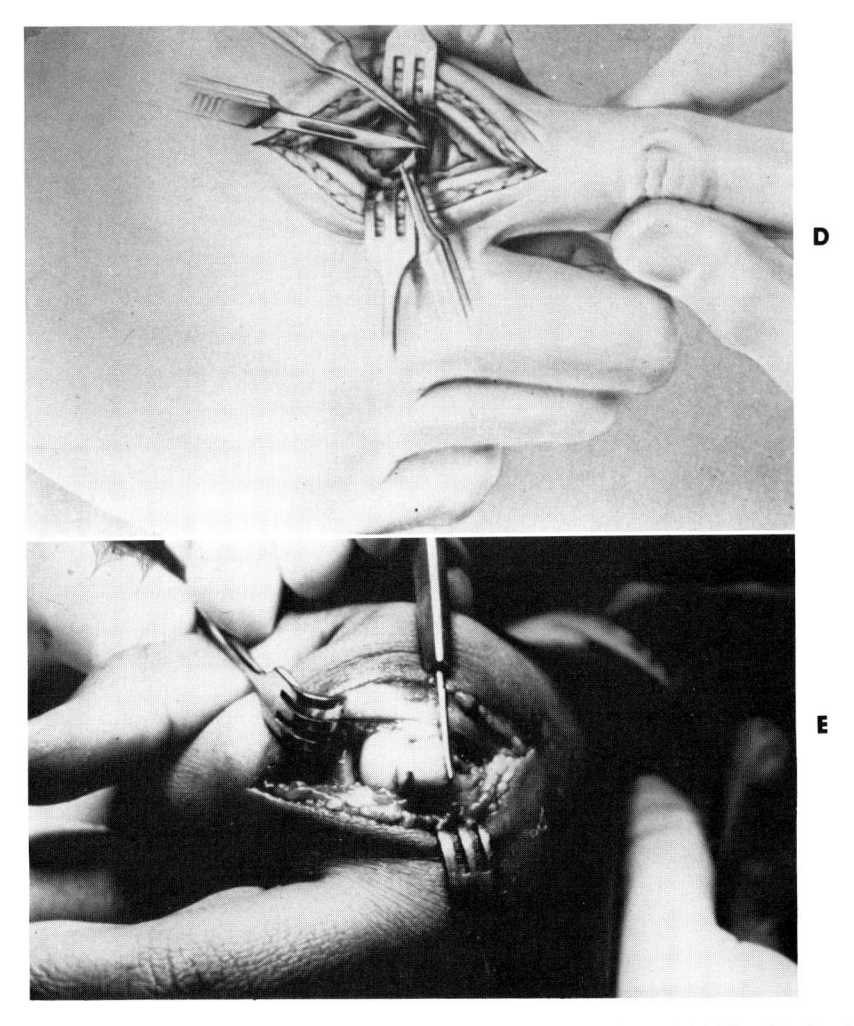

FIG. 14-1, cont'd. B and **C,** X-ray views show fracture-dislocation of MCP joint. **D,** Dorsal approach for MCP joint dislocation. Volar plate is incised longitudinally, and joint reduces easily. **E,** Fractured metacarpal head is well exposed for Kirschner wire fixation.

SECTION 4 BONE PROBLEMS

DISPLACED METACARPAL FRACTURE WITHOUT DISLOCATION
Case 2

A 19-year-old man was working with a meat grinder and sustained an injury to his hand. A roentgenogram showed a fracture of the metacarpal at the neck level with 180 degrees of rotation so that the articular surface was in opposition with the fractured end of the proximal portion of the metacarpal. This was a closed injury (Fig. 14-2). The suggested treatment was open reduction and fixation of the metacarpal head in an anatomic position.

Discussion

Any fracture that involves a joint should be reduced to an anatomic position for healing and restoration of joint motion. The fracture of the metacarpal head can be exposed through a dorsal longitudinal incision and the metacarpal head fixed with Kirschner wires.

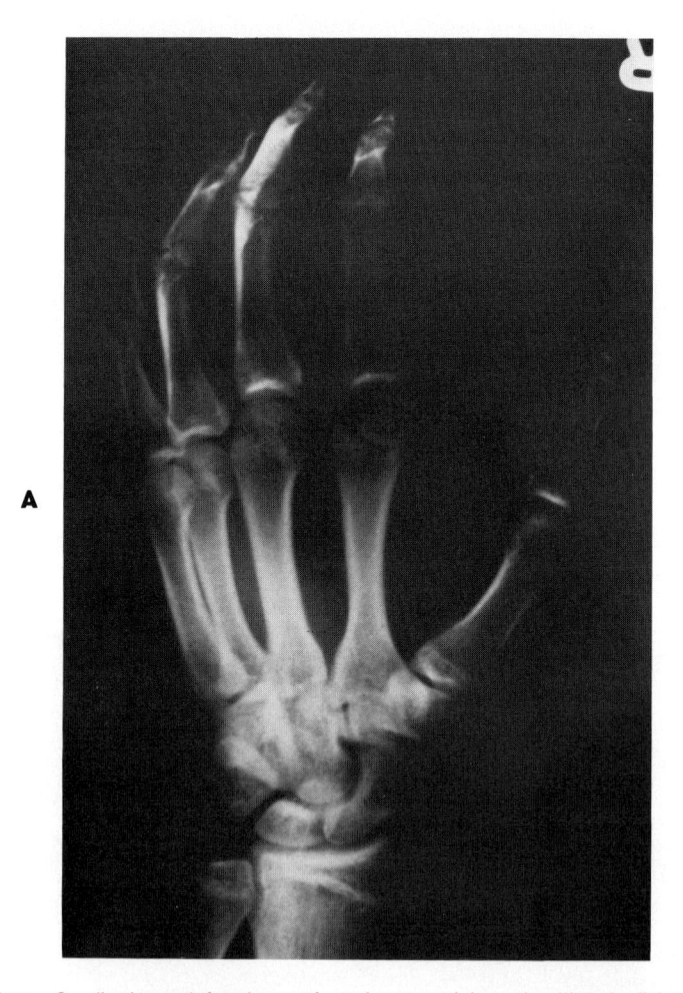

FIG. 14-2. Case 2: displaced fracture of metacarpal head without dislocation. **A,** Initial roentgenogram of fracture of metacarpal head. **B,** After reduction with Kirschner wire fixation.

CHAPTER 14 COMPLEX FRACTURES OF THE FINGER METACARPALS

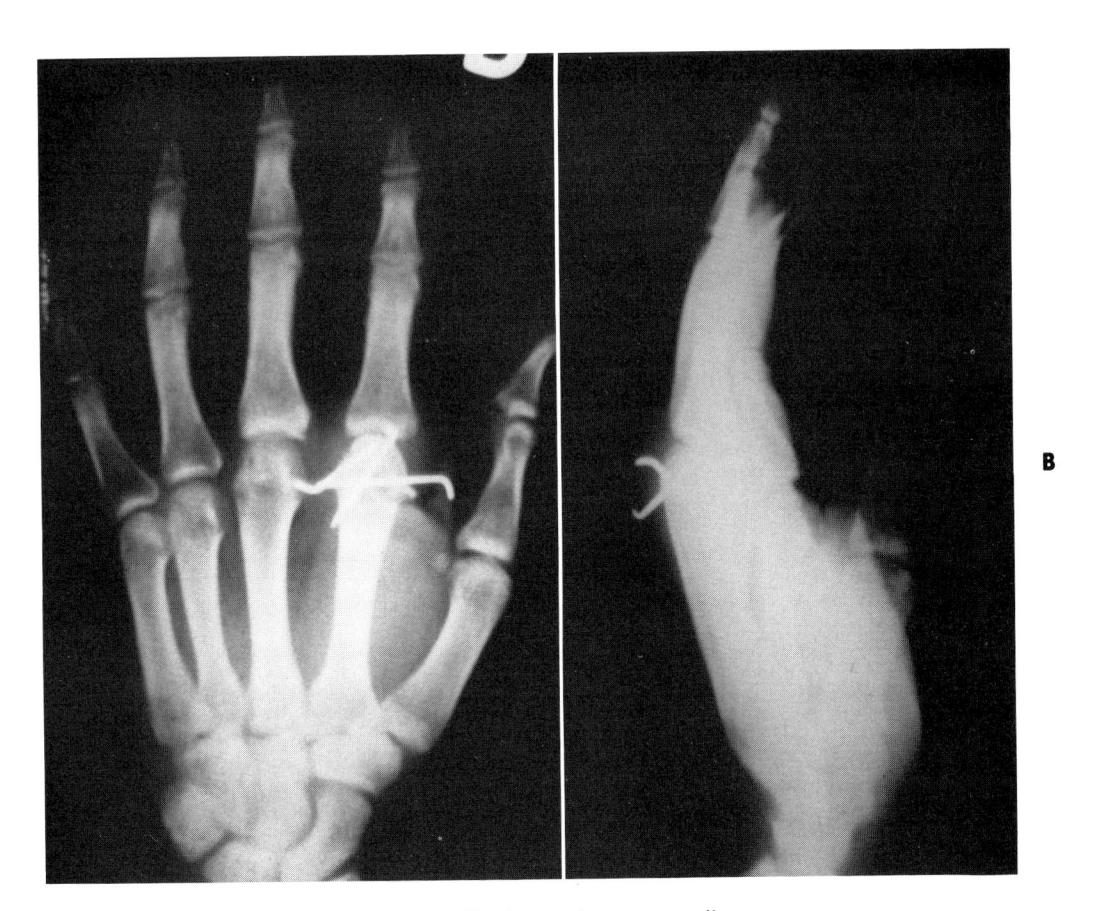

FIG. 14-2, cont'd. For legend see opposite page.

119

SECTION 4 BONE PROBLEMS

DISPLACED FRACTURE OF METACARPAL EPIPHYSIS
Case 3

An 11-year-old boy was playing ball and fell. He injured his right hand. A roentgenogram showed a fracture of the epiphysis of the index metacarpal with complete displacement (Fig. 14-3). The suggested treatment was closed reduction and cast immobilization.

Discussion

Displaced epiphyseal fractures of the metacarpal should be reduced to an anatomic position if possible. They usually can be held in a short-arm cast. However, it is important to check the position of the fracture by a roentgenogram each week for 3 weeks to check for any redisplacement. Proper rotation of the fingers and metacarpal head should be maintained. Further growth may correct an angulation deformity but will not correct a rotation deformity.

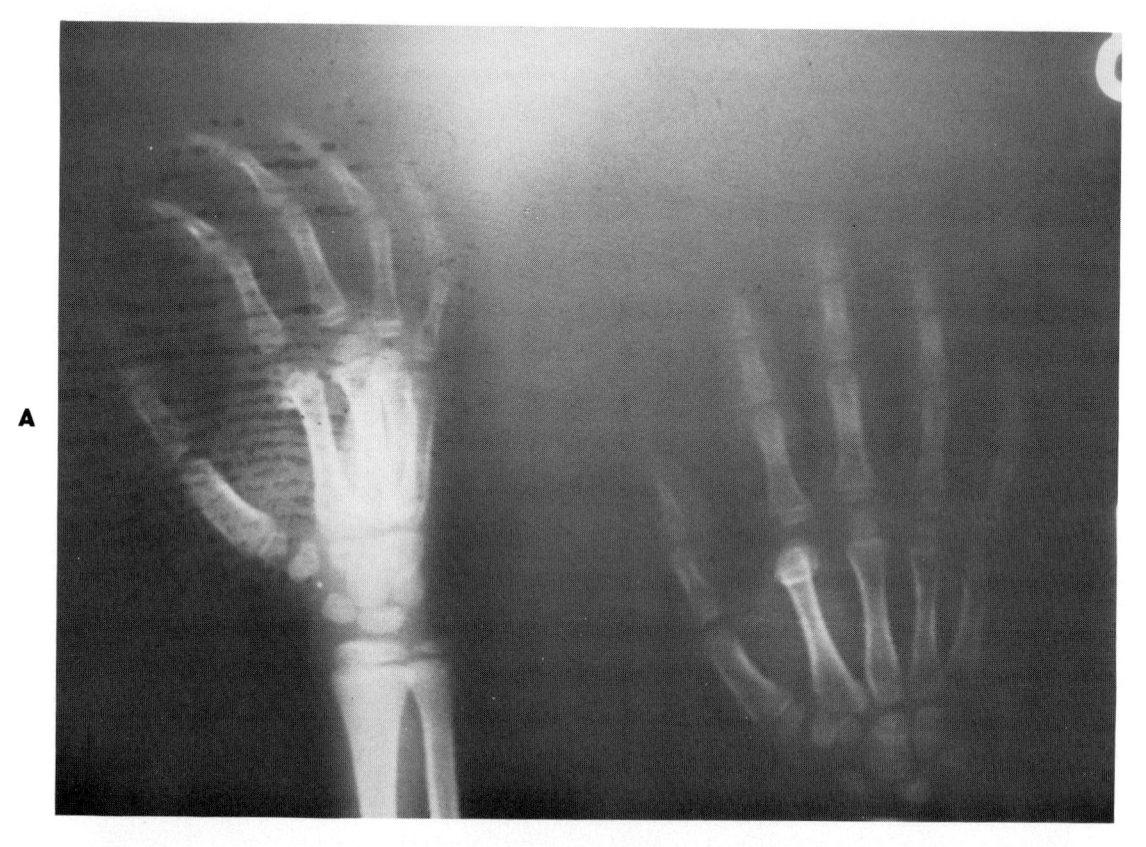

FIG. 14-3. Case 3: **A,** Initial roentgenogram of fracture of metacarpal epiphysis with volar displacement of metacarpal head. **B,** Roentgenogram of reduced epiphyseal fracture of metacarpal in cast.

CHAPTER 14 COMPLEX FRACTURES OF THE FINGER METACARPALS

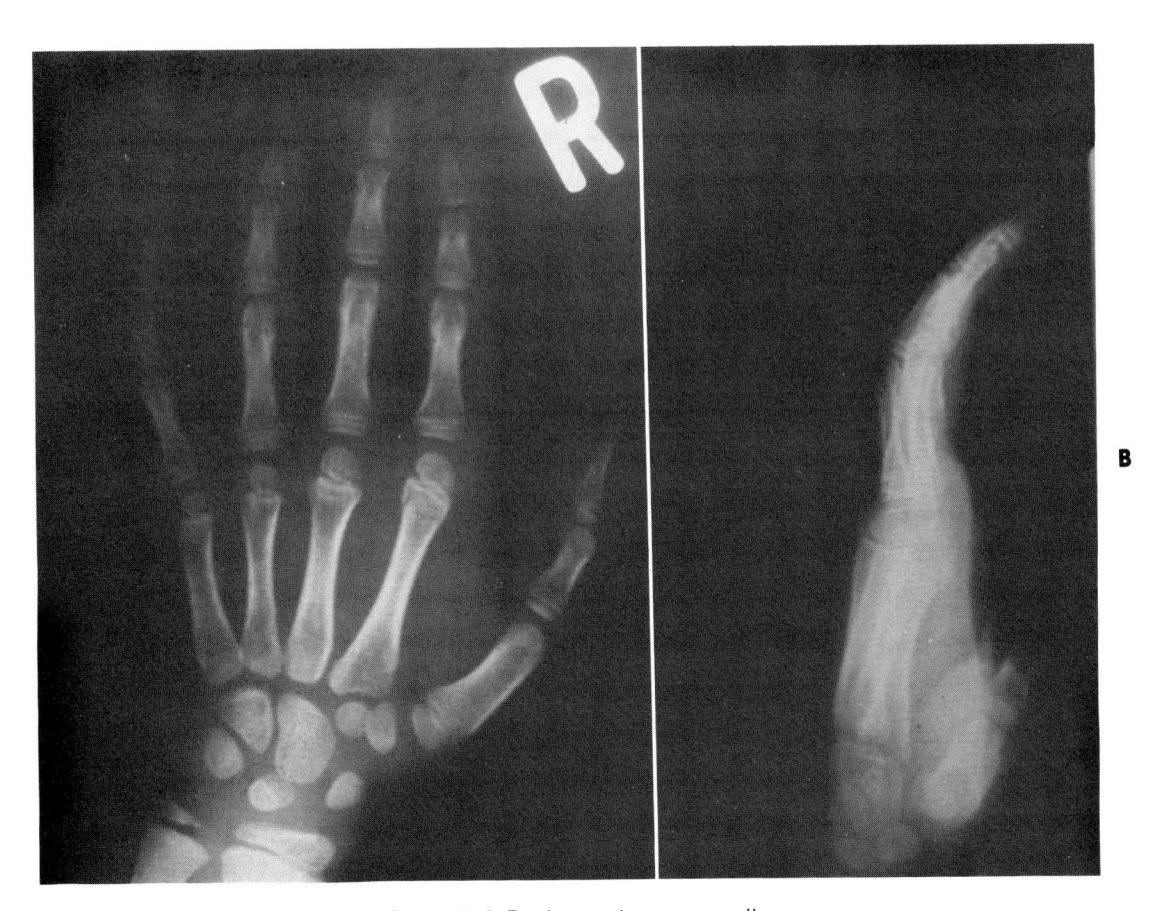

FIG. 14-3, cont'd. For legend see opposite page.

SECTION 4 BONE PROBLEMS

FRACTURE OF FIFTH METACARPAL NECK (BOXER'S FRACTURE)
Case 4

An angry young man hit a wall with his fist. The hand was swollen and tender over the metacarpal of the little finger. The knuckle was depressed. A roentgenogram of the hand showed a fracture of the fifth metacarpal neck with dorsal angulation (boxer's fracture) (Fig. 14-4). The suggested treatment was closed reduction and cast immobilization.

Discussion

The angulated fracture of the fifth metacarpal neck—so-called boxer's fracture—most often can be managed by closed reduction and immobilization in a short-arm cast. The plaster is well molded about the volar surface of the metacarpal head. Up to 40 degrees of angulation of the fifth metacarpal is an acceptable reduction for good

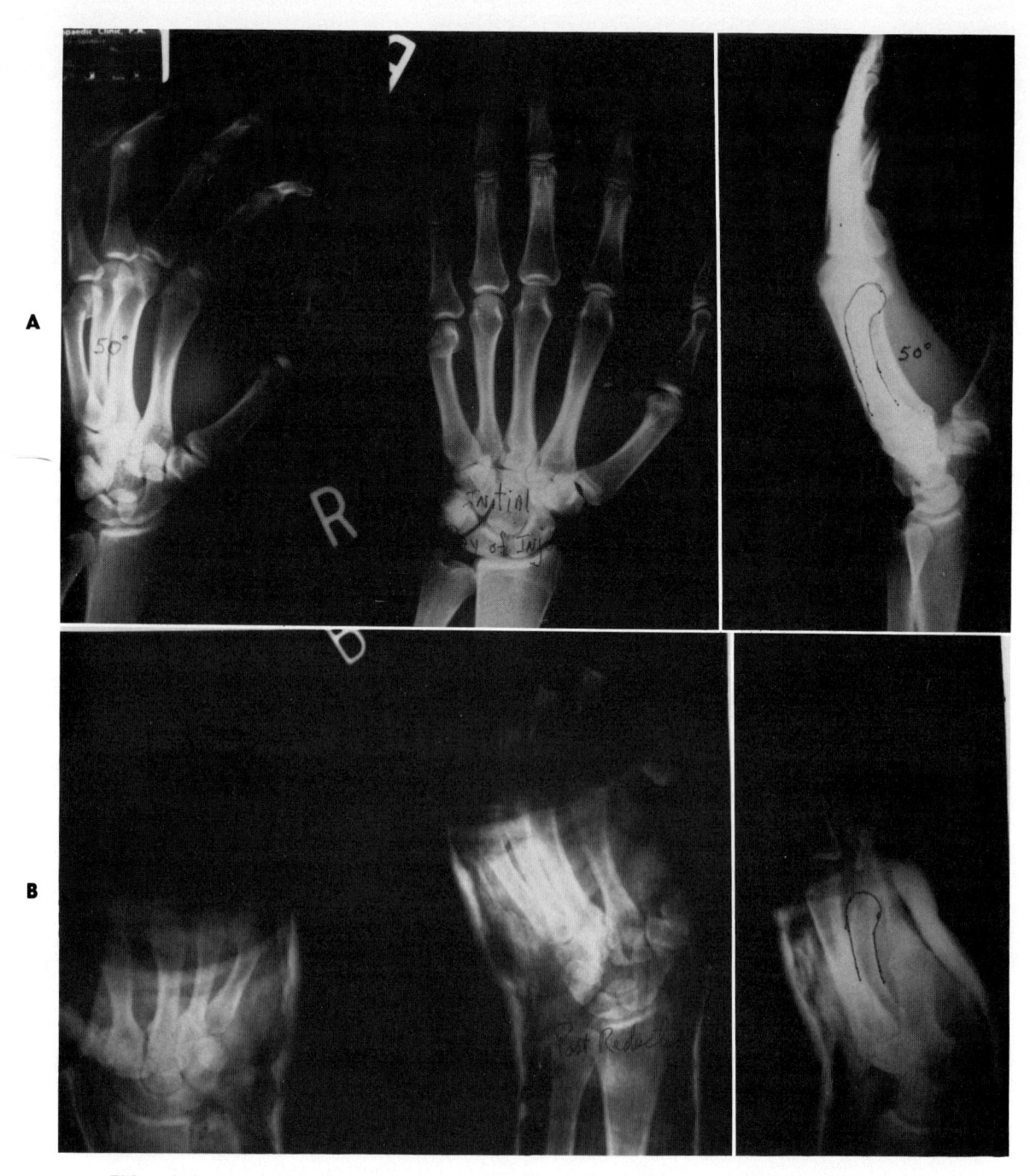

FIG. 14-4. Case 4: roentgenograms showing fracture of fifth meacarpal neck with dorsal angulation of 50 degrees. **(A)**, fracture of fifth metacarpal neck after closed reduction and cast application **(B)**.

CHAPTER 14 COMPLEX FRACTURES OF THE FINGER METACARPALS

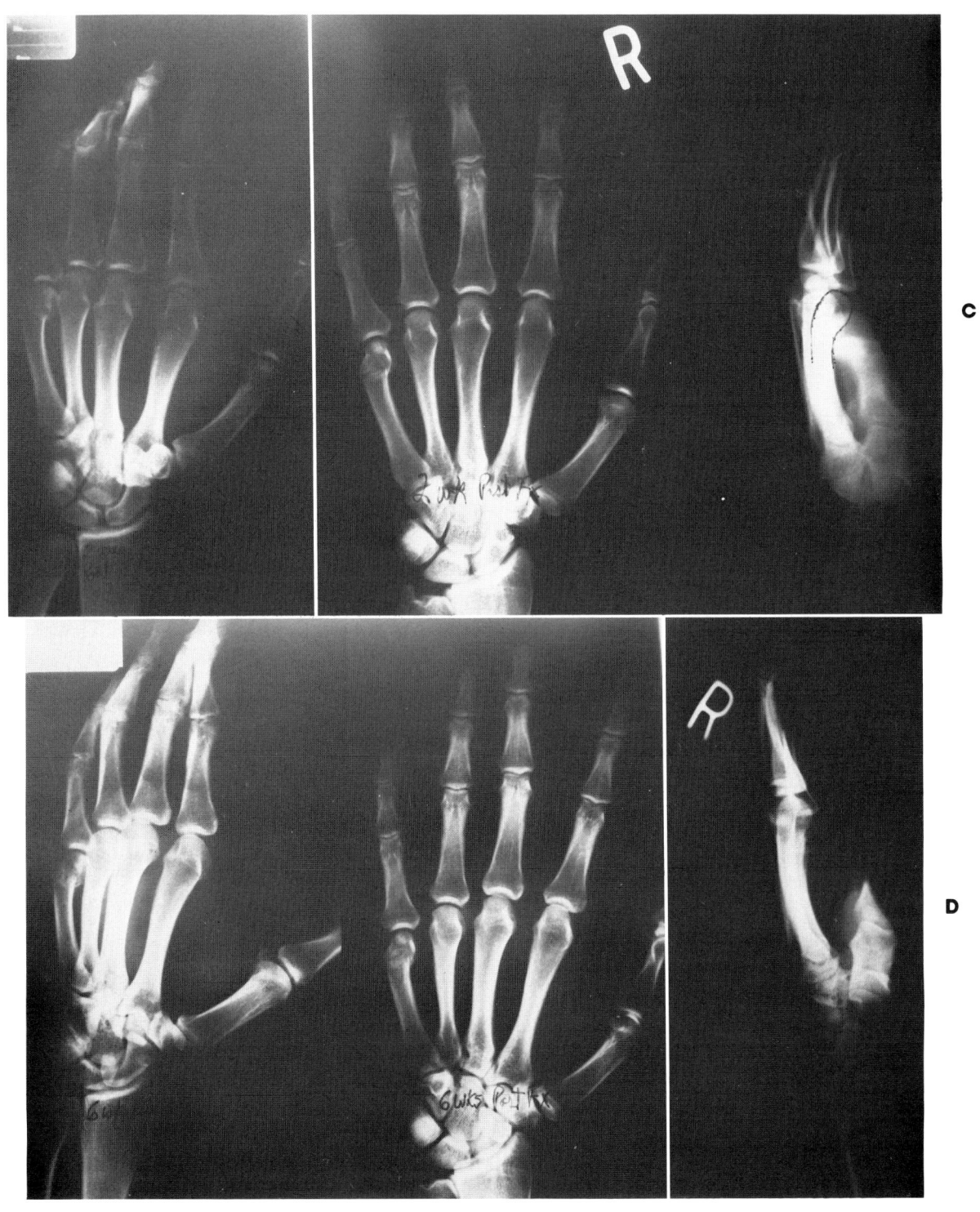

FIG. 14-4, cont'd. Fracture of fifth metacarpal neck, 2 weeks after reduction, with 25 degrees of angulation **(C)**, and fracture of fifth metacarpal neck, 6 weeks after reduction, with 25 degrees of angulation **(D)**.

SECTION 4 BONE PROBLEMS

hand function. It is important to recheck the position by radiographs, and if the angulation cannot be corrected and maintained to less than 40 degrees of dorsal angulation, then reduction and Kirschner wire fixation should be considered. Proper rotation of the finger is important at the time of reduction. The hand is held in a cast with the fingers held in flexion. At the end of 10 days of cast immobilization the cast should be removed, and active flexion and extension of the fingers should be observed for any rotation deformity. If a deformity results in overlapping of the fingers, then remanipulation or open reduction should be considered. Pure dorsal angulation of a metacarpal fracture of less than 40 degrees of or slight shortening is compatible with good hand function. However, a rotation deformity results in overlapping of digits.

DISPLACED FRACTURE OF METACARPAL SHAFT
Case 5

A 22-year-old man was working in an industry, and his hand was crushed between two pipes. Roentgenograms showed a displaced transverse fracture of the midshaft of the fifth metacarpal (Fig. 14-5). The suggested treatment was open reduction and intramedullary Kirschner wire fixation of the metacarpal fracture.

Discussion

A displaced fracture of the midshaft of the metacarpal usually requires open reduction and can be fixed by an intramedullary Kirschner wire. If the fractures are not reduced and fixed, then the arch configuration of the hand is lost, and the finger of the fractured metacarpal may rotate or angulate, resulting in overlapping of the fingers when making a fist.

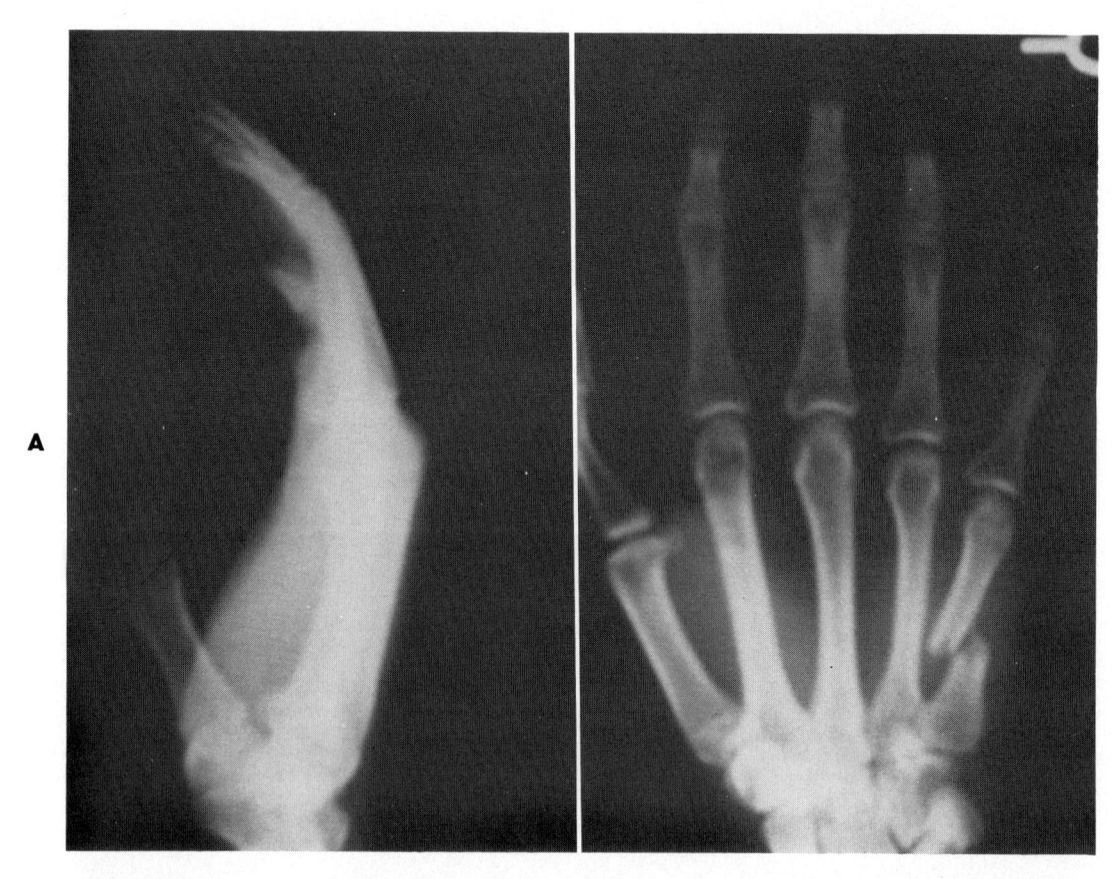

FIG. 14-5. Case 5: roentgenograms of displaced fracture of metacarpal shaft **(A)** and after open reduction and intramedullary Kirschner wire fixation.

Metacarpal shaft fractures, either oblique or transverse, that have minimal or no displacement or angulation may be treated by cast immobilization alone for 6 weeks, with good results.

CONCLUSION

A group of cases showing complex fractures of the finger metacarpal bones is presented here to demonstrate that the surgeon must be aware of the specific requirements for proper care of fractures of the finger metacarpals at various levels. The most disabling complication following treatment of finger metacarpals is malrotation resulting from inadequate reduction or loss of reduction. Therefore the complex fracture of the finger metacarpals may require open reduction and internal fixation.

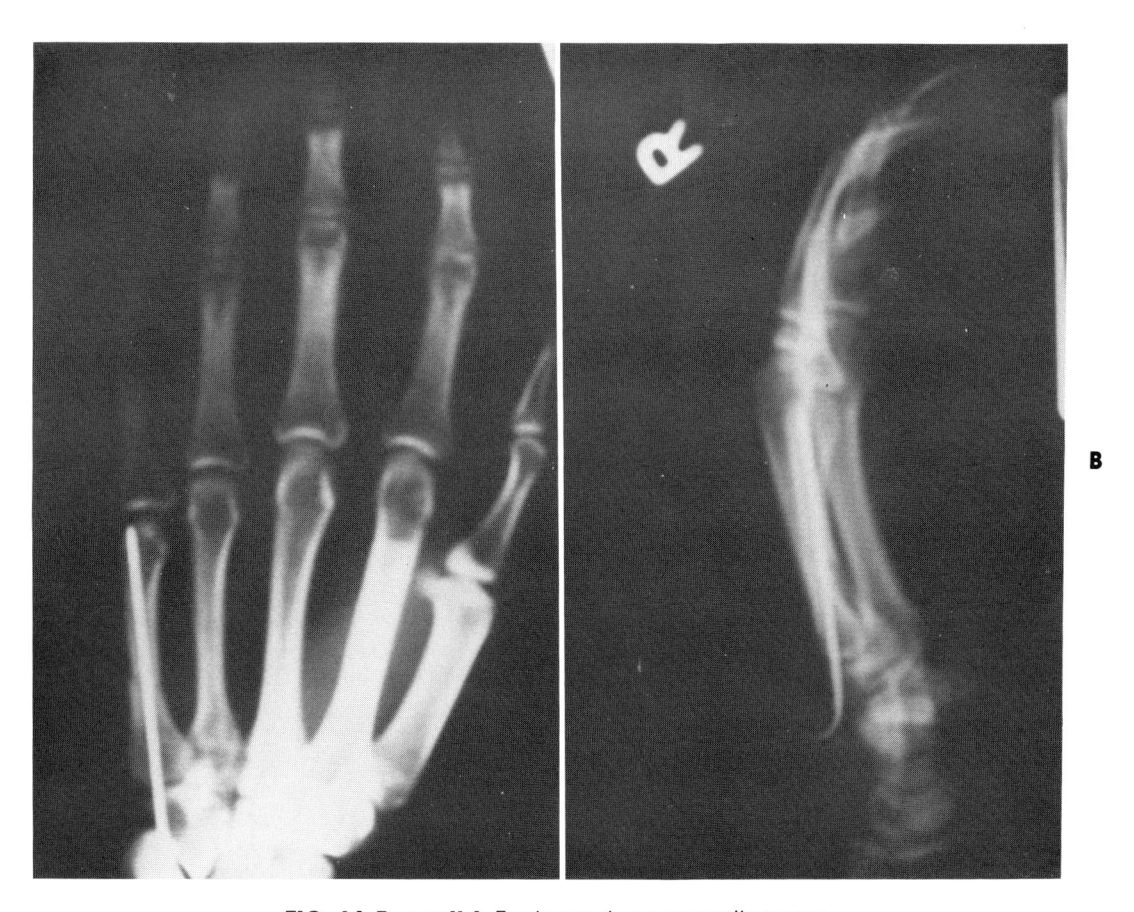

FIG. 14-5, cont'd. For legend see opposite page.

Chapter 15 Factors influencing digital performance after phalangeal fracture

James W. Strickland

James B. Steichen

William B. Kleinman

Noreen Flynn

Bunnell[6] states that finger fractures are so frequent and result in so much disability that they cause about as much compensation expense as do fractures of the long bones. Others have recognized that phalangeal fractures are common and that the frequency of malunion and stiffness of the fingers after these injuries indicates the importance of the problem.[20]

This chapter reviews the various factors that influence the final performance of a finger after phalangeal fracture and indicates the relative importance of each factor based on clinical experience, the reported findings of others, and data from a retrospective study of phalangeal fractures in our own practice. It must be emphasized at the outset that the phalangeal fractures in our study group represent those seen in a practice devoted entirely to hand surgery; they are therefore of considerably greater severity than those which are routinely encountered in an emergency room.

RETROSPECTIVE STUDY

From 1418 tubular bone fractures, 178 distal phalangeal tuft and 217 metacarpal fractures were deleted from the study. Another 711 fractures were deleted because of insufficient follow-up analysis, secondary management, or primary amputation or arthrodesis. This left 312 cases with 415 phalangeal fractures available for the extraction of pertinent information for analysis.

Eighty-three percent of the patients in this group were male, and the average age was 32.2 years. Fracture distribution between the hands was almost equal, and the three central digits incurred fractures with similar frequency. Excluding tuft fractures, fractures of the proximal and middle phalanges were more frequent than those of the distal phalanx and were approximately equal in occurrence (Fig. 15-1).

Some 50.9% of the fractures resulted from crushing injuries, whereas a direct blow was responsible for 29.8%, and rotational or longitudinal trauma resulted in 9.7%. Of the fractures in this series, 9.5% were attributed to other causes.

An indication of the severity of the fractures in this specialized study is that 68% of the fractures were open, 45% exhibited marked displacement, and comminuted and transverse fractures were the most frequent. Sixty-nine percent of the fractures had associated injuries, with 60% involving skin and 44% having either flexor or extensor tendon damage. Open fixation was required in 67% of the cases in this study.

An additional part of this study involved the isolation of 101 nonarticular fractures of the proximal phalanges to

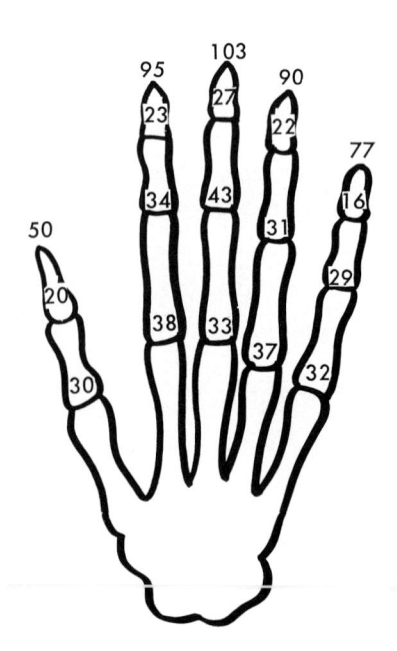

FIG. 15-1. Distribution of fractures of both hands: greatest percentage was in middle three digits with fairly equal distribution between proximal and middle phalanges.

try to create a more accurate evaluation of the influence of various factors. Although reducing any of these factors to a pure form was impossible, it was hoped that meaningful information would result from confining the study to one anatomic area without joint involvement.

To evaluate digital performance after fracture, the average total active motion (TAM) was determined, and a percent of the normal TAM was computed using 140 degrees as a normal value for the thumb and 260 degrees for the other four digits. For purposes of clarity all TAM values in this chapter are expressed as a percentage of normal.

The average digital motion after all fractures of the index, long, ring, and small fingers in this study was 73% of normal. Substantially worse results were seen in the thumb, where function was decreased to 59%. The average TAM of the entire group was 71.4% of normal.

FACTORS INFLUENCING DIGITAL FUNCTION AFTER PHALANGEAL FRACTURE

In considering the factors that influence the final result after phalangeal fractures, three general categories should be recognized: (1) patient factors, (2) fracture factors, and (3) management factors. Unfortunately the surgeon can exercise control over only one of these three important categories, that being the management of the fracture itself. Factors unique to the injury and the particular patient will have a pronounced effect on the ultimate digital function after phalangeal fracture. Although these fracture and patient factors by virtue of their prognostic importance are worth consideration, there is very little that can be done to alter their influence on the final performance of a given finger. The importance of various factors following phalangeal fractures is reviewed in the following sections.

Patient factors

Patient factors include age, associated diseases, socioeconomic factors, and patient understanding and motivation.

It is well recognized that older patients tend to develop joint stiffness more rapidly after phalangeal fractures than do younger patients. Our study of the influence of age on fracture performance indicated that the percentage of digital motion returned following nonarticular proximal phalangeal fractures dropped from a TAM of 70% of normal to 51% of normal after the age of 50. The results were 88% of normal in the first two decades and 70% for the third, fourth, and fifth decades, with a substantial drop in the last two decades studied (Fig. 15-2).

Chronic debilitating diseases, particularly those with vascular or metabolic alterations, also may have a prejudicial effect on digital performance by delaying fracture healing and increasing the potential for infection and adhesion formation. Socioeconomic factors on occasion may influence the patient's decisions with regard to the selection of medical management and the ability to properly carry out the treatment program.

A failure to appreciate the full ramifications of the injury and to adhere closely to professional advice with regard to digital immobilization and subsequent mobilization also may have an extremely detrimental effect. Finally, and perhaps most important, the motivation of the patient is an extremely important ingredient in the

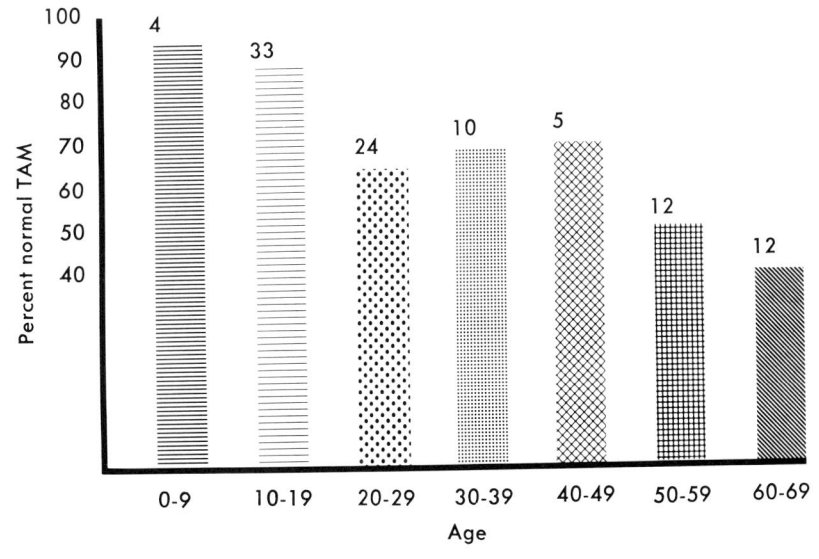

FIG. 15-2. Nonarticular phalangeal fractures of proximal phalanx: breakdown by age groups.

SECTION 4 BONE PROBLEMS

restoration of digital function after phalangeal fractures. Particularly with regard to the patient's approach to the rehabilitative process after fracture healing, determination and willingness to enthusiastically participate in splinting and exercise programs will have a substantial impact on finger and hand performance. Although the surgeon in some instances can increase the patient's participation in his or her own care and stimulate the rehabilitative efforts, unfortunately many patients will prove to be refractory to advice and encouragement.

Fracture factors

Fracture factors influencing digital performance after phalangeal injuries include the location, type, displacement, and stability of the fracture and also the presence of associated soft tissue injuries to skin, joint ligaments, tendons, nerves, and vessels. The most troublesome phalangeal fractures have been described by Stark[23] and include dorsal intraarticular fractures of the distal interphalangeal (DIP) joint, oblique intraarticular fractures of the DIP joint, oblique intraarticular fractures of the proximal interphalangeal (PIP) joint, spiral fractures of

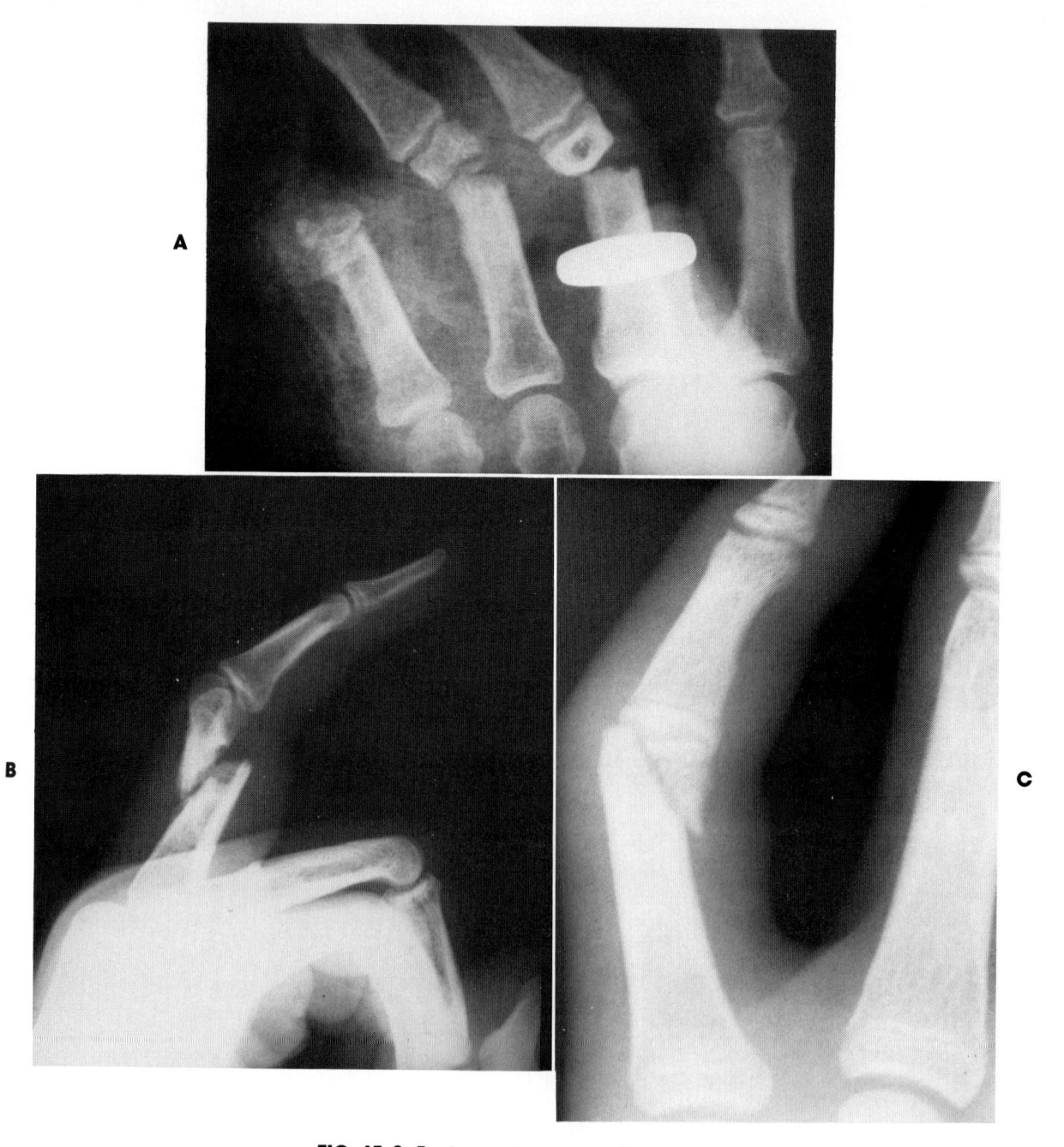

FIG. 15-3. For legend see opposite page.

the proximal phalanx, intraarticular fractures of the base of the middle phalanx, fractures of the dorsal lip of the middle phalanx, and fractures of the volar base of the middle phalanx (Fig. 15-3).

It is obvious that injuries resulting in comminuted or widely displaced fractures with their obligatory injury to adjacent soft tissue will have a more compromising effect on ultimate digital performance than will undisplaced or minimally displaced fractures. Fractures located adjacent to or involving joints also will have a prejudicial effect on function, as will injuries to adjacent tendons, nerves, vessels, and joint ligaments. The relative impact of these fracture factors is considered in the following sections.

Fracture type, stability, and displacement. James[13] and James and Wright[14] stated that flexion contractures of the PIP joint occurred in almost all the 58 unstable fractures and that loss of full flexion secondary to stiffness of the interphalangeal (IP) joints occurred commonly. A surprising finding in this study was that after 75 unstable closed fractures of the phalanges only 17 fingers had full recovery, whereas the other 58 lost motion. Wright[24] stated that unstable fractures returned 64.5% of normal function in his series.

In our series fracture type also was evaluated, and it was found that transverse fractures of the four digits returned 76% of normal function, whereas comminuted fractures of the same digits returned only 62% (Fig. 15-4). There was a similar (18%) drop in thumb motion when comparing comminuted with transverse fractures.

In our study we attempted to delimit the influence of displacement on final range of motion by narrowing our focus to nonarticular fractures of the proximal phalanx without tendon injuries. This isolated field of fractures indicated a clear deterioration in results as severity of displacement increased, with an average TAM of 88% for undisplaced fractures, 80% for minimally displaced fractures, and 74% for the markedly displaced category (Fig. 15-5).

Joint involvement. Huffaker, Wray, and Weeks[12] attempted to analyze factors influencing the final range of motion in the fingers after fractures of the hand and found that for the entire fracture group the median TAM without joint involvement was 220 degrees, whereas the

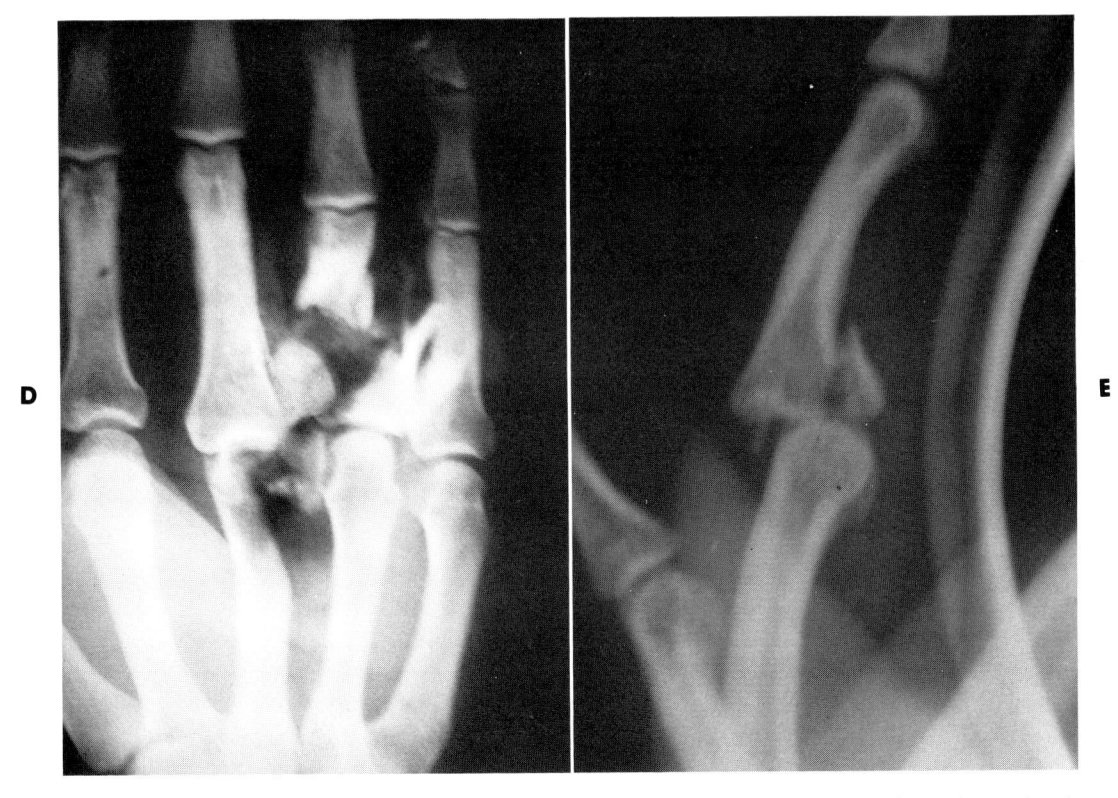

FIG. 15-3. Difficult fractures of phalanges. **A,** Widely displaced fractures through proximal phalangeal necks of long and ring fingers; amputation of fifth finger. **B,** Dorsally displaced short oblique fractures through proximal phalangeal neck. **C,** Proximally displaced oblique intraarticular fracture of proximal phalanx. **D,** Severely comminuted proximal phalangeal fracture with intraarticular component. **E,** Fracture-dislocation of base of middle phalanx with displaced volar fragment.

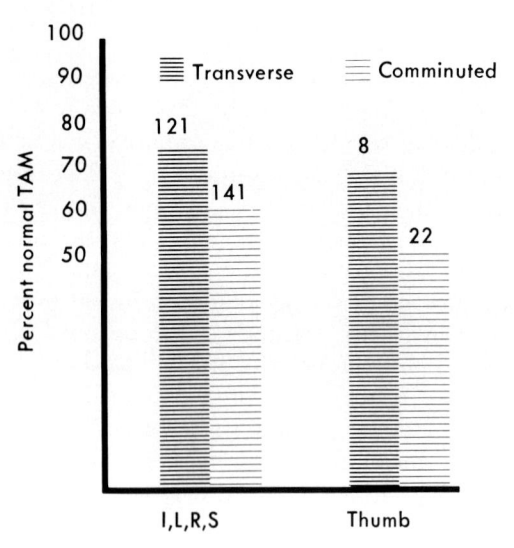

FIG. 15-4. Comparison of transverse and comminuted phalangeal fractures, indicating substantial deterioration with comminution. *I,* Index; *R,* ring; *L,* long; *S,* small finger.

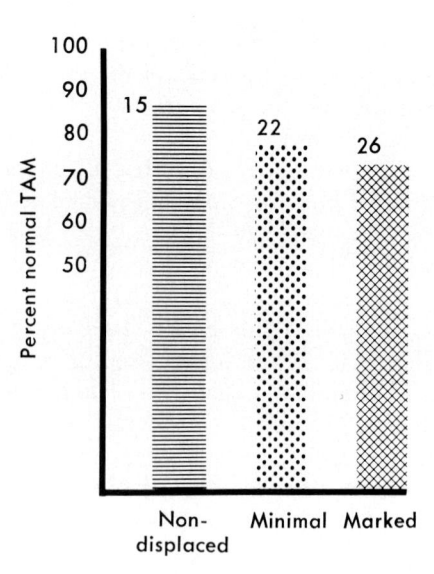

FIG. 15-5. Influence of displacement on nonarticular fractures of proximal phalanx with no tendon injury, indicating only slight deterioration in minimally and markedly displaced groups compared with nondisplaced fractures.

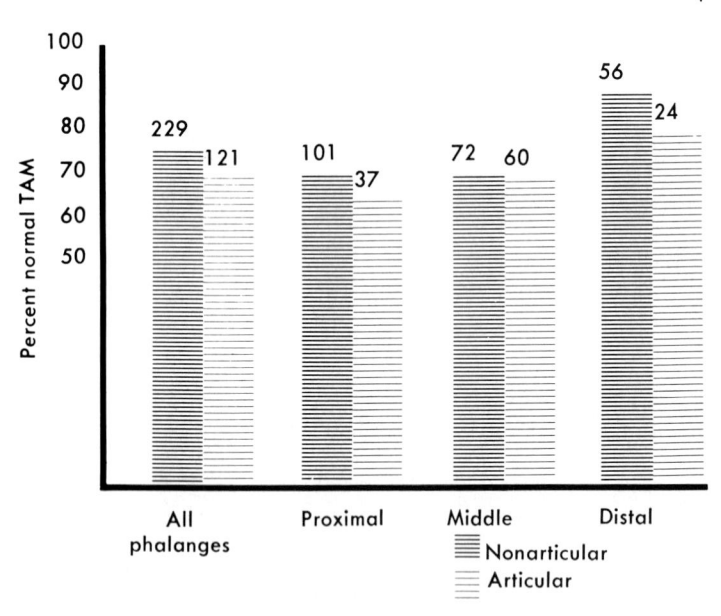

FIG. 15-6. Comparison of performance of phalangeal fractures in index, long, ring, and small fingers with and without articular involvement, indicating only moderate additional functional loss resulting from joint involvement.

range with joint injury was 175 degrees. Simple fractures with no joint involvement had a median return of 256 degrees, decreasing to 224 degrees with joint injury. Crushing injuries with joint involvement returned 150 degrees, compared with those with no joint involvement, which returned 206 degrees.

In our series nonarticular fractures were found to have 5% (12.3 degrees) better functional recovery than their counterparts with injury to the articular surfaces. The maximum difference in return between articular and nonarticular fractures was 9% (24 degrees) in the distal phalangeal group, and nonarticular proximal and middle phalangeal fractures returned 70% of normal compared with 64% and 70%, respectively, with articular involvement (Fig. 15-6).

Soft tissue injuries. James[13] stated that the results of fractures of the proximal and middle phalanges of the fingers are clearly related to the degree of soft tissue wounding, including skin, vessels, tendons, and joints. Flatt[9] pointed out that damage to soft tissues is inevitable in any fracture of the hand and that in some instances this damage is relatively slight, whereas in others it may be far more important than the fracture. He emphasized that many fractures of the hand are of the com-

CHAPTER 15 FACTORS INFLUENCING DIGITAL PERFORMANCE AFTER PHALANGEAL FRACTURE

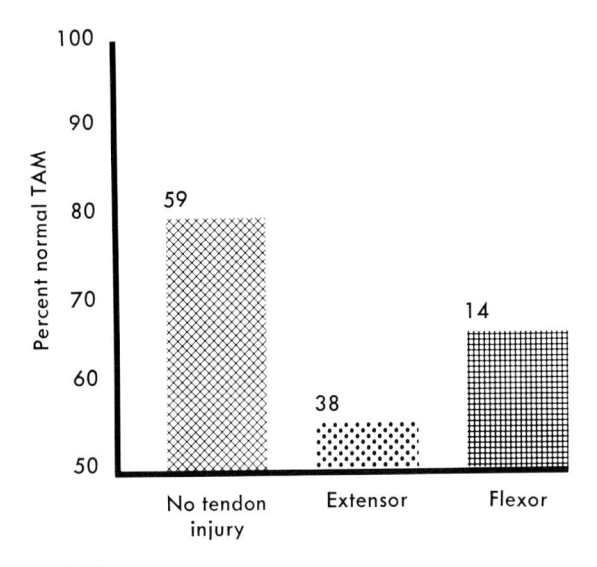

FIG. 15-7. Graph indicating significant influence of tendon injuries on nonarticular fractures of proximal phalanx, with extensor tendon injuries being more prejudicial than flexor tendon injuries in this series.

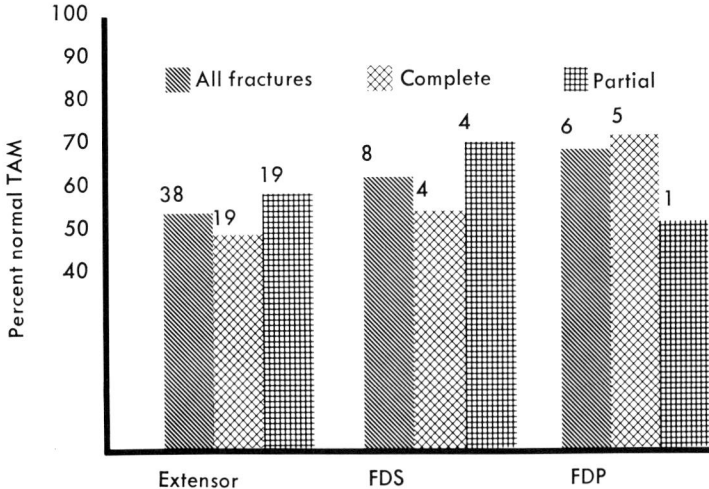

FIG. 15-8. Comparison of performance of complete or partial lacerations of extensor tendon, flexor digitorum superficialis (FDS), and flexor digitorum profundus (FDP) tendons in nonarticular fractures of proximal phalanx. Poorest function is seen in complete extensor tendon injuries, followed by complete lacerations of flexor digitorum superficialis.

pression type in which there is "injury in depth." First, the skin is damaged, then the deeper structures are damaged, and finally the bone is shattered. "A finger injured in this way may be so crippled that even if the skin wound could be closed and the fracture reduced, the final result would be a healed fracture surrounded by a stiff, insensitive cylinder of skin."[9]

Phalangeal fractures associated with significant overlying skin wounds usually carry a poorer prognosis than the closed fractures, which often result from injuries of less magnitude. Concomitant involvement of digital nerves and vessels also may have a detrimental effect on finger function, although their exact impact on fracture healing is unclear.

The influence of associated tendon injuries on final digital performance after phalangeal fractures has been recognized. James[13] stated that "wounding of the extensor apparatus of the dorsum of the phalanges in association with fracture presents one of the most difficult of all problems of the hand." He further stated that in his experience involvement of a joint or tendon almost certainly would result in the loss of function. Huffaker, Wray, and Weeks[12] also indicated that associated flexor tendon injuries with or without joint involvement had a poor final result and that only a fair result was achieved when associated extensor tendon injuries were seen. They found that flexor tendon injuries in association with phalangeal fractures reduced the median return to 44 degrees, and associated extensor tendon injuries returned 184 degrees. It was their conclusion that associated flexor tendon injuries caused more functional loss than did extensor tendon injuries.

In our study the effect of tendon injuries on the performance of the PIP joint after nonarticular fractures was significant. The TAM was found to be 79% of normal in those fractures without tendon injuries but dropped to 55% with concomitant tendon injury. Complete severance of an extensor tendon resulted in a TAM of only 49% of normal with an improvement to 60% for partial lacerations. An average TAM of 63% resulted from superficialis interruption, with a 69% return found after profundus tendon damage (Figs. 15-7 and 15-8).

131

SECTION 4 BONE PROBLEMS

Management factors

The surgeon entrusted with the management of phalangeal fractures will find that there are many factors that must be considered in formulating a successful approach to the return of digital function. These factors include the following:
1. Recognition of injury
2. Tissue management
3. Fracture reduction
4. Maintenance of reduction
5. Mobilization of joints
6. Management of complications

Recognition of injury and tissue management. The accurate diagnosis of the specific injury should always include a careful physical examination, followed by an anteroposterior and true lateral roentgenogram and an oblique view when the injury is close to a joint. Proper wound care and the repair of associated tendon, vessel, and nerve injuries should be carried out in a manner that prevents additional tissue damage.

Fracture reduction and maintenance. The goals of fracture reduction include the correction of the deformity and the achievement of stability. If a stable fracture with proper alignment and rotation can be accomplished

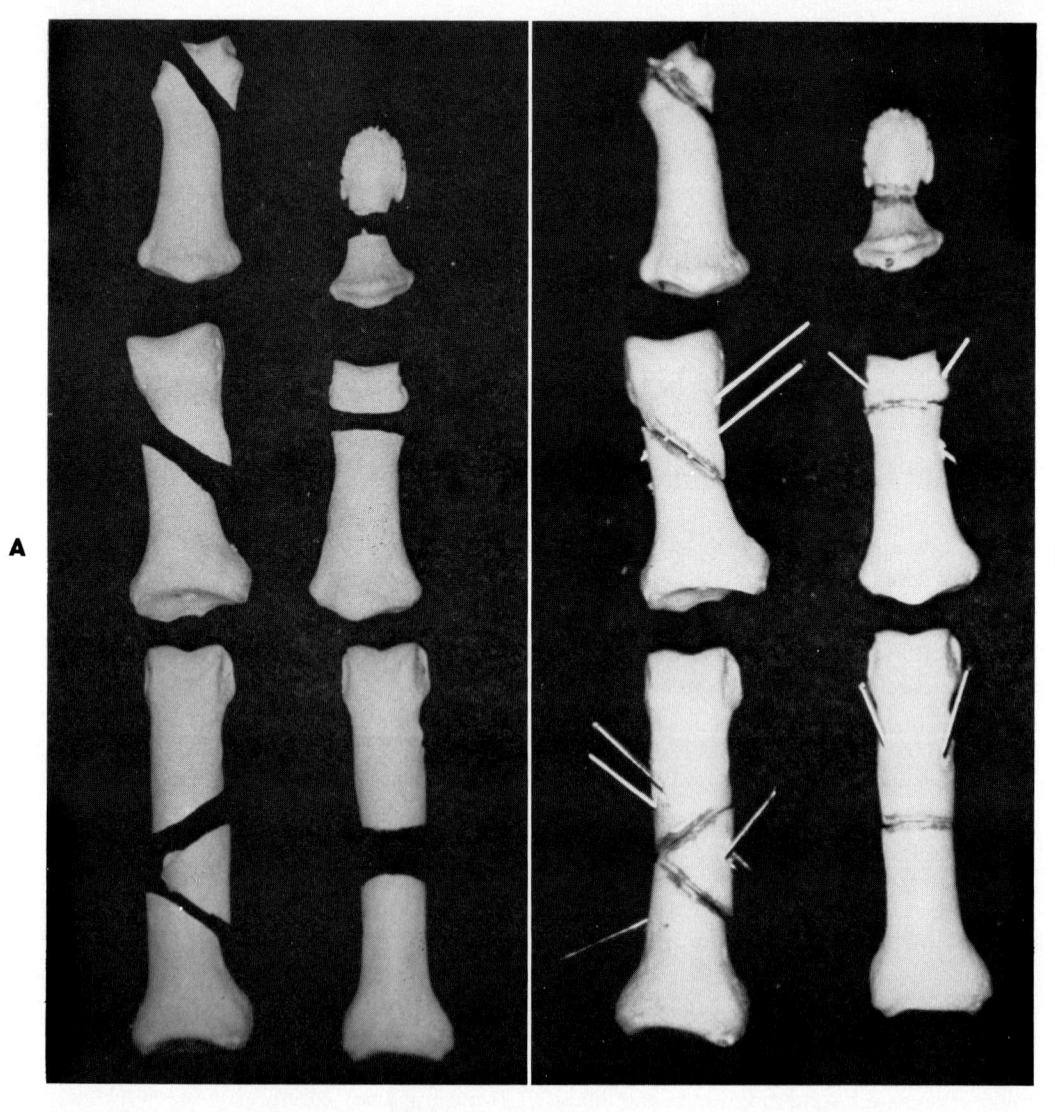

FIG. 15-9. Difficult fractures of phalanges. **A,** Appearance of several types of phalangeal fractures, which are often unstable and difficult to manage without open fixation: oblique intraarticular fracture of distal portion of middle phalanx, oblique midshaft fracture of middle phalanx, comminuted midshaft fracture of proximal phalanx, transverse fracture of distal phalanx (often open), transverse fracture of neck of middle phalanx, and transverse fracture of midshaft of proximal phalanx. **B,** Possible methods of securing stability by means of Kirschner wire internal fixation.

by closed techniques, simple splinting in a "balanced position" is appropriate for a 3-week period. With the exception of fractures that were undisplaced when initially seen, all stable, reduced phalangeal fractures should be maintained in a plaster cast or cast-splint combination that immobilizes the wrist in a partially extended position. It is important that immediate postoperative radiographs confirm the maintenance of reduction, and frequent x-ray checks should be carried out to ensure that no loss of position has occurred.

The indications for internal fixation of phalangeal fractures have been listed by Robins[21] and include the following:
1. Fractures of the shaft of the phalanges if closed treatment has failed to achieve satisfactory position
2. Fractures with displacement close to or involving a joint
3. In certain cases to afford stability after major hand fractures

James[13] stated that the principal indication for internal fixation was an oblique fracture of a condyle and that unstable fractures were being managed increasingly by internal fixation. In our practice open reduction is indicated when satisfactory reduction cannot be achieved or when the fracture remains unstable following reduction. Intraarticular, periarticular, comminuted, multiple-level, and some transverse or oblique midshaft fractures are examples of fractures that frequently require internal fixation (Fig. 15-9).

FIG. 15-10. Lateral view of digital phalanges indicating tubular nature of diaphyses with proximal and distal metaphyseal widening.

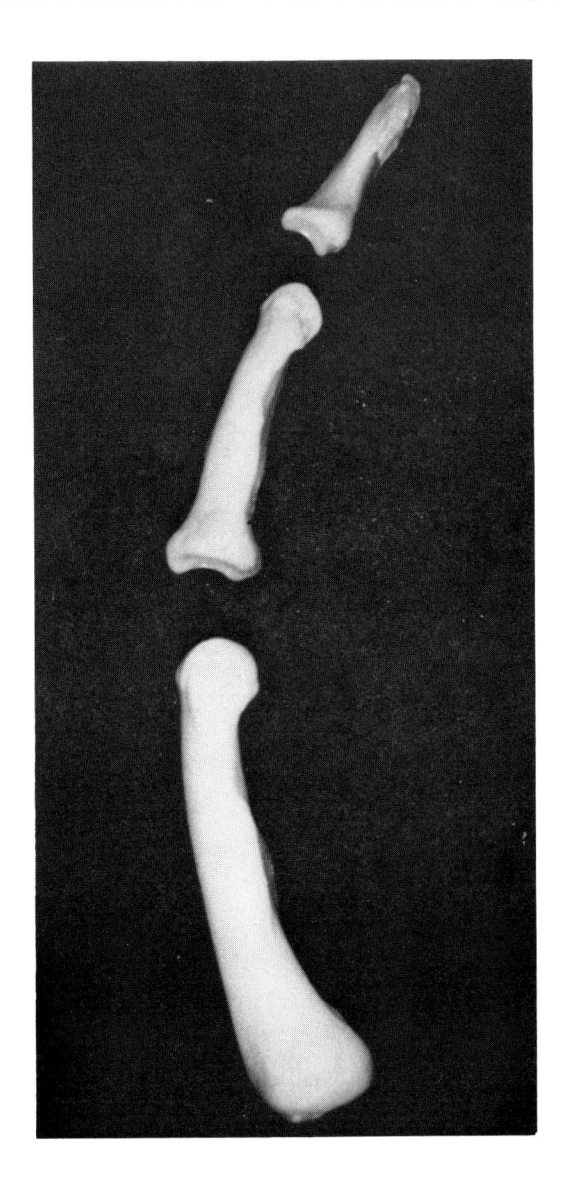

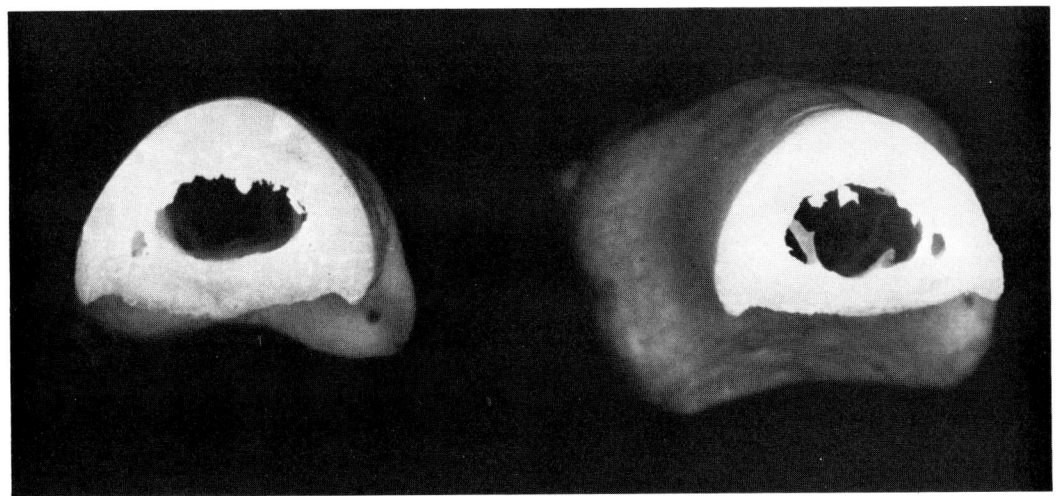

FIG. 15-11. End-on view of transversely sectioned midshafts of middle and proximal phalanges, respectively, depicting thick cortices and small medullary canals.

SECTION 4 BONE PROBLEMS

Techniques for open reduction usually include a dorsal surgical approach with fixation achieved by means of Kirschner wires, interosseous wires, screws, or occasionally plates. The technique selected should be compatible with the skill and experience of the surgeon and should result in the least possible trauma to digital soft tissues. When correctly used, Kirschner wire fixation is perhaps the least damaging and most effective, and the use of motorized pin drivers has greatly facilitated pin placement. The technique requires a thorough understanding of the tubular anatomy of the phalangeal bones with their small medullary canals (Figs. 15-10 and 15-11). It is also important that Kirschner wire fixation be carried out so as not to cross joints and impede the opportunity to begin joint mobilization before fracture healing and pin removal. Transverse fractures are best

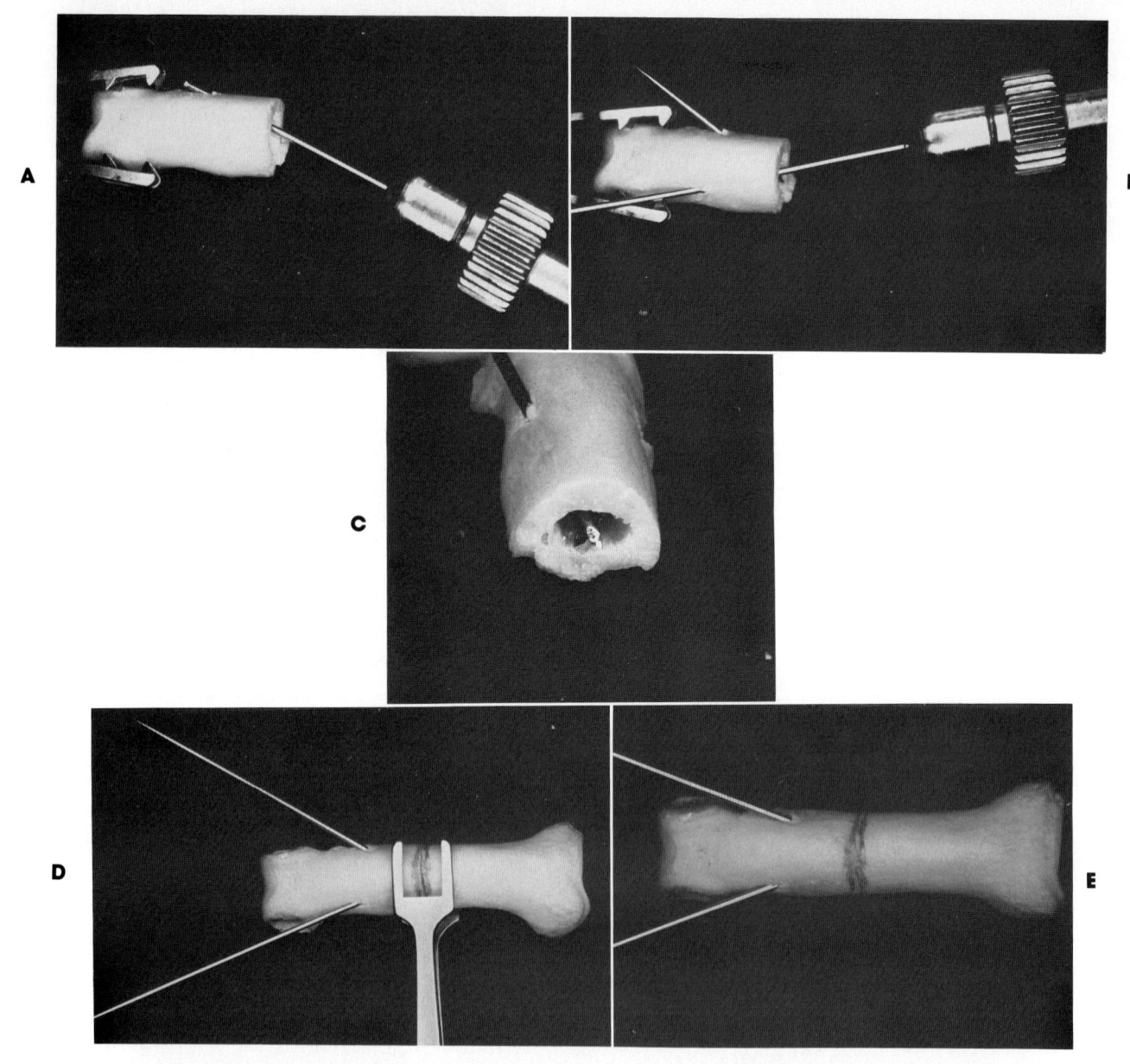

FIG. 15-12. Technique of Kirschner wire fixation for transverse midshaft fracture. **A,** Placement of pins from inside medullary canal of distal fragment through diaphyseal cortex using motorized drill. **B,** Placement of second oblique pin through opposite cortex. **C,** Appearance of pin tips in medullary canal of distal fragment prior to phalangeal reduction and retrograde pin placement. **D,** Reduction of phalangeal fragment in preparation for final pin placement. **E,** Securely fixed phalangeal fracture after retrograde pin placement.

CHAPTER 15 FACTORS INFLUENCING DIGITAL PERFORMANCE AFTER PHALANGEAL FRACTURE

secured by means of crossed Kirschner wires introduced first into the medullary canal of one fragment and then passed across into the other fragment after reduction (Figs. 15-12 and 15-13). Although some comminuted fractures may be better managed without an effort at internal fixation, pins often may be used to reestablish the position of major fragments. Individualized placement of pins for spiral, oblique, and articular fractures may be necessary, and under x-ray control percutaneous techniques may be applicable in some instances (Fig. 15-14).

Mobilization of joints. After open or closed reduction, decisions must be made as to the proper timing for joint mobilization, and the exact techniques to be used must be carefully considered. It is the policy of most surgeons to initiate at least gentle active and passive motion pro-

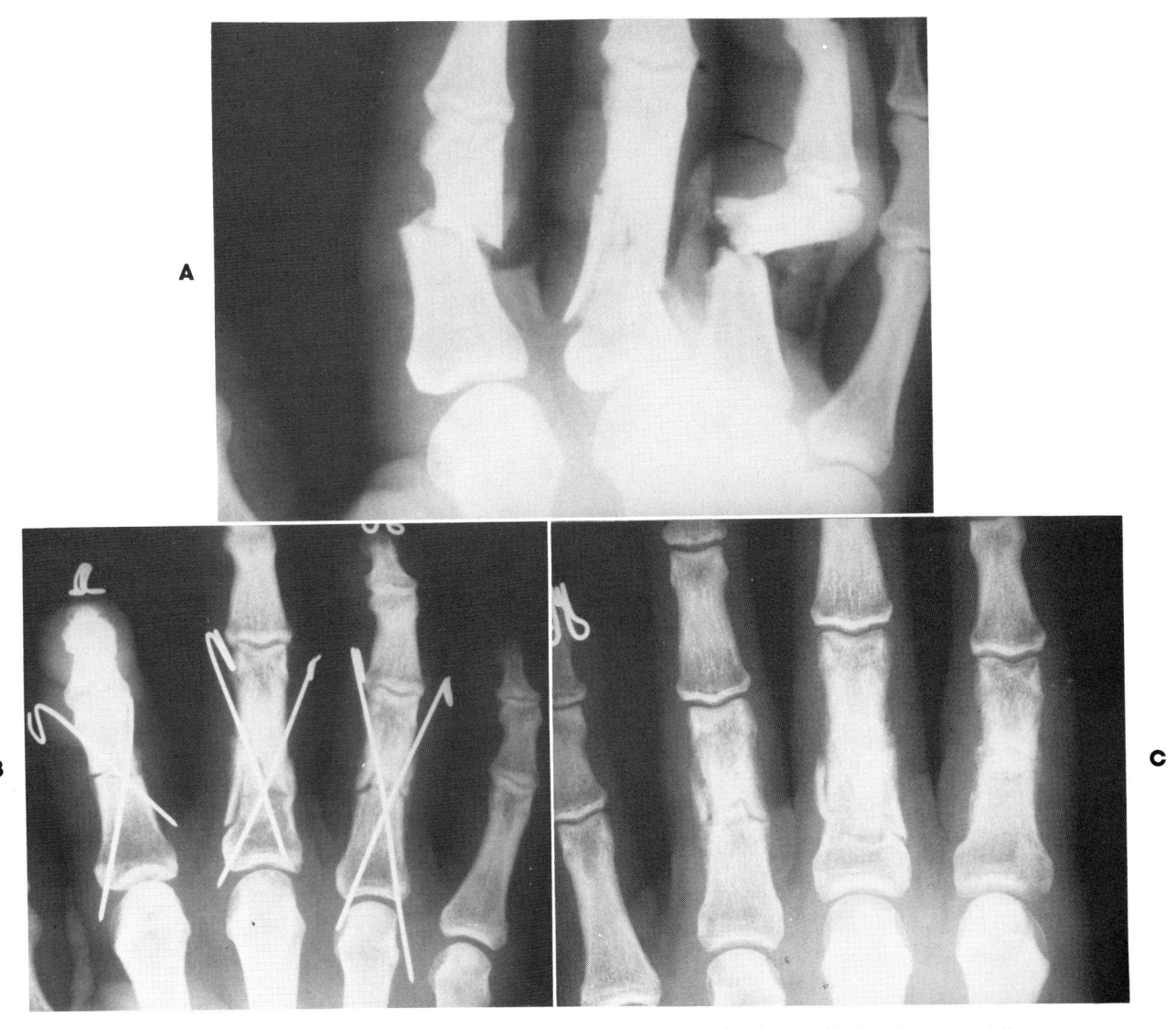

FIG. 15-13. Example of Kirschner wire fixation of phalangeal fractures of index, long, and ring fingers. **A,** Open unstable fractures through midshaft of proximal phalanges of index and ring fingers and proximal third of long finger. **B,** Appearance of fractures after crossed Kirschner wire fixation. Note nonarticular placement of Kirschner wires. **C,** Appearance of fractures after satisfactory healing and pin removal.

SECTION 4   BONE PROBLEMS

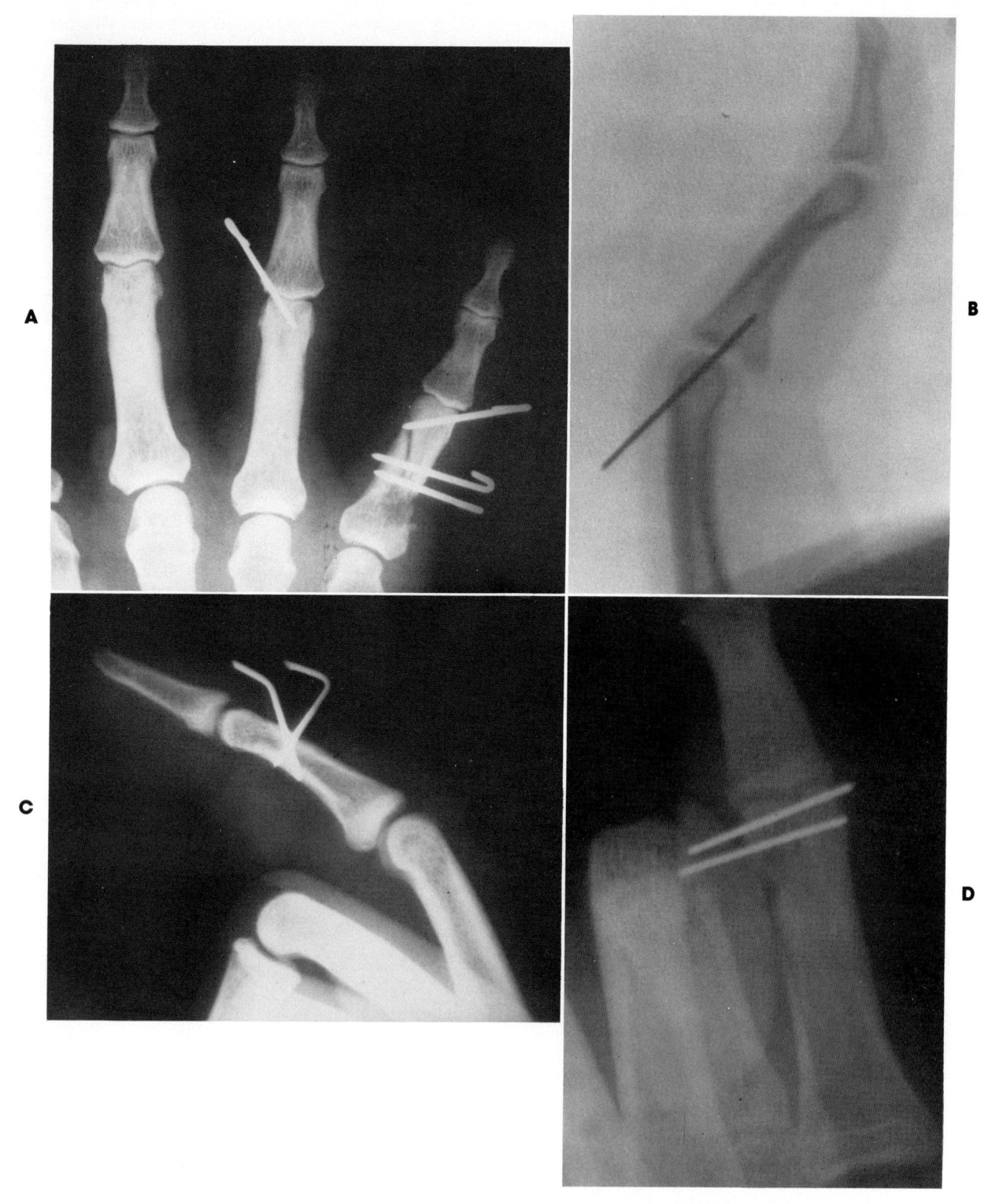

FIG. 15-14. Additional internal fixation technique for difficult phalangeal fractures. **A,** Transverse and oblique pin fixation of long oblique fracture of proximal phalanx of small finger with single pin fixation of articular fracture of proximal phalanx of ring finger. **B,** Kirschner wire used to maintain reduced position of middle phalanx after fracture-dislocation with large volar fragment. **C,** Two-pin dorsal fixation of long oblique fracture of middle phalanx. **D,** Percutaneous fixation of articular fracture of proximal phalanx using two pins.

grams as soon as soft tissue healing will permit, with an effort made to begin motion by at least the third week after fracture regardless of the x-ray appearance of the fracture. In severe fractures the use of nonarticular Kirschner wires to provide phalangeal stability will be helpful in initiating early motion before solid bony union occurs.

Ruedi, Burri, and Pfeiffer[22] stated that prolonged immobilization of fractured phalanges led to joint stiffness and dystrophy of soft tissues. Although some[10,18] have advocated early digital mobilization following fracturing, others[9] have felt that excessive early motion and unwise operative intervention may produce rather than prevent permanent crippling of the hand. Most authors* believe that approximately 3 weeks of immobilization following phalangeal fracture are appropriate, and many† have emphasized that more than 3 weeks of immobilization may be severely detrimental to digital function. Wright[24] maintained that immobilization for periods longer than 3 weeks, regardless of the type of splintage, resulted in the loss of movement at the MCP and interphalangeal (IP) joints.

In our study there was found to be no meaningful difference in the ultimate performance of fractured digits following mobilization during each of the first 4 weeks after fracture, with a return of function between 75% and 80% of normal achieved. A decisive drop to 66% was seen in those fractures in which mobilization was initiated later than 4 weeks (Fig. 15-15).

---

*References 2, 5, 13, and 15-17.
†References 5, 15, 17, 19, and 24.

Complications. Complications of phalangeal fractures include joint stiffness,[13] nonunion, malunion, infection, reflex dystrophy, sensory loss, tendon adherence with the limiting effect on the excursion of distal digital joints, and pain sufficient to warrant amputation.* The management of these complications includes procedures well known to the hand surgeon, such as tenolysis, capsulectomy, osteotomy, arthroplasty, arthrodesis, and amputation.

In this series complications occurred in 19.04% of all phalangeal fractures. The percentage of the entire complication group is summarized in the following list:

Angulatory deformity	29%
Delayed union	22%
Malunion	13%
Nonunion	12%
Rotation deformity	12%
Infection and osteomyelitis	8%
Other	4%

Combined factors

The influence of both displacement and immobilization was studied, and it was found that undisplaced fractures returned to 90% of normal function after immobilization during the first 4 weeks (Fig. 15-16). A precipitous fall to 65% occurred when mobilization was delayed beyond 4 weeks. In minimally displaced fractures there was a gradual drop from 98% in the first week to 74% when mobilized after the fourth week. Markedly dis-

---

*References 1, 3, 4, 7, 8, 11, and 20.

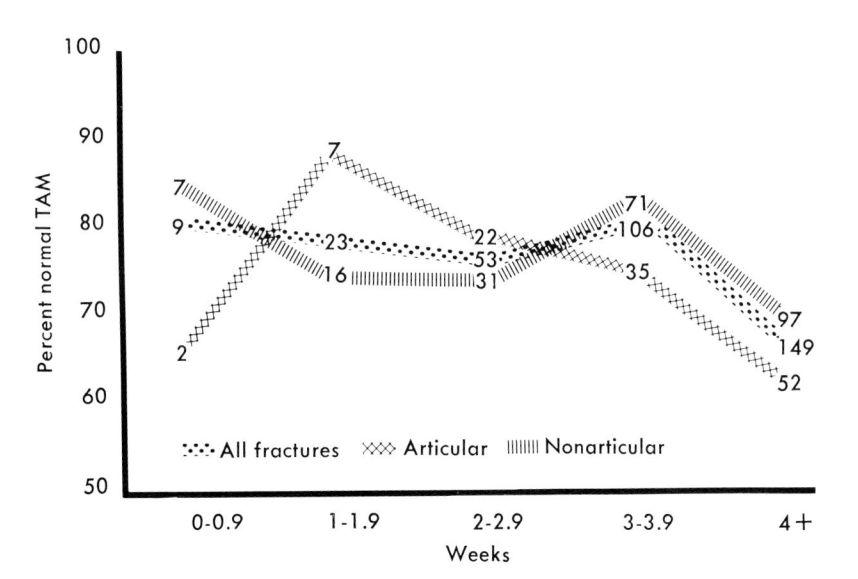

FIG. 15-15. Effect of immobilization on all fractures, articular fractures, and nonarticular fractures of phalanges. Little meaningful difference in final TAM occurs in those fractures mobilized during any of the first 4 weeks after fracturing, although there is marked decline of function in those fractures mobilized after fourth week.

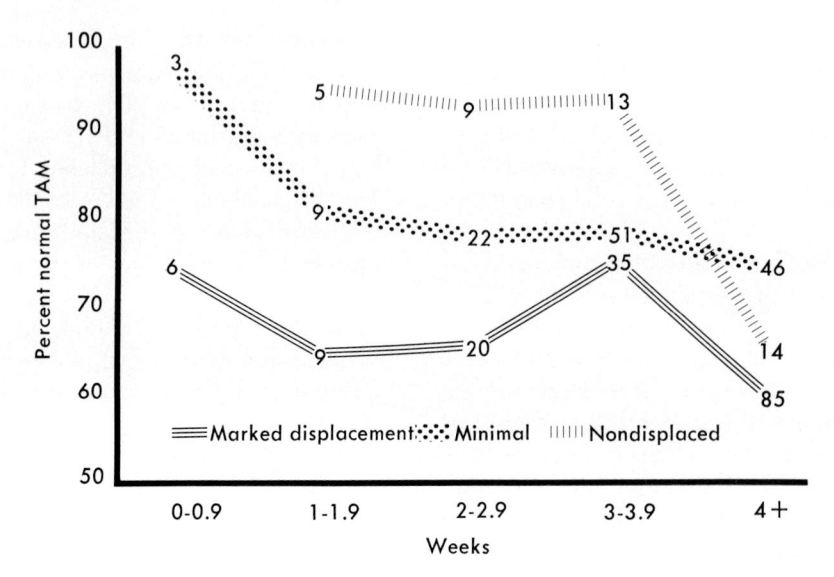

FIG. 15-16. Study of effect of immobilization and displacement on final digital performance after phalangeal fracturing. Best performance occurred in nondisplaced fractures mobilized before fourth week, with minimally displaced and markedly displaced fractures performing worse. In all cases there was decline of function if immobilization was continued beyond third week.

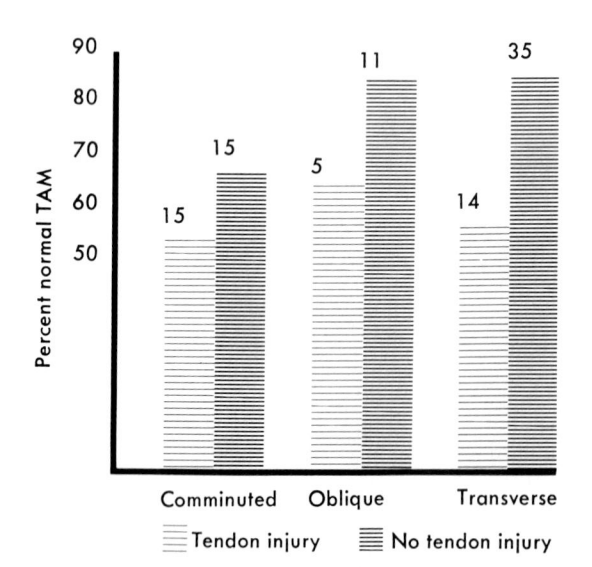

FIG. 15-17. Comparison of performance of nonarticular proximal phalanx oblique, transverse, and comminuted fractures with and without tendon injury. Comminuted fractures with tendon injury gave worst performance, with comminuted transverse and oblique fractures also returning poor function. Best finger function returned after oblique or transverse fractures without tendon injury.

placed fractures produced a drop from 75% in the first week to 65% for the second and third weeks before rising to 74% for the digits mobilized during the fourth week. Again there was a steep decline to 61% after 4 weeks.

Additional studies were carried out to determine the influence of fracture type and tendon injuries on combined factors of digital performance. Worse results occurred in comminuted fractures with tendon injuries where a 52% return occurred compared with 68% in the same type of fracture without tendon involvement (Fig. 15-17).

SUMMARY

The surgeon confronted with severe phalangeal fractures should be aware of the fracture, patient, and management factors that will influence the final result. Because the surgeon exercises direct control on only the management of fractures, it is important that careful attention be given to the injured digit and the best techniques selected to provide phalangeal healing and the restoration of digital motion. The influence of various factors on the ultimate performance of the digit after phalangeal fracture is discussed in this chapter, drawing from the published work of others, our own experience, and data from a retrospective study of these injuries in a hand surgery practice.

In comparing our results with the impressions and

studies of others, we are in agreement that vigorous efforts to produce early digital joint motion during the first 3 weeks after a phalangeal fracture may be unwarranted. However, it does appear to be extremely important that mobilization efforts are instituted by at least the fourth week to prevent a rather precipitous decline in performance. It also has been shown that concomitant injuries to tendons are extremely detrimental to final digital performance, and in our study extensor tendon injuries were more detrimental than were flexor tendon injuries. Increasing patient age also has been shown to have a significant aggravating effect on finger performance following phalangeal fracture, and a lesser influence is exerted by comminution and phalangeal displacement.

Even though it is emphasized that the phalangeal fractures in this study represent those seen in a practice devoted entirely to surgery of the hand and are therefore more severe than those from a normal emergency room, it is hoped that this discussion will provide at least prognostic help to the surgeon dealing with these difficult injuries.

REFERENCES

1. Barton, N.: Fractures of the phalanges of the hand, Hand **9**:1, 1977.
2. Bloem, J.J.A.M.: The treatment and prognosis of uncomplicated dislocated fractures of the metacarpals and phalanges, Arch. Chir. Neerl. **23**:55, 1971.
3. Bordon, J.: Complications of fractures and ligamentous injuries of the hand, Orthop. Rev. **1**:29, 1972.
4. Borgeskov, S.: Conservative therapy for fractures of the phalanges and metacarpals, Acta Chir. Scand. **133**:123, 1967.
5. Brooks, A.L.: Principles and problems of phalangeal fracture treatment, J. La. State Med. Soc. **113**:432, 1961.
6. Bunnell, S.: The injured hand: principles of treatment, Indust. Med. Surg. **22**:251, 1953.
7. Butt, W.D.: Fractures of the hand. II. Statistical review, Can. Med. Assoc. J. **86**:775, 1962.
8. Conolly, W.B.: Complications following the early treatment of hand injuries: an analysis of 100 cases, Aust. N.Z. J. Surg. **42**:145, 1972.
9. Flatt, A.E.: Closed and open fractures of the hand: fundamentals of management, Postgrad. Med. **39**:17, 1966.
10. Green, D.P., and Anderson, J.R.: Closed reduction and percutaneous pin fixation of fractured phalanges, J. Bone Joint Surg. **55A**:1651, 1973.
11. Howard, L.D., Jr.: Fractures of the small bones of the hand, San Francisco, 1960, L.D. Howard, Jr.
12. Huffaker, W.H., Wray, R.C., Jr., and Weeks, P.M.: Factors influencing final range of motion in the fingers after fractures of the hand, Plast. Reconstr. Surg. **63**:82, 1979.
13. James, J.I.P.: Fractures of the proximal and middle phalanges of the fingers, Acta Orthop. Scand. **32**:401, 1962.
14. James, J.I.P., and Wright, T.A.: Fractures of metacarpals and proximal and middle phalanges of the finger, J. Bone Joint Surg. **48B**:181, 1966.
15. Joshi, B.B.: Percutaneous internal fixation of fractures of the proximal phalanges, Hand **8**:86, 1976.
16. McNealy, R.W., and Lichtenstein, M.E.: Fractures of the bones of the hand, Am. J. Surg. **50**:563, 1940.
17. Namba, K.: Statistical study of fractures of phalanges, J. Bone Joint Surg. **46A**:214, 1964.
18. Nemethi, C.E.: Phalangeal fractures treated by open reduction and Kirschner-wire fixation, Indust. Med. Surg. **23**:148, 1954.
19. Nichols, H.M.: Manual of hand injuries, ed. 2, Chicago, 1960, Year Book Medical Publishers, Inc.
20. Roberts, N.: Fractures of the phalanges of the hand and metacarpals, Proc. R. Soc. Med. **31**:793, 1938.
21. Robins, R.H.C.: Injuries and infections of the hand, London, 1961, Edward Arnold Publishers, Ltd.
22. Ruedi, T.P., Burri, C., and Pfeiffer, K.M.: Stable internal fixation of fractures of the hand, J. Trauma **11**:381, 1971.
23. Stark, H.H.: Troublesome fractures and dislocations of the hand. In American Academy of Orthopaedic Surgeons: Instructional Course Lectures, vol. 19, St. Louis, 1970, The C.V. Mosby Co.
24. Wright, T.A.: Early mobilization in fractures of the metacarpals and phalanges, Can. J. Surg. **11**:491, 1968.

Chapter 16 The role of tenolysis after phalangeal fractures

Warren B. Burrows
Robert H. Hartwig
William B. Kleinman
James W. Strickland

THE PROBLEM

The intimate relation of extensor and flexor tendons to the digital phalanges is predisposed to excursion-limiting adhesions after fracture. To minimize the loss of joint motion resulting from these adhesions, some[7] have advocated immediate joint exercise programs, whereas others[13] believe that the majority of phalangeal fractures require at least 3 weeks of immobilization to allow early bone healing. Secondary contracture of joint capsules and ligaments may further limit digital motion, and attempts at joint mobilization by vigorous therapeutic manipulation or dynamic splinting may result in tendon attenuation or rupture rather than the anticipated stretching of adhesions. The object of this chapter is to analyze the problem of tendon-bone adhesions after phalangeal fractures and to demonstrate the effectiveness of tenolysis[5] in regaining joint mobility.

THE BIOLOGIC BASIS OF FRACTURE-TENDON ADHESIONS

After phalangeal fracture there is a predictable sequence of events, beginning at the moment of injury and leading ultimately to healing and scar formation. These events include hemorrhage, inflammation, collagen synthesis, collagen maturation, and remodeling. Fracture hematoma easily gains access to the flexor and extensor tendons and provides the potential mechanism for fracture-tendon adhesions.

During the first 3 days after injury an inflammatory response occurs, and fracture hematoma is invaded by neutrophils and monocytes, which release vasoactive substances, such as histamine and serotonin, and phagocytize dead cells and debris. During the third and fourth days there is an ingrowth of fibroblasts, and on the fifth and sixth days collagen synthesis begins. The formation of collagen is at its peak at the end of the second week; from the second to fourth weeks collagen maturation occurs. At this time there is a gain in linear strength created by the development of covalent cross-linking bonds between tropocollagen molecules and the ionic bonding between fibrils. Although scar remodeling continues for 6 months, tendon-to-bone adhesions that develop during this early stage may become very dense and refractory to any therapeutic efforts to stretch or separate them.

The close relation of the dorsal apparatus and the flexor digitorum superficialis tendon to the proximal phalanx is demonstrated in Fig. 16-1. The lateral bands, distal extensor tendon, and flexor digitorum profundus tendon have a similar intimate relation to the middle phalanx.[14] These are the most common areas of adhesion formation after phalangeal fracture. Of great clinical significance are those adhesions which develop between the fractured proximal phalanx and the overlying dorsal apparatus, consisting of the extensor digitorum communis and contributions from the intrinsic tendons on both sides (Fig. 16-2). Adhesions developing in this area

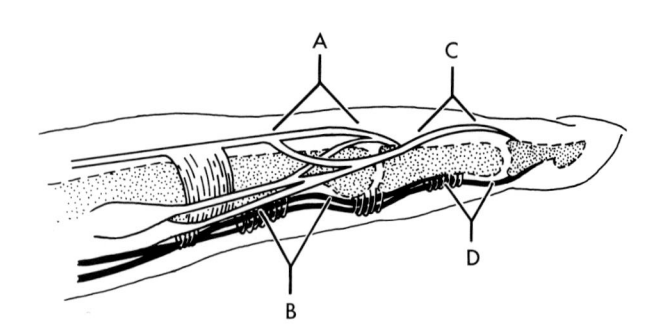

FIG. 16-1. Anatomic relationship of dorsal apparatus *(A)* and flexor digitorum superficialis *(B)* to proximal phalanx, and terminal extensor tendon *(C)* and flexor digitorum profundus *(D)* to middle phalanx, is shown diagrammatically.

serve as flexion-limiting check-reins at the proximal interphalangeal (PIP) joint (Fig. 16-3), which are often very difficult to overcome by therapy alone.[17] Secondary extension contracture of the PIP joint may complicate the situation, and concomitant fracture adhesions to the flexor digitorum superficialis may further inhibit flexion efforts at that joint.

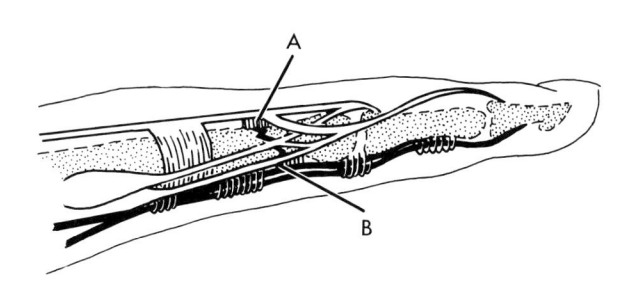

FIG. 16-2. After proximal phalangeal fracture, dense adhesions can form between fracture and dorsal apparatus (*A*) or between fracture and extrinsic flexor tendons (especially flexor digitorum superficialis [*B*]).

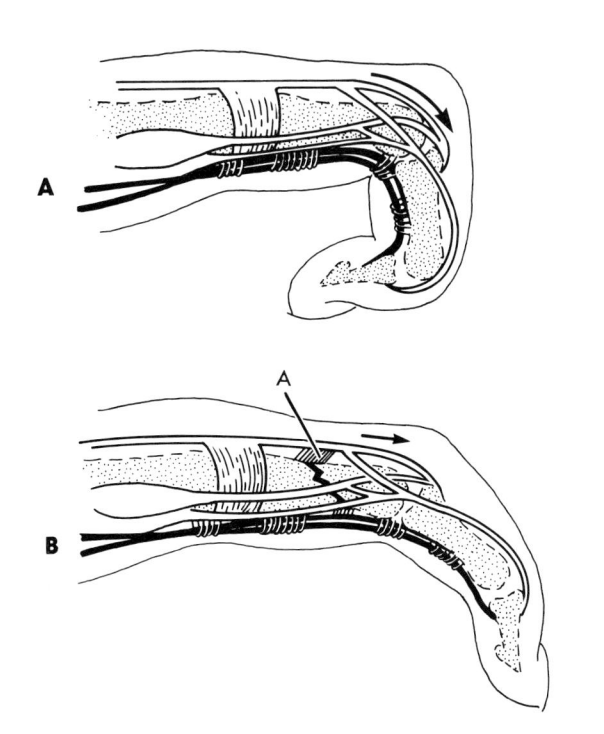

FIG. 16-3. A, Normal excursion of dorsal apparatus in absence of fracture adhesions. **B,** Check-rein effect of scar formation precludes full active or passive range of motion of distal joints of digit *(A)*.

TECHNIQUES OF TENOLYSIS AND CAPSULOTOMY AFTER PHALANGEAL FRACTURE

Improvement of joint motion after tenolysis is predicated not only on the extent of the original injury and the underlying pathologic condition but also on the patient's own understanding and acceptance of the procedure. Efforts should be made to thoroughly inform the patient of what is expected from the surgery and to provide motivation for maintenance of the increased motion that will result. These procedures should be done rarely in children younger than 10 years of age because of the difficulties associated with carrying out satisfactory postoperative therapy. Without a highly motivated patient, mobilization of a stiff finger by tenolysis is doomed to failure.

There are three basic operations for regaining motion in stiff digits after phalangeal fracture (Fig. 16-4): extensor tenolysis, flexor tenolysis, and capsulotomy. Extensor tenolysis is simply the surgical lysis of all restricting adhesions between the dorsal apparatus and the underlying bone. Flexor tenolysis includes the mobilization of the flexor digitorum superficialis and the flexor digitorum profundus tendons along the fibro-osseous canal. Finally, dorsal or volar capsulotomy with excision of portions of the joint capsule and collateral ligaments may be necessary to regain small joint motion. Detailed descriptions of extensor tenolysis,[8] flexor tenolysis,[4,11,17,18] and capsulotomy* have been published, and certain features of each of these techniques should be reviewed prior to clinical application.

---

*References 2, 3, 6, 9, 12, and 16.

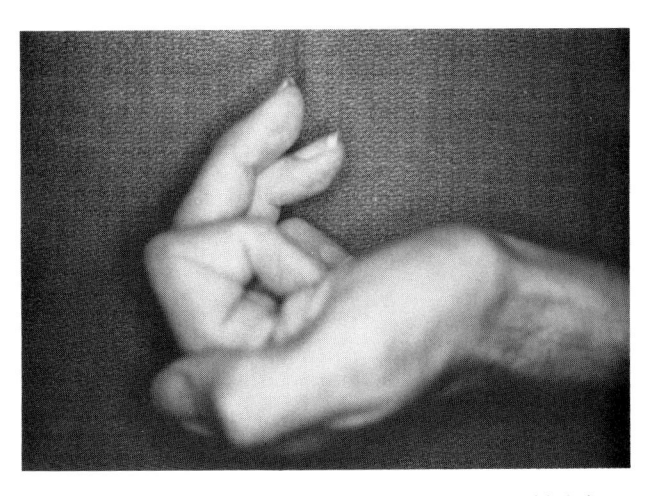

FIG. 16-4. Extension contractures and decreased total active flexion in middle and ring fingers following healed proximal phalangeal fractures and example of check-rein effect.

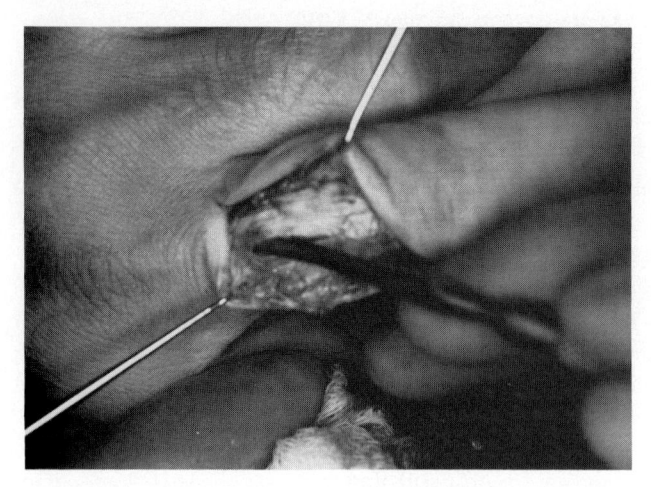

FIG. 16-5. Tenolysis of dorsal apparatus is performed through dorsal curvilinear incision. Central tendon and lateral bands must be individually freed from scar tissue.

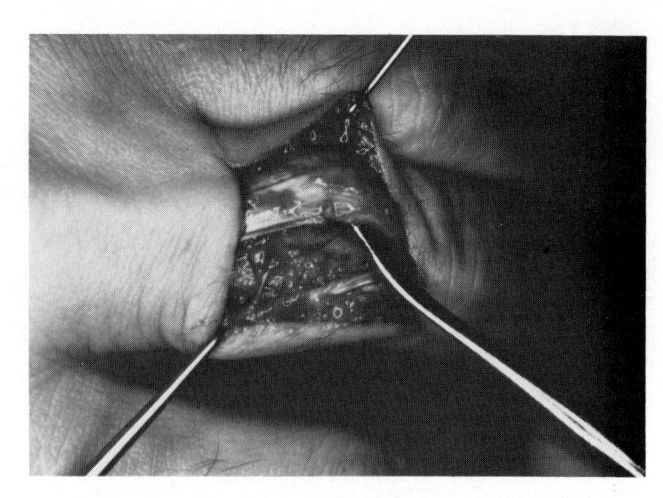

FIG. 16-6. Care must be taken during tenolysis of dorsal apparatus not to damage insertion of central tendon onto dorsal base of middle phalanx.

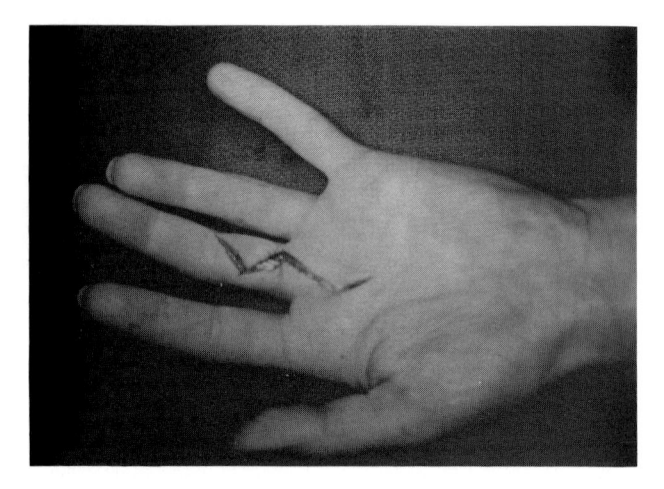

FIG. 16-7. Flexor tenolysis can be performed by either midlateral incision or Bruner zigzag incision (above).

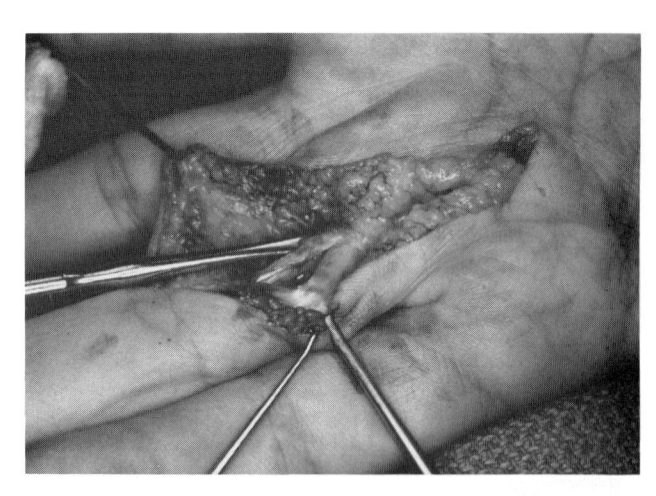

FIG. 16-8. Tenolysis of flexor digitorum superficialis from adhesions to bone, as well as of intertendinous adhesions between superficialis and profundus tendons, is performed with great care taken to preserve annular pulleys of fibroosseous canal.

Extensor tenolysis

Depending on the site of previous phalangeal fracture, extensor tenolysis is performed on the dorsum of the finger through a curvilinear incision. This incision can be extended to the metacarpophalangeal (MCP) joint or to the distal interphalangeal (DIP) joint as necessary; further extension of the dissection may be required to free the extensor tendons over the dorsum of the hand or the wrist. Using a small elevator, the surgeon frees the dorsal apparatus from the underlying periosteum and callus (Fig. 16-5). Care must be taken to ensure that the lateral bands also are mobilized. In severe cases this procedure may have to be carried out over the entire length of the finger. In freeing the dorsal apparatus, care must be taken not to avulse the central tendon from its insertion on the dorsal base of the middle phalanx (Fig. 16-6).

The procedure is best done with the patient under local anesthesia and awake. This method allows the patient to actively demonstrate the ability to fully flex and extend the fingers during surgery. The use of local anesthesia also allows the patient to visualize the motion obtained and what he or she must strive for during postoperative therapy. If the patient is under general anesthesia during tenolysis, a traction flexor check should be done at the wrist to ensure that there are no adhesions present along the entire flexor system.

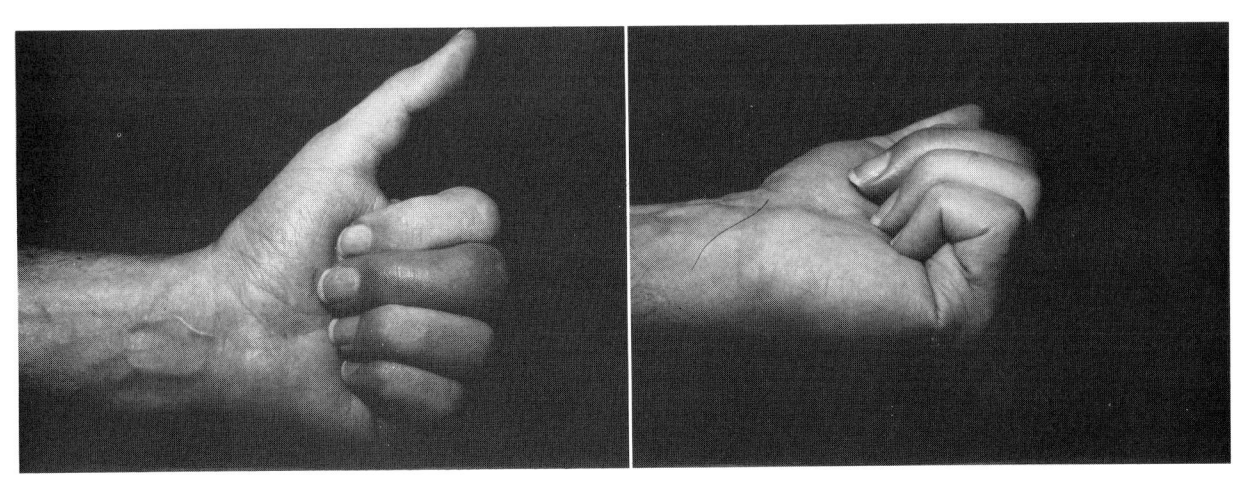

FIG. 16-9. TAM of patient in Fig. 16-4 after tenolysis shows elimination of check-rein effect of dorsal apparatus and improved excursion of extrinsic flexor tendons.

Flexor tenolysis

Flexor tenolysis is performed by exposing the flexor tendons throughout their length in the fibro-osseous canal either by a volar zigzag (Bruner) or midlateral incision[10,11,15,18] (Fig. 16-7). This procedure necessitates the isolation and protection of the neurovascular bundles and careful preservation of all possible pulleys. An elevator is passed along the flexor tendons to divide adhesions in the area of the phalangeal fracture (Fig. 16-8). Although the injury may have been local, adhesions can form throughout the length of the fiberosseous canal; care should be taken to ensure that all restricting adhesions are lysed. If a specific pulley is not salvageable, pulley reconstruction can be performed. Again, there is a distinct advantage in performing flexor tenolysis with the patient awake so that he or she can demonstrate the recovery of function and obviate the need for a proximal wrist flexor check.

Capsulotomy

Joint capsulotomy can be performed through either dorsal or volar approaches, depending on the nature of the contracture and which portions of the joint capsule require release. In cases of extension contracture the dorsal capsule and dorsal portions of the collateral ligaments are incised. Flexion contractures are managed by excision of the proximal (check-rein) portions of the volar plate and the accessory collateral ligaments. The retrovolar space between the proximal volar plate and the distal condyles of the proximal phalanx may be obliterated by fibrous connective tissue and should be reopened to restore proper joint motion. Local anesthesia again is recommended to ensure the patient's ability to actively move the digit through a full arc of motion.

Postoperative management

For each of these procedures active and passive motion is initiated the day after surgery. Dynamic splints are used as needed to maintain extension and flexion. Careful individual monitoring of finger performance is mandatory to make appropriate alterations in splinting and therapy (Fig. 16-9). Extension lag at the PIP joint is a frequent postoperative problem and can be best managed by extension splinting between exercise sessions.

RESULTS OF TENOLYSIS

In a review of patients who underwent tenolysis after phalangeal fracture there was a significant gain in total active motion (TAM)[1] in 20 of 27 patients (74%). (See Chapter 15.) The final gain in TAM for all patients was 43 degrees. For those patients who did improve, the average gain was 67.7 degrees, which represented a 49% increase in the total arc of motion (with a mean preoperative TAM of 139 degrees and mean postoperative TAM of 207 degrees). Forty percent of the patients who improved demonstrated an improvement of greater than 75% TAM with an average increase of 110 degrees. The greatest gain was 155 degrees in one finger.

Seven of the 27 patients (26%) did not improve. These failures could be attributed to the severity of the original fracture, to infection, or to a lack of patient cooperation.

Comminuted fracture	Transverse fracture	Oblique fracture	With extensor tendon injury	Without extensor tendon injury
60.0 degrees	19.2 degrees	25.8 degrees	57.0 degrees	50.3 degrees

In this study it was difficult to establish a correlation between the type of fracture and the results of tenolysis. Although comminuted fractures returned a poor range of motion after fracture, they demonstrated greater gains in TAM than did other fracture types, such as the above.

Fingers without concomitant tendon laceration showed an average increase of 50.3 degrees TAM after tenolysis; those with tendon injuries showed an increase of 57 degrees. Those patients who underwent tenolysis within 16 weeks of injury had an increased arc of motion of 52.4 degrees, whereas those with tenolysis performed after 16 weeks had an average increase in total arc of motion of 30 degrees.

CONCLUSIONS

Adhesions between bone callus and adjacent flexor or extensor tendons are frequently overlooked causes of motion loss after phalangeal fracture. Overenthusiastic splinting or exercise programs for these fingers may actually do more harm than good by stretching or rupturing tendons distal to the area of adherence. When the motion of the digital joints has plateaued at an unacceptable total arc, consideration should be given to tenolysis, combined with capsulotomy if necessary. In this chapter we have shown that lysis of tendon-bone adhesions can be an effective method of regaining lost motion after phalangeal fracture. It is clear that appropriately selected patients can benefit significantly from these procedures even after severe digital injuries. It is important that the surgeon be thoroughly familiar with the techniques of tenolysis and capsulotomy and that the patient be well motivated and understand the rationale for these procedures.

REFERENCES

1. American Society for Surgery of the Hand: The hand: examination and diagnosis, Aurora, Colo., 1978, American Society for Surgery of the Hand.
2. Curtis, R.M.: Capsulectomy of the interphalangeal joints of the fingers, J. Bone Joint Surg. **36A:**1219, 1954.
3. Drury, B.: Para-articular fusion of the proximal interphalangeal joint of the hand, Cal. Med. **90:**37, 1958.
4. Fetrow, K.O.: Tenolysis in the hand and wrist: a clinical evaluation of 220 flexor and extensor tenolyses, J. Bone Joint Surg. **49A:**667, 1967.
5. Hurst, L.N., McCain, W.G., and Lindsay, W.K.: Results of tenolysis: a controlled evaluation in chickens, Plast. Reconstr. Surg. **52:**171, 1973.
6. McCormack, R.M.: Stiffness of the injured hand, J. Trauma **4:**581, 1964.
7. McMurtry, R.V., and Murray, J.F.: Management of phalangeal fractures, J. Hand Surg. **6:**295, 1981.
8. Peacock, E.E., Jr., and Van Winkle, W., Jr.: Wound repair, ed. 2, Philadelphia, 1976, W.B. Saunders Co.
9. Pratt, D.R.: Joints of the hand and fingers—their stiffness, splinting and surgery, Cal. Med. **66:**22, 1947.
10. Schneider, L.H., and Hunter, J.M.: Flexor tenolysis. In American Academy of Orthopaedic Surgeons: Symposium on Tendon Surgery in the Hand, St. Louis, 1975, The C.V. Mosby Co.
11. Schneider, L.H., and Mackin, E.J.: Tenolysis. In Hunter, J.M., et al., editors: Rehabilitation of the hand, St. Louis, 1978, The C.V. Mosby Co.
12. Sprague, B.L.: Proximal interphalangeal joint contractures and their treatment, J. Trauma **16:**259, 1976.
13. Strickland, J.W., et al.: Phalangeal fractures in a hand surgery practice: a statistical review and in-depth study of the management of proximal phalangeal shaft fractures, J. Hand Surg. **4:**285, 1979.
14. Tubiana, R., and Valentin. P.: The physiology of the extension of the fingers, Surg. Clin. North Am. **44:**907, 1964.
15. Verdan, C.E., Crawford, G.P., and Martini-Benkedache, Y.: The valuable role of tenolysis in the digits. In Cramer, L.M., and Chase, R.A., editors: Symposium on the hand, vol. 3, St. Louis, 1971, The C.V. Mosby Co.
16. Weckesser, E.C., Littler, J.W., Stack, H.G., et al.: Panel discussion: mobilization of the stiffened proximal interphalangeal joint, J. Bone Joint Surg. **46:**917, 1964.
17. Weeks, P.M., and Wray, R.C.: Management of acute hand injuries, ed. 2, St. Louis, 1978, The C.V. Mosby Co.
18. Whitaker, J.H., Strickland, J.W., and Ellis, R.K.: The role of flexor tenolysis in the palm and digits, J. Hand Surg. **2:**462, 1977.

SUGGESTED READINGS

Craver, J.M., Madden, J.W., and Peacock, E.E., Jr.: The effect of sutures, immobilization and tenolysis on healing of tendons: a method for measuring work of digital flexion in a chicken's foot, Surgery **64:**437, 1968.

Potenza, A.D.: Critical evaluation of flexor-tendon healing and adhesion formation within artificial digital sheaths, J. Bone Joint Surg. **45A:**1217, 1963.

Wray, R.C., Jr., Moucharafieh, B., and Weeks, P.M.: Experimental study of the optimal time for tenolysis, Plast. Reconstr. Surg. **61:**184, 1978.

SECTION FIVE INFECTION PROBLEMS

Chapter 17 The management of difficult infections of the hand

Thomas L. Greene
James W. Strickland

The symptoms, signs, and principles of treatment of common infectious processes in the hand are generally well known to most physicians. In a medical practice partially or exclusively devoted to surgery of the hand, however, one will encounter infections with unusual and difficult diagnostic and/or treatment problems. These occur either as a result of initial diagnostic or treatment failure or from complications of surgical procedures that in their own right are considered difficult hand surgery problems.

Many of these difficult infections are chronic. They may have been treated previously by one or more physicians, frequently without adequate diagnostic procedures to identify the causative organism. To further complicate the situation, injudicious or limited surgical procedures may increase the tissue destruction and spreading of the infection before definitive care can be obtained. Delay by the patient in seeking medical care also can result in a more extensive disease process when first seen.

Most infections, including many discussed here, are caused by common organisms. The bacteriology and antimicrobial susceptibility of these organisms are generally well established and are not discussed in detail. It is beyond the scope of this chapter to discuss in detail the numerous unusual or difficult infections that could be encountered. Discussion therefore is limited primarily to tuberculosis, the sequelae of neglected common infections, necrotizing fasciitis, and infections complicated by the presence of systemic diseases or implanted foreign material.

MYCOBACTERIAL INFECTIONS

Certain organisms are, by their nature, slow growing and typically lead to a chronic and clinically occult infectious process. *Mycobacterium tuberculosis* may cause slowly progressive, painless tensosynovitis about the wrist and palm. Synovitis or arthritis of the joints of the wrist and hand also can occur and leads to extensive joint destruction (Figs. 17-1 and 17-2). Diagnosis is established by the presence of granulomas and mycobacteria in the tissues. Treatment consists of thorough debridement of all involved tissues, and on occasion arthrodesis may be necessary when there is severe joint destruction.[5] Depending on the extent of disease and the degree of clinical suspicion that *M. tuberculosis* is present, administration of one or more antituberculotic drugs is begun promptly, since confirmation by culture may take up to 6 weeks.[5]

Infections caused by nontuberculotic mycobacteria—*M. avium*, *M. kansasii*, and *M. marinum*—are being recognized with greater frequency.[3] They are usually the result of direct inoculation of the hand and may present as chronic ulcerations that may involve tendon sheaths, bursae, or joints.[3] Isolation of *M. marinum* by culture requires incubation at 30° to 32° C, as opposed to other mycobacteria that are grown at 37° C.[8]

Treatment of nontuberculotic mycobacterial infections also involves thorough debridement of involved tissues. Specific drug therapy is determined by sensitivity testing of the organism, since the nontuberculotic mycobacteria, especially *M. marinum*, may be resistant to the usual antituberculotic drugs: isoniazid, aminosalicylic acid, and streptomycin.[8]

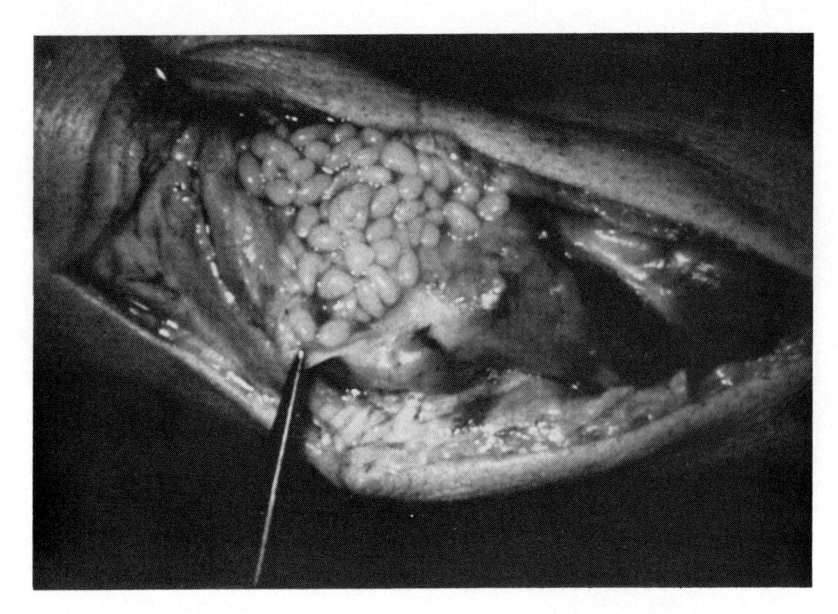

FIG. 17-1. Synovitis of wrist caused by *M. tuberculosis,* demonstrating abundant rice body formation. Differentiation from rheumatoid synovitis is made by presence of typical granulomas and mycobacteria in histologic sections and by culture of organism.

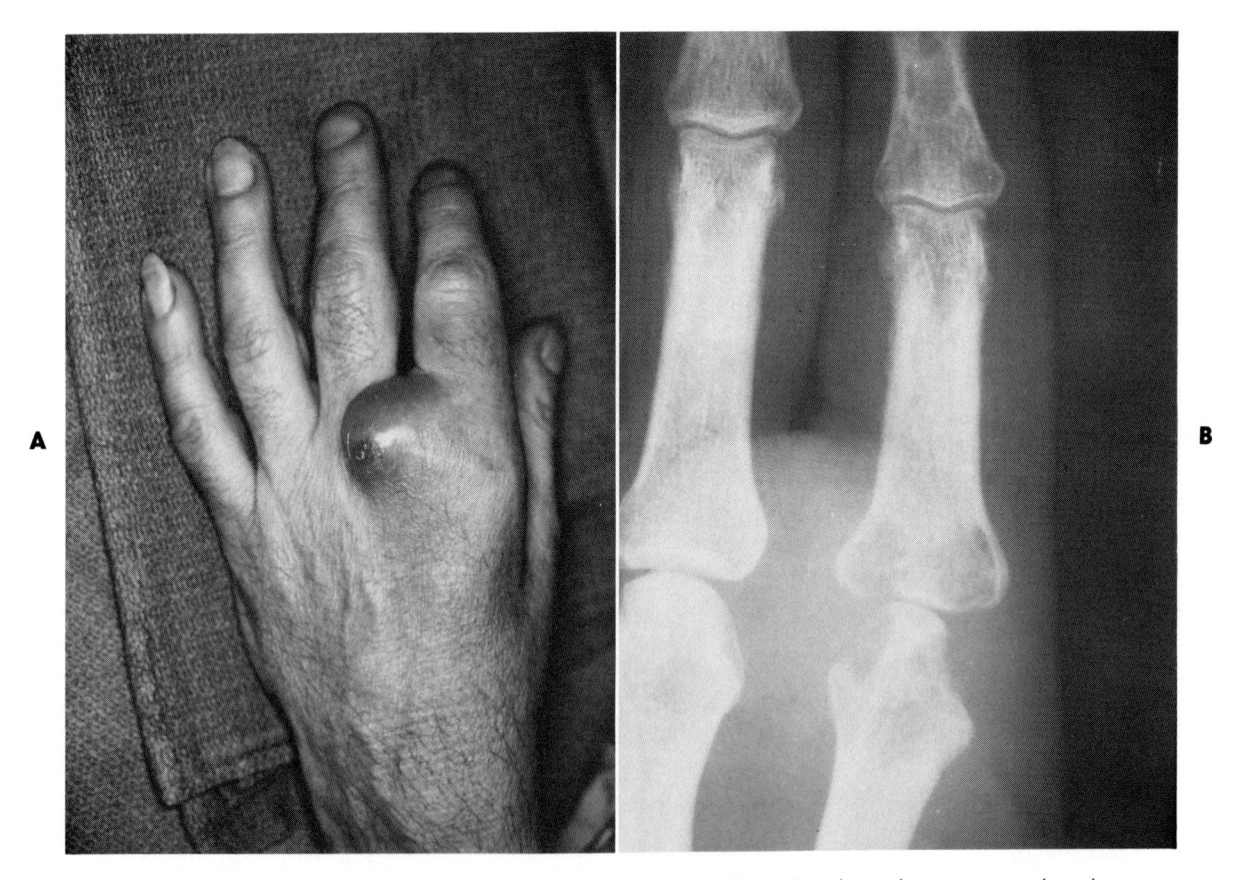

FIG. 17-2. A, Slowly enlarging mass and soft tissue swelling developed over second metacarpophalangeal joint. **B,** Radiograph demonstrates considerable erosion of most of adjacent surfaces of joint. Excision of soft tissue mass and complete synovectomy of joint led to diagnosis of tuberculosis. Isoniazid was given for 3 months. Excellent range of motion of joint resulted, and there was no recurrence of tuberculous arthritis.

NEGLECTED INFECTIONS

It is distressing that we continue to see severe infections that began as common, readily treated diseases and evolved into extensive destructive lesions with a guarded prognosis for normal functional recovery. Limited treatment by inexperienced personnel, compounded in some cases by patient neglect, is all too often the summary of events.

Infections about the fingertips (paronychia and felon in particular) are quite common. Adequate drainage and antistaphylococcic antibiotics can predictably result in cure. Inadequate drainage and delay in the hope that the infection will resolve can lead to extensive spread along the soft tissues of the digit and invasion of bone or tendon sheath, occasionally compromising the viability of the digit. Treatment of such infections requires wide and thorough drainage and debridement of necrotic tissues, including tendon and bone when necessary (Fig. 17-3). Specific antibiotics for the organisms cultured should be given in sufficient dosages until the tissues are healed, which may require up to 6 weeks if osteomyelitis has occurred. Hospitalization for intravenous antibiotic administration should be routine for these severe infections. Amputation of nonviable parts or of digits destroyed beyond hope of useful function should be considered early in the course of treatment (Fig. 17-4).

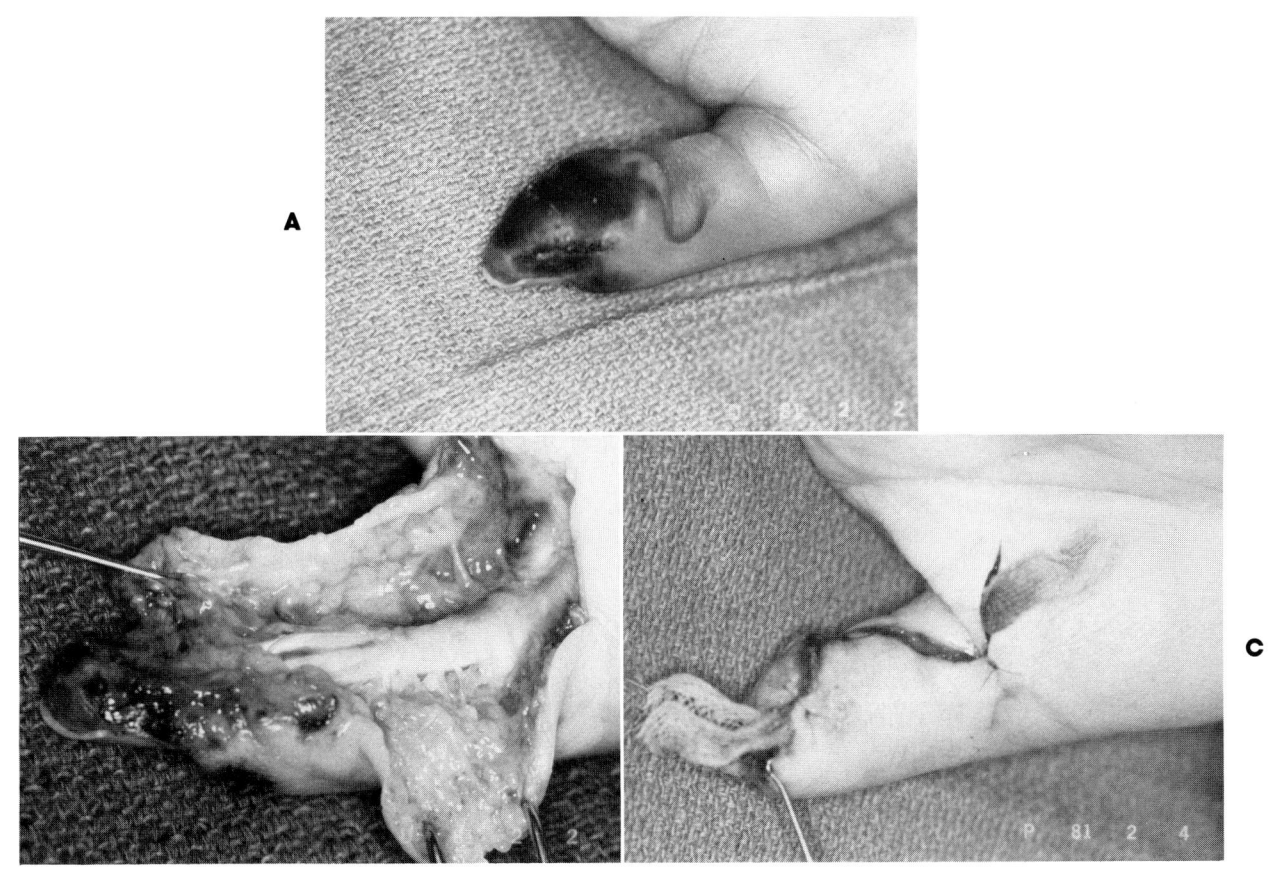

FIG. 17-3. A 36-year-old hairdresser developed acute pain and swelling of tip of left thumb without definite history of injury. Twenty-four hours later, attempt at drainage of pulp through two lateral incisions was made. Infection continued to develop, and necrosis of pulp became evident **(A)**, at which point she was referred for further care. Extensive volar incision allowed drainage of soft tissue abscess and flexor sheath, which also had become involved **(B)**. Necrotic distal phalanx was removed, and wound was closed loosely over drains **(C)**. Cultures grew *S. aureus.* Intravenous antibiotics and wound care resulted in prompt resolution of infection.

SECTION 5 INFECTION PROBLEMS

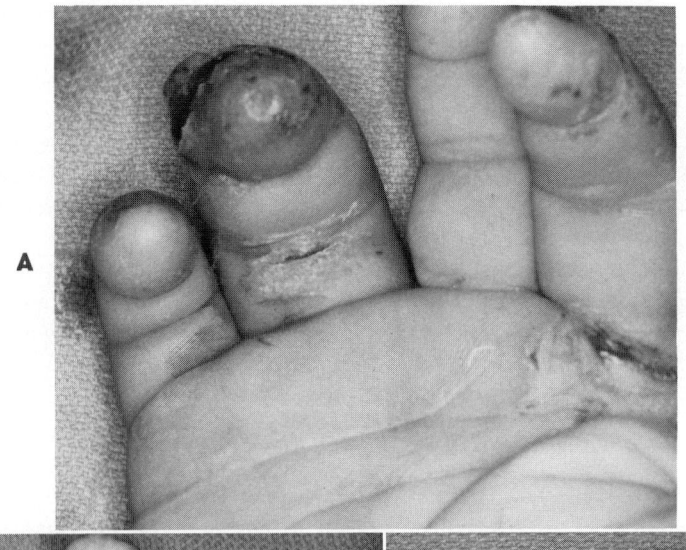

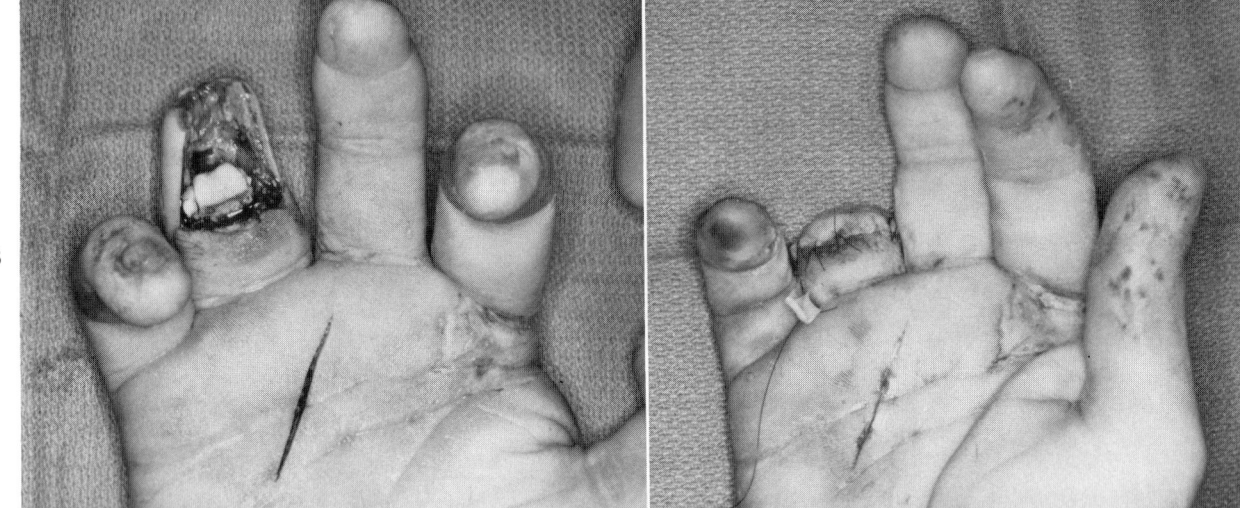

FIG. 17-4. Crush injury to distal phalanx of right ring finger was neglected by otherwise healthy 50-year-old meat cutter. When first evaluated, digit was massively swollen and diffusely fluctuant, and distal phalanx was deformed, necrotic, and draining abundant purulent material **(A)**. Primary open amputation through proximal interphalangeal (PIP) joint and excision of necrotic flexor tendons from digit and palm were performed **(B)**. *S. aureus* was cultured and was resistant to penicillin. Delayed primary closure 5 days later **(C)** along with continued antibiotic therapy resulted in subsidence of infection.

NECROTIZING FASCIITIS

Although most soft tissue infections of the hand are caused by common gram-positive organisms, significant exceptions occur. A variety of gram-negative organisms may be responsible, particularly after injury involving contaminated organic materials.[1]

Necrotizing fasciitis is a rapidly spreading infection of the superficial fascia of the skin and produces necrosis extending to the subcutaneous adipose tissue and eventually the overlying skin[4] (Fig. 17-5). The investing fascia of the muscles may be involved in the necrotic process. Myonecrosis, typical of clostridial gas gangrene, does not occur, but some of the offending organisms may produce gas in the soft tissues. The infection appears as areas of erythema, pain, and edema that progress to form central patches of purple with serosanguineous bullae[4]. The central areas of skin develop necrosis in several days. The infection tends to spread rapidly along subcutaneous tissue planes. The patient is systemically ill, and sepsis or metastatic infection may ensue.

Streptococcus pyogenes classically have been the or-

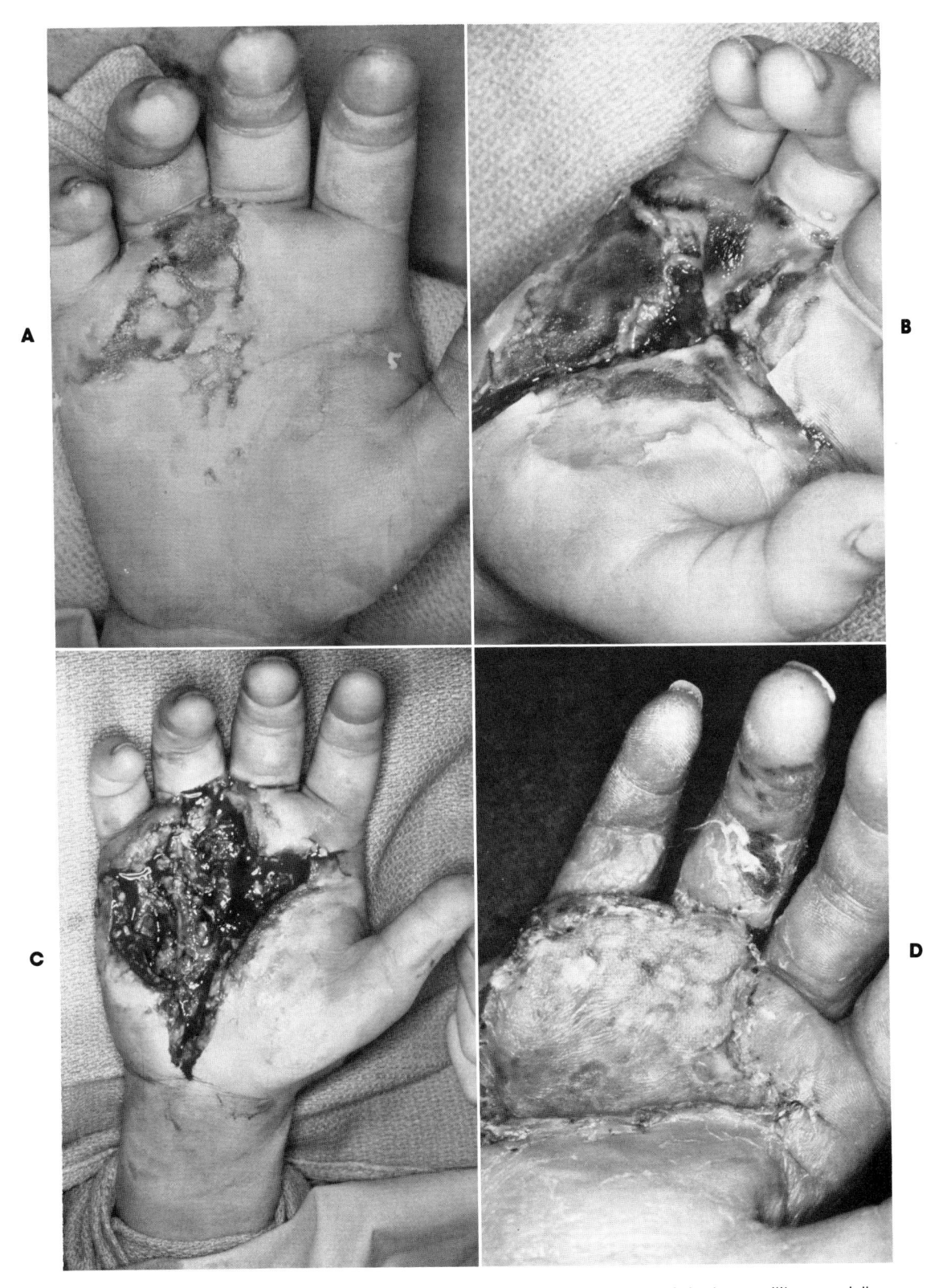

FIG. 17-5. A 22-year-old woman, who had brittle juvenile onset diabetes mellitus, rapidly developed extensive cellulitis of right palm with bullae and areas of early skin necrosis **(A)**. Incision and drainage of palm were followed by continued spread of infection and more extensive skin necrosis **(B)**. Debridement of all necrotic and infected tissues **(C)** was followed by delayed split-thickness skin grafting **(D)**. Cultures grew *S. aureus* and group A beta-hemolytic streptococci.

ganisms responsible for this severe infection,[7] but more recently a variety of aerobic, anaerobic, and facultative anaerobic organisms has been isolated from these wounds.[2] Typically more than one organism is recovered. A synergism between the facultative anaerobic organisms frequently isolated, such as streptococci and *Enterobacteriaceae* organisms, and anaerobic bacteria, usually bacteroides or *Fusobacterium* organisms, has been implicated in this infectious process.[2]

Early recognition of this entity is essential. Gram stain of the bullous fluid or wound aspirate will help in choosing the appropriate antibiotic therapy. Cultures for anaerobic as well as aerobic organisms are mandatory. Radical excision and debridement of all the involved skin, subcutaneous tissue, and fascia are the most important parts of treatment.[4]

Anaerobic bacteria are being isolated more frequently with the advent of improved culture techniques. The presence of anaerobic organisms should be suspected and appropriate antibiotic coverage begun when purulent drainage has the characteristic fetid odor or when the Gram stain smear demonstrates their presence.

SYSTEMIC DISEASE COMPLICATING INFECTION

In dealing with extensive infections, one should be alert for the possibility that a predisposing systemic disease or circulatory problem exists. Diabetes mellitus, especially when under poor control, can be a major factor contributing to the extensive nature of an infection and its resistance to treatment.[6] In some instances diabetes may have been previously undiagnosed. Serum glucose studies should be a routine procedure for patients with an infectious process.

During the course of a severe infection occult hematologic malignancies also may be detected for the first time by the presence of neutropenia or thrombocytopenia. Circulatory compromise from conditions such as Raynaud's disease, thromboangiitis obliterans (Buerger's disease), atherosclerotic disease of the major vessels, and emboli can lead to spreading of the infection and ineffectiveness of the antibiotic therapy. These problems should be recognized by appropriate history taking or physical examination. Unfortunately their presence may preclude successful treatment by anything short of amputation.

FOREIGN MATERIALS AND INFECTIONS

Retained foreign material often can lead to an infectious process and remain as a cause of chronicity and resistance to treatment if not recognized. The possibility of a foreign body must be considered for injuries caused by metal or wooden objects. The possibility of unusual foreign bodies should be considered when an infection does not respond to antibiotics and drainage procedures (Fig. 17-6).

A foreign material commonly used in hand surgery is silicone rubber in its various prosthetic forms. Infections following implantation of these devices are usually caused by common organisms, and the presence of infection ultimately may require removal of the prosthesis, which may be detrimental to the results of the initial procedure. Silicone prostheses are commonly used as replacements for certain carpal bones (trapezium, scaphoid, and lunate) and as interpositional arthroplasties in the metacarpophalangeal and PIP joints. When infection develops about these implants, either early or late in the postoperative period, removal of the prosthesis, thorough and continued drainage of purulent material, and appropriate antibiotic therapy will usually result in a cure. In spite of removal of the prosthesis, a satisfactory result can occur, particularly in the carpal bones. Here the abundant scar tissue that forms can make possible a table resection arthroplasty (Fig. 17-7).

Use of silicone rubber prostheses to prepare a suitable tissue bed for tendon graft procedures is accepted as routine. Purulent tenosynovitis may ensue if secure anchorage of the distal aspect of the prosthesis is not accomplished and erosion through the skin occurs. These can be quite devastating infections and may completely obviate the possibility of further tendon reconstruction if prompt and aggressive treatment is not initiated. Initial incision and drainage of the tendon sheath combined with intermittent irrigation through catheters occasionally may be successful; but for more established infections removal of the prosthesis should be a part of the drainage procedure. In an attempt to salvage the pseudosheath for future tendon grafting a heavy gauge, nonreactive suture such as Prolene may be placed in the sheath and secured proximally and distally. Postoperatively tendon sheath irrigation may be continued. Once the infection has resolved, a free-tendon graft may be placed in the newly created tendon sheath, its course having been preserved by the suture, dilating the sheath as needed for easy passage of the graft.

SUMMARY

Acute or chronic infections can be expected to be encountered by the hand surgeon. Knowledge of unusual types of organisms and conditions encountered is required for prompt recognition and treatment. An aggressive management approach involving appropriate microbial cultures and antibiotic sensitivity determinations, followed by the initiation of specific antibiotic therapy and thorough surgical drainage and debridement procedures, can be expected to result in the cure of a high percentage of infections while maintaining the functional capability of the hand.

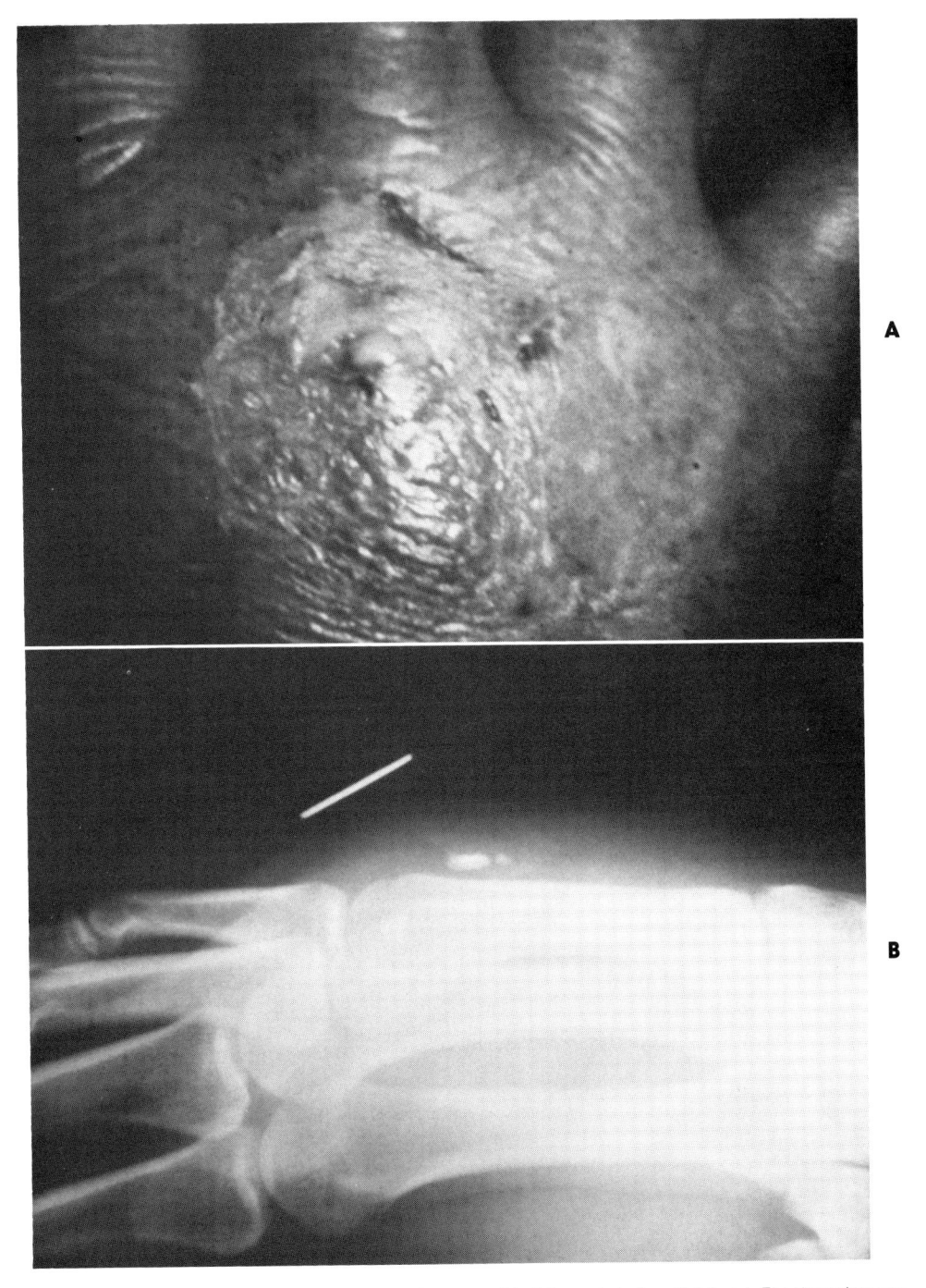

CHAPTER 17 THE MANAGEMENT OF DIFFICULT INFECTIONS OF THE HAND

FIG. 17-6. Young male sustained injury to dorsum of left hand during fist fight. Fluctuant mass developed over dorsum of hand, which was treated with two limited incision and drainage procedures that were not successful. At time of referral, sinus-draining purulence was present over third metacarpal dorsally **(A)**. Radiograph was obtained with metallic marker over sinus. Radiopaque foreign body can be seen over dorsum of metacarpal **(B)**. Wide incision and drainage and removal of large fragment of dental cap eventually led to resolution of infection.

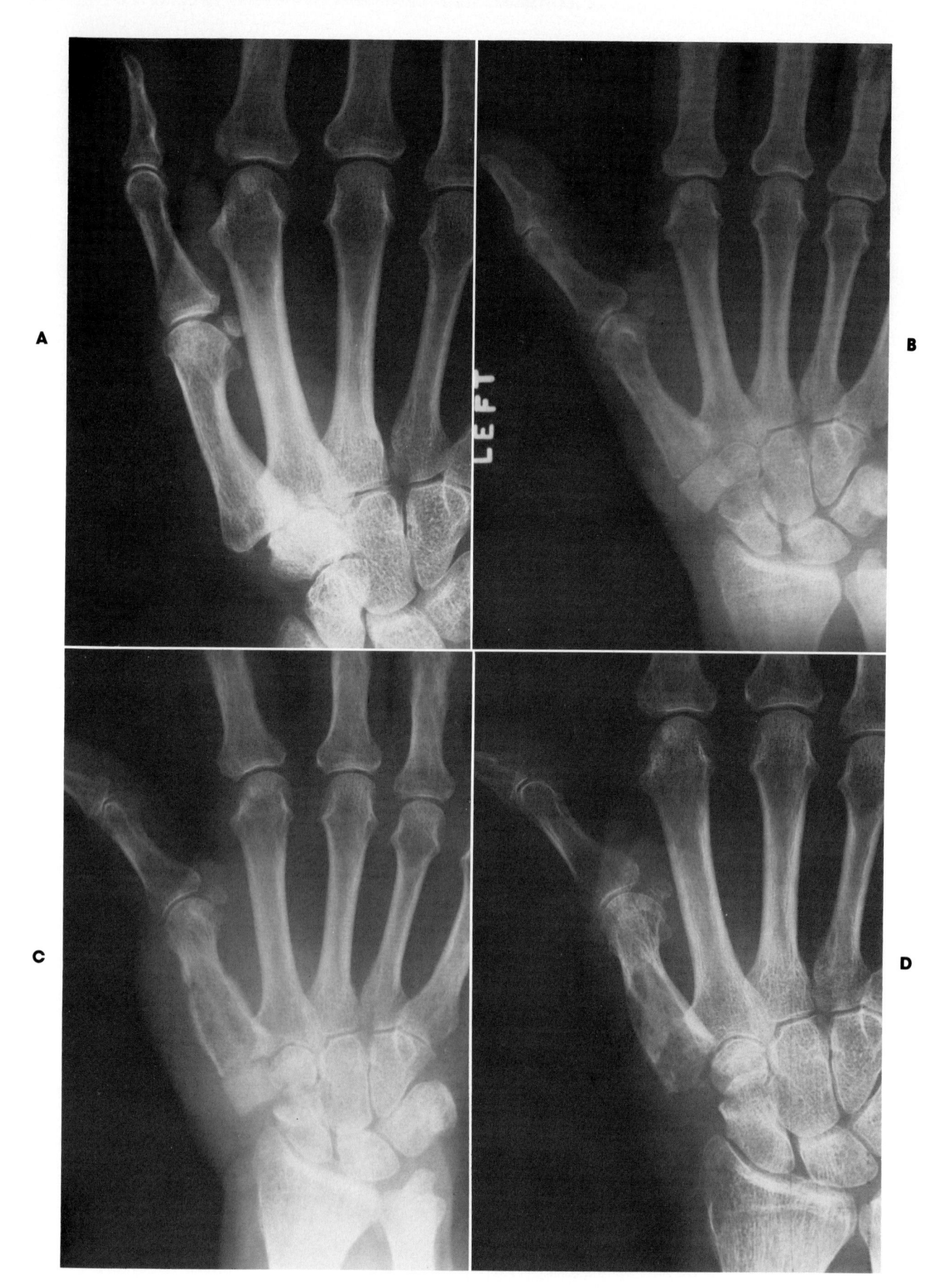

FIG. 17-7. For legend see opposite page.

FIG. 17-7. Pantrapezial degenerative arthritis of thumb **(A)** was treated by silicone replacement arthroplasty of trapezium **(B)**. Three months postoperatively pain and swelling developed about thumb. Radiograph **(C)** at that time demonstrated dislocation of prosthesis from scaphoid and expansion and erosion of intramedullary canal of first metacarpal with diffuse periosteal reaction. Treatment consisted of removal of prosthesis, thorough debridement of area, open-wound management, and intravenous antibiotics. In follow-up radiograph **(D)** osteomyelitis had resolved with maintenance of space between first metacarpal and scaphoid. Thumb was stable and pain free and had good mobility.

REFERENCES

1. Fitzgerald, R.H., et al.: Bacterial colonization of mutilating hand injuries and its treatment, J. Hand Surg. **2**:85, 1977.
2. Giuliano, A., et al.: Bacteriology of necrotizing fasciitis, Am. J. Surg. **134**:52, 1977.
3. Gunther, S.F., et al.: Experience with atypical mycobacterial infection of the deep structures of the hand, J. Hand Surg. **2**:90, 1977.
4. Koehn, G.G.: Necrotizing fasciitis, Arch. Dermatol. **114**:581, 1978.
5. Linscheid, R.L., and Dobyns, J.H.: Common and uncommon infections of the hand, Orthop. Clin. North Am. **6**:1063, 1975.
6. Mandel, M.A.: Immune competence and diabetes mellitus: pyogenic human hand infections, J. Hand Surg. **3**:458, 1978.
7. Meleney, F.L.: Hemolytic streptococcus gangrene, Arch. Surg. **9**:317, 1924.
8. Williams, C.S., and Riordan, D.C.: *Mycobacterium marinum* (atypical acid-fast bacillus) infections of the hand, J. Bone Joint Surg. **55A**:1042, 1973.

Chapter 18 Difficult infections of the hand

Lawrence H. Schneider

There is no question that hand infections, particularly those of a more serious nature, are decreasing in incidence. The systemically ill patient with a life-threatening hand infection is rare. Many busy clinics have reported that, although they continue to see hand infections, the serious deep palmar abscesses are almost unknown. This has been attributed to the improved local care given by physicians to all wounds in general and the availability of specific antibiotic therapies that may prevent major infections from developing from those of a relatively minor nature. There are still occasions when the surgeon is confronted with a difficult infection problem, and the application of the most basic principles of good extremity surgery will be tested. Those who treat infections of the hand stand in great debt to the work of Kanavel[12] and his associates.[13,16] Even though the patient's life rarely is threatened, the ravages of hand infection still can be very disabling to function of the hand. Preservation of function is the goal when difficult infections are encountered.

When reviewing the case histories of patients with more serious infection problems, it is clear that there are several factors, not all under the control of the surgeon, that come into play in determining the functional result.

DIAGNOSIS

The presence of infection is usually clearly discernible, but the diagnosis must be confirmed by laboratory methods. Cultures have to be adequate, and in the difficult infection more than the routine aerobic culture may be needed. In cases that respond poorly the presence of anaerobes must be suspected. In the chronic problem the possibility of fungi or acid-fast bacilli must be considered. Rheumatoid arthritis, gout, calcific tendinitis, and tumors in their various presentations all have been treated as infection, with the reverse also being true.

ADEQUACY OF PRIOR TREATMENT

The use of antibiotics in adequate dosage is recommended after culture. In the acute infection the use of synthetic penicillins, effective against penicillinase-producing staphylococci, must be considered. However, one must not rely solely on antibiotic therapy in a localized infection. Surgical drainage must be used and used adequately with respect for the rules regarding incisions in the hand. Repeat drainage must be performed if early drainage proves inadequate in detering the progress of the infectious process. Drainage also produces material for culture necessary for definitive diagnosis.

THE NATURE OF THE ORGANISM

Some bacterial species are observed to be more virulent than others, especially in synergistic combinations or in the patient weakened by disease. This includes patients immunologically debilitated by the use of systemic steroids. The injection of local steroids may lower resistance on a local basis.

Now, in the antibiotic era, difficult hand infections still are encountered, as illustrated in the following case studies.

SECTION 5 INFECTION PROBLEMS

SEPTIC TENOSYNOVITIS

Deep infections such as palmar space abscesses being rare, the most common infection that significantly threatens hand function is flexor tenosynovitis. The causative organism is usually a *Staphylococcus* organism entering the sheath via a puncture or other open wound. When this condition is recognized, treatment is straightforward. Very early in the disease, antibiotics and splinting of the hand can be justified if close observation is possible. If there is any suggestion that purulent material is present in the tendon sheath, then drainage is recommended. Although authors[2,20] have washed out the sheath and installed tubes for closed irrigation, an open technique is preferred. A midlateral incision in the finger to drain the sheath between the pulleys, combined with a transverse opening in the palm, will allow satisfactory drainage. Preservation of the pulleys is necessary for later function. Active motion is started to maintain mobility when drains are removed at 24 to 48 hours. Although most fingers can be returned to full function, at times, because of delay or a particularly virulent organism, the result can be catastrophic.

Case 1

A 40-year-old man lacerated the volar aspect of his right index finger on a power saw blade. The wound was cleansed and closed in an accident ward on the day of injury. Despite antibiotic therapy, infection in the flexor tendon sheath supervened and did not respond to two operative drainage attempts. Cultures revealed the presence of *Staphylococcus epidermidis,* and when transferred to our service 31 days after injury, the patient exhibited

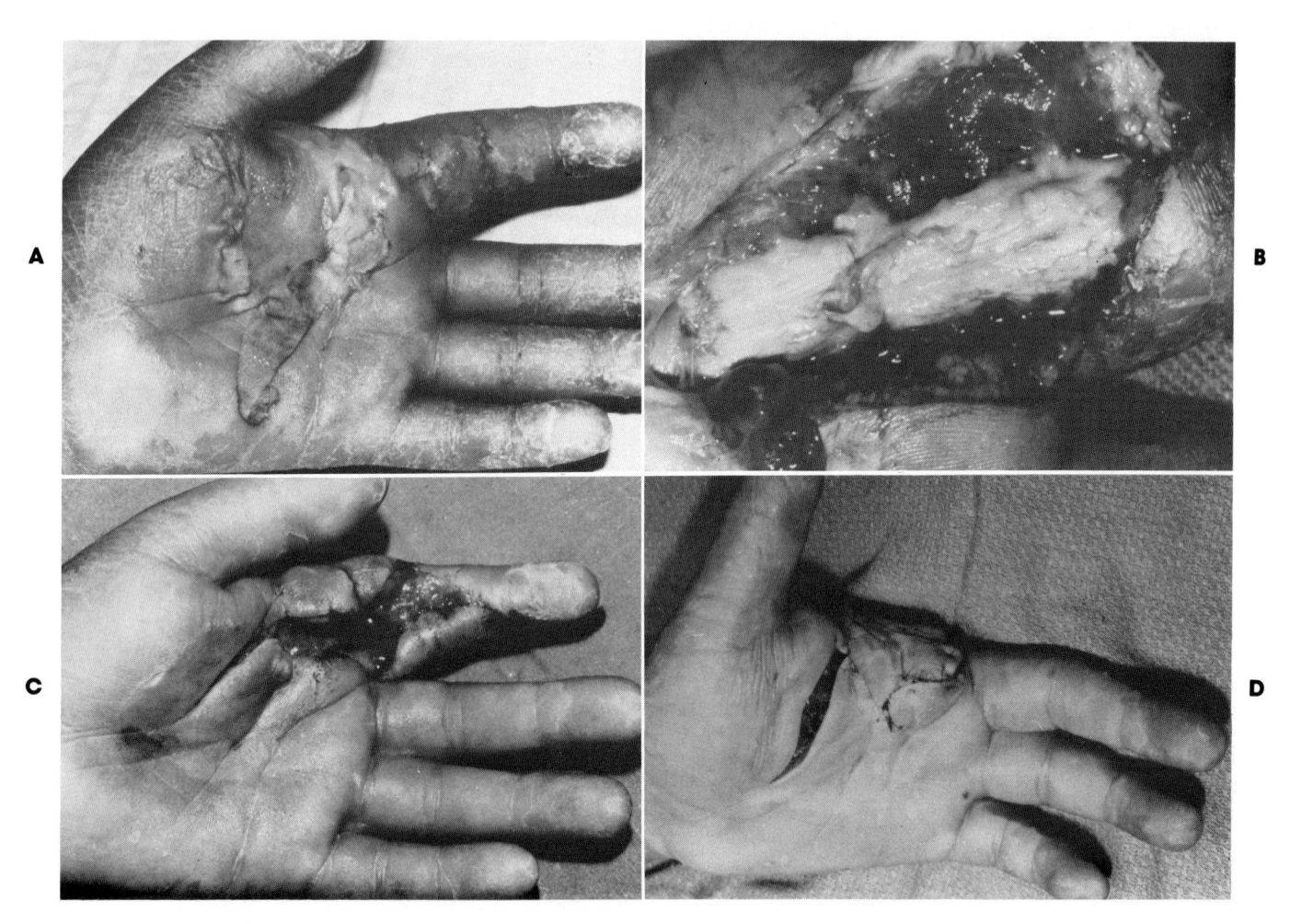

FIG. 18-1. Septic tenosynovitis. **A,** There was massive destruction of soft tissue plus bone infection at 31 days after injury. **B,** Close-up of flexor tendon shows marked involvement by infection. **C,** Necessary debridement of grossly involved tissues left finger with no chance for reasonable function. **D,** Ray resection soon after allowed patient to mobilize his remaining digits. **E** and **F,** Function attained 6 weeks later.

destruction of the soft tissues of the index finger and osteomyelitis involving the proximal phalanx (Fig. 18-1, *A* and *B*). His hand was stiff, with motion limited at all joints. Immediate debridement of all infected tissue (Fig. 18-1, *C*) with cultures revealed the presence of *Eikenella corrodens*. With a functionally nonviable finger, ray resection (Fig. 18-1, *D*) soon after enabled the patient to enter an intensive hand therapy program, which salvaged function in what was the uninvolved portion of his hand (Fig. 18-1, *E* and *F*).

Comment. An unusual combination of pathogens combined with soft tissue destruction by the original trauma led to the loss of this finger. If an aggressive surgical program had not finally evolved, this patient would have suffered a functional loss of much of his hand.

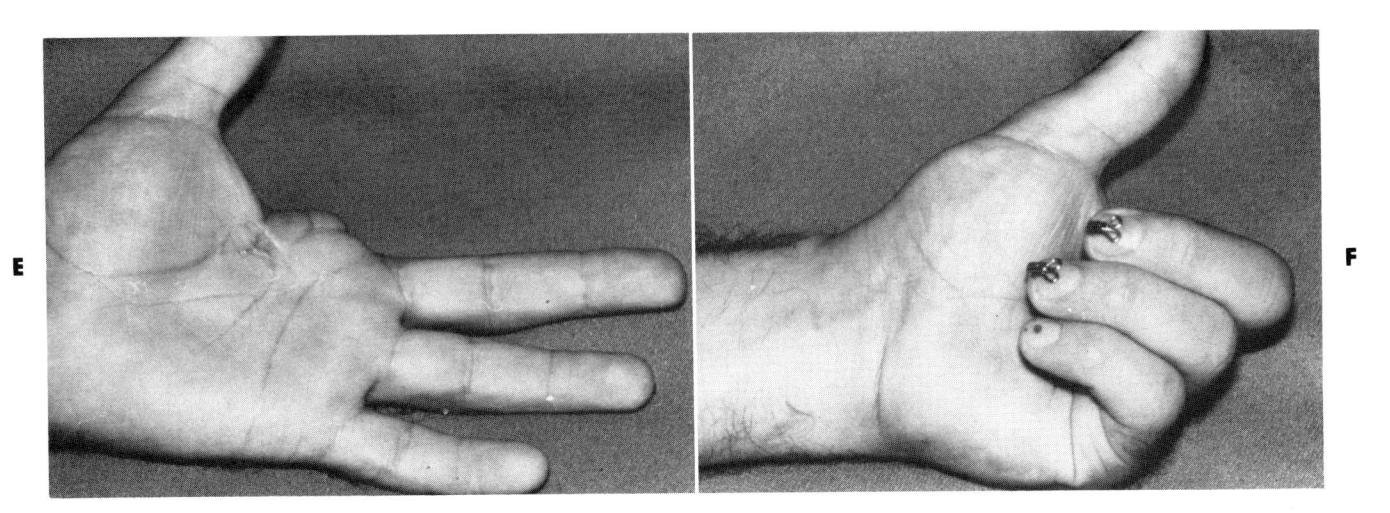

FIG. 18-1, cont'd. For legend see opposite page.

SECTION 5   INFECTION PROBLEMS

FUNGAL INFECTION IN THE HAND

It is rare to find a fungus as the causative agent in deep hand infection. Problems, when seen, are usually cutaneous or subcutaneous, but there are only sporadic reports of deeper involvement in the hand.[5,6,8,11] When fungal infections are systemic, there often is a debilitated patient or one compromised by immunosuppressant agents or steroids. In patients with chronic infection in the hand, fungal cultures may be indicated, especially if the infection is associated with a patient undergoing chemotherapy or one weakened by chronic disease.

Case 2

A 65-year-old physician had chronic tenosynovitis on the dorsum of his hand (Fig. 18-2, *A*). This had begun spontaneously and had not responded to self-administered injections of hydrocortisone into the dorsum of the hand. The patient deferred surgery, and his condition deteriorated, until, 8 months and approximately 40 hydrocortisone injections later, exploration and synovectomy were carried out (Fig. 18-2, *B*). Cultures showed no bacterial growth. Fungal cultures grew an organism finally identified as *Phialophora gougerotii*. The wound healed slowly with maximal interference by the patient (Fig. 18-2, *C*). Six months later a second, more radical excision of the synovium ultimately brought the condition under control (Fig. 18-2, *D*).

Comment. An unusual contaminant found a steroid-enriched area in which it thrived. Only radical debridement brought the condition under control. There is no satisfactory practical drug therapy when this particular organism is localized in the synovial tissues of the hand.

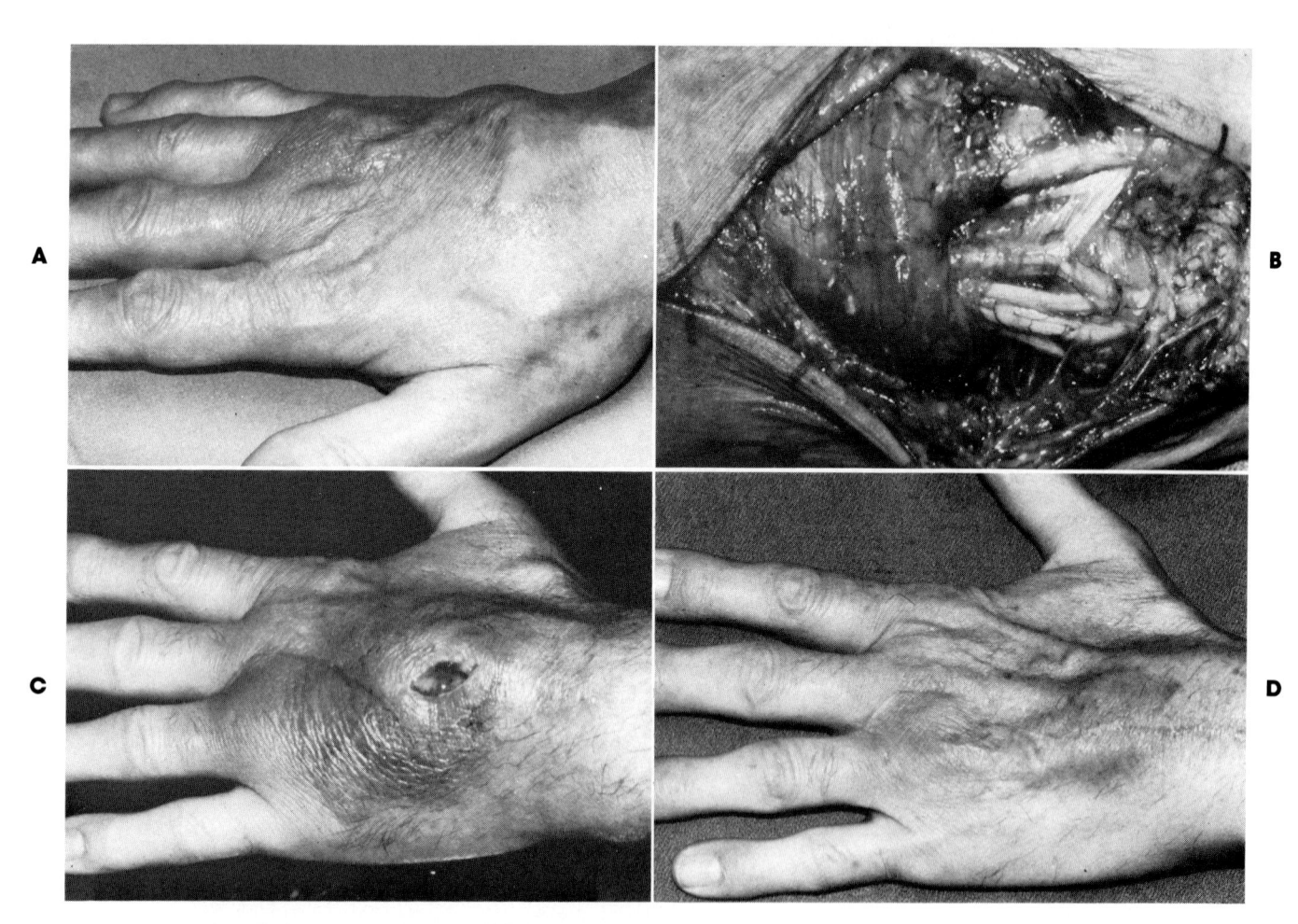

FIG. 18-2. Fungal infection. **A,** Chronic tenosynovitis at dorsum of hand, self-treated with injections of hydrocortisone. **B,** Marked involvement of tenosynovium is seen at synovectomy carried out after 8 months and 40 injections. **C,** Area healed slowly with maximal interference by patient. **D,** Second, more radical excision of tenosynovium ultimately controlled condition. Patient recovered full range of motion.

CHAPTER 18 DIFFICULT INFECTIONS OF THE HAND

INFECTION CAUSED BY HUMAN TOOTH

It is now generally recognized that a hand wound caused by a human tooth must be treated vigorously. Debridement, proper cultures, antibiotics, and open treatment of the wound usually will preserve function. Early papers on this subject stressed the importance of fusiform bacilli and spirochetes[10] as causative agents in these infections. Later reports[7,15] stated that streptococci in combination with these organisms as well as S. aureus were the significant offenders. Also seen in combination with the streptococci were various gram-negative bacteria thought to be acting synergistically with the gram-positive cocci.

Mann, Hoffeld, and Farmer,[15] in a recent publication, reviewed the literature and presented 136 human bite wounds as well as an extensive bibliography on the subject. Their cases most commonly involved infections by streptococci and staphylococci. S. aureus was most frequently seen in the wounds that did poorly. Their recommended treatment includes hospital admission and extensive surgical debridement with all wounds left open. They use a penicillinase-resistant analogue of penicillin and gentamicin. The antibiotics are adjusted when bacteriologic studies so suggest. The hand is rested in a splint, and at about 48 hours active motion is begun. When the infection is seen to be under control, the patient is released to outpatient care.

Goldstein and associates[7] stress the importance of anaerobic and 10% CO_2 cultures along with the aerobic cultures. Their cases showed mainly streptococci and staphylococci, but 60% of the small series also had anaerobic bacteria present. These included bacteroides and *Eikenella corrodens*.[1] This last pathogen is interesting in that, although sensitive to penicillin, it usually is resistant to the synthetic penicillins. This prompted the authors to suggest the use of both penicillin and a penicillinase-resistant penicillin as initial empiric therapy of "clenched fist" injuries pending results of the cultures.

Even with the best treatment the frequent delays in reaching care seen in these patients often preclude a good functional result.

Case 3

A 25-year-old man sustained a laceration over the long finger metacarpophalangeal joint from an opponent's tooth during an altercation. He was admitted for treatment 24 hours later in pain, with the wound surrounded by edema and erythema (Fig. 18-3, *A*). There was a watery discharge. The patient was hospitalized and the wound debrided and packed open. Intravenous penicillin was given, and the extremity was elevated and rested on a splint. One day later he was started on intermittent open soaks and active motion. Cultures revealed the presence of *S. aureus*. He was discharged with oral antibiotic medication on the fifth day to be monitored on an outpatient basis. He gradually recovered function over the next month (Fig. 18-3, *B* and *C*).

Comment. Early care resulted in satisfactory functional recovery in a potentially serious problem.

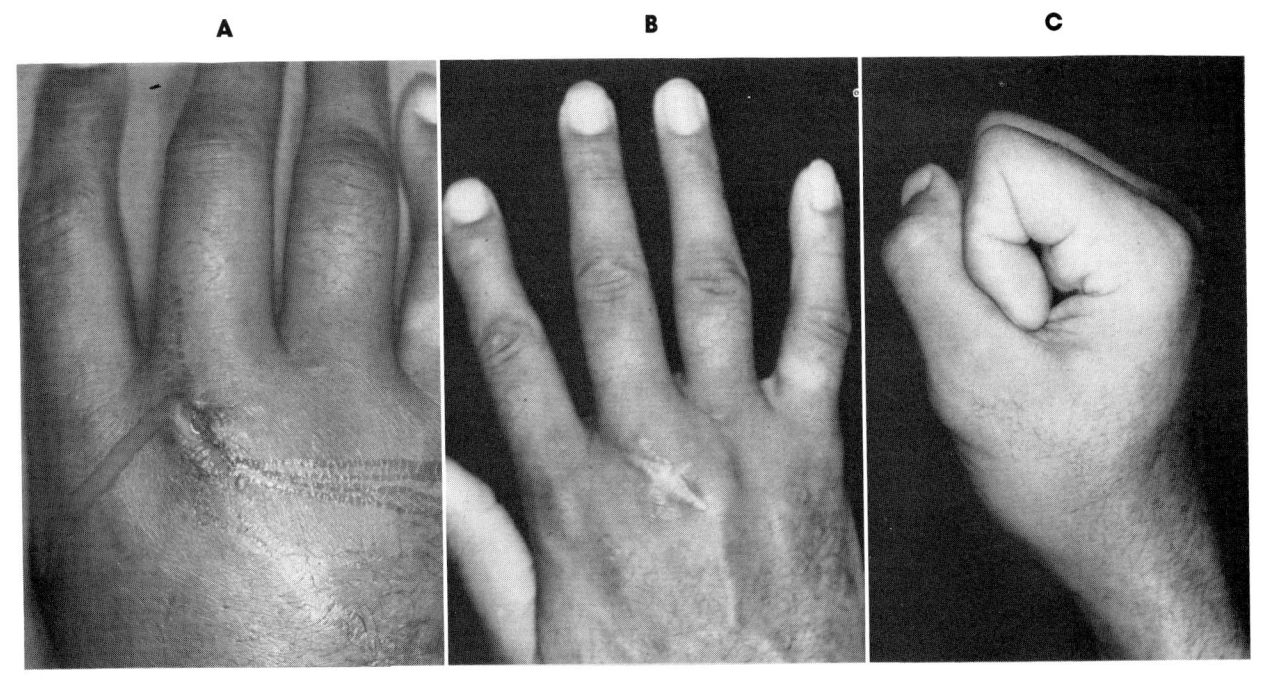

FIG. 18-3. Human tooth infection. **A,** Twenty-four hours after wound from human tooth to dorsum of hand, there is a serous discharge noted. **B** and **C,** After debridement and antibiotic therapy, wound healed, and patient gradually recovered function over next month.

SECTION 5 INFECTION PROBLEMS

INFECTIOUS GANGRENE

Infectious gangrene, originally described by Meleney[17] as a lesion of the abdominal wall as well as in the extremities caused by an invasion by anaerobic hemolytic streptococci can occur after a trivial injury.[21] Meleney[18,19] later added cases in which the streptococci were joined by *S. aureus*, acting synergistically to destroy the soft tissues usually in laparotomy incisions. Other authors[4,22,24] added experiences with infections that had similar characteristics with a combination of bacteria implicated as causative organisms. Terms such as *synergistic necrotizing cellulitis* or *necrotizing fasciitis* were used. Many times the anaerobic streptococci were found to be associated with a gram-negative rod such as *Escherichia coli* or *Proteus* or *Klebsiella* organisms.

The treatment is dependent on early appreciation of the severity of the problem. This is difficult, since at times the wound may be regarded as minor. Surgical intervention must be radical with incision and/or excision of the gangrenous tissues. The wounds are left open, and high-dosage specific antibiotic therapy is necessary. Amputation may be an inevitable sequela to this problem.

Case 4

A 9-year-old boy fell, sustaining a forearm fracture. The radius was compounded from within, a small laceration being present in the midforearm. The patient was taken to the operating room where local debridement was carried out along with closed reduction of the fractures. The wound was not sutured, and broad-spectrum antibiotics were given. At 24 hours the patient became febrile, and at 48 hours the wound again was debrided in the operating room, when it became apparent that infection was present. Cultures yielded gram-negative rods, later identified as *E. coli*, and *S. aureus*. Despite appropriate antibiotic therapy and two more debridements, the infection could not be controlled. The patient was transferred to our service at 28 days. He appeared chronically ill, and his wound encompassed the entire forearm (Fig. 18-4, *A*). On debridement all volar and dorsal soft tissues were found to be necrotic except for a 2.5-cm wide bridge of skin on the dorsal forearm (Fig. 18-4, *B*). High forearm amputation preserved elbow function.

Comment. An innocuous wound, undoubtedly treated properly initially, developed into a massive problem. The lesion apparently was not recognized or recognizable at 48 hours when a more radical debridement might have saved the extremity. This is speculative, since at times, despite the most heroic therapy, the limb or life is lost.

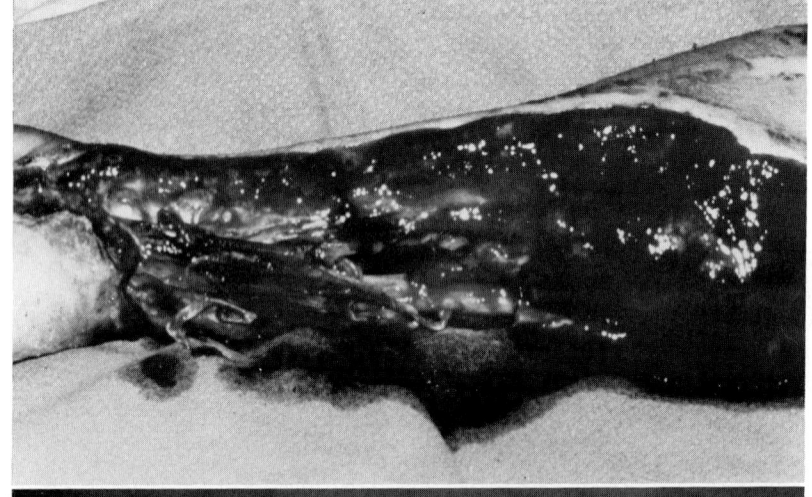

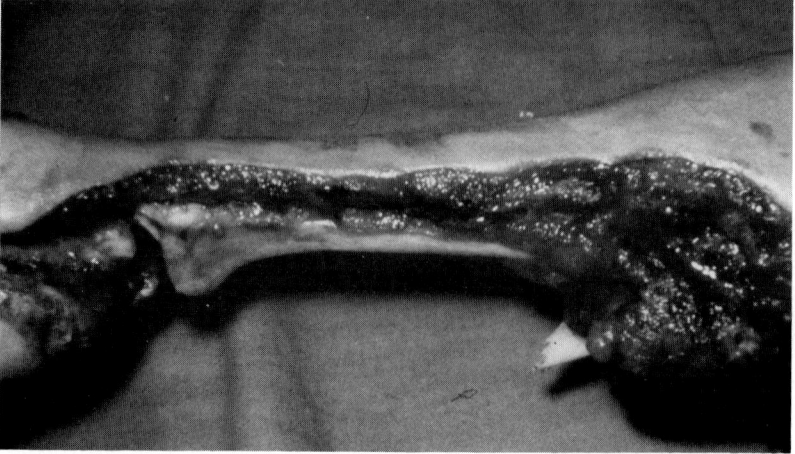

FIG. 18-4. Infectious gangrene. **A,** At 28 days after injury, massive wound encompassed entire forearm. There was no viable muscle, nerve, or tendon in forearm. **B,** After debridement it was obvious extremity was not salvageable, and high-forearm amputation was carried out.

ACID-FAST DISEASE IN THE HAND
Mycobacterium tuberculosis[14,23]

Infections caused by the *Mycobacterium tuberculosis* are being seen with less frequency, along with the general decline in the pulmonary form of the disease. Cases do occur on occasion, and the surgeon must be suspicious in the presence of a chronic low-grade inflammation, usually involving the tenosynovium of the hand or wrist but also seen in the osseous structures. In the soft tissue infection the differential diagnosis includes rheumatoid arthritis, and biopsy and cultures are necessary for a definitive diagnosis. It is interesting to note that prior to diagnosis many of these lesions are mistakenly treated by antiinflammatory agents, including steroid injections (Fig. 18-5). At the time of tenosynovectomy, smears for acid-fast bacilli are studied along with routine cultures as well as acid-fast cultures and fungal studies. It is important, when there is a chance of mycobacterial infection, to culture at 30° as well as 37° C to allow the growth of *M. marinum*. If clinical suspicion warrants, the patient should be administered antituberculotic medications while awaiting confirmation by culture.

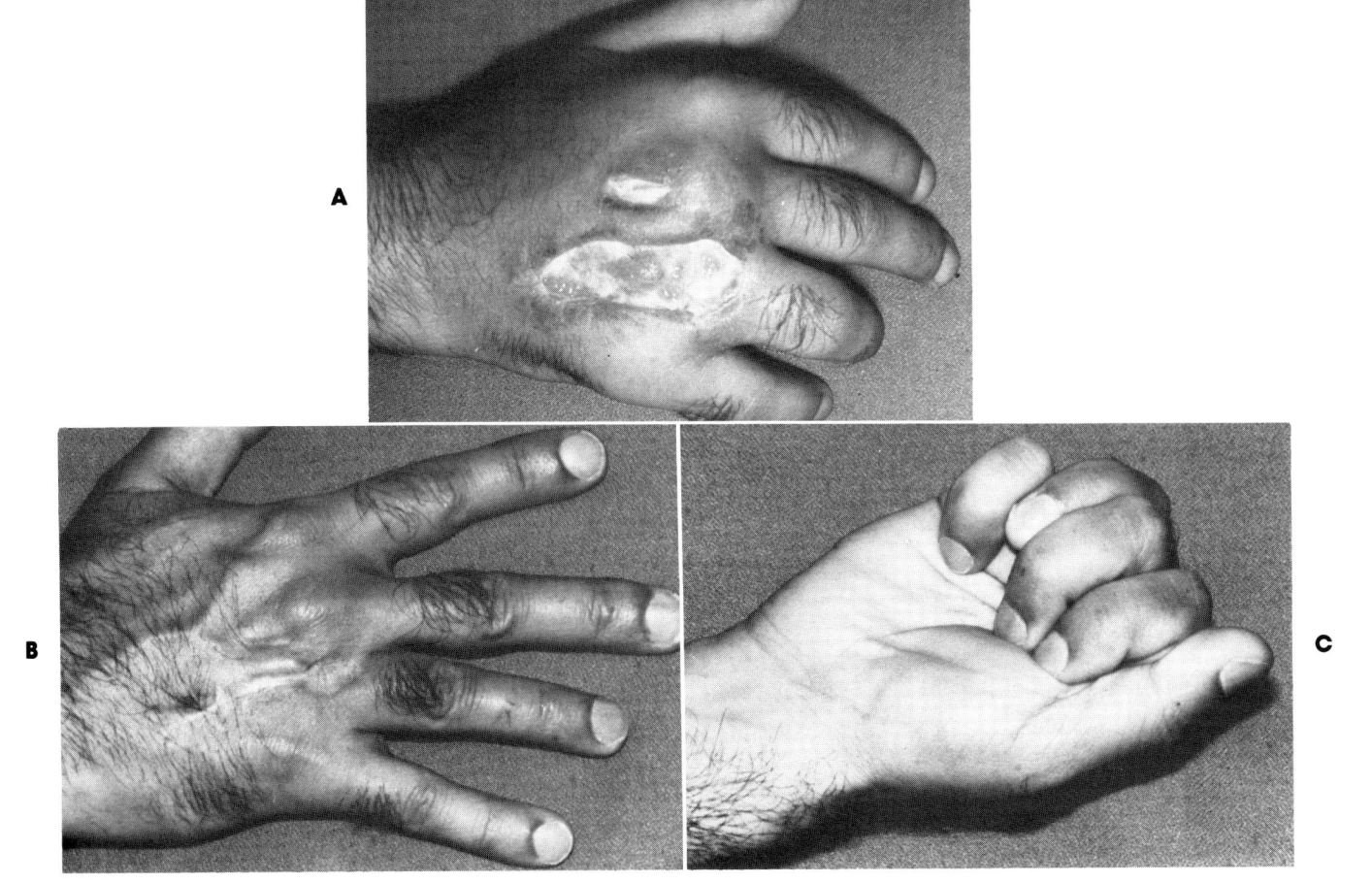

FIG. 18-5. Acid-fast disease. **A,** A 35-year-old pharmacist had several steroid injections for "nonspecific tenosynovitis." Advancing infection had destroyed skin on dorsum of hand. Tissue removed at debridement revealed *M. tuberculosis.* **B** and **C,** Under prolonged antituberculotic drug therapy, wound healed, and these photographs taken 6 years later show limited but useful ring finger function.

SECTION 5 INFECTION PROBLEMS

M. marinum[3,9,25]

Usually associated with skin lesions (swimming pool granuloma), *M. marinum* has now been recognized with greater frequency as a cause of infection in the deeper structures of the hand. This is because more laboratories are becoming proficient in the identification of the organism.

Case 5

A 27-year-old salesman had a 6-month history of swelling of his right long finger; no history of trauma was elicited. He had been treated with various antibiotics with no improvement. A recent hydrocortisone injection was followed by an increase in symptoms and prompted hand surgery consultation. At this point the finger was markedly swollen and restricted in motion at all joints (Fig. 18-6, *A*). A diagnosis of mycobacterial infection was entertained in the differential diagnosis, and surgical exploration was undertaken. The finger was drained of a creamy material (Fig. 18-6, *B*), and the wounds on both the dorsum of the finger and the volar aspect of the palm were left open. Smears revealed acid-fast bacteria, later identified as *M. marinum*. The finger responded very slowly to ethambutol and rifampin, and, although the wound ultimately healed, the finger had little active function at the interphalangeal joints.

Comment. A long delay in diagnosis contributed to the poor functional result in this patient with an unusual infection.

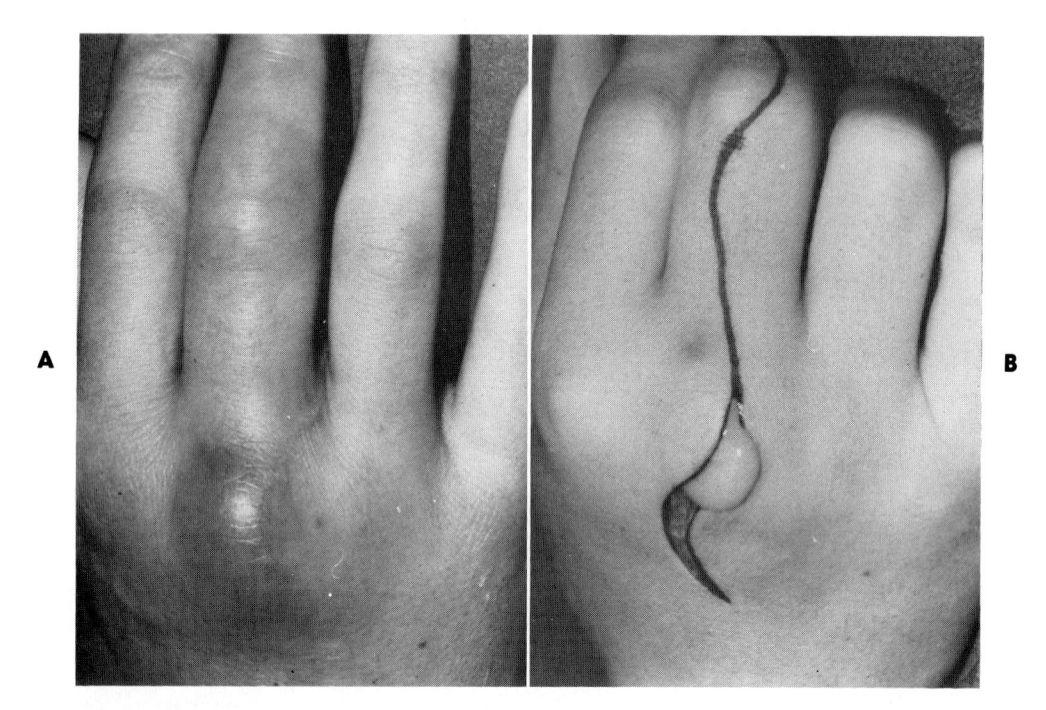

FIG. 18-6. Atypical acid-fast disease. **A,** Six-month history of swelling and pain in long finger. **B,** At incision and drainage, creamy material exuded. Smears and cultures revealed acid-fast bacteria identified as *M. marinum*.

SUMMARY

The difficult infection is still with us. We are better equipped to deal with these problems than were our predecessors, with improved culture techniques and better antibacterial medications. The medications, although helpful, should not be relied on too heavily; rather a good balance of clinical judgment and surgical skill is needed to get the best functional result possible in these difficult problems.

REFERENCES

1. Brooks, G.F., O'Donoghue, J.M., Rissing, J.P., Soapes, K., and Smith, J.W.: *Eikenella corrodens*, a recently recognized pathogen, Medicine **53**:325, 1974.
2. Carter, S.J., Burman, S.O., and Mersheimer, W.L.: Treatment of digital tenosynovitis by irrigation with peroxide and oxytetracycline, Ann. Surg. **163**:645, 1966.
3. Cortez, L.M., and Pankey, G.A.: *Mycobacterium marinum* infections of the hand, J. Bone Joint Surg. **55A**:363, 1973.
4. Crosthwait, R.W., Jr., Crosthwait, R.W., and Jordan, G.L.: Necrotizing fasciitis, J. Trauma **4**:149, 1964.
5. Duran, R.J., Coventry, M.B., Weed, L.A., and Kierland, R.R.: Sporotrichosis: a report of 23 cases in the upper extremity, J. Bone Joint Surg. **39A**:1330, 1957.
6. Goldman, S., Lipscomb, P.R., and Ulrich, J.A.: Geotrichum tunefaction of the hand, J. Bone Joint Surg. **51A**:587, 1969.
7. Goldstein, E.J.C., Miller, T.A., Citron, D.M., and Finegold, S.M.: Infections following clenched fist injury: a new prospective, J. Hand Surg. **3**:455, 1978.
8. Green, W.O., and Adams, T.E.: Mycetoma in the United States, Am. J. Clin. Pathol. **42**:75, 1964.
9. Gunther, S.F., Elliot, R.C., Brand, R.L., and Adams, J.P.: Experience with atypical mycobacterial infection in the deep structures of the hand, J. Hand Surg. **2**:90, 1977.
10. Hennessey, P.H., and Fletcher, W.: Infections with the organisms of Vincent's angina following man bite, Lancet **2**:127, 1920.
11. Iverson, R.E., and Vistnes, L.M.: Coccidiodomycosis tenosynovitis in the hand, J. Bone Joint Surg. **55A**:413, 1973.
12. Kanavel, A.B.: Infections of the hand, Philadelphia, 1939, Lea & Febiger.
13. Koch, S.L.: Acute rapidly spreading infections following trivial injuries of the hand, Surg. Gynecol. Obstet. **69**:277, 1934.
14. Leung, P.C.: Tuberculosis of the hand, Hand **10**:285, 1978.
15. Mann, R.J., Hoffeld, T.A., and Farmer, C.B.: Human bites of the hand: 20 years of experience, J. Hand Surg. **2**:97, 1977.
16. Mason, M.L.: Symposium on surgical infections: infections of the hand, Surg. Clin. North Am. **22**:455, 1942.
17. Meleney, F.L.: Hemolytic streptococcus gangrene, Arch. Surg. **9**:317, 1924.
18. Meleney, F.L.: Hemolytic streptococcus gangrene, J.A.M.A. **92**:2009, 1929.
19. Meleney, F.L.: Treatise on surgical infections, New York, 1948, Oxford University Press, Inc.
20. Neviaser, R.J.: Closed tendon sheath irrigation for pyogenic flexor tenosynovitis, J. Hand Surg. **3**:462, 1978.
21. Quintiliani, R., and Engh, G.A.: Overwhelming sepsis associated with group a beta hemolytic streptococci, J. Bone Joint Surg. **53A**:1391, 1971.
22. Rea, W.J., and Wyrick, W.J.: Necrotizing fasciitis, Ann. Surg. **172**:957, 1970.
23. Robins, R.H.C.: Tuberculosis of the wrist and hand, Br. J. Surg. **54**:211, 1967.
24. Stone, H.H., and Martin, J.D.: Synergistic necrotizing cellulitis, Ann. Surg. **175**:702, 1972.
25. Williams, D.S., and Riordan, D.C.: *Mycobacterium marinum* infections of the hand, J. Bone Joint Surg. **55A**:1042, 1973.

SECTION SIX JOINT PROBLEMS

Chapter 19 The thumb axis joints: a biomechanical model

Ronald L. Linscheid

The most unique aspect of the human wrist is the shape and position of the scaphoid bone. In the popular description of the functional anatomy of the carpus as consisting of a proximal and distal row, the scaphoid is considered a connecting link between the two. In another concept of the anatomy, as proposed by Navarro and cited by Taleisnik,[15] the wrist may be divided into three columns: ulnar rotation, middle flexion-extension, and opposition or radial. The latter supports the thumb, which by virtue of the mated saddle articular surfaces of the trapezium and first metacarpal is capable of a circumduction movement that permits the important act of opposition. In the neutral position the longitudinal axes of the scaphoid, trapezium, and first metacarpal are essentially colinear. Whereas the trapezium, firmly fixed to the distal row, is static, the position of the scaphoid and first metacarpal is dependent on wrist position and thumb position, respectively. This complex represents a multilinked, cantilevered system that is acted on by the thenar intrinsic muscle forces of the adductor pollicis, flexor pollicis brevis, opponens, first dorsal interosseous, and abductor pollicis. The extrinsic muscles are abductor pollicis longus, extensor pollicis brevis, extensor pollicis longus, and flexor pollicis longus. These forces are largely compressive across the first metacarpotrapezial joint.[5,13]

The scaphotrapezial joint is acted on by the flexor pollicis longus, extensor pollicis longus, flexor carpi radialis, extensor carpi radialis brevis and longus, abductor pollicis longus, and extensor pollicis brevis muscles. To a lesser extent, the extrinsic muscles of the finger and other wrist movers also contribute. The intrinsic muscles acting on the thumb represent 48% of the intrinsic muscle mass of the hand. Those muscles acting directly on the thumb axis represent 10% of the muscle mass crossing the wrist.

Static force analysis of a three-dimensional thumb model suggests a scalar force of 6 to 13 times the output force generated at the thumb tip.[4] An adult man averages appositional pinch force of 10 to 16 kg and a female 6 to 10 kg. The compressive forces are well balanced in general, but in an imbalanced situation the component of force tangential to the articular surface of the trapezium and scaphoid presents a shearing force on the articular cartilage and a translational force that must be borne by the capsular ligaments. Constraining shear forces range from 0.06 to 2.66 times the output force.

The concave distal surface of the trapezium is aligned at an 80-degree angle to the plane of the palm in the coronal plane.[7,9] The radius of curvature is such as to minimize translational forces in the arc of normal motion in this plane of approximately 35 to 40 degrees. In a plane parallel to the palm the concave surface of the base of the first metacarpal retains an excursion arc of approximately one radian. Axial rotation is restrained by the capsular ligaments and the opposed hyperbolic surfaces.[7,12,13]

The trapezium is cantilevered from a shallow notch composed by the base of the second metacarpal and the trapezoid and stabilized by strong ligamentous attachments.[5]

The metacarpotrapezial joint is especially vulnerable to degenerative arthrosis. Pathomechanics are assumed to consist of a chain of events in which there is cartilaginous erosion on the radiopalmar surface of the first metacarpal, radiodorsal translation of the first metacarpal, and hypertrophic changes of the periphery.* Endochondral ossification occurring in the ulnar shoulder of the trapezium increases the slope of the trapezium and the subluxation of the metacarpal. The moment arm on which the compressive force of the metacarpal acts is increased as well.

The attitude of the trapezium relative to the second metacarpal and trapezoid may play a part in this process as well (Fig. 19-1). Even slight rotation of the trapezium from the base of the second metacarpal, occasioned by laxity of the suspensory ligaments, may encourage radiodorsal translation of the metacarpal base and alter the contact characteristics with the scaphoid.[5] This is suggested by the less common, isolated scaphotrapezial degenerative joint disease in which the zigzag collapse of the thumb axis is apparent on lateral roentgenograms (Fig. 19-2).

---

*References 1, 7, 10, 11, and 14.

SECTION 6 JOINT PROBLEMS

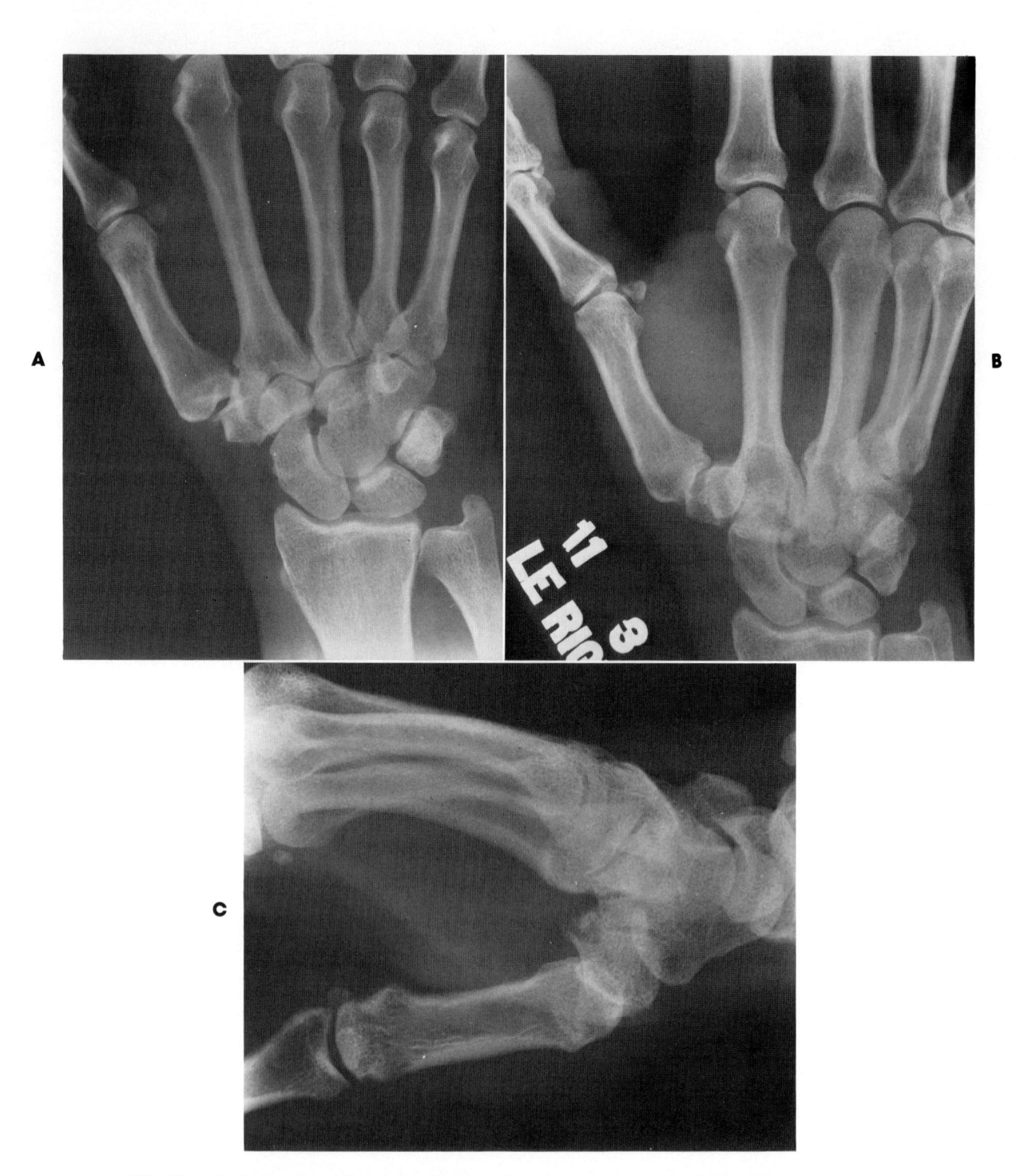

FIG. 19-1. Early degenerative joint disease of metacarpotrapezial joint of thumb in 44-year-old housewife with weak and painful thumbs. **A,** Anteroposterior view shows good joint space with radial translation of first metacarpal base and radial osteophyte from trapezium. **B,** Oblique view suggests, in addition, that trapezium has rotated counterclockwise from its articulation with second metacarpal base. **C,** Lateral view shows irregularly along ulnar margin of trapezium, consistent with osseoligamentous tensile reaction. There was probable spread between trapezium and second metacarpal.

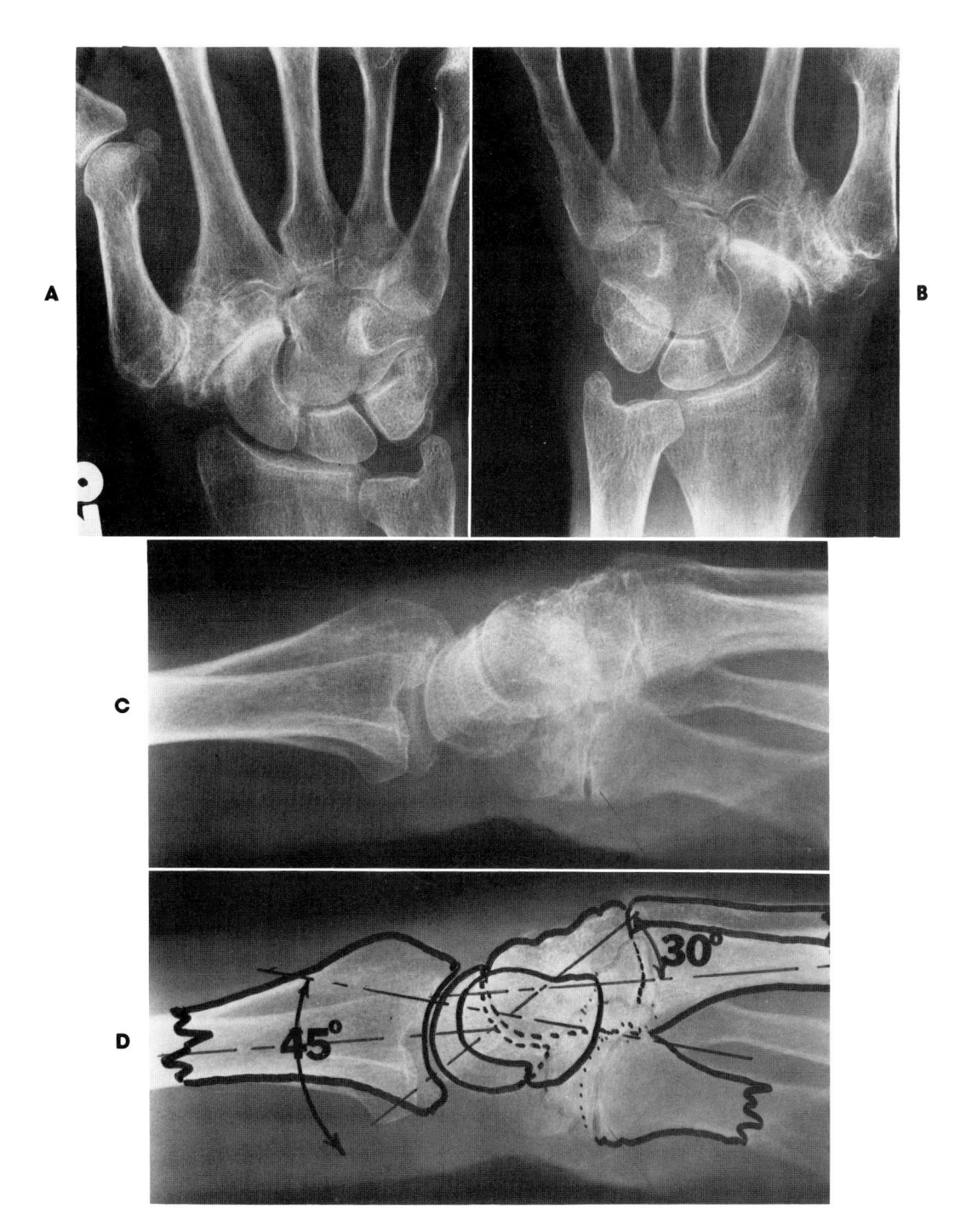

CHAPTER 19 THE THUMB AXIS JOINTS: A BIOMECHANICAL MODEL

FIG. 19-2. Pantrapezial degenerative joint disease with marked scaphotrapeziotrapezoidal component. **A** and **B,** Right and left thumb axes with hyperextension of metacarpophalangeal joint and degenerative joint disease of metacarpotrapezial and scaphotrapeziotrapezoidal joints. Note radial subluxation of first metacarpal and ulnar subluxation of distal pole of scaphoid from apparent rotation of trapezium clockwise on left and counterclockwise on right. **C** and **D,** Lateral view suggests that compressive force across scaphotrapeziotrapezoidal joint has caused dorsiflexion of scaphoid and diminished scapholunate angle (45 degrees). There is also evidence of intercarpal collapse with dorsiflexion instability of lunate (capitolunate angle is 30 degrees). This pattern suggests that early instability of trapezium (Fig. 16-1) may progress to this marked deformity.

CLINICAL APPLICABILITY

Metacarpotrapezial degenerative joint disease has been treated with a variety of surgical approaches, including capsulorrhaphy, arthrodesis, trapezial excision, and arthroplasty.* Osteotomy to correct alignment has received only cursory attention. The advantages and disadvantages of the various procedures are the subject of some controversy, but the plethora of procedures attests to the prevalent incomplete satisfaction with one procedure. The goals of treatment should be to abolish pain, increase pinch strength, retain normal motion, and prevent later complications. To accomplish this in the late case requires joint modification and thumb axis realignment. Prophylactic treatment could include trapezial realignment by osteotomy or arthrodesis as well as capsulorrhaphy.

The consequences of total trapeziectomy include metacarpal subluxation, intercalary collapse of the carpus, diminished pinch strength, and metacarpal instability in some instances. Retention of a stable trapezium combined with surface arthroplasty is an optional approach.

The scaphotrapezial joint has received scant attention. Osteochondral fractures and degenerative joint disease occur here as well. Arthrosis of this joint impairs wrist rather than thumb motion. Surface replacement arthroplasty and arthrodesis are the present treatment modalities. The latter significantly reduces carpal excursion and may stress the remaining open joints. The former is difficult and fraught with complications. It likewise fails to adequately support the thumb axis, but trapezial stabilization with or without surface arthroplasty may be a viable alternative.

This chapter has stressed the biomechanical factors of understanding the thumb axis. Although I do not propose a new treatment modality, the stabilization of the second metacarpotrapeziotrapezoidal complex as a point of departure is suggested.

*References 2, 3, 5, 6, 8, 9, 11, and 14.

REFERENCES

1. Burton, R.I.: Basal joint arthrosis of the thumb, Orthop. Clin. North Am. 4:331, 1973.
2. Carroll, R.E., and Hill, N.A.: Arthrodesis of the carpometacarpal joint of the thumb, J. Bone Joint Surg. **55B:** 292, 1973.
3. Chuinard, R.G., et al.: Interposition arthroplasty of the first metacarpal-trapezial joint, Presented at American Society for Surgery of the Hand Meeting, New Orleans, 1976.
4. Cooney, W.P., and Chao, E.Y.S.: Biomechanical analysis of static forces in the thumb during hand function, J. Bone Joint Surg. **59A:**27, 1977.
5. Crosby, E.B., Linscheid, R.L., and Dobyns, J.H.: Scaphotrapezial trapezoidal arthrosis, J. Hand Surg. 3:223, 1978.
6. Dell, P.C., Brushart, T.M., and Smith, R.J.: Treatment of trapeziometacarpal arthritis: results of resection arthroplasty, J. Hand Surg. 3:243, 1978.
7. Eaton, R.G., and Littler, J.W.: A study of the basal joint of the thumb: treatment of its disabilities by fusion, J. Bone Joint Surg. **51A:**661, 1969.
8. Froimson, A.: Tendon arthroplasty of the trapeziometacarpal joint, Clin. Orthop. 70:191, 1970.
9. Haines, R.W.: The mechanism of rotation at the first carpo-metacarpal joint, J. Anat. 78:44, 1944.
10. Lasserre, C., et al.: Osteoarthritis of the trapeziometacarpal joint, J. Bone Joint Surg. **31B:**534, 1949.
11. Leach, R.E., and Bocton, P.E.: Arthritis of the carpometacarpal joint of the thumb: results of arthrodesis, J. Bone Joint Surg. **50A:**1171, 1968.
12. Napier, J.R.: The form and function of the carpometacarpal joint of the thumb, J. Anat. **89:**362, 1955.
13. Pieron, A.P.: The mechanism of the first carpometacarpal (CMC) joint: an anatomical and mechanical analysis, Acta Orthop. Scand. (Suppl.) **1:**1, 1973.
14. Swanson, A.: Flexible implant resection arthroplasty in the hand and extremities, St. Louis, 1973, The C.V. Mosby Co.
15. Taleisnik, J.: Personal communication, 1978.

Chapter 20 Management of posttraumatic arthritis of the proximal interphalangeal joint with silicone implant arthroplasty

James W. Strickland

J. Anthony Dustman

Leo Stelzer

William B. Stromberg, Jr.

James B. Steichen

John L. Bell

Restoring pain-free motion in posttraumatic disabilities of the proximal interphalangeal (PIP) joint is one of the most challenging problems in reconstructive hand surgery (Fig. 20-1). Joints rendered painful, unstable, angulated, or stiff by articular fracture, dislocation, or crushing historically have been managed by arthrodesis or resection arthroplasty procedures. The loss of joint motion necessitated by arthrodesis is an obvious disadvantage, and the results of resection arthroplasty procedures have been unpredictable, often with residual instability or pain.[3,4]

The use of inert materials to carry out interpositional or prosthetic replacement arthroplasty has been increasingly explored. Burman[2] reported in 1940 on the use of a Vitallium cap in one PIP joint with good initial results. Brannon and Klein[1] in 1959 described the use of a titanium hinge prosthesis in 12 joints with satisfactory results in eight. In 1968 Swanson and Yamauchi[18] reported on the use of an intramedullary stemmed silicone rubber implant for the replacement of destroyed digital joints, with encouraging findings with regard to pain relief and motion. Subsequent studies[6,11-17] on the use of this flexible implant have indicated that it has provided an acceptable alternative to other management options.

Although other similar flexible implants have been designed,[8,9] the Swanson silicone rubber implant has remained the most popular, and improvements in the design and material of that prosthesis have evolved. A high-performance silicone rubber prosthesis was developed and released in 1973 and has had greatly increased durability.

The excellent relief from pain and preservation of motion after silicone rubber replacement arthroplasty in patients with rheumatoid arthritis and erosive osteoarthritis have further substantiated the merits of this technique as an alternative to arthrodesis in the traumatically damaged and painful PIP joint.[15] After an initial presentation of the combined results of the hand surgery services at St. Vincent Hospital in Indianapolis and Passavant Hospital in Chicago to the American Society for Surgery of the Hand in 1974,[10] an ongoing study was completed on 100 patients undergoing silicone rubber replacement arthroplasty for posttraumatic arthritis of the PIP joint. This chapter describes the surgical techniques for this procedure and reports on the postoperative performance of the involved joints in this group of patients.

SECTION 6 JOINT PROBLEMS

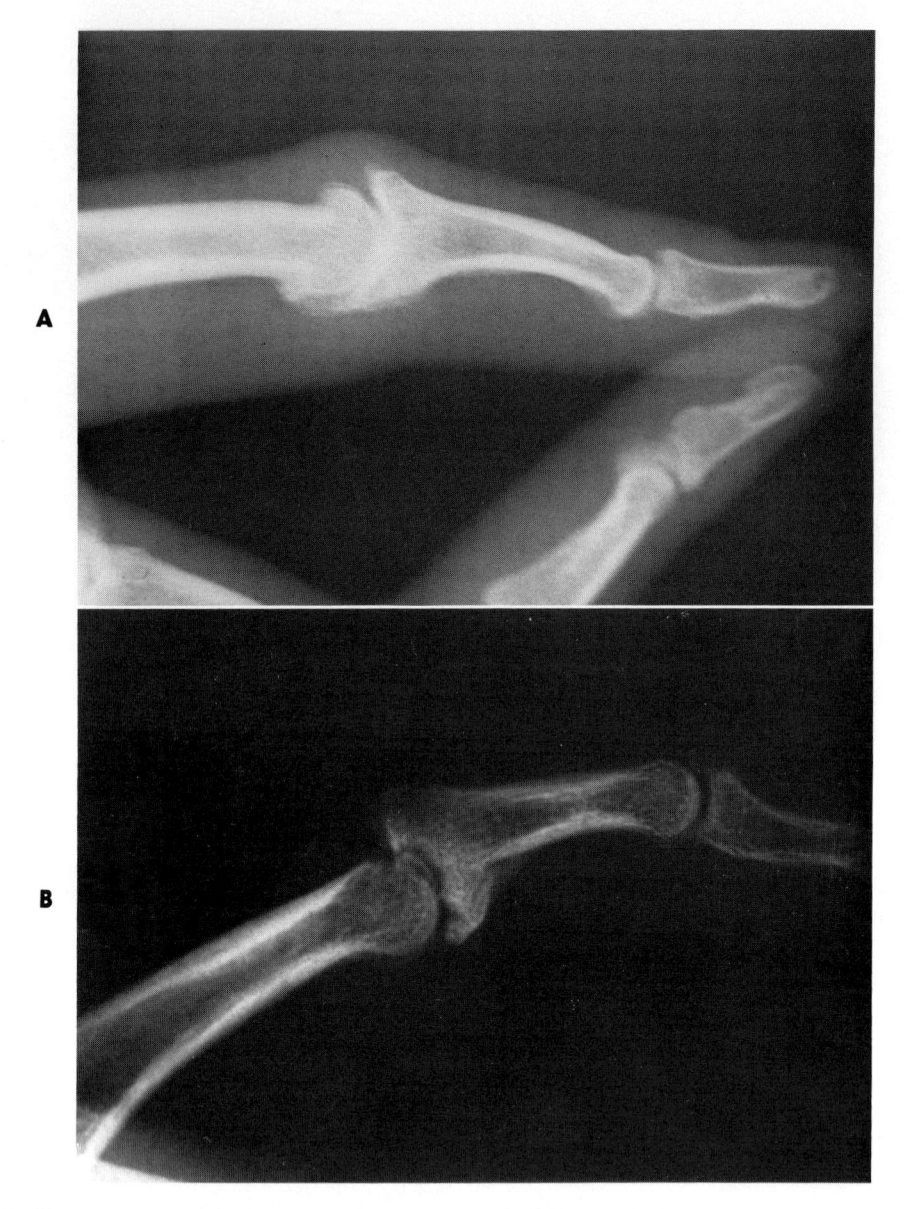

FIG. 20-1. Examples of posttraumatic disabilities of PIP joint. **A,** Posttraumatic arthritic deterioration of PIP joint after crush. **B,** Traumatic arthritic destruction with dorsal subluxation of middle phalanx after fracture-dislocation.

MATERIAL

In the 10-year period included in this study 100 silicone interpositional arthroplasties were carried out in 91 patients with posttraumatic disabilities of the PIP joint. The study group consisted of 59 males and 32 females, and the digital frequency distribution was as follows:

Index finger	23
Long finger	28
Ring finger	29
Small finger	20
TOTAL	100

Articular fracture or fracture-dislocation was the most common mechanism of injury (57%), with crush (34%) and dislocation (9%) being less common precursors of traumatic arthritis.

The interval from injury to surgery averaged 30 months with the longest being 25 years and the shortest 7 days. With one exception all patients had preoperative pain in the involved joint, with 26% having severe, 54% moderate, and 19% mild discomfort. The average preoperative extension loss was 27 degrees, with flexion to 47 degrees and an arc of 20 degrees. The average arc of

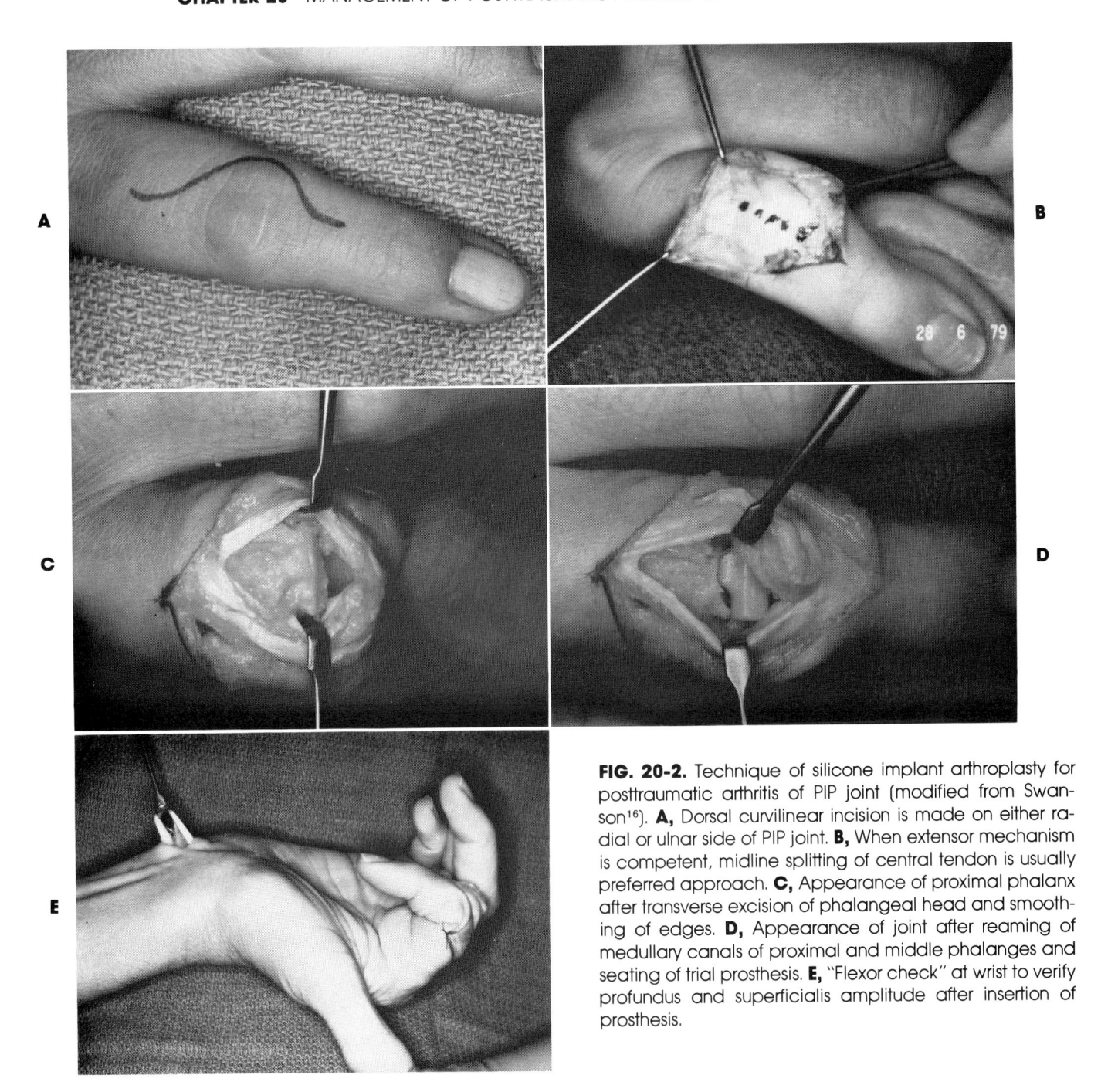

CHAPTER 20 MANAGEMENT OF POSTTRAUMATIC ARTHRITIS OF THE PROXIMAL INTERPHALANGEAL JOINT

FIG. 20-2. Technique of silicone implant arthroplasty for posttraumatic arthritis of PIP joint (modified from Swanson[16]). **A,** Dorsal curvilinear incision is made on either radial or ulnar side of PIP joint. **B,** When extensor mechanism is competent, midline splitting of central tendon is usually preferred approach. **C,** Appearance of proximal phalanx after transverse excision of phalangeal head and smoothing of edges. **D,** Appearance of joint after reaming of medullary canals of proximal and middle phalanges and seating of trial prosthesis. **E,** "Flexor check" at wrist to verify profundus and superficialis amplitude after insertion of prosthesis.

motion was 25 degrees after dislocation, 20 degrees after fracture, and 19 degrees after crushing injuries.

In the final evaluation all patients lost to follow-up analysis before 3 months were omitted. Follow-up studies in this patient group ranged from 3 months to 4 years with an average of 7.4 months. At the time of the final follow-up analysis all joints were evaluted with regard to pain, stability, and range of motion.

OPERATIVE TECHNIQUE

With occasional modifications, the technique described by Swanson[16] was used throughout this series. Through a dorsal curvilinear incision (Fig. 20-2, A) the PIP joint is approached either through (Fig. 20-2, B) or lateral to the extensor tendon, or the extensor tendon is divided transversely near its insertion if reconstruction of the central extensor tendon is required. The appropriate amount of proximal phalangeal head is transversely excised (Fig. 20-2, *C*). Beveling is carried out to overcome angular deformities, and excess bone that might limit motion or damage the prosthesis is excised. After the medullary canals are prepared by means of a small awl and motorized bur, the appropriate size implant is selected and seated (Fig. 20-2, *D*), and an attempt is made to return the finger to its normal resting posture with a full range of passive motion.

When necessary, the central extensor tendon is reconstructed by shortening and advancement into the retained cuff at the base of the middle phalanx[5] or by Matev's technique[7] using the lateral bands. The presence of adequate flexor tendon excursion is verified either by active flexion under local anesthesia or by a small distal palmar or wrist incision (Fig. 20-2, *E*), which allows proximal retraction of the flexor tendons. In a few cases in which satisfactory flexor amplitude cannot be demonstrated, tenolysis is indicated.

The postoperative regimen is varied, depending on whether a repair of the extensor tendon has been carried out. When the extensor tendon is intact, active and passive motion is initiated at approximately 3 days, and static extension splinting is alternated with dynamic flexion splinting. If the extensor mechanism is reconstructed, extension splinting is continued for 3 weeks to allow tendon healing, after which static extension and dynamic flexion splinting is begun.

RESULTS

The most significant finding in this review of 100 procedures was consistent relief from pain. Seventy-five percent of patients reported that there was no pain, and 23% described only mild discomfort, whereas two patients still reported substantial pain.

The range of motion in the replaced joints, shown in Table 20-1, indicates an average lack of full extension of 20 degrees with flexion to 63 degrees and an arc of 43 degrees. When compared with preoperative motion, there was a 7-degree average improvement in extension and a 16-degree improvement in flexion, with an increased arc of 23 degrees. The greatest postoperative arc of motion was 90 degrees, and the smallest was 0 degrees. Twenty-two joints demonstrated an increase in joint motion from 61 to 90 degrees (Fig. 20-3), with 32 joints improving from 31 to 60 degrees and 37 from 0 to 30 degrees. Six joints were unchanged, and three experienced a motion loss.

A study of the etiologic subgroups (Table 20-2) indicated that the most improvement (28 degrees) followed articular fracture, with a 21-degree average improvement seen after dislocation and a 19-degree improvement after crush (Fig. 20-4). Five patients in this series complained of lateral instability, and passive laxity in excess of 10 degrees was demonstrated in four. A study of age as an influence on final motion was carried out with no significant correlation discovered.

The eight complications in this series included two infections, one patient with persistent severe pain resulting in amputation, two joints with instability sufficient to require revision, and three fractured implants, all of which occurred in prostheses implanted prior to the development of high-performance silicone. Severe bone erosion occurred on one occasion, resulting in joint collapse and the need for arthrodesis (Fig. 20-5).

Pseudocapsulectomy consisting of the excision of the thick dorsal tissue were carried out in nine joints in an effort to improve flexion (Fig. 20-6). The average preoperative arc of motion in these joints was 20 degrees and improved to 47 degrees, an average increase of 27 degrees.

To determine if surgical experience and technical refinements produced an improvement in performance, the first 70 arthroplasty procedures were compared with the last 30 (Table 20-3). It was apparent that satisfaction with the procedure had led to broader indications, with an average preoperative arc of 29 degrees in the last 30 joints compared with 16 degrees in the first 70. Although the average arc of postoperative motion was 6 degrees better in the last 30 cases, the average improvement was only 18 degrees compared with 25 degrees in the first 70 joint replacements, largely because the preoperative arc was less in that group. These studies imply that indications for the procedure were increasing and that performance was improving with the passage of time.

Text continued on p. 181.

Table 20-1. Comparative PIP motion

	Preoperative (degrees)	Postoperative (degrees)	Change (degrees)
Extension	27	20	+7
Flexion	47	63	+16
Arc	20	43	+23

Table 20-2. Motion of subgroups

Mechanism of injury	Number	Preoperative (degrees)	Postoperative (degrees)	Change (degrees)
Fracture	57	20	48	+28
Dislocation	9	25	46	+21
Crush	34	19	38	+19

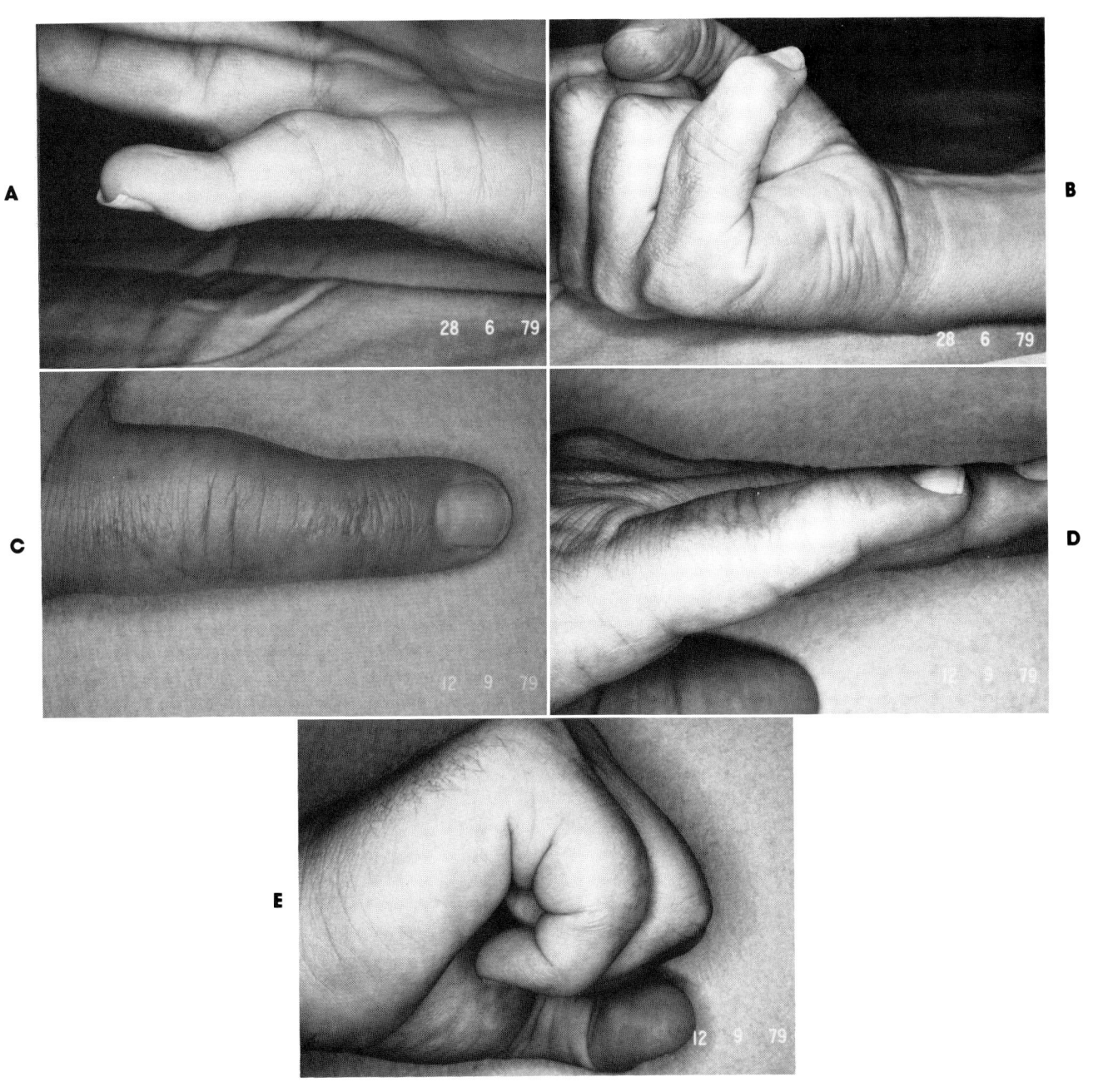

CHAPTER 20 MANAGEMENT OF POSTTRAUMATIC ARTHRITIS OF THE PROXIMAL INTERPHALANGEAL JOINT

FIG. 20-3. Example of silicone replacement arthroplasty for posttraumatic arthritis of PIP joint. **A,** Appearance of small finger with severe posttraumatic arthritis of PIP joint after fracture-dislocation. **B,** Same finger in attempted flexion. **C,** Appearance of dorsal aspect of finger at 3 months. **D,** Digital extension at 3 months. **E,** Excellent PIP joint flexion at 3 months after replacement arthroplasty.

SECTION 6 JOINT PROBLEMS

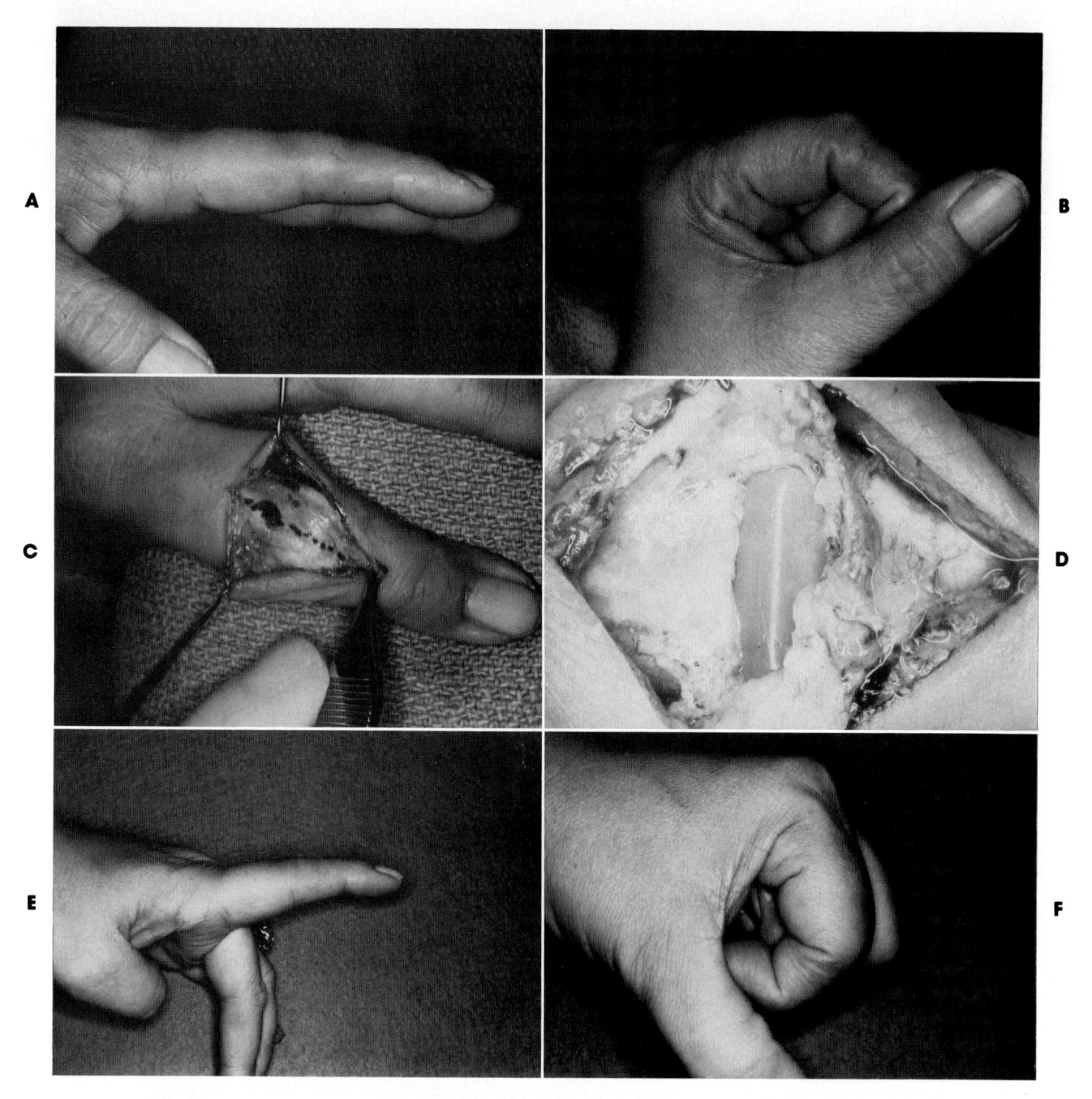

FIG. 20-4. Silicone rubber replacement arthroplasty of PIP joint of index finger for pain and motion loss following crushing injury. **A,** Preoperative extension. **B,** Preoperative flexion. **C,** Operative approach with linear splinting of extensor mechanism. **D,** Appearance of seated silicone rubber implant. **E,** Postoperative extension of index finger. **F,** Postoperative flexion. This patient is now pain free, and index stability is sufficient to allow strong pinch.

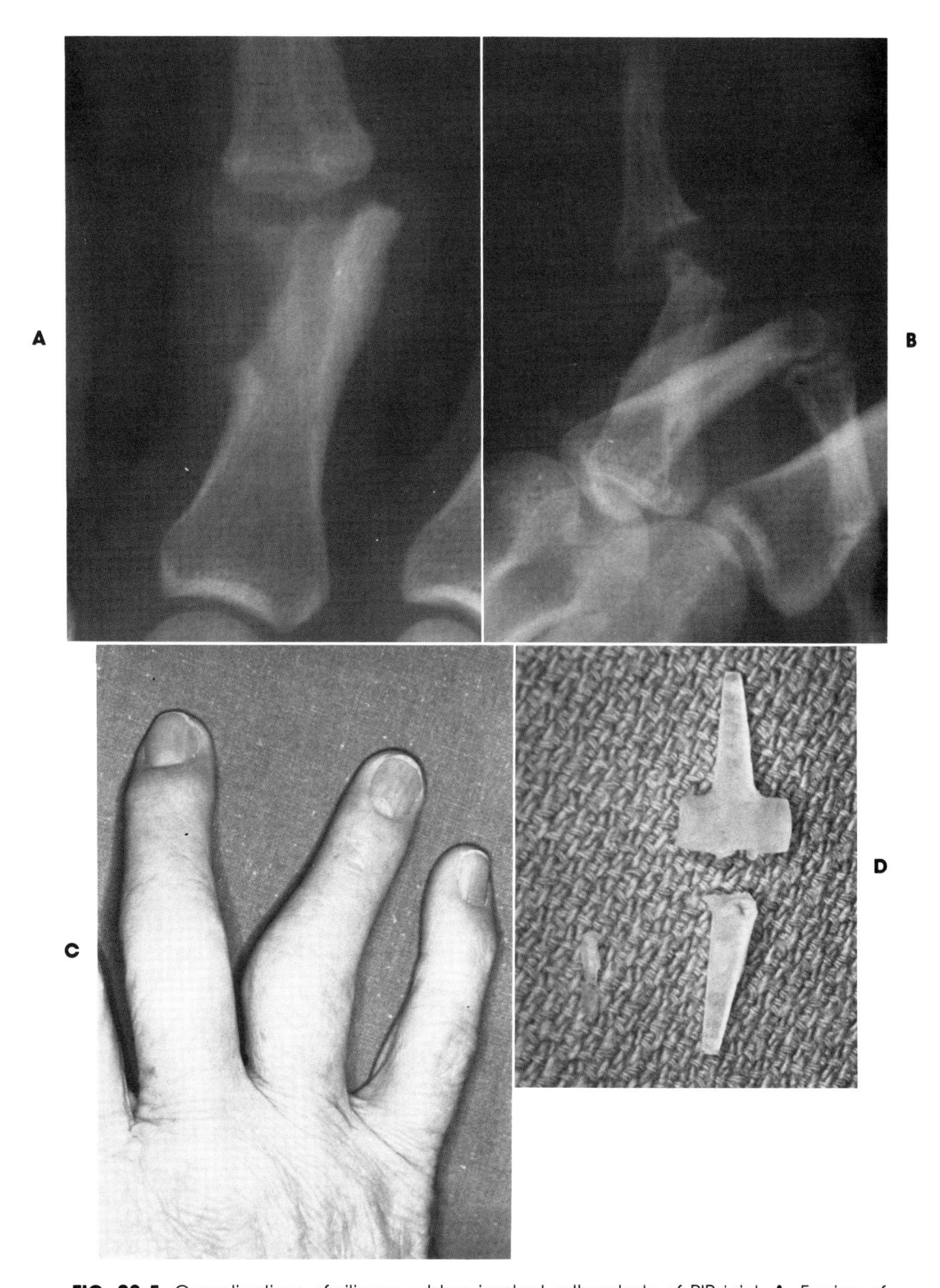

CHAPTER 20 MANAGEMENT OF POSTTRAUMATIC ARTHRITIS OF THE PROXIMAL INTERPHALANGEAL JOINT

FIG. 20-5. Complications of silicone rubber implant arthroplasty of PIP joint. **A,** Erosion of lateral cortex of distal portion of proximal phalanx after excessive thinning at time of medullary canal reaming. Significant angular deformity developed. **B,** Lateral appearance of same joint with dorsal subluxation of middle phalanx. **C,** Angulated appearance of ring finger 9 months after silicone rubber implant arthroplasty. **D,** Fractured prosthetic implant from C, which had resulted in loss of stability and angulation. This prosthesis was not made with the high-performance silicone rubber currently available.

SECTION 6 JOINT PROBLEMS

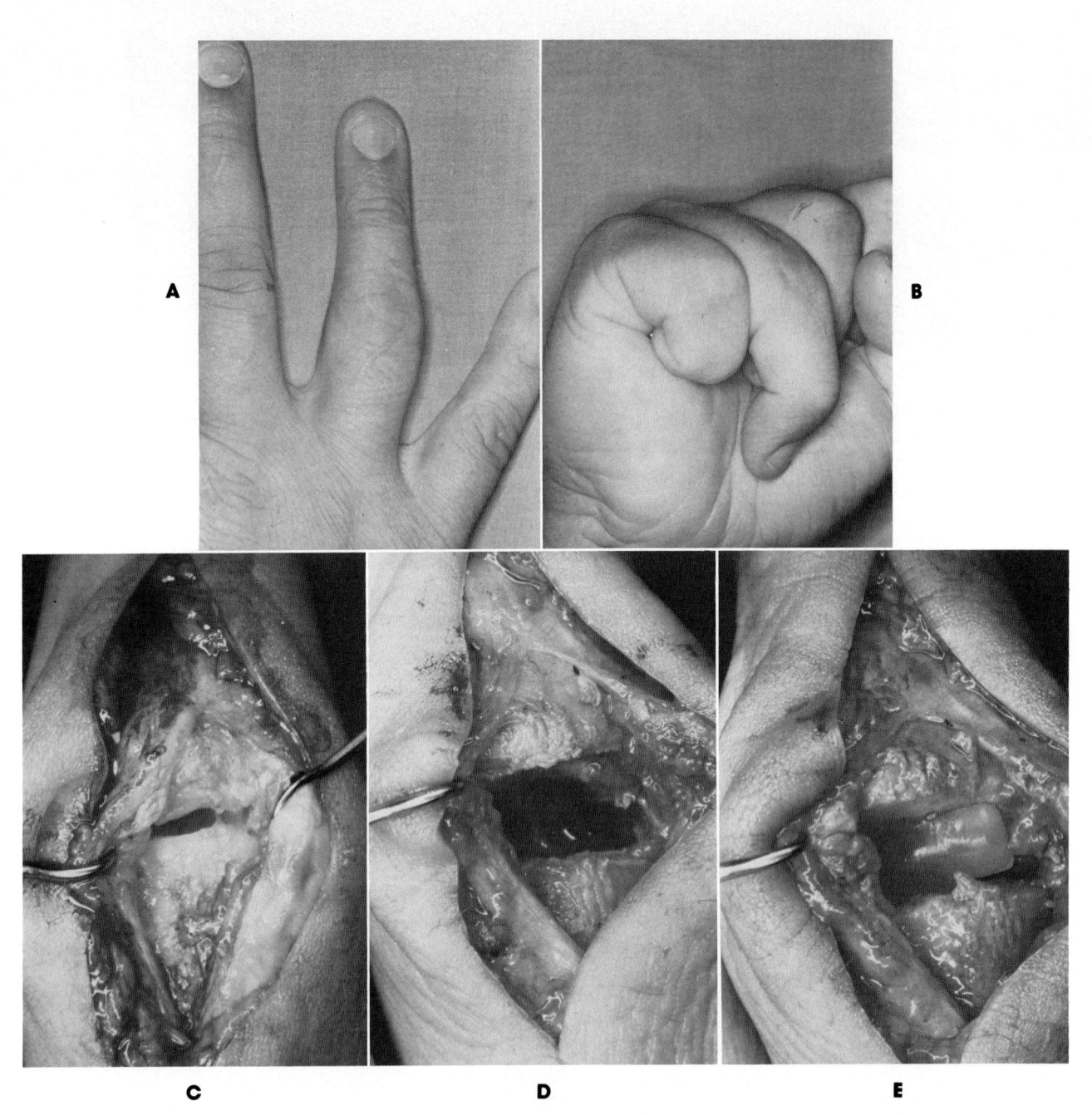

FIG. 20-6. Unsatisfactory motion of PIP joint after silicone replacement arthroplasty 2 years previously. Pseudocapsulectomy was carried out in an effort to improve function. **A,** Satisfactory alignment and PIP joint extension preoperatively. **B,** PIP joint flexion to only 35 degrees. **C,** Appearance of thick pseudocapsule at time of dorsal reexploration and implant removal. **D,** Appearance of interphalangeal defect after excision of thick dorsal pseudocapsule and some overhanging bone. **E,** Joint appearance after seating of new implant. **F,** Slight flexion deformity of ring finger after pseudocapsulectomy. **G,** Excellent restoration of PIP joint flexion after this procedure.

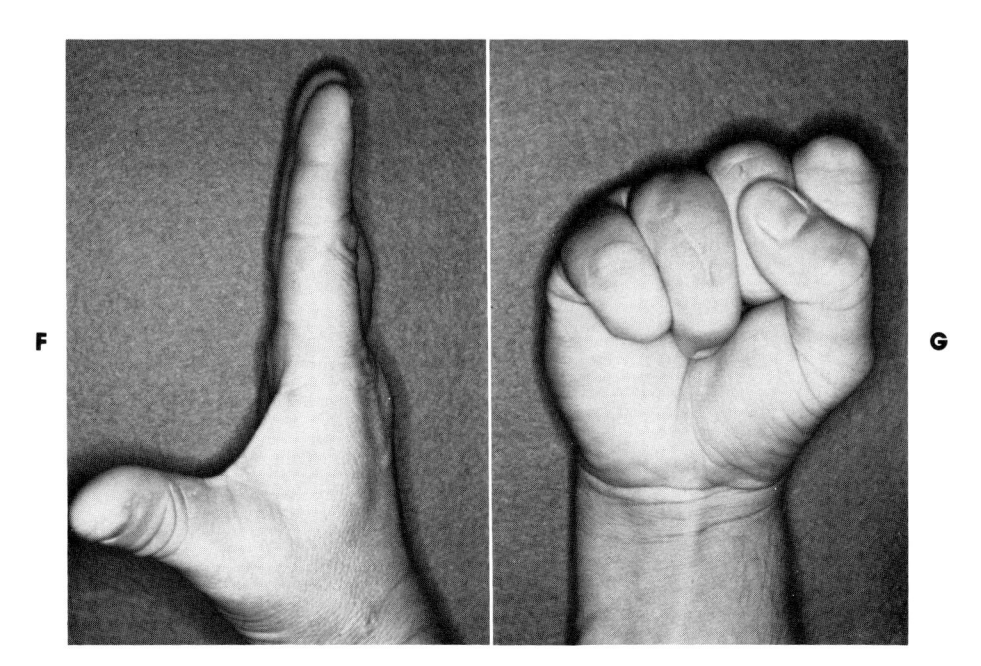

FIG. 20-6, cont'd. For legend see opposite page.

Table 20-3. Performance change (first 70 patients compared with last 30)

	Extension (degrees)	Flexion (degrees)	Arc (degrees)
Preoperative			
70	25	41	16
30	32	61	29
Postoperative			
70	18	59	41
30	24	71	47
Difference			
70	+7	+18	+25
30	+8	+10	+18

DISCUSSION

Severe traumatic damage to the PIP joint always has been a difficult problem to satisfactorily manage, and the result is often one of pain, stiffness, angular deformity, or instability. The gratifying use of a flexible silicone rubber implant designed by Swanson in the management of arthritic destruction of the PIP joint for patients with rheumatoid arthritis and erosive osteoarthritis inevitably led to the clinical trial of this prosthesis for those patients whose arthritis was secondary to trauma. Concern was expressed by many as to whether this prosthesis would prove to be sufficiently durable to withstand the significantly greater stresses produced by patients who were often younger and stronger than those afflicted with nontraumatic arthritic disease.

In 1973 Swanson[15] reported on the use of the silicone rubber implant for posttraumatic disabilities of the PIP joint in 41 joints with an average preoperative arc of motion of 12 degrees. In his series the postoperative arc of motion improved to 51 degrees, and there was consistent relief from pain. Iselin[6] in 1975 described the results of silicone arthroplasty (Swanson design) in 45 PIP joints after trauma and stated that 75% (34 out of 45) of his patients were satisfied with their surgeries, 58% had "fair mobility" (more than 40% range of motion), 22% (10 out of 45) had "little but useful mobility," and 20% (nine arthroplasties) were considered failures. Our results are generally in accord with those of Swanson and Iselin: relief from pain was consistently achieved by silicone implant arthroplasty.

Complications following this procedure have been minimal, and for the most part the joints are sufficiently stable for use in normal hand function. The results obtained in this series would indicate that this procedure is a suitable alternative to other salvage techniques. Using the technique described by Swanson, one should be able to achieve a stable, pain-free joint with approximately 20 degrees improvement in the arc of motion in the majority of digits managed by this procedure.

SUMMARY

It can be seen that this study is in fact a short-term evaluation of the performance of the flexible silicone rubber implant. Long-term evaluation and documentation will be necessary before it can be truly determined if the motion achieved during the early postoperative follow-up period can be maintained on a long-term basis and whether the prosthesis is sufficiently durable to resist fracturing under the stress of repetitious use over many years. Further improvements in prosthetic design and material stability and durability undoubtedly will occur and result in a substantial improvement over the results presented here. Nonetheless the performance of the implants at this time would appear to be quite encouraging and represents a distinct improvement over other salvage techniques in properly selected patients.

REFERENCES

1. Brannon, E.W., Klein, G.: Experiences with a finger-joint prosthesis, J. Bone Joint Surg. **41A**:87, 1959.
2. Burman, M.S.: Vitallium cap arthroplasty of metacarpophalangeal and interphalangeal joints of the fingers, Bull. Hosp. Joint Dis. **1**:79, 1940.
3. Carroll, R.E., and Taber, T.H.: Digital arthroplasty of the proximal interphalangeal joint, J. Bone Joint Surg. **36A**:912, 1954.
4. Dobyns, J.H.: Articular fractures of the hand, J. Bone Joint Surg. **48A**:610, 1966.
5. Elliott, R.A.: Injuries to the extensor mechanism of the hand, Orthop. Clin. North Am. **1**:335, 1970.
6. Iselin, F.: Arthroplasty of the proximal interphalangeal joint after trauma, Hand **7**:41, 1975.
7. Matev, I.B.: Transposition of the lateral slips of the aponeurosis in treatment of long-standing "boutonniere deformity" of the fingers, Br. J. Plast. Surg. **17**:281, 1964.
8. Niebauer, J.J.: Dacron-silicone prosthesis for the metacarpophalangeal and interphalangeal joints. In Cramer, L.M., and Chase, R.A., editors: Symposium on the hand, St. Louis, 1971, The C.V. Mosby Co.
9. Niebauer, J.J., Shaw, J.L., and Doren, W.W.: The silicone-Dacron hinge prosthesis: design, evaluation and application, J. Bone Joint Surg. **50**:634, 1968.
10. Strickland, J.W., Stromberg, W.B., and Bell, J.L.: Silastic replacement arthroplasty in post traumatic disabilities of the proximal interphalangeal joint, J. Bone Joint Surg. **56A**:1096, 1974.
11. Swanson, A.B.: Arthroplasty in traumatic arthritis in the joints of the hand, Orthop. Clin. North Am. **1**:285, 1970.
12. Swanson, A.B.: Implant arthroplasty in the hand. In Cramer, L.M., and Chase, R.A., editors: Symposium on the hand, St. Louis, 1971, The C.V. Mosby Co.
13. Swanson, A.B.: The results of silicone rubber implant arthroplasty in the digits, J. Bone Joint Surg. **53A**:807, 1971.
14. Swanson, A.B.: The use of flexible implants in orthopaedic surgery, J. Bone Joint Surg. **53A**:1657, 1971.
15. Swanson, A.B.: Flexible implant resection arthroplasty in the hand and extremities, St. Louis, 1973, The C.V. Mosby Co.
16. Swanson, A.B.: Reconstructive surgery in the arthritic hand and foot, Clin. Symp. **31**:1, 1979.
17. Swanson, A.B., Matev, I.B., and Waller, T.: The proximal interphalangeal joint in arthritic disabilities and experiences in the use of silicone rubber implant arthroplasty, J. Bone Joint Surg. **52A**:1265, 1970.
18. Swanson, A.B., and Yamauchi, Y.: Silicone rubber implants for replacement of arthritic or destroyed joints, J. Bone Joint Surg. **50A**:1272, 1968.

Chapter 21 Controversies in hand surgery: resection arthroplasty versus silicone replacement arthroplasty for trapeziometacarpal osteoarthritis

Richard J. Smith

Peter C. Amadio

Osteoarthritis of the trapeziometacarpal joint is most common in postmenopausal women.[2,4,34] In its early stages there is mild synovitis within the joint, which causes pain during pinching or grasping. X-ray examination usually will reveal soft tissue swelling, joint narrowing, and sclerosis of the subchondral bone. A small osteophyte often is seen at the ulnar side of the distal aspect of the trapezium.

As the disease progresses, articular cartilage is lost, and the joint space progressively narrows. As the osteophyte enlarges, the base of the first metacarpal subluxates radially and dorsally. Often the first metacarpal develops a fixed flexion-adduction contracture with secondary hyperextension of the metacarpophalangeal joint.[3,4]

Patients with trapeziometacarpal arthritis often complain of pain at the base of the trapezium, which is exacerbated by weather change, manual activities, and relatively mild trauma. Examination will reveal swelling and tenderness of the involved joint, limitation of abduction and pronation of the thumb, and weakened pinch strength. Pain is reproduced by passive circumduction of the first metacarpal base while compressing the metacarpal against the trapezium. This is known as a positive *grind* test[38] (Fig. 21-1). If the metacarpal is subluxated, it can be reduced by traction on the extended thumb and digital pressure to the dorsum of its base.

In most patients conservative measures will relieve the pain.[9,26] A short C-splint may be used intermittently throughout the day to immobilize the trapeziometacarpal joint. Salicylates, indomethacin, and ibuprofen are often helpful in treating the pain of synovitis. With more advanced arthritis, conservative measures may be ineffective, and surgical treatment may be required.

Many operative procedures have been recommended for the treatment of painful trapeziometacarpal osteoarthritis. They may be subdivided into three general categories.

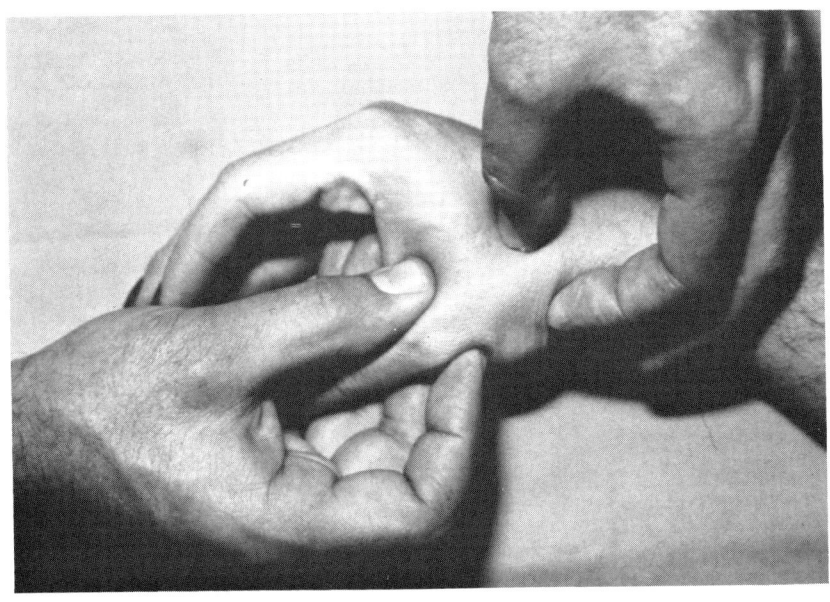

FIG. 21-1. *Grind* test: passive circumduction of metacarpal base while compressing metacarpal against trapezium reproduces patient's pain.

TRAPEZIOMETACARPAL ARTHRODESIS

Trapeziometacarpal arthrodesis[6,27,30,33] can restore excellent alignment to the thumb in which the first metacarpal is flexed and adducted because of subluxation of the trapeziometacarpal joint. With successful arthrodesis there is complete relief from pain in the trapeziometacarpal joint. Occasionally there may be difficulty in achieving arthrodesis in view of the relatively poor blood supply of the trapezium. Pseudarthrosis rates of 10%[12] to 50%[30] have been reported. With loss of motion at the base of the first metacarpal, many patients will complain postoperatively of limited thumb adduction and flexion.[15,40,42] Although some rotation may occur at the trapezioscaphoid joint, pronation usually is limited. In addition, from 30% to 86% of patients with trapeziometacarpal arthritis also have arthritic changes between the trapezium and the scaphoid, the trapezium and the second metacarpal, or the trapezium and the trapezoid.[20,24,37,38] In these patients, pain may persist even with solid trapeziometacarpal arthrodesis.[17,37,40,42]

TRAPEZIOMETACARPAL ARTHROPLASTY

In patients with early osteoarthritis, ligament reconstruction at the trapeziometacarpal joint may relieve pain and restore strength and stability.[13] In more advanced cases the distal articular surface of the trapezium or the proximal end of the metacarpal may be resected and the joint resurfaced either with fascia or plastic.* A metallic prosthesis fixed to the bone with methyl methacrylate also has been used to reconstruct this joint.[9] Many authors[1,22,43] have reported excellent results with interpositional arthroplasty at the trapeziometacarpal joint. Others have reported fracture of the plastic interpositional material in 5% to 33% of patients.[2,7] With lax trapeziometacarpal ligaments the metacarpal base may dislocate.[24] If arthritis exists at the other articular surfaces of the trapezium, trapeziometacarpal interpositional arthroplasty may fail to achieve a pain-free thumb.[24,38]

RESECTION ARTHROPLASTY

Resection of the entire trapezium was advocated in 1949 by Gervis.[18] Since that time many techniques of resection arthroplasty have been performed. Some† have recommended the interposition of fascia or tendon, permitting a new joint to form between the base of the first metacarpal and the distal pole of the scaphoid. Others[8] describe a metal and ceramic implant. Still others[11,14,36,38] have advocated interposition of a silicone implant with a stem inserted into the proximal metacarpal shaft. The silicone implant is designed to fill the gap left by the trapezial resection. No motion is permitted between the implant and the metacarpal except for passive axial rotation, and the implant functions as an extension of the metacarpal to the distal pole of the scaphoid.

Good results with trapezium resection without silicone replacement have been reported.* Yet silicone replacement has been said to restore greater strength.[11,15,38] Some clinics have reported subluxation of the silicone replacement in over 20% of patients† and dislocation in from 5% to 19%.[20] Many of these patients require reoperation.[28,41]

To better stabilize the implant, various techniques have been recommended, including partial resection of the trapezoid and scaphoid,[14,31] tenodesis of the flexor carpi radialis through the metacarpal base,[3,4,14,38] tendon graft reconstruction of intercarpal and carpometacarpal ligaments,[21] a hole placed through the implant through which a tendon is passed,[11] a Dacron tie passing from the implant above the base of the second metacarpal,[16,36] and postoperative Kirschner wire fixation.[39] In some clinics it is reported that stability of the implant can be confidently expected after use of one or more of these reconstructive procedures.[11,39]

It is difficult to compare results of different operative techniques in the treatment of painful trapeziometacarpal osteoarthritis. Many controversies remain: should the trapezium be excised or resurfaced or the trapeziometacarpal joint fused? If the trapezium is excised, should it be replaced with silicone? Is there a difference in results if trapezial resection is followed by fascial arthroplasty as compared with silicone replacement arthroplasty?

To control as many variables as possible in a clinical study, we have concentrated on only one of these controversies: compared with trapezial resection for postmenopausal osteoarthritis of the trapeziometacarpal joint, how do the results of fascial arthroplasty and silicone replacement arthroplasty differ?

A COMPARISON OF TRAPEZIAL RESECTION ARTHROPLASTY WITH AND WITHOUT SILICONE REPLACEMENT

Some of the potential advantages and disadvantages to fascial arthroplasty and silicone replacement arthroplasty after excision of the trapezium are the following:

A. Trapezial excision arthroplasty without silicone replacement
　1. Potential advantages
　　a. Technically easier to do; shorter operative time

---

*References 1, 10, 23, 25, 35, and 43.
†References 5, 9, 17, 29, 32, and 34.

*References 7, 10, 17, 19, and 34.
†References 20, 28, 36, 39, and 41.

b. Less expensive (avoids cost of implant)
   c. No foreign body inserted
   d. No risk of implant fracture or dislocation
   e. Does not require tendon transfer for stabilization
   f. Good thumb motion anticipated since new joint (metacarposcaphoid) is "loose"
   g. Does not require osteotomy of adjacent trapezoid, metacarpal, or scaphoid
   h. Does not require fixation with Kirschner wire
   2. Potential disadvantages
   a. First ray shortened, causing relative lengthening of flexors and extensors
   b. Does not correct flexion-adduction deformity of first metacarpal
   c. Unstable first metacarpotscaphoid joint with weakness of pinch
   d. Late collapse with secondary metacarposcaphoid arthritis
B. Trapezial excision arthroplasty with silicone replacement
   1. Potential advantages
   a. Maintains normal length of first ray
   b. Provides stable interposition between metacarpal and scaphoid
   c. Restores stability at thumb base
   d. Restores strong painless pinch
   2. Potential disadvantages
   a. Risks
   (1) Breakage
   (2) Infection (usually requires removal of implant)
   (3) Local tissue reaction
   b. With failure of stabilization, subluxation or dislocation of implant may occur

We have reviewed these techniques in two parallel series. A retrospective analysis was done of trapezial excision arthroplasty in all postmenopausal women with trapeziometacarpal osteoarthritis from two clinics. In one clinic a rolled tendon interposition was inserted for reconstruction after trapeziectomy ("fascial" arthroplasty); in the other a Swanson-design silicone replacement implant was used. The results of these two series were compared.

Indications for resection arthroplasty without silicone interposition

Trapezial resection arthroplasty with tendon interposition was performed in all postmenopausal patients with painful, disabling osteoarthritis of the trapeziometacarpal joint if the following conditions existed:
   1. The patient did not respond to conservative treatment.
   2. The patient did not have severe flexion-adduction deformity of the first metacarpal. With severe flexion-adduction deformity, the patient was treated with metacarpal osteotomy with or without trapeziometacarpal arthrodesis.

Trapezial resection was not used for young workers nor if posttraumatic osteoarthritis was the result of the malunion of a Bennett fracture. These patients usually were treated by resection of the base of the first metacarpal with insertion of a Kessler-type silicone implant. Resection rarely was performed in patients with rheumatoid arthritis, particularly if there was ulnar translocation of the radiocarpal joint.

Techniques of resection arthroplasty without silicone interposition

Trapezial resection arthroplasty was performed by a dorsal J-shaped or longitudinal incision. The longitudinal portion of the incision lies over the dorsal base of the first metacarpal and the trapezium. When the J-shaped incision is used, the volar portion curves anteriorly in the thenar crease. Care is taken to identify and protect the superficial branches of the radial nerve. The abductor pollicis longus is transected 1 to 1.5 cm proximal to its insertion and retracted proximally and distally. The trapeziometacarpal and trapezioscaphoid joints are identified and the joint capsule incised longitudinally. By subperiosteal dissection, the trapezium is freed anteriorly and posteriorly. Whenever possible, the trapezium is removed in one piece.

Occasionally the deep portion of the trapezium is removed piecemeal. If exposure is difficult, the origin of the thenar muscles is freed from the trapezium and scaphoid anteriorly.

The palmaris longus is removed by two or three transverse incisions in the forearm. Muscle belly and tendon are folded several times and placed in the defect created by excision of the trapezium. If there is no palmaris longus on either hand, a plantaris tendon or absorbable gelatin sponge (Gelfoam) is placed in the joint space. The capsule is closed with interrupted nonabsorbable sutures. The abductor pollicis longus tendon is overlapped and shortened 1 to 1.5 cm. Postoperatively the thumb is held in a plaster cast in abduction and opposition for 3 weeks. A short C-splint is used for protection for an additional 3 weeks thereafter. The patient is instructed to remove the splint four times per day for active exercises of the thumb.

Results of trapezial resection without silicone interposition

Eighteen thumbs of 17 postmenopausal patients with trapeziometacarpal arthritis (one bilateral) were treated by resection of the trapezium without silicone arthroplasty. They were reviewed 6 to 72 months after surgery. In one patient there were complications from an axillary block anesthesia that resulted in painful paresthesia of the limb for several months. This patient had a poor result and continued to complain of pain at the base of the thumb. Of the remaining 16 patients, the average range of pronation was 45 degrees, abduction was 51 degrees, and all could flex to touch the head of the fifth metacarpal. Mean average pinch pressure was 5.0 kg. The average grip pressure of the operated hand was 17 kg. Aside from the previously noted patient and one other who had weakness following proximal interphalangeal arthroplasties, all patients stated that they were pleased with the operation, and all agreed that they would undergo the operation again if it were necessary (Fig. 21-2). Five patients noted some pain with heavy use of the thumb. Three patients developed pain in the first dorsal compartment of the wrist within 1 year of

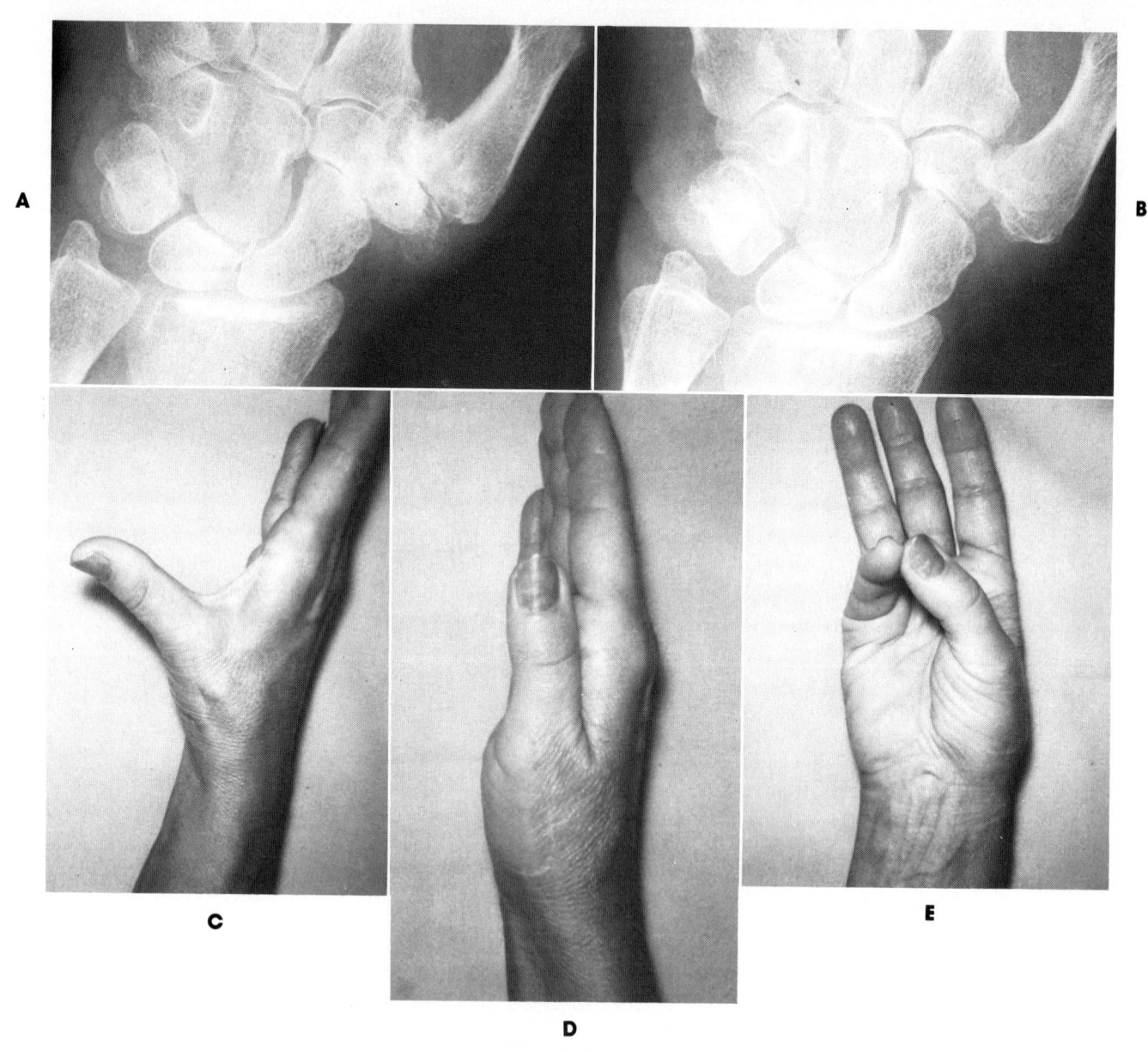

FIG. 21-2. A, Preoperative roentgenogram of patient with painful trapeziometacarpal arthritis. Joint space is narrowed, and there is large osteophyte at distal ulnar surface of trapezium. Metacarpal base is subluxated. **B,** Three months after trapezial resection and palmaris longus interposition, new joint space is preserved. Patient was pain free. One year after trapezial resection there is excellent abduction **(C),** adduction **(D),** and opposition **(E).**

operation. Each had complete pain relief after release of the dorsal retinacular ligament. The shortened abductor pollicis longus appears to have caused late nonseptic tenosynovitis. One patient with bilateral resection arthroplasty won a golf tournament 1 year after her surgery. She stated that she had no pain during athletics.

Comparison with silicone replacement arthroplasty

The group of patients just discussed was compared with similar cases in the literature of trapeziometacarpal arthroplasty for osteoarthritis. The results are presented in Tables 21-1 and 21-2.

All the reviewed series included both men and women. Only Swanson[38] reported results separately according to sex, so that although the pinch and grip strengths listed in the Swanson series are for women only, all other results combine both sexes.

For the series with silicone replacement, average key pinch strength ranged from 4.0 to 5.7 kg. Abduction varied from 33 to 50 degrees. Pronation was reported in one series as ranging from 30 to 50 degrees. Grip varied from 18.0 to 23.2 kg. Overall, 18% (48 of 290) of the implants were subluxated and 6% (13 of 214) dislocated at the time of the reviews.

DISCUSSION

The ideal arthroplasty is one that restores normal strength and normal motion and provides a pain-free joint without significant risk of complications. As yet, the ideal arthroplasty has not been developed for the trapeziometacarpal joint. With resection arthroplasty excellent results can be obtained by silicone replacement of the trapezium. Yet many authors report difficulties with implant subluxation despite the many modifications made in the surgical technique of trapezial replacement over the last several years. Tenoplasty and ligament reconstruction may result in decreased range of motion.

We have found resection of the trapezium *without* silicone interposition, and with the insertion of a palmaris longus tendon graft as a collagen interposition, to be a dependable procedure that predictably relieves pain, maintains motion, and has little risk of complication. It does not appear to have the potential problems of significantly decreased pinch strength or instability if proper operative technique and postoperative management are followed and the patient is properly selected. In view of the potential problem of late first dorsal compartment pain after abductor pollicis longus shortening, release of the dorsal retinacular ligament is now recommended at the time of arthroplasty.

CONCLUSIONS

For postmenopausal, painful trapeziometacarpal osteoarthritis unrelieved by conservative measures, trapezial resection without silicone interposition usually results in a pain-free strong, and mobile thumb. The results, as judged by pain relief, range of motion, and pinch strength, appear comparable to the results of silicone replacement arthroplasty. The operation appears most suitable for the postmenopausal osteoarthritic patient without significant flexion-adduction deformity of the first metacarpal, particularly if there is evidence of pantrapezial osteoarthritis. The operation is safe, rapid, and reliable.

Table 21-1. Resection arthroplasty without silicone replacement

	Our series	Sims and Bentley[37]	Murley[34]
Key pinch strength	5.0 kg (83%)*	63%*	75%*
Abduction	51 degrees		75%*
Pronation	45 degrees (73%)*		80%*
Grip strength	17.0 kg	56%*	66%*
Subluxation	None		
Dislocation	None		

*Refers to strength or motion of opposite side.

Table 21-2. Resection arthroplasty with silicone replacement (literature review)

	Poppen and Niebauer[36]	Eaton[11]	Ferlic, Busbee, and Clayton[16]	Swanson[38]	Swanson, Watermeier, and Swanson[39]
Key pinch strength	100%*	5.7 kg	4.0 kg (84%)*	4.5 kg	Not noted
Abduction	35 degrees	Not noted	33 degrees (83%)*	48.3 degrees	50 degrees
Pronation	Not noted	Not noted	30 to 50 degrees	Not noted	Not noted
Grip strength	100%*	Not noted	23.2 kg (87%)*	18.0 kg	Not noted
Subluxation	4/14	2/50	2/11	9/45	31/150
Dislocation	2/14†	3/50	None	None	8/150

*Refers to strength or motion of opposite side.
†Three others were removed for synovitis.

REFERENCES

1. Ashworth, C.R., Blatt, G., Chuinard, R., and Stark, H.: Silicone-rubber interposition arthroplasty of the carpometacarpal joint, J. Hand Surg. **2**:345, 1977.
2. Aune, S.: Osteoarthritis of the first carpometacarpal joint, Acta Chir. Scand. **118**:488, 1959.
3. Braun, R.M.: Stabilization of Silastic implant arthroplasty at the trapeziometacarpal joint, Clin. Orthop. **121**:263, 1976.
4. Burton, R.I.: Basal joint arthrosis of the thumb, Orthop. Clin. North Am. **4**:331, 1973.
5. Carroll, R.E.: Fascial arthroplasty for the carpometacarpal joint of the thumb, Orthop. Trans. **1**:15, 1978.
6. Carroll, R.E., and Hill, N.A.: Arthrodesis of the carpometacarpal joint of the thumb, J. Bone Joint Surg. **55B**:292, 1973.
7. Crawford, G.P.: Interposition arthroplasty of the carpometacarpal joint of the thumb, Hand **9**:130, 1977.
8. De la Caffiniere, J.Y., and Aucoutorier, P.: Trapeziometacarpal arthroplasty by total prosthesis, Hand **11**:41, 1979.
9. Dell, C., Brushart, T.M., and Smith, R.J.: Treatment of trapeziometacarpal arthritis: results of resection arthroplasty, J. Hand Surg. **3**:243, 1978.
10. Dickson, R.A.: Arthritis of the carpometacarpal joint of the thumb, treatment, silicone sponge interposition arthroplasty, Hand **8**:197, 1976.
11. Eaton, R.G.: Replacement of the trapezium for arthritis of the bone articulations, J. Bone Joint Surg. **61A**:76, 1979.
12. Eaton, R.G., and Littler, W.J.: A study of the basal joint of the thumb, J. Bone Joint Surg. **51A**:661, 1969.
13. Eaton, R.G., and Littler, W.J.: Ligament reconstruction for the painful thumb carpometacarpal joint, J. Bone Joint Surg. **55A**:1655, 1973.
14. Eiken, O.: Prosthetic replacement of the trapezium, Scand. J. Plast. Reconstr. Surg. **5**:131, 1971.
15. Eiken, O., and Carstam, N.: Functional assessment of the thumb, Scand. J. Plast. Reconstr. Surg. **4**:122, 1970.
16. Ferlic, D.C., Busbee, G.A., and Clayton, M.L.: Degenerative arthritis of the carpometacarpal joint of the thumb: a clinical follow-up of 11 Niebauer prostheses, J. Hand Surg. **2**:212, 1977.
17. Froimson, A.I.: Tendon arthroplasty of the trapeziometacarpal joint, Clin. Orthop. **70**:191, 1970.
18. Gervis, W.H.: Excision of the trapezium for osteoarthritis of the trapeziometacarpal joint, J. Bone Joint Surg. **31B**:537, 1949.
19. Gervis, W.H.: A review of excision of the trapezium for osteoarthritis of the trapeziometacarpal joint after 25 years, J. Bone Joint Surg. **55B**:56, 1973.
20. Haffajee, D.: Endoprosthetic replacement of the trapezium for arthrosis in the carpometacarpal joint of the thumb, J. Hand Surg. **2**:141, 1977.
21. Jackson, I.T., and St. Onge, R.A.: The use of palmaris longus tendon to stabilize trapezium implants, Hand **9**:42, 1977.
22. Kessler, I.: Silicone arthroplasty of the trapeziometacarpal joint, J. Bone Joint Surg. **55B**:285, 1973.
23. Kessler, I., and Axer, A.: Arthroplasty of the first carpometacarpal joint with a silicone implant, Plast. Reconstr. Surg. **47**:252, 1971.
24. Kessler, I., Baruch, A., Hecht, O., and Amit, S.: Osteoarthritis at the base of the thumb, Acta Orthop. Scand. **47**:361, 1976.
25. Kofman, S.: Zur Frage der Nearthrosenbildung am Koxalgelenk, Zentralbl. Chir. **39**:1162, 1923.
26. Lasserre, C., Pauzat, D., and Derennes, R.: Osteoarthritis of the trapeziometacarpal joint, J. Bone Joint Surg. **31B**:534, 1949.
27. Leach, R.E., and Bolton, P.E.: Arthritis of the carpometacarpal joint of the thumb, J. Bone Joint Surg. **50A**:1171, 1968.
28. Lister, G.D., Kleinert, H.E., Kutz, J.E., and Atasoy, E.: Arthritis of the trapezial articulations treated by prosthetic replacement, Hand **9**:117, 1977.
29. Marmor, L., and Peter, J.: Osteoarthritis of the carometacarpal joint of the thumb, Am. J. Surg. **117**:632, 1969.
30. Mattson, H.S.: Arthrodesis of the first carpometacarpal joint for osteoarthritis, Acta Orthop. Scand. **49**:602, 1969.
31. McGrath, M.H., and Watson, H.K.: Arthroplasty of the carpometacarpal joint of the thumb in arthritis, Orthop. Rev. **8**:127, 1979.
32. Mosher, J.F.: The "anchovy" procedure. Orthop. Rev. **8**:63, 1979.
33. Muller, G.M.: Arthrodesis of the trapeziometacarpal joint for osteoarthritis, J. Bone Joint Surg. **31B**:540, 1949.
34. Murley, A.H.G.: Excision of the trapezium in osteoarthritis of the first carpometacarpal joint, J. Bone Joint Surg. **42B**:502, 1960.
35. Patterson, R.: Carpometacarpal arthroplasty of the thumb, J. Bone Joint Surg. **5**:249, 1933.
36. Poppen, N.K., and Niebauer, J.J.: "Tie-in" trapezium prosthesis: long-term results, J. Hand Surg. **3**:445, 1978.
37. Sims, C.D., and Bentley, G.: Carpometacarpal osteoarthritis of the thumb, Br. J. Surg. **57**:442, 1970.
38. Swanson, A.B.: Disabling arthritis of the base of the thumb, J. Bone Joint Surg. **54A**:456, 1972.
39. Swanson, A.B., Watermeier, J.J., and de Goot Swanson, G.: Trapezium implant arthroplasty: long term evaluation, Orthop. Trans. **1**:15, 1978.
40. Weilby, A.: Surgical treatment of osteoarthritis of the carpometacarpal joint of the thumb, Scand. J. Plast. Reconstr. Surg. **5**:136, 1971.
41. Weilby, A., and Sondorf, J.: Results following removal of silicone trapezium metacarpal implants, J. Hand Surg. **3**:154, 1978.
42. Weinman, D.T., and Lipscomb, P.: Degenerative arthritis of the trapeziometacarpal joint: arthrodesis or excision? Mayo Clin. Proc. **42**:276, 1967.
43. Wilson, J.N.: Arthroplasty of the trapeziometacarpal joint, Plast. Reconstr. Surg. **49**:143, 1972.

Chapter 22 Carpometacarpal dislocations (excluding the thumb)

Thomas L. Greene

James W. Strickland

Dislocations and fracture-dislocations of the medial four carpometacarpal (CMC) joints are uncommon injuries. Multiple reports of one or a few such injuries have occurred in the literature, with practically every conceivable pattern of dislocation, either single or combination, dorsal or volar, having been described.*

A review of the pertinent regional anatomy and the basic principles of management of these injuries is presented here.

*References 1, 4-6, and 9-14.

ANATOMY

The CMC joints of the medial four digits are an interlocking, multifaceted arrangement of articulations (Fig. 22-1), which provide the stable and comparatively immobile part of the hand that is necessary for power grasp and to which the mobile thumb opposes.[8] The stability of these joints is provided by the configuration of the articular surfaces, the capsuloligamentous structures (both volar and dorsal), interosseous ligaments that bind the bases of the metacarpals together, and the deep transverse metacarpal ligaments that restrict lateral movement at these joints.

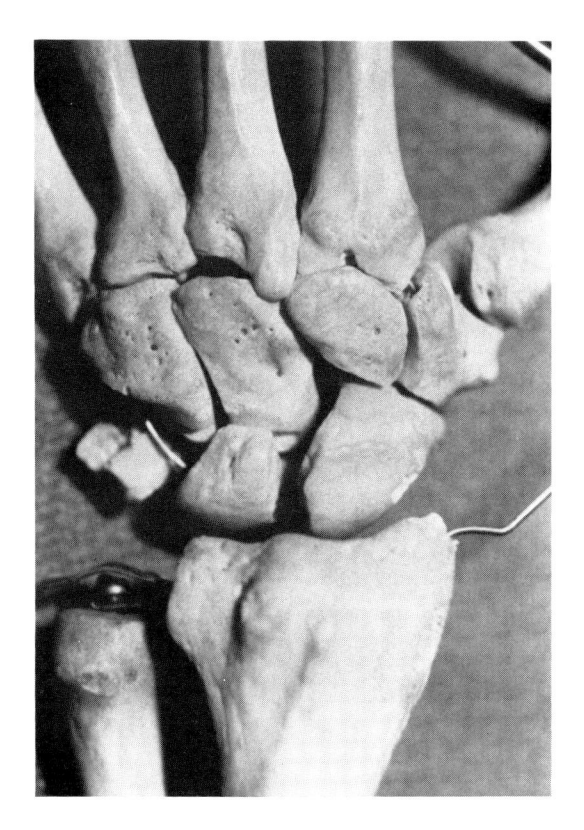

FIG. 22-1. Distal row of carpal bones and bases of metacarpals form interlocking arrangement of articulations, providing relatively immobile medial four CMC joints.

SECTION 6 JOINT PROBLEMS

The largest articular facet on the base of the second metacarpal has an inverted V configuration that corresponds to a reciprocal surface on the trapezoid. A radial facet articulates with the trapezium and an ulnar one with the base of the third metacarpal. The extensor carpi radialis longus and flexor carpi radialis insert onto its dorsal and volar bases, respectively. The base of the third metacarpal has its major articulation with the capitate. A prominent styloid process on its dorsoradial surface also articulates with the capitate. Radial and ulnar facets correspond to reciprocal surfaces on the adjacent second and fourth metacarpals. The extensor carpi radialis brevis inserts onto the base of the third metacarpal and the ulnar portion of the second metacarpal. The second and third CMC joints are essentially immobile and are important for maintaining the stable longitudinal arch of the hand.

The distal surface of the hamate is divided into radial and ulnar portions by a small vertical ridge. The fourth metacarpal articulates with this radial facet and also has a radial lateral facet for the third metacarpal base. The arrangement of the fourth CMC joint allows approximately 15 degrees of flexion-extension movement.[5] The fifth CMC joint more closely resembles the saddle configuration of the trapeziometacarpal joint of the thumb, being reciprocally concavoconvex, and as such it allows 25 to 30 degrees of flexion-extension movement and some rotation.[1] The extensor carpi ulnaris and the flexor carpi ulnaris (by way of the pisometacarpal ligament) insert onto the dorsal and volar bases of the fifth metacarpal, respectively.

The medial four CMC joints are further strengthened by strong dorsal and lesser volar ligaments that span the joints in an A-frame fashion, binding the metacarpals to their adjacent carpal bones.[5] Short, stout, intermetacarpal ligaments are present at the bases of adjacent metacarpals and serve to prevent lateral gliding and angulation.

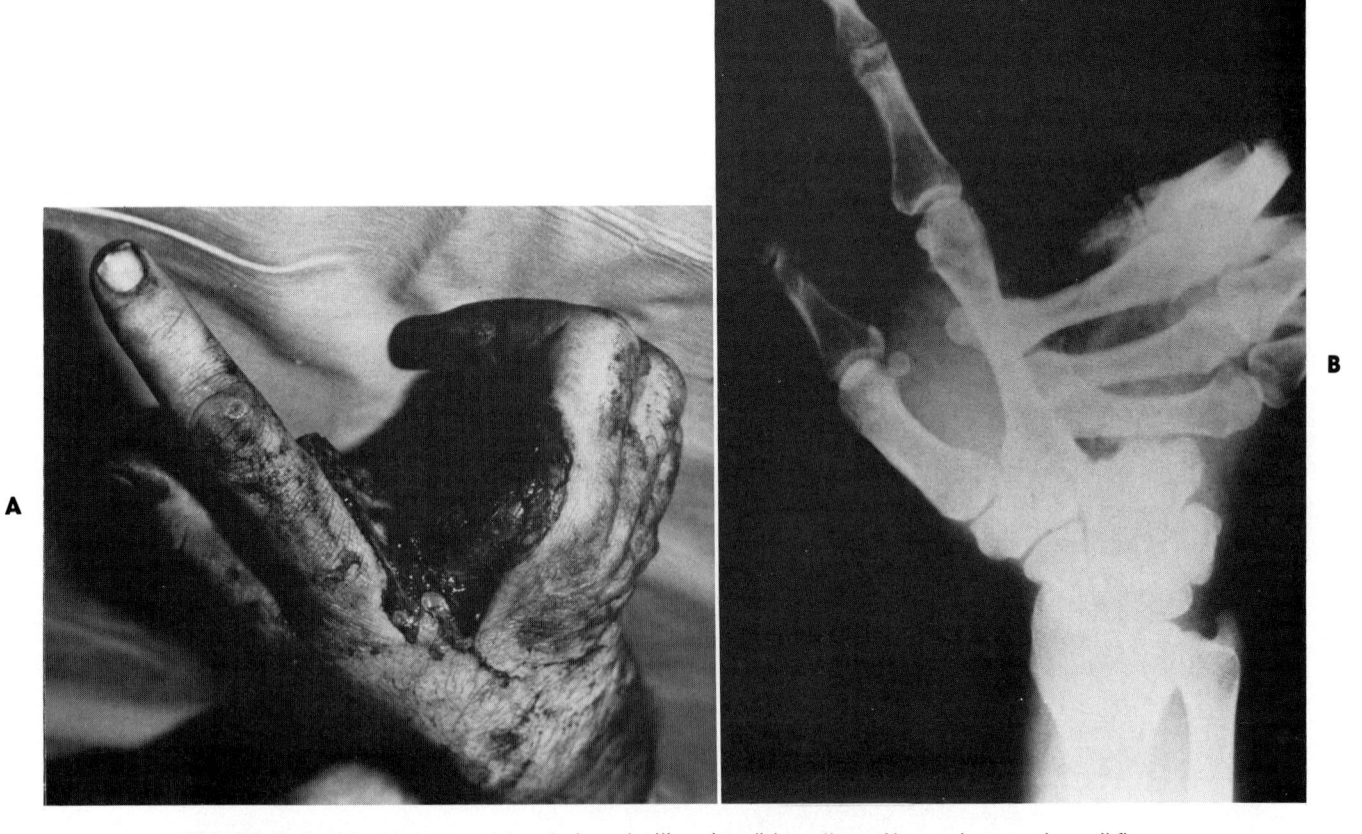

FIG. 22-2. A, Extensive open injury to hand with volar dislocation of long, ring, and small finger CMC joints, resulting from high speed vehicular accident. **B,** Radiograph of hand demonstrates dislocation of medial three CMC joints as a unit.

CHAPTER 22 CARPOMETACARPAL DISLOCATIONS (EXCLUDING THE THUMB)

MANAGEMENT OF THE ACUTE DISLOCATION

The mechanism of injury is either a direct blow to the base of the metacarpal or an axially directed force along the metacarpal shaft. The number of joints involved and the directions in which the dislocations occur are dependent on the magnitude of the force and the direction it is applied.

Recognition of the injury may be difficult because of the swelling of the hand that can occur. A careful review of the radiographs, including oblique views if needed, will demonstrate the pattern of dislocation. Fractures about the bases of the metacarpals may coexist because of the strong ligamentous attachments in this area.

These injuries often will be the result of high-impact trauma with multiple organ system injuries. Within the hand itself one must be alert to the possibility of concomitant injury to other osseous or soft tissue structures (Fig. 22-2). A careful assessment of neural function is

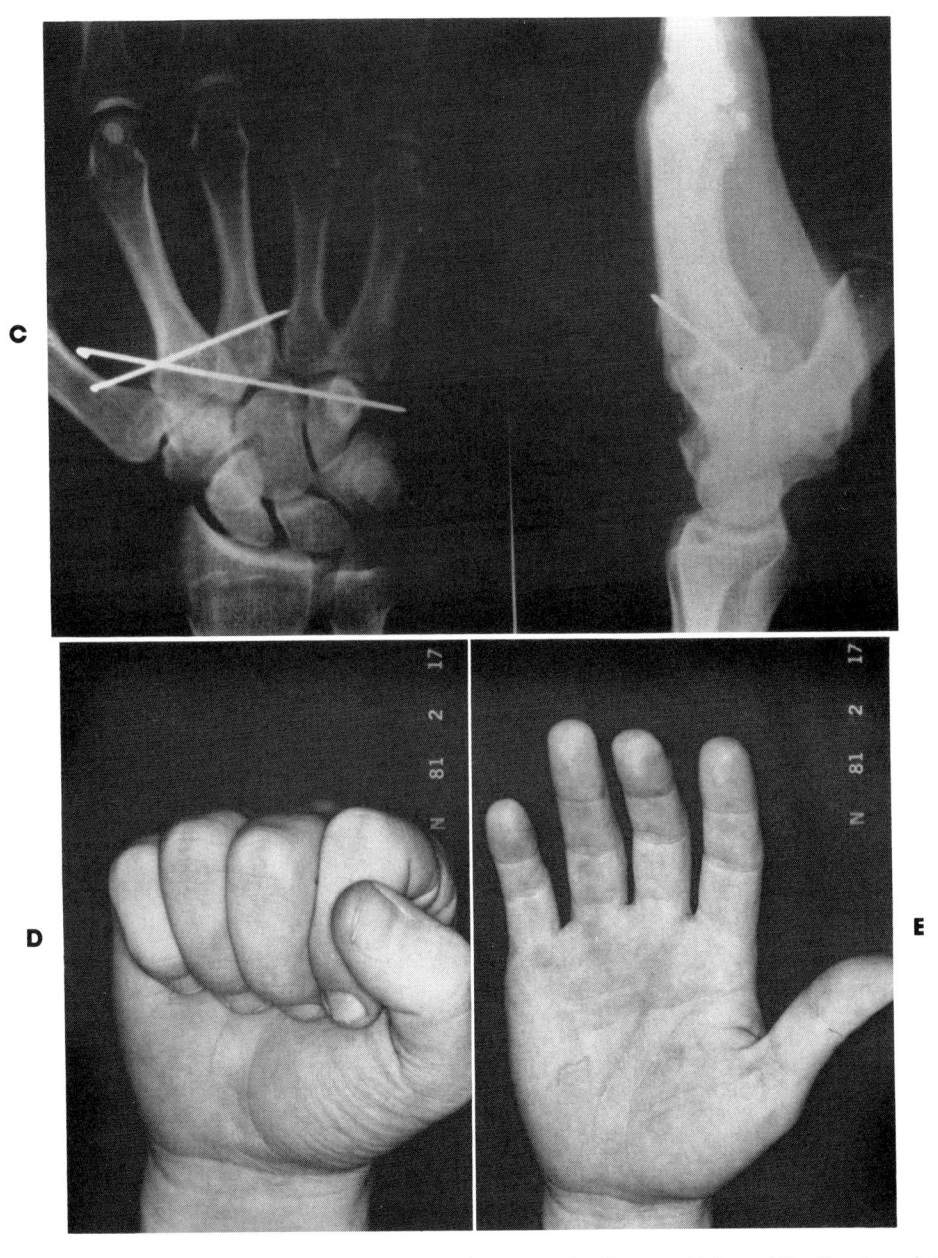

FIG. 22-2, cont'd. C, Treatment consisted of open reduction and internal fixation to uninjured second metacarpal base. **D** and **E,** Several months after injury patient has excellent, stable pain-free motion of hand with correct rotational alignment of fingers.

SECTION 6 JOINT PROBLEMS

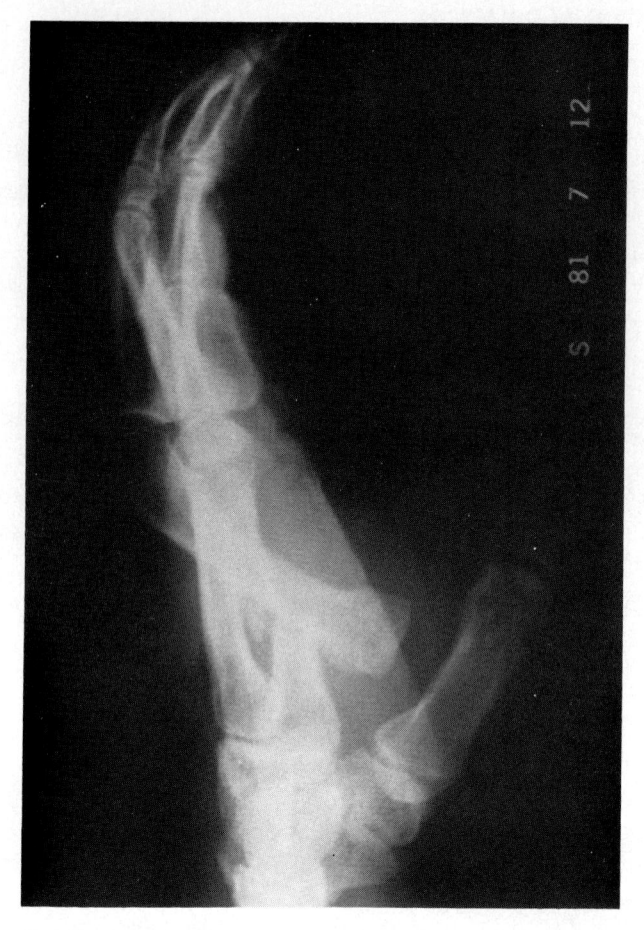

FIG. 22-3. Volar dislocation of base of third metacarpal with displaced fracture of second metacarpal. Volar dislocations may result in median or ulnar nerve injury.

needed in view of the reports of median[15] and ulnar[2] nerve injury following dislocation, particularly volar dislocation (Fig. 22-3).

The more mobile fourth and fifth CMC joints (Fig. 22-4) are probably dislocated more frequently than the second and third. Dislocations of these joints, either singly or, more frequently, in various combinations, have occurred, with dorsal dislocations being more common than volar ones.[3]

An accurate reduction of the articular surfaces and secure fixation to prevent redisplacement are the essential components of successful treatment.[6] Incomplete reductions can lead to an imbalance of the flexor and extensor systems with claw deformity of the digits,[6] weakness of grip,[1] or traumatic arthritis.

It has been frequently recognized that reduction of these dislocations, when they are acute, is relatively easy to accomplish with longitudinal traction and manual pressure over the dislocated bases.[3] Maintenance of reduction has been more difficult to achieve, however.[6] External immobilization with casts or splints has been unreliable in maintaining the reduction. Closed reduction and percutaneous pinning of the dislocated metacarpals to adjacent uninjured metacarpals or to the carpus will prevent loss of reduction.[1,6,11] Early mobilization of the digits is encouraged to prevent stiffness. The pins are removed at 6 weeks, allowing time for sufficient soft tissue healing to occur. The results of this method of treatment have been excellent.[1,6,11]

Open reduction may be needed occasionally if the patient is seen after several days when soft tissue swelling makes closed reduction difficult or when soft tissue or bone is interposed in the joints, preventing reduction. Again the reduction is held for 6 weeks by percutaneous pin fixation with mobilization of the digits begun shortly after surgery.

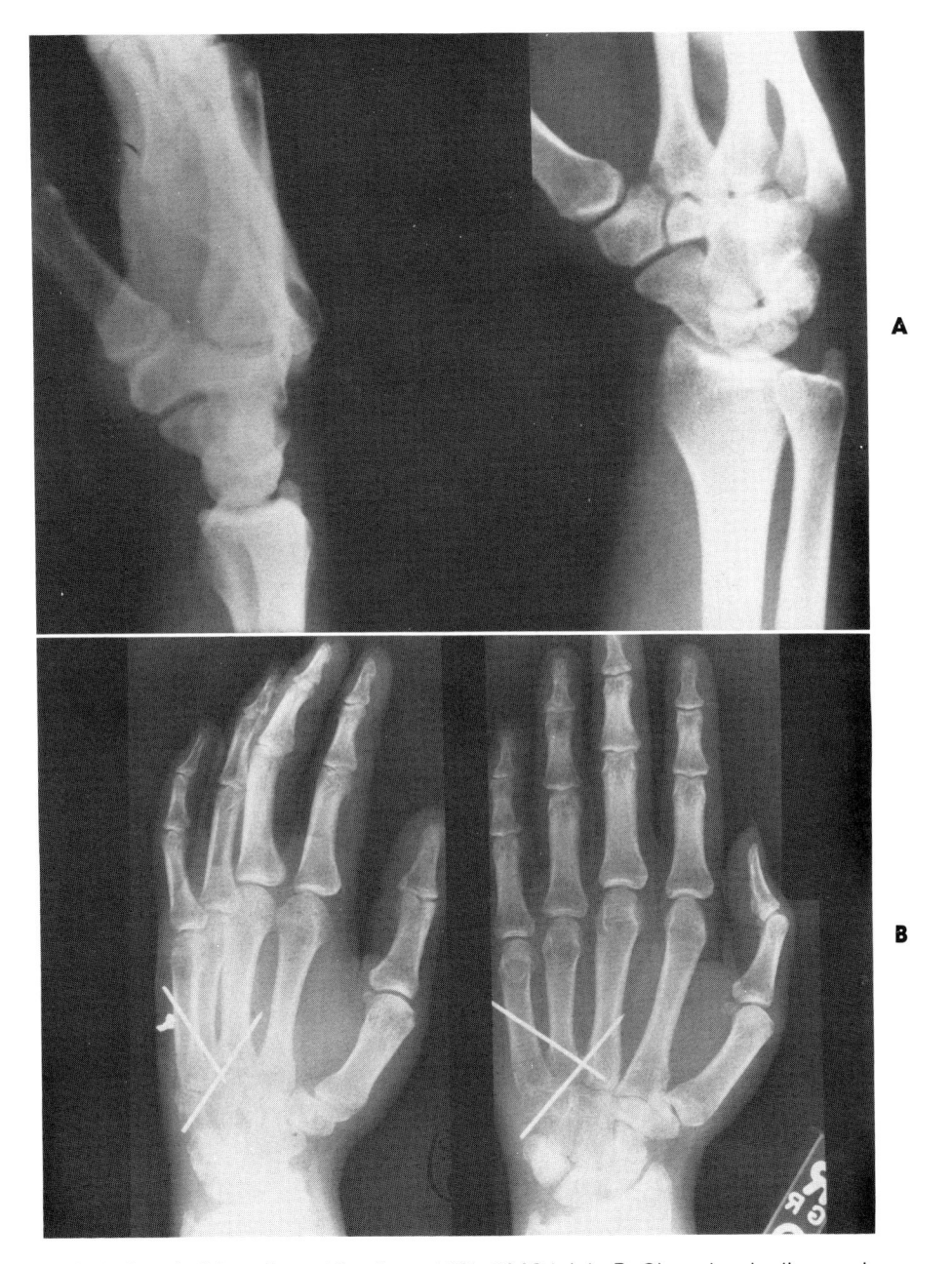

CHAPTER 22 CARPOMETACARPAL DISLOCATIONS (EXCLUDING THE THUMB)

FIG. 22-4. A, Doral dislocation of fourth and fifth CMC joints. **B,** Closed reduction and percutaneous Kirschner wire fixation of dislocated metacarpal bases to carpus and third metacarpal.

SECTION 6 JOINT PROBLEMS

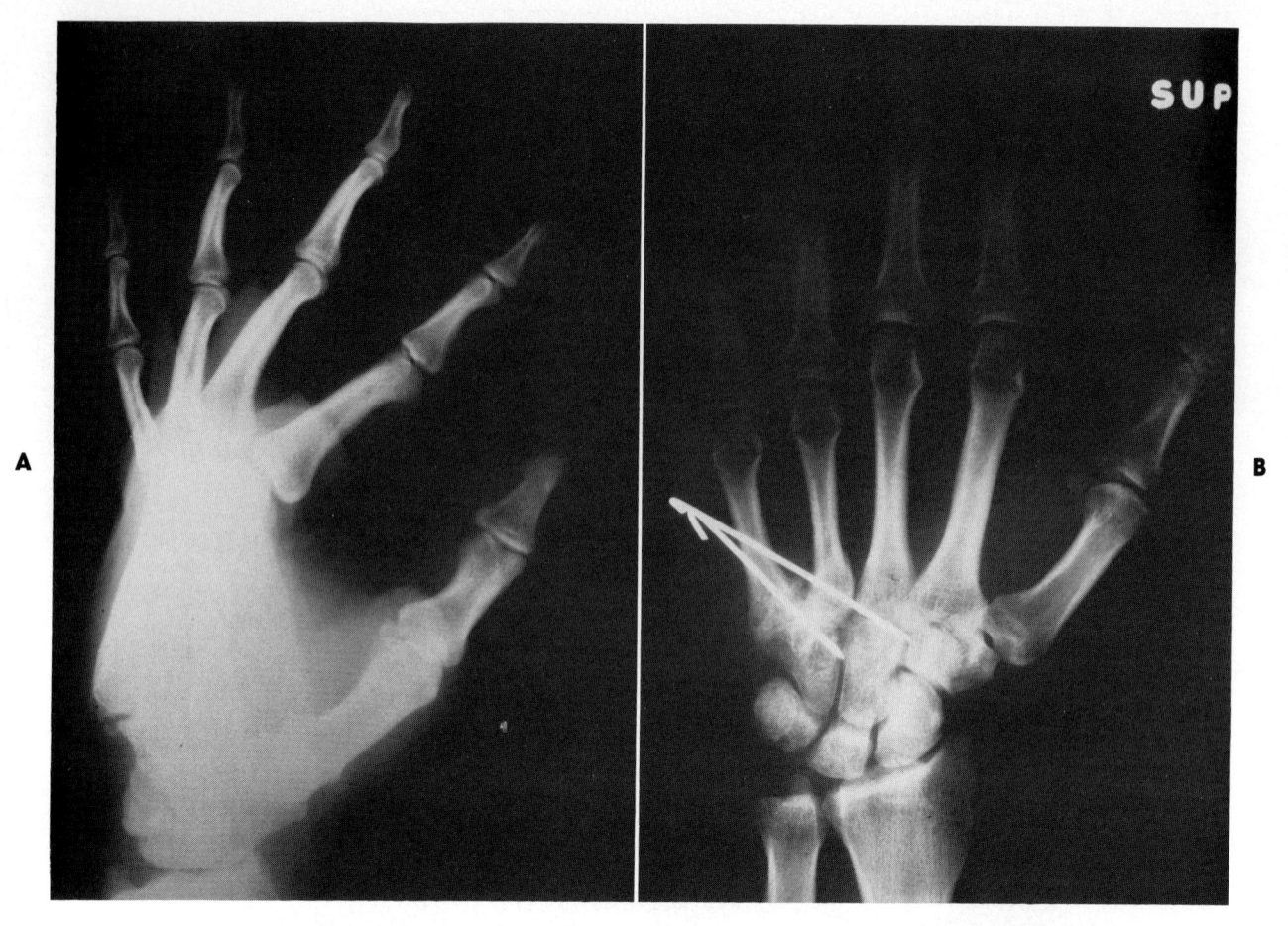

FIG. 22-5. A, Chronic dislocation of fourth and fifth CMC joints resulted in painful arthrosis and weakness of grip. **B,** Open reduction and arthrodesis of fourth and fifth metacarpals to hamate were performed. Fusion of CMC joints, especially more mobile fourth and fifth ones, does not appear to significantly alter function of hand.

MANAGEMENT OF THE CHRONIC DISLOCATION

Occasionally a dislocation may go untreated for weeks or months because of patient neglect or physician oversight. If the patient is seen relatively early, reduction, usually by open means, can be accomplished. If degenerative changes in the articular surfaces have begun, arthrodesis of the involved joints will be needed (Fig. 22-5). Arthrodesis of the relatively more mobile fourth and fifth CMC joints, although eliminating their motion, does not seem to significantly alter the function of the hand.[7]

SUMMARY

Dislocations of the medial four CMC joints represent uncommon injuries to these joints. An accurate, stable reduction is the goal of treatment. When the dislocations are recognized and seen early, closed reduction and percutaneous pinning are the treatment methods of choice. Open reduction and internal fixation may be necessary if soft tissue or bony fragments prevent closed reduction. When the injury is seen late, arthrodesis of the involved joints is preferred and has not caused a significant impairment of function of the hand.

REFERENCES

1. Bora, F.W., and Didizian, N.H.: The treatment of injuries to the carpometacarpal joint of the little finger, J. Bone Joint Surg. **56A:**1459, 1974.
2. Gore, D.R.: Carpometacarpal dislocation producing compression of the deep branch of the ulnar nerve, J. Bone Joint Surg. **53A:**1387, 1971.
3. Green, D.P., and Rowland, S.A.: Fractures and dislocations in the hand. In Rockwood, C.A., Jr., and Green, D.P., editors: Fractures, vol. 1, Philadelphia, 1975, J.B. Lippincott Co.

4. Hartwig, R.H., and Louis, D.S.: Multiple carpometacarpal dislocations: a review of four cases, J. Bone Joint Surg. **61A**:906, 1979.
5. Harwin, S.F., Fox, J.M., and Sedlin, E.D.: Volar dislocation of the bases of the second and third metacarpals: a case report, J. Bone Joint Surg. **57A**:849, 1975.
6. Hsu, J.D., and Curtis, R.M.: Carpometacarpal dislocations on the ulnar side of the hand, J. Bone Joint Surg. **52A**:927, 1970.
7. Joseph, R.B., et al.: Chronic sprains of the carpometacarpal joints, J. Hand Surg. **6**:172, 1981.
8. Kaplan, E.B.: Functional and surgical anatomy of the hand, ed. 2, Philadelphia, 1965, J.B. Lippincott Co.
9. Ker, H.R.: Dislocation of the fifth carpo-metacarpal joint, J. Bone Joint Surg. **37B**:254, 1955.
10. Kleinman, W.B., and Grantham, S.A.: Multiple volar carpometacarpal joint dislocation: case report of traumatic volar dislocation of the medial four carpometacarpal joints in a child and review of the literature, J. Hand Surg. **3**:377, 1978.
11. Nalebuff, E.A.: Isolated anterior carpometacarpal dislocation of the fifth finger: classification and case report, J. Trauma **8**:1119, 1968.
12. Shephard, E.S., and Solomon, D.J.: Carpo-metacarpal dislocation: report of four cases, J. Bone Joint Surg. **42B**:772, 1960.
13. Shorbe, H.B.: Carpometacarpal dislocations: report of a case, J. Bone Joint Surg. **20**:454, 1938.
14. Waugh, R.L., and Yancey, A.G.: Carpometacarpal dislocations, with particular reference to simultaneous dislocation of the bases of the fourth and fifth metacarpals, J. Bone Joint Surg. **30A**:397, 1948.
15. Weiland, A.J., Lister, G.D., and Villarreal-Rios, A.: Volar fracture dislocations of the second and third carpometacarpal joints associated with acute carpal tunnel syndrome, J. Trauma **16**:672, 1976.

SECTION SEVEN RHEUMATOID ARTHRITIS PROBLEMS

Chapter 23 The caput ulnae syndrome: update

Mack L. Clayton

The wrist is the key joint in the hand. It is the final spatial positioning point for the hand for all functions. Any pain in the wrist greatly reduces grip strength.

In rheumatoid arthritis of the wrist area, synovitis involves all the various carpal and radioulnar joints. The various dorsal tendon compartments may be involved. The majority of cases have varying degrees of involvement of both tendons and joints.[2,4] The most common clinical problem concerns the radioulnocarpal complex of the triangular fibrocartilage and the sling of ligaments to the triquetrum and lateral portion of the wrist (Fig. 23-1). The extensor carpi ulnaris tendon is functionally a part of the complex, and it runs through a loose bursa (rather than a snug tunnel) at the head of the ulna; in pronation it is an ulnar deviator; in supination it is a good dorsiflexor, since it rotates to the dorsum of the wrist. With progressive synovial destruction of the radioulnocarpal complex the ulnar head displaces dorsally (caput-ulnae syndrome)[1] as the first deformity. The carpus supinates, and the ulnar border descends. Tenosynovitis of the extensor carpi ulnaris further aggravates the problem, since it displaces volarward, along with the carpus, and loses its ulnar deviating power (it may even become a flexor). This predisposes the patient to radial rotation of the wrist (which further predisposes him or her to ulnar drift of fingers).[3] Other extensor compartments are involved often, with the abductor and short extensor being least involved.

Tenosynovitis can cause local pain. Tendons can rupture from several causes: (1) erosion from bony spicules at the ulnar head, (2) compression by the dorsal carpal ligament, (3) direct invasion of the tendon by synovium, and (4) aseptic necrosis of the tendon because of constrictive tenosynovium.

With pain (the patient's main concern) and the typical swelling of tenosynovitis, early surgery is indicated to relieve pain, preserve function, and prevent tendon rupture.

It is rare that one does only an excision of the distal ulna or just a tenosynovectomy or synovectomy; if bony destruction is too pronounced, then arthroplasty or arthrodesis is indicated. The usual operation is described here but can be varied according to the pathologic condition.

The procedure consists of dorsal tenosynovectomy, distal ulna excision, radiocarpal synovectomy, and radioulnocarpal complex reconstruction; occasionally less than the full procedure is performed.

With the patient under tourniquet control, a long (10 to 14 cm) incision over the dorsum of the wrist, beginning slightly to the ulnar side and extending distally to just beyond base of third metacarpal, is made. The incision is mildly wavy and long enough that retraction is gentle. Dorsal veins should be preserved as much as possible. Dorsal sensory nerves also are easily protected, since the incision is made between them. Skin incision should proceed directly to the dorsal carpal ligament, and all fat is gently reflected with the skin. Skin and soft tissues are often very atrophic and thin (like toilet tissue) and must be handled gently. Wide exposure is necessary. The dorsal carpal ligament is reflected like the page of a book from over the ulnar border in a sheet about 5 cm wide,[2] opening the compartments of the finger ex-

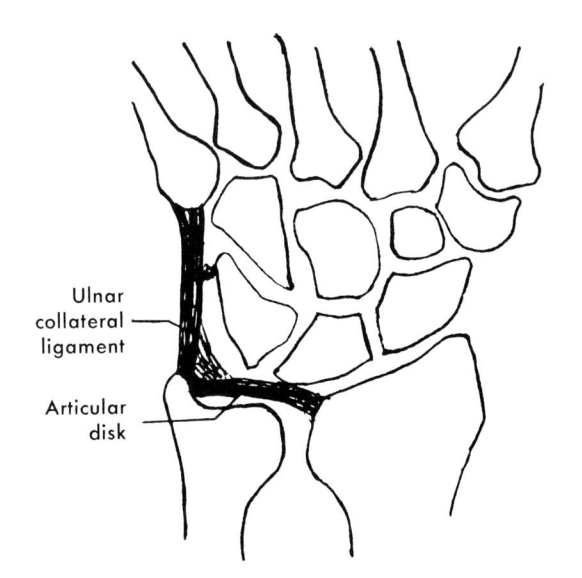

FIG. 23-1. Normal distal radioulnocarpal complex.

SECTION 7 RHEUMATOID ARTHRITIS PROBLEMS

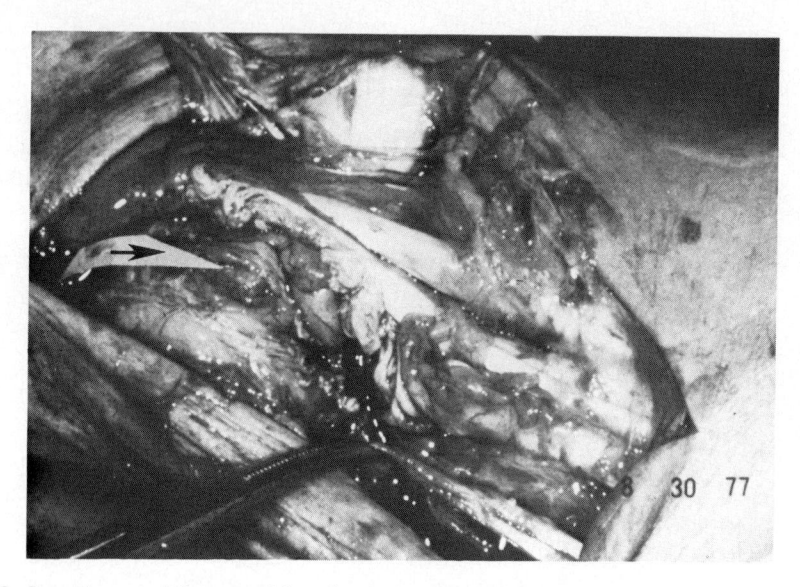

FIG. 23-2. Dorsal carpal ligament is reflected radially. Note arrow on distal aspect of ulna and almost complete rupture of ring extensor with fraying and ruptured extensor communis five; hemostat was placed on ruptured proprius to small finger.

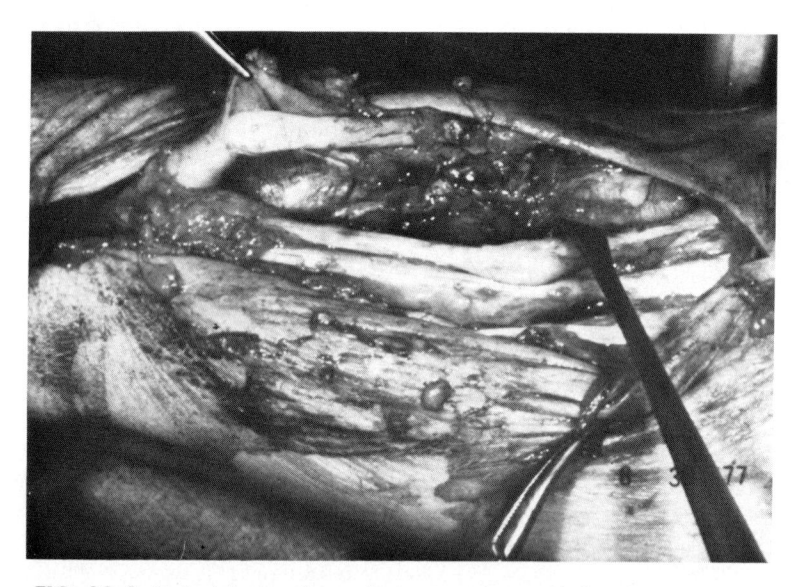

FIG. 23-3. Note intratendinous lesions and constrictive tenosynovitis.

tensors and the long thumb extensor (Fig. 23-2). The wrist extensor compartment is inspected and simply incised if involved. The dorsal carpal ligament also is reflected ulnarward, exposing the extensor carpi ulnaris. Tenosynovectomy is performed, removing the involved area and excising intratendinous involvement (Fig. 23-3). Complete, meticulous removal is not necessary, since the tendons will rest in a bed of healthy fat, and the tendons will heal in the altered environment. Rheumatoid synovium does not proliferate and invade tendons in healthy fat.

The distal aspect of the ulna is exposed subperiosteally, and the distal 1.4 to 2 cm is excised and smoothed. The radioulnar disk usually is destroyed. Traction on the fingers will distract the wrist, and radiocarpal synovectomy is performed with a small rongeur. In more advanced cases (with intercarpal ligamentous disruption, complete loss of cartilage, or moderate bony destruction)

CHAPTER 23 THE CAPUT ULNAE SYNDROME: UPDATE

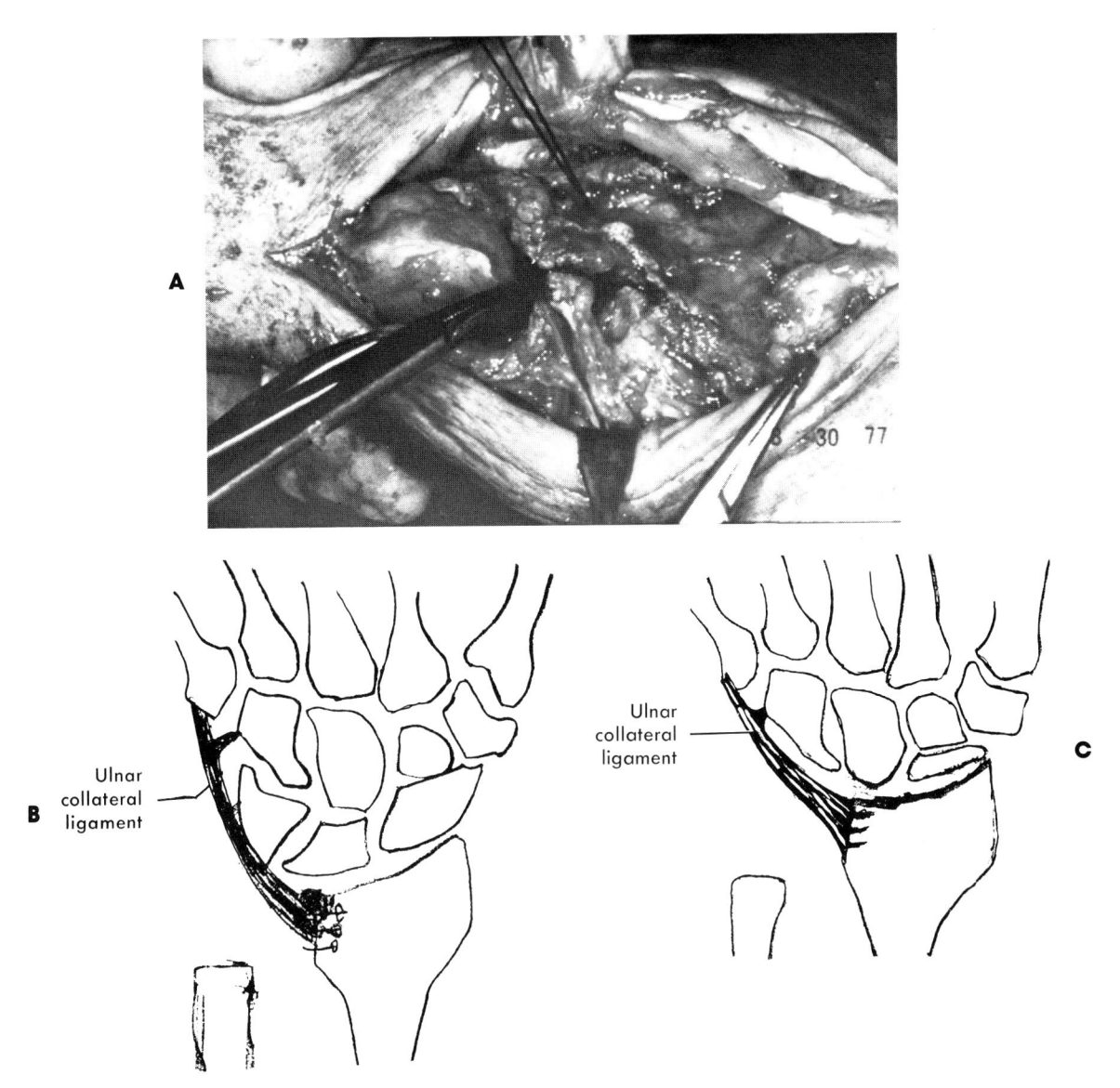

FIG. 23-4. A, Key suture in reconstruction of distal radioulnocarpal complex. Retractor is placed under extensor carpi ulnaris. Central hemostat on dorsal carpal ligament is passed beneath extensor carpi ulnaris, and ligament and lateral capsule are sutured to dorsoulnar edge of radius (after ulnar head excision). This corrects ulnar sliding and supination rotatory deformity. **B,** Reconstruction of distal radiocarpal complex by suture of ulnar collateral ligament capsule and retinaculum to dorsal distal radius, correcting supination deformity and preventing ulnar slide of carpus, and distal aspect of ulnar has been excised. (Articular disk had been destroyed in process.) Note how in normal and in reconstructed complexes there is continuance of "hammock" from radius to lateral aspect of wrist. **C,** Same type of reconstruction as in *B* after proximal row carpectomy.

the dorsal capsule of the wrist is reflected from the radius distally, and a proximal row carpectomy (proximal half of scaphoid, lunate, and triquetrum) is performed, including a synovectomy. The capsule is resutured to the radius. (An additional benefit of proximal row carpectomy may be decompression of the joints of the fingers by shortening the bone.)

The key point of the reconstruction consists of passing the ulnar retinaculum beneath the extensor carpi ulnaris and suturing the retinaculum and the ulnar volar capsule to the dorsum of the distal radius (Fig. 23-4). This reconstructs the radioulnocarpal complex and helps prevent later ulnar sliding and supination deformity. If the wrist is unstable radially, the radiocarpal ligaments are tight-

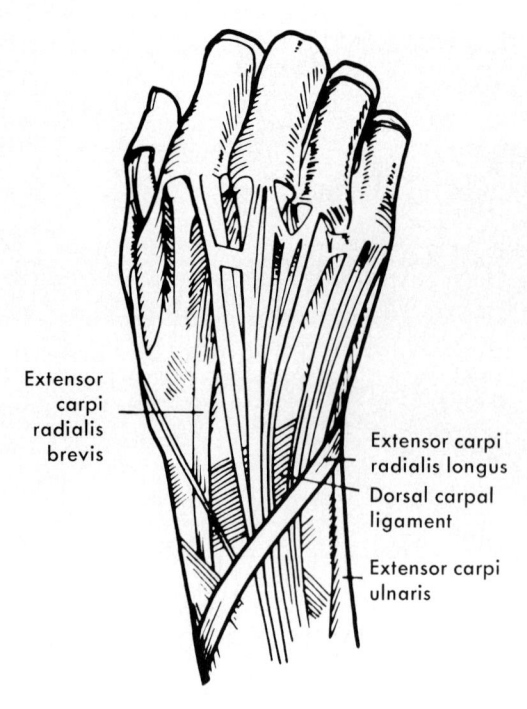

FIG. 23-5. Transfer of extensor carpi radialis brevis to extensor carpi ulnaris is indicated when good extensor carpi ulnaris reconstruction cannot be obtained.

ened by bringing a strip of volar capsule upward across the bare area of the scaphoid and suturing it to the dorsum of the radius; this is done only for proximal row carpectomy.

The proximal retinaculum beneath the extensor carpi ulnaris is passed over the distal ulna and sutured to the periosteum along the edge of the radius. The dorsal carpal ligament is passed beneath the thumb and finger extensors and overlapped along the ulnar "sliding" of the wrist, but too much excision leaves a "floppy" end. Silicone capping of the ulna is unnecessary. A small portion of the dorsal ligament is fashioned to make a sling pulley to hold the extensor carpi ulnaris close to the dorsum of the ulna and restore its function for wrist balance. If it is ruptured or attenuated, then the extensor carpi radialis longus can be transferred to the distal extensor carpi ulnaris to balance rotation and correct supination deformity (descent of the fourth and fifth metacarpals) (Fig. 23-5).[3]

If digital extensors are ruptured, tendon transfers are performed. For a single rupture usually a side-to-side suture to the neighboring extensor is sufficient. For the extensor pollicis longus, the extensor indicis proprius is the choice. The extensor carpi radialis longus also is available for transfer. The extensor carpi radialis brevis and extensor carpi ulnaris should not be sacrificed. The transfers depend on the surgeon's preference and experience. Transfer of the superficialis to the ring and long fingers also can be done.

The tourniquet should be released, bleeders controlled, and drains used, and skin closure with staples is now our choice. Nonadherent dressing and a thick layer of Dacron batting with light compression using a bias-cut stockinette are applied. A volar plaster splint, immobilizing the wrist in the neutral position with slight ulnar deviation, is incorporated into the dressing. (Dorsiflexion would allow extensor tendons to push against the incision). Proximal interphalangeal joint motion is started in a few days. Metacarpal motion is added later while the wound is healing. The wrist is immobilized for about 2 weeks, and several daily range of motion exercises are started. Staples are removed at 3 weeks, since healing is slow and tendons move beneath the incision.

I have had only one case of extensor tendon rupture after 174 wrist synovectomies. Other long-term reports also have good results. In the cases that progress, salvage by arthroplasty or arthrodesis can still be performed.

REFERENCES

1. Backdahl, M.: The caput-ulnae syndrome in rheumatoid arthritis, Acta Rheum. Scand. (Suppl.) **5:**1, 1963.
2. Clayton, M.L.: Surgical treatment at the wrist in rheumatoid arthritis: a review of 37 patients, J. Bone Joint Surg. **47A:**741, 1965.
3. Clayton, M.L., and Ferlic, D.C.: Tendon transfer for radial rotation of the wrist in rheumatoid arthritis, Clin. Orthop. **100:**176, 1974.
4. Clayton, M.L., and Ferlic, D.C.: The wrist in rheumatoid arthritis, Clin. Orthop. **106:**192, 1975.

Chapter 24 Flexor tenosynovitis in the rheumatoid hand

Donald C. Ferlic

Mack L. Clayton

FLEXOR TENOSYNOVITIS IN THE FINGER

Flexor tenosynovitis in the rheumatoid finger may cause pain, triggering, decreased motion, ulnar drift, and rupture of flexor tendons. In the rheumatoid patient, flexor tendons may rupture at their insertion, within the tendon sheath, or at the wrist, and diagnosing the location of a rupture is sometimes difficult. Decreased motion of the finger as a result of flexor synovitis is characterized by the examiner being able to palpate the boggy synovium in many cases and to note that passive flexion is possible through a greater range of motion than is active flexion. One must first ascertain that the flexor tendons are intact. For the problems of pain, triggering, and decreased motion, generally conservative measures are instituted. This consists of making certain the patient is under adequate medical control, perhaps using one steroid injection into the digital theca and then a program of range of motion exercises. For the trigger finger in the patient with rheumatoid arthritis the usual operation of releasing the proximal pulley may not be proper for two reasons: (1) the triggering may be more distal because of an intratendinous nodule restricting motion at one of the distal pulleys; and (2) there is a greater chance of ulnar drift occurring after the proximal pulley system is divided.

There has been much debate about the cause of ulnar drift, and many contributing factors have been listed. Most authors think that it begins with metacarpophalangeal (MCP) synovitis, leaving the MCP joint vulnerable to outside forces acting on the joint. Among these forces are those of the long flexor tendons. Smith, Juvinall, and Bender[5] have shown how the flexor tendons entering the tendon sheath at the MCP joint are supported by the metacarpal glenoidal ligament system and that the flexor tendons make an ulnar bend as they enter the tendon sheath. Therefore the flexor tendons subluxate to the ulnar side when the metacarpal glenoidal ligament system is damaged either by rheumatoid invasion of the system or by surgically releasing the proximal pulley system. Flatt[3] has demonstrated an increase in ulnar torque if the proximal tendon sheath is cut, thereby increasing the ulnar bend of the flexor tendon sheath, pulling the finger into ulnar deviation. We therefore feel that, for the trigger finger in the rheumatoid patient, one should not release the proximal pulley but instead should reduce the contents of the flexor tendon sheath.[2] In doing this procedure a volar zigzag incision from the distal interphalangeal (DIP) joint into the palm is made, and a tenosynovectomy is carried out, but the pulley system is meticulously preserved. The ulnar slip of the superficialis tendon is excised from its insertion to the palm, thereby increasing the cross-sectional area of the tendon sheath. The procedure is carried out with the patient under wrist block or intravenous lidocaine (Xylocaine) anesthesia so that active motion equal to passive motion can be demonstrated on the operating table. Motion of the fingers is started on the second or third postoperative day. In the series of patients on whom we have performed this procedure, we have only experienced two problems. One finger needed a tenolysis, since motion was not started until 2 weeks after surgery, and a second patient had a marked recurrence of flexor tenosynovitis that necessitated a secondary tenosynovectomy.

In addition to the ulnar bend of the flexor tendons contributing to ulnar drift, Shapiro[4] has discussed the association of radial deviation of the wrist with ulnar drift of the fingers, and it can be shown that radial deviation of the wrist will increase the ulnar torque of the flexor tendons. Therefore one must consider correcting the radial rotation of the metacarpals when attempting to correct ulnar drift. A tendon transfer for this problem has been described,[1] which consists of transferring the extensor carpi radialis longus to the extensor carpi ulnaris. It is indicated in patients who cannot actively deviate their wrist in an ulnar direction.

FLEXOR TENOSYNOVITIS AT THE WRIST

Flexor tenosynovitis at the wrist may cause limitation of finger motion, carpal tunnel syndrome, triggering of the fingers at the wrist, and rupture of the tendons. The indication for flexor tenosynovectomy is significant synovial disease in the tendons in spite of adequate medical management. Some authors have condemned flexor tenosynovectomy at the wrist because of the severe limitation of motion that may follow this procedure. We have not found this to be true if motion is started on the second or third day after operation, and we do not hesitate to recommend this procedure.

In dealing with median nerve compression at the wrist in the rheumatoid patient, the most common complication of flexor tenosynovitis, two factors must be kept in mind. One is the normal anatomic variation of the branches of the nerve; second, the nerve and its branches are more susceptible to iatrogenic damage because the nerve may be displaced or rotated by the flexor synovitis. Another important consideration in carpal tunnel syndrome is to observe the floor of the carpal canal to ensure the synovium has not ruptured through the volar wrist ligaments compromising the space in the carpal canal.

Although ruptured flexor tendons at the wrist are not as common a problem as tendon ruptures on the dorsum of the wrist, they certainly do occur. The tendon most commonly ruptured is the flexor pollicis longus, followed by the profundus tendon to the index finger. The location of the rupture of the tendon may not be obvious, but if the thumb flexor is ruptured, look carefully for a rupture of the superficialis or profundus tendon of the index finger. If this combination is present, one may be certain that the rupture is at the wrist level. The location of the rupture often can be diagnosed by palpating the tendon sheaths and ascertaining the area of greatest tenosynovitis.

For the rheumatoid patient with a ruptured flexor tendon the most important recommendation that can be made is flexor tenosynovectomy. After this has been done, then consideration should be given to the specific problem. For the ruptured flexor pollicis longus the case should be handled individually. If the thumb has extremely bad joints, arthrodesis of the interphalangeal joint is all that is necessary. If there is minimal tenosynovitis and minimal involvement of the thumb, a tendon graft may work quite adequately. In the treatment of ruptured finger flexors the problem again needs to be individualized. Tenosynovectomy to prevent further tendon rupture is again the most important part of the surgical treatment. If a lone profundus tendon is ruptured, stabilization of the distal joint should be carried out by tenodesis or arthrodesis with no attempt at tendon grafts or transfers. If only a superficialis tendon is ruptured, only a tenosynovectomy should be carried out, with no attempt to correct the ruptured tendon. If both profundus and superficialis tendons are ruptured, the finger is very disabled. In such a case, after the flexor tenosynovectomy, if the wrist is not too severely involved, tendon transfer may be carried out, but motion needs to be started soon after surgery. Tendon grafting has not been satisfactory. If the joints in the finger are stiff, or if there is marked tenosynovitis with serious potential tendon adhesions, then only arthrodesis or tenodesis of both the DIP and the proximal interphalangeal joints is the best salvage procedure.

REFERENCES

1. Clayton, M.L., and Ferlic, D.C.: Tendon transfer for radial rotation of the wrist in rheumatoid arthritis, Clin. Orthop. **100**:176, 1974.
2. Ferlic, D.C., and Clayton, M.L.: Flexor tenosynovectomy in the rheumatoid finger, J. Hand Surg. **3**:364, 1978.
3. Flatt, A.E.: Some pathomechanics of ulnar drift, Plast. Reconstr. Surg. **37**:295, 1966.
4. Shapiro, J.S.: A new factor in the etiology of ulnar drift, Clin. Orthop. **68**:32, 1970.
5. Smith, E.M., Juvinall, R.C., and Bender, L.F.: Role of the finger flexors in rheumatoid arthritis of the metacarpophalangeal joints, Arthritis Rheum. **7**:467, 1964.

Chapter 25 Complex arthritic disabilities of the thumb

James W. Strickland

William B. LaSalle

Subsequent to the excellent descriptions by Bunnell,[3] Clayton,[4] and Brewerton[2] of the thumb in rheumatoid arthritis patients, numerous important contributions describing the incidence and pathomechanics of deformity and methods of treatment have appeared in the literature. Hand surgeons and rheumatologists have come to recognize that the restoration of function to a painful, unstable, or deformed thumb often will provide the patient with long-term functional benefits exceeding those obtained by other, more elaborate procedures on the wrist or digital joints.

Various studies* have indicated that the thumb is involved in approximately 60% of all patients with rheumatoid arthritis affecting the hand. Because of the capricious nature of the rheumatoid process, which may attack any of the joints or tendons of the thumb, there is wide variation in the type of deformity that may result. Although isolated disease involving destruction of either the metacarpophalangeal (MCP) or interphalangeal (IP) joint of the thumb may occur, the most difficult management problems involve complex deformities resulting from either simultaneous arthritic involvement of several joints or the imbalance of the three-joint osseous chain created by the collapse of one of its joints secondary to direct invasion or tendon loss. The development of reciprocal deformity in the joints adjacent to those with primary involvement then is perpetuated by the strong, axially applied forces acting on the thumb.[29] The pathomechanics of these deformities must be well understood to carry out procedures that will best restore painless thumb stability and mobility.

Numerous descriptions and classification of the deformities of the rheumatoid thumb have been provided.[14,19,21,30] Nalebuff[19,21] described the type 1 deformity as one of MCP joint flexion and IP joint extension without involvement of the carpometacarpal (CMC) joint. Type 2 and 3 deformities involve destruction of the CMC joint with secondary MCP flexion–IP hyperextension or MCP extension–IP flexion combinations, depending on the pattern of compensatory collapse. Swanson and Swanson[30] described rheumatoid thumb disease as postural; unstable, stiff, or painful; or involving tendon disabilities, and they simplified the classification of complex lesions into boutonniere and swan-neck deformities.

BOUTONNIERE DEFORMITY

The boutonniere lesion (Fig. 25-1) (Nalebuff[19,21] type 1) is the most common thumb deformity in rheumatoid arthritis patients and is estimated to occur in 57% of rheumatoid arthritics with hand involvement.[30] This deformity arises secondary to synovitis of the MCP joint with subsequent attenuation of the dorsal capsule and the extensor apparatus around MCP joint. The extensor pollicis longus and adductor expansion are displaced to the ulnar side of the MCP joint, and a similar radial displacement of the thenar expansion occurs. The extensor pollicis brevis also becomes attenuated, and after the loss of these dorsal support structures a volar subluxation

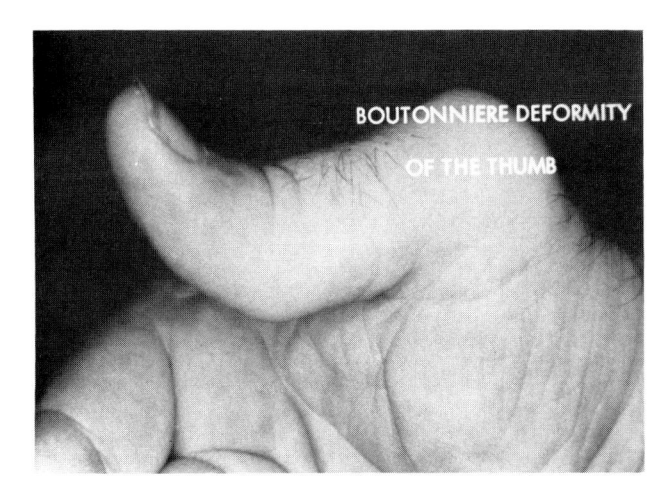

FIG. 25-1. Boutonniere deformity of rheumatoid thumb with severe flexion deformity at MCP joint and reciprocal hyperextension at IP joint.

---
*References 2, 21, 23, and 27-30.

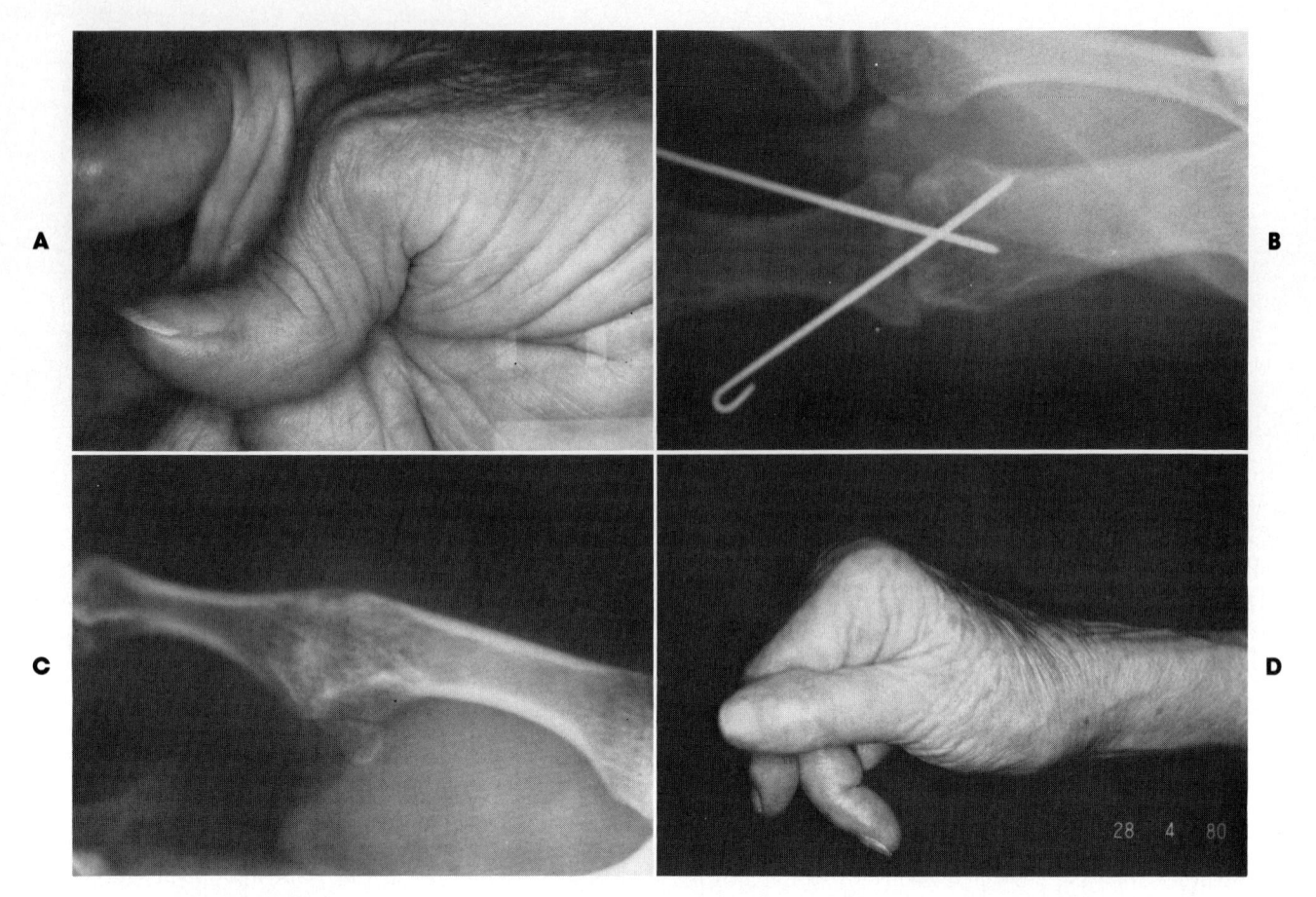

FIG. 25-2. Management of boutonniere deformity. **A,** Severe MCP flexion–IP extension combination (Nalebuff[19,21] type 1). **B,** Arthrodesis of MCP joint. **C,** Appearance of MCP joint after arthrodesis. **D,** Improved position, stability, and function of thumb after MCP joint arthrodesis with restored balance at IP joint level.

of the proximal phalanx occurs. A dynamic aggravation of the deformity results when the extensor pollicis longus and intrinsic tendons attempt to extend the thumb. This additional IP joint extension forces the MCP joint to sublux further. A vicious cycle is created wherein MCP joint flexion and IP joint extension accentuate each other. Ultimately a fixed contracture will develop at one or both distal joints, and articular destruction may occur.

The boutonniere deformity is quite disabling in that it limits the breadth of grasp, and the contact surfaces of the distal aspect of the thumb for pinching and grasping are substantially altered. In rare instances when there is concomitant CMC joint involvement and collapse (Nalebuff[19,21] type 2), the functional sequelae can be even more disabling.

Although rebalancing procedures have been described for the early boutonniere deformity,[12,16] they have not always proved to be of long-term benefit. Because the deformity is usually seen at a fairly advanced stage, arthrodesis of the MCP joint has been recommended by most authors* as the best form of treatment (Fig. 25-2). Stabilization of the MCP joint often will balance the hyperextended IP joint by increasing the tension on the flexor pollicis longus and decreasing the overpull of the extensor pollicis longus. It is occasionally necessary to manipulate the IP joint into flexion and to temporarily maintain its position with a longitudinally placed Kirschner wire at the time of MCP arthrodesis. Swanson[29] and Swanson[30] recommend a hemitenodesis of the IP joint for the persistent flexible hyperextension deformity.

On occasion deformity and instability at the IP joint level may be the most disabling features of the boutonniere deformity of the rheumatoid thumb, and in these instances it may be preferable to perform an arthrodesis at that level. If IP joint arthrodesis is carried out, the MCP joint may be left alone, managed by tendon and soft tissue reconstruction,[12,16,19] subjected to interposi-

---

*References 4, 6, 13, 19, 21, and 23.

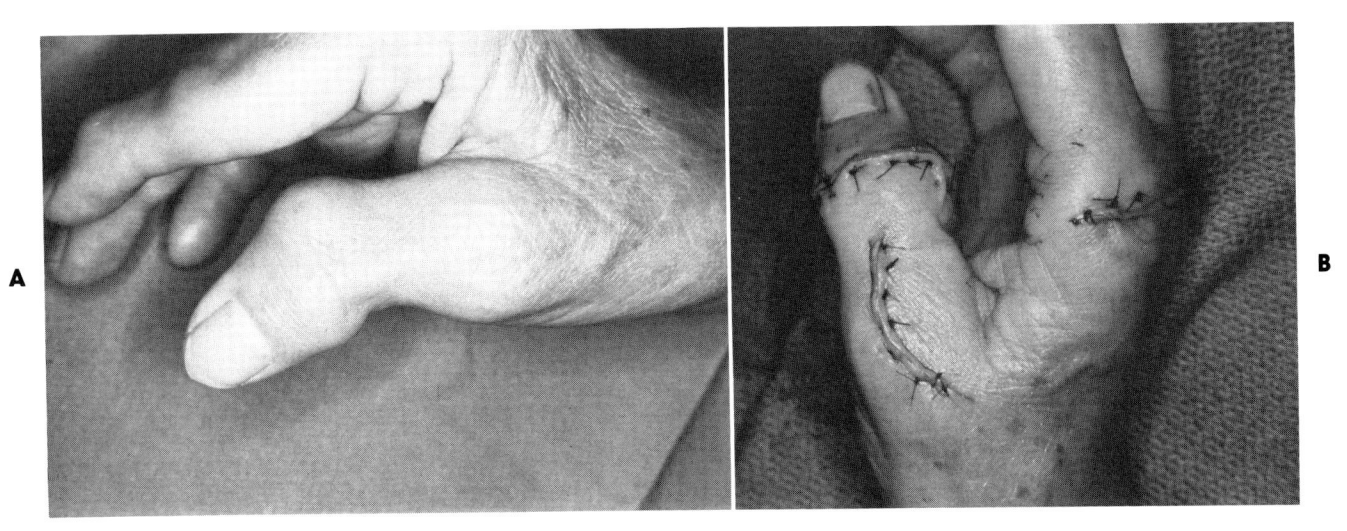

FIG. 25-3. A, Boutonniere lesion of rheumatoid thumb with angular deformity at IP joint. **B,** Management by arthrodesis of IP joint and dorsal rebalancing of MCP joint.

tional arthroplasty,[17,27,32] or treated by arthrodesis, depending on the severity of the deformity. If the MCP joint is stable and flexible with minimal articular damage, it may be rebalanced to some extent by the obligatory tightening of the extensor pollicis longus resulting from correction of the IP joint hyperextension deformity. If additional rebalancing is necessary, a proximal dorsal transfer of the intrinsic wing tendons[12] or extensor pollicis longus "rerouting"[16,20] may prove to be beneficial (Fig. 25-3). Fusion of both the MCP and IP joints after severe destruction and instability at both levels may be infrequently necessary for the restoration of satisfactory function.[4,6,13,16]

Although favored by some,[17,27,32] the use of a flexible silicone rubber implant at the MCP joint of the thumb is worrisome. The procedure would seem to have the advantage of maintaining useful motion and facilitating prehension of small objects. Even the proponents of arthroplasty, however, concede that one should immobilize the MCP joint until lateral stability occurs with an obligatory decrease in motion in the flexion-extension plane.[16] If the procedure must be modified to provide stability at the expense of motion, it would seem to have little advantage over arthrodesis.

On occasion one will be confronted with severe thumb deformities in patients with arthritis mutilans or psoriatic arthritis in which substantial bone resorption has resulted in total loss of stability at the MCP or IP joints or both. Arthrodesis should be carried out in these cases but will require the use of generous blocks of iliac bone graft to restore length and stability.[8] In several instances when grafts have failed, we have reconstructed these flaccid thumbs successfully with an interpositional threaded Steinmann pin and methyl methacrylate (Fig. 25-4).

BOUTONNIERE DEFORMITY WITH CMC COLLAPSE

Boutonniere deformity of the rheumatoid thumb in combination with destruction of the basilar thumb joint (Nalebuff[19,21] type 2) is thought to result from a different sequence of events than those leading to the isolated boutonniere deformity. Synovitis and capsular stretching originate at the CMC level, which ultimately subluxates and dislocates. The first metacarpal will then adduct, and this is followed by a shortening of the adductor pollicis brevis. The first metacarpal ultimately will become fixed in adduction, and, as the patient repeatedly attempts to bring the thumb away from the palm for wide grasp and pinch activities, a hyperextension deformity will occur at the IP joint. Ultimately a flexion deformity at the MCP joint will be produced as the forces of pinch come into action.[20,22] The role of adductor spasm* has been debated, and it would appear to have, if not an initiating, at least a perpetuating influence on this deformity.

Management of the boutonniere deformity with basilar joint collapse can best be carried out by arthroplasty of the CMC joint with mobilization of the first metacarpal and occasionally adductor release and first web space deepening. Although CMC arthrodesis was once considered appropriate,[21] the functional limitation imposed by this procedure, particularly when there is concomitant MCP and IP joint deformity, and the development of

---

*References 4, 6, 13-15, and 17.

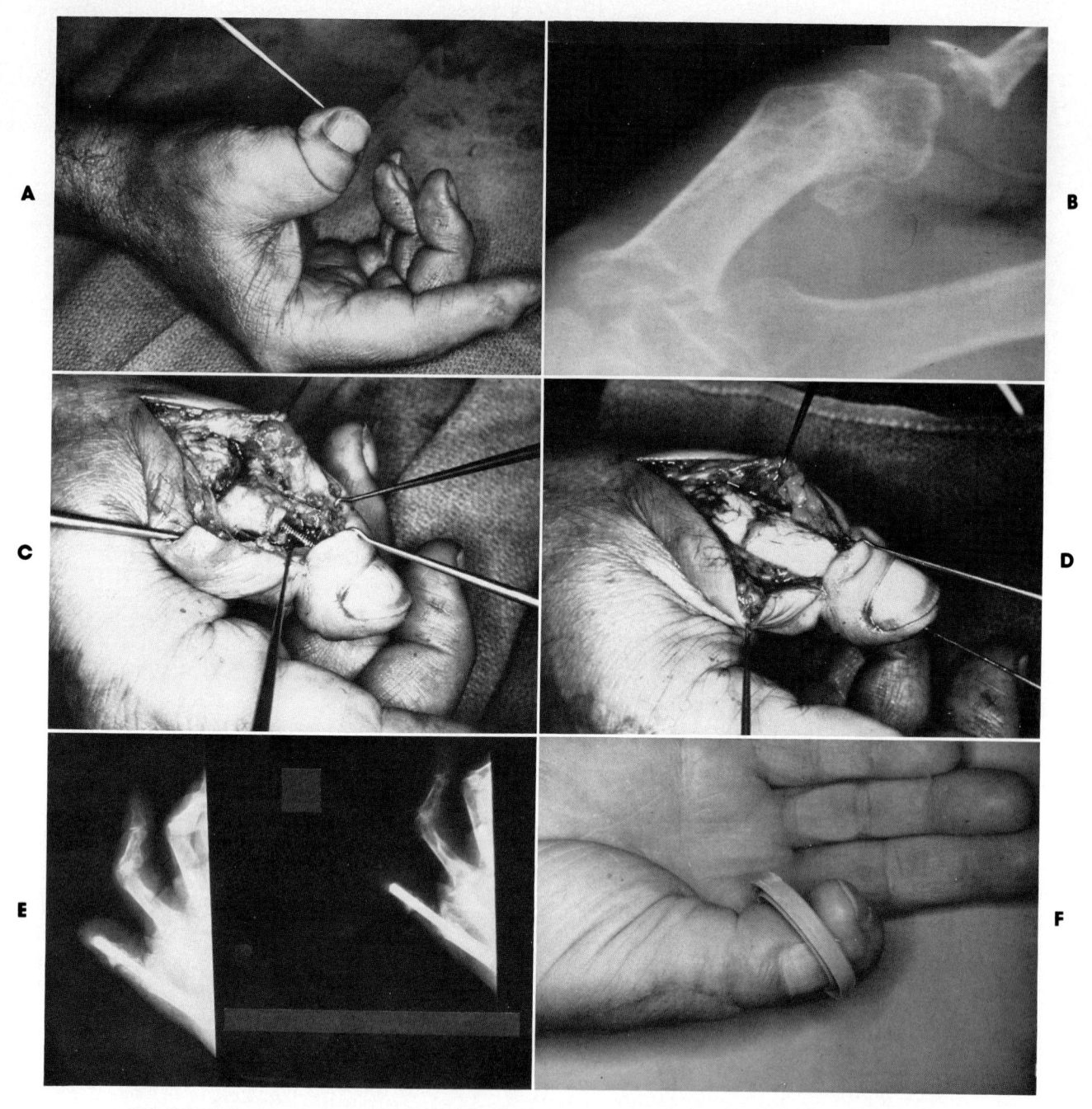

FIG. 25-4. A, Severe instability of IP joint of right thumb with extensive bony resorption of distal aspect of proximal phalanx. **B,** X-ray appearance indicating extent of bony loss. **C,** Thumb reconstruction by restoration of length and maintenance of position with threaded Steinmann pin. **D,** Interpositional plug of methyl methacrylate surrounding Steinmann pin. **E,** X-ray appearance of reconstructed thumb. **F,** Markedly improved length and pinch stability after this procedure.

improved arthroplasty techniques have greatly reduced its applicability to reconstruction of the rheumatoid hand. A detailed description of the techniques of basilar joint arthroplasty is given in the section devoted to swan-neck deformity. Management of the MCP and IP joints is accomplished in a manner similar to that described for boutonniere deformity without CMC involvement.

SWAN-NECK DEFORMITY

The swan-neck thumb deformity (Nalebuff[19,21] type 3) is estimated to occur in 9% of all hands afflicted with rheumatoid arthritis[25-32] and consists of destruction of the basilar thumb joint with lateral dislocation of the first metacarpal base and adduction of the first metacarpal combined with hyperextension of the MCP joint and a flexion deformity of the IP joint (Fig. 25-5). According to Vainio[33] adduction contracture develops as a result of osseous or fibrous ankylosis of the trapzeiometacarpal joint, whereas others[4,6,15] believe that the deformity is caused primarily by spasm of the adductor muscle. It has been postulated that this deformity is again a result of the efforts of the patient to extend the thumb in the presence of an adduction contracture of the first metacarpal and that the laxity of the volar structures of the MCP joint allows hyperextension to occur at that level rather than at the IP joint level.[21] As a result, the proximal phalanx assumes an extended position and may dislocate with an obligatory reciprocal flexion deformity occurring at the IP joint level.

An advanced swan-neck deformity will render the rheumatoid thumb almost functionless by virtue of its inability to reach around large objects, pinch to the index finger, or provide strong counterpressure. Management of this deformity again involves arthroplasty of the CMC joint, occasionally combined with a deepening of the first web space by Z-plasty.[13]

Trapezial excision arthroplasty has been advocated by some[9,10,18] and can provide excellent relief from pain with the restoration of satisfactory stability and pinch strength.[5] Soft tissue interpositional arthroplasty[7] has also gained considerable popularity and is a relatively simple procedure involving removal of the trapezium and the use of a tendon or muscle to fill the resulting space. As with other excisional techniques, this procedure consistently produces a pain-free basilar joint, although the mobility of the first metacarpal base is somewhat variable.

Interpositional implant arthroplasty using silicone implants* has enjoyed increasing popularity for the management of these problems. The implant designed by Swanson[29] adequately maintains the space created by trapezial excision, and the development of a supportive pseudocapsule provides mobility and consistent relief from pain.[24] The current technical recommendations by Swanson[29] are quite exacting and involve the use of the flexor carpi radialis tendon to reinforce the palmar capsule. The abductor pollicis longus tendon is employed as a lateral reinforcement to ensure the stability of the implant, and a Kirschner wire is used to maintain the prosthesis's position during the early stages of healing.[29]

A personal modification of the technique for silicone interpositional arthroplasty[24] involves the retention of a small wafer of the volar aspect of the trapezium with its edges trimmed away from the scaphoid and first meta-

---

*References 1, 11, 22, 24, and 26-32.

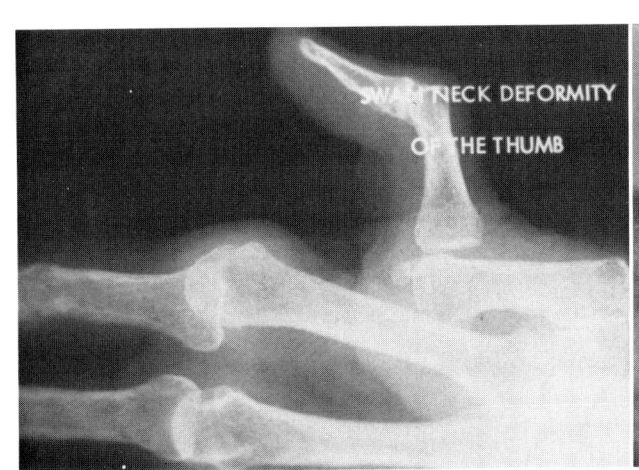

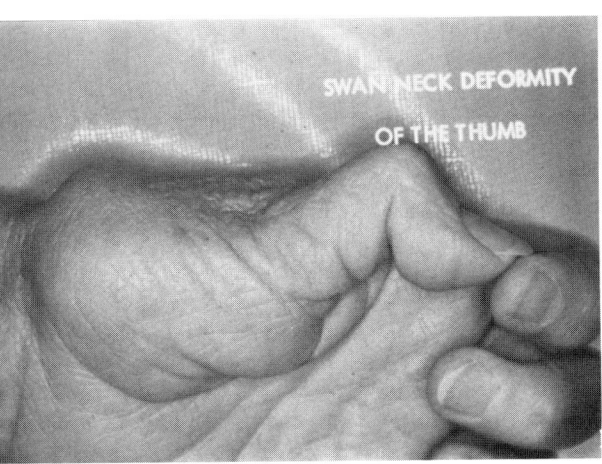

FIG. 25-5. Swan-neck deformity of thumb. **A,** X-ray appearance indicating complete collapse at CMC joint with adduction contracture of first metacarpal, hyperextension dislocation of MCP joint, and flexion deformity at IP joint. **B,** Clinical appearance of swan-neck deformity of rheumatoid thumb.

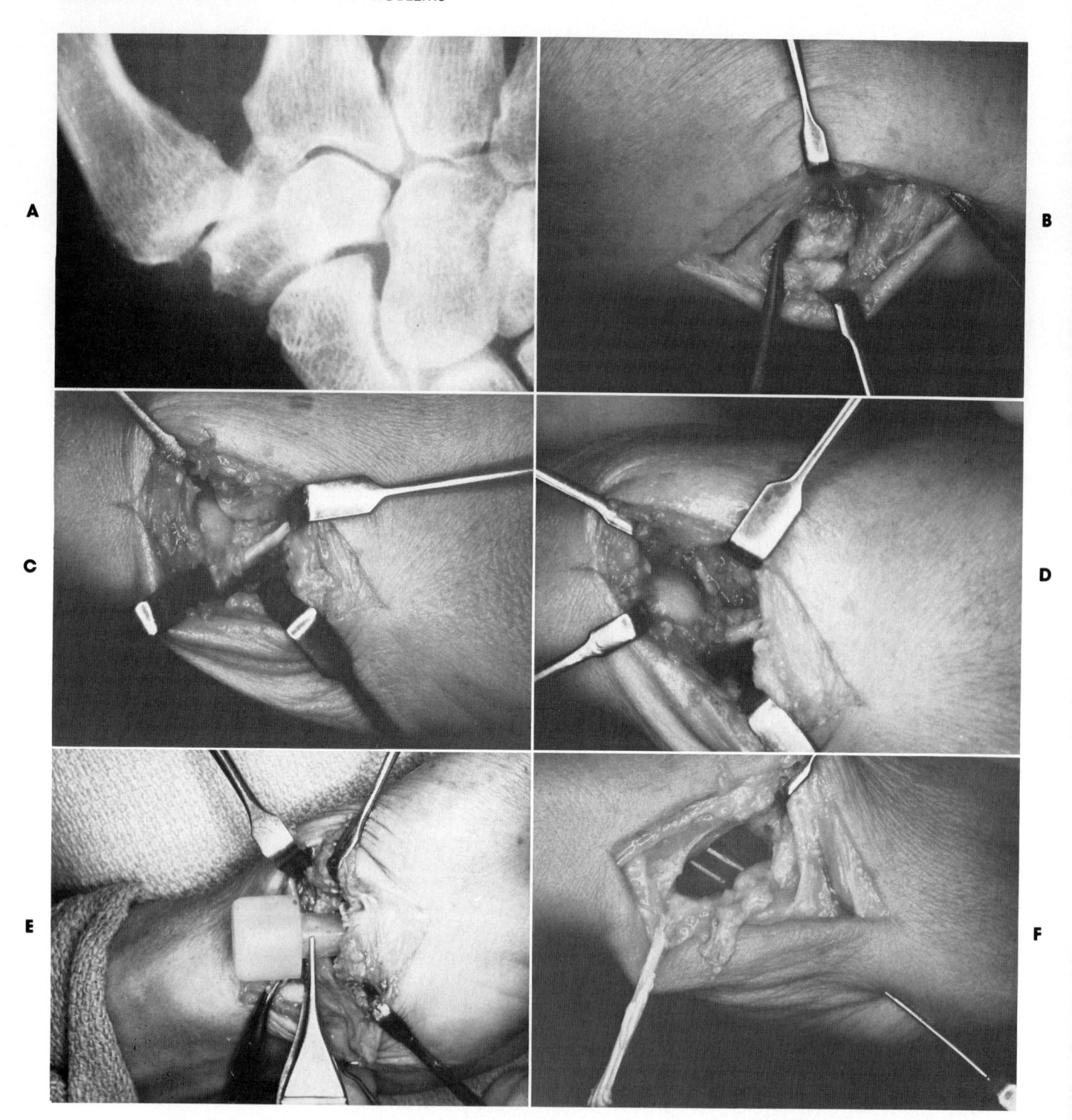

FIG. 25-6. Our technique of silicone replacement arthroplasty (Swanson[29]) of basal thumb joint. **A,** Preoperative appearance of arthritically subluxed basilar thumb joint. **B,** Delineation of trapezial margins after division of capsule. **C,** Following excision of trapezium (with exception of small volar wafer depressed by bottom retractor) flexor carpi radialis tendon is seen and dome of scaphoid is noted to be covered on its entire medial slope by base of trapezoid. **D,** Exposure of entire dome of scaphoid following excision of overlapping medial portion of trapezoid. **E,** Insertion of prosthesis by placement of stem into medullary canal of first metacarpal. **F,** Prosthesis in place with pin fixation and preparation for lateral capsule reinforcement by use of strip of abductor pollicis longus.

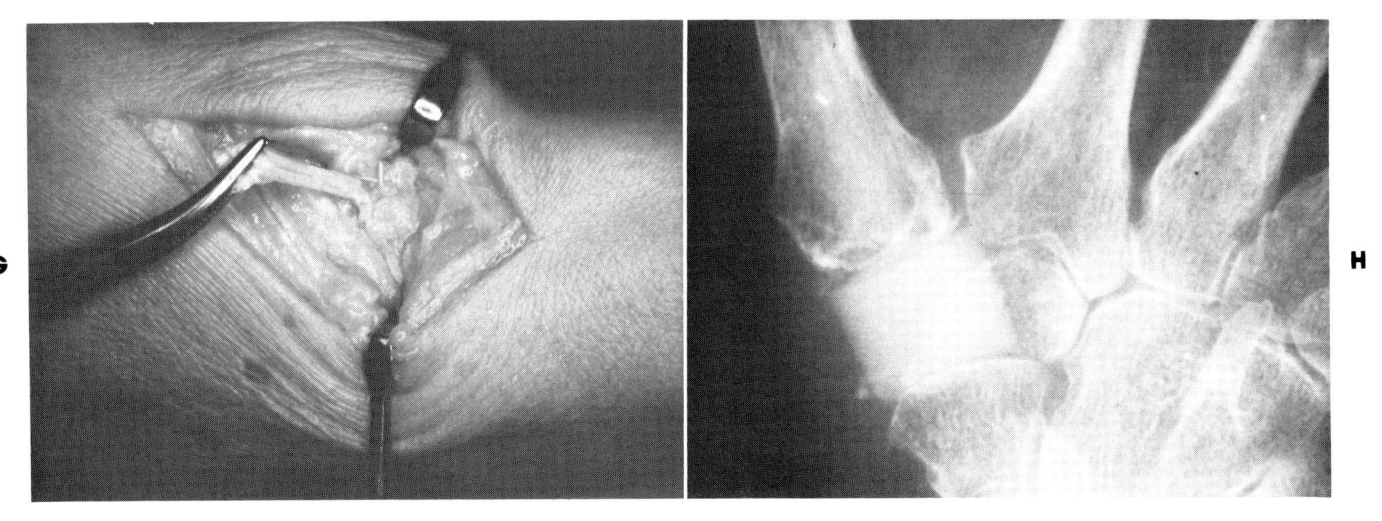

FIG. 25-6, cont'd. G, Completion of lateral reinforcement by capsular imbrication. **H,** X-ray appearance of well-seated trapezial implant.

carpal base. This wafer provides support for the implant and obviates the need for wrist flexor reinforcement. In addition, the wedge-shaped portion of the trapezoid overlying the medial downslope of the scaphoid dome is excised to allow stable seating of the concave base of the prosthesis. At the time of closure the lateral capsule is reefed with a strip of the abductor pollicis longus, and a transfixing wire as described by Swanson[29] is usually employed. These technical modifications have provided consistently predictable and satisfactory results following 6 weeks of immobilization for the development of the pseudocapsule. The procedure is particularly applicable for basilar joint destruction in the rheumatoid thumb, and concomitant arthrodeis at a distal level can be easily carried out (Fig. 25-6).

At the time of arthroplasty, mobilization of the first metacarpal may be indicated with occasional release of the adductor aponeurosis,[13] the adductor muscle,[6,19,21] or both (Fig. 25-7). Some[17] believe that after trapezial excision a formal adductor release is rarely necessary. Mild hyperextension of the MCP joint may spontaneously correct after repositioning of the first metacarpal, without the need for any reconstruction at that level. A volar tenodesis may be helpful in some instances to reinforce the attenuated volar plate.[29] In most cases, however, the deformity is severe and fixed, and arthrodesis of the MCP joint in 20 degrees of flexion and slight abduction is the procedure of choice (Fig. 25-8).

The procedures at the CMC and MCP joint levels should correct or improve the IP joint flexion deformity, although gentle manipulation may be indicated. On rare instances where there is sufficient instability and joint destruction, arthrodesis of both the MCP and IP joints may be carried out at the same time as basilar joint arthroplasty. It should be recognized, however, that fusion of both joints places greater stress at the CMC area and that the arthroplasty of that joint must be carefully protected for several months.

DEFORMITIES SECONDARY TO TENDON RUPTURES

Functional loss in the rheumatoid thumb may result from rupture of the extensor pollicis longus, flexor pollicis longus, or extensor pollicis brevis tendons, and each will have a significant functional effect on thumb performance. It is important that a rupture of the flexor pollicis longus not be confused with the hyperextension deformity of the IP joint seen in the boutonniere deformity. Similarly, the loss of IP joint extension secondary to extensor pollicis longus rupture should not be confused with the swan-neck deformity. When rupture of the flexor or extensor pollicis longus tendons is an isolated phenomenon resulting from wrist synovitis, with little associated IP joint pathosis, it may be appropriate to carry out a tendon transfer using the extensor indicis proprius to return thumb extension or the brachioradialis or a superficialis tendon to reactivate the flexor pollicis longus. Long-standing ruptures with concomitant arthritis of the IP joint are better managed by arthrodesis. Rupture or attenuation of the extensor pollicis brevis is a frequent occurrence in rheumatoid arthritis patients. However, it usually occurs at the MCP joint in association with substantial synovitis, and its loss contributes to the development of a boutonniere deformity and need not be discussed separately.

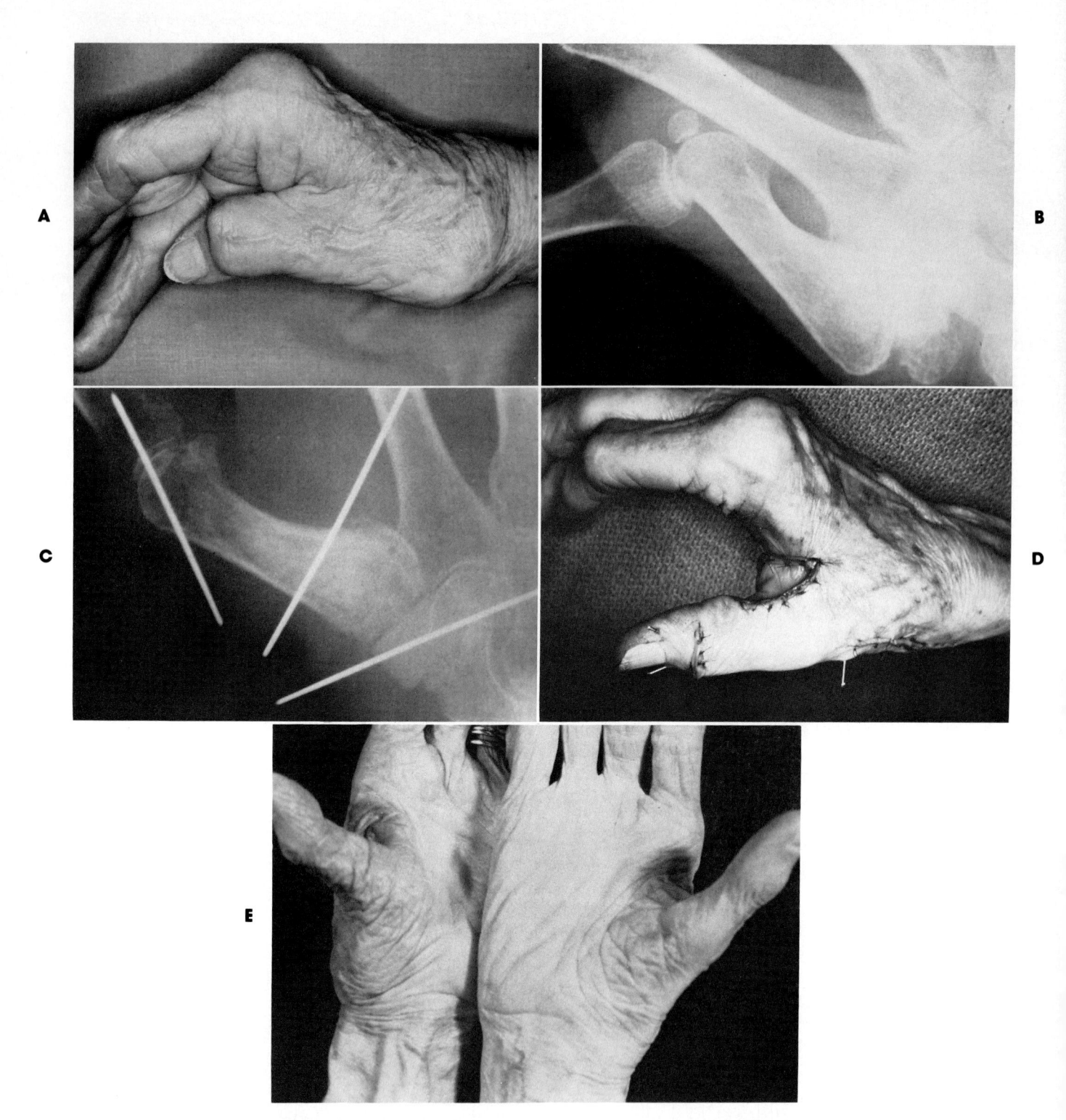

FIG. 25-7. Reconstruction of swan-neck deformity of rheumatoid thumb. **A,** Clinical appearance with lateral subluxation of base of first metacarpal, severe adduction contracture of first metacarpal, hyperextension deformity of MCP joint, and flexion deformity of IP joint. **B,** X-ray appearance of severely collapsed first metacarpal in swan-neck deformity. **C,** X-ray appearance of thumb after reconstruction using silicone rubber replacement arthroplasty of basilar thumb joint and release of adducted first metacarpal. **D,** Appearance of reconstructed thumb at conclusion of operative procedure, which included IP joint arthrodesis and MCP rebalancing. **E,** Appearance of reconstructed right thumb at 6 months, compared with unoperated swan-neck deformity on left.

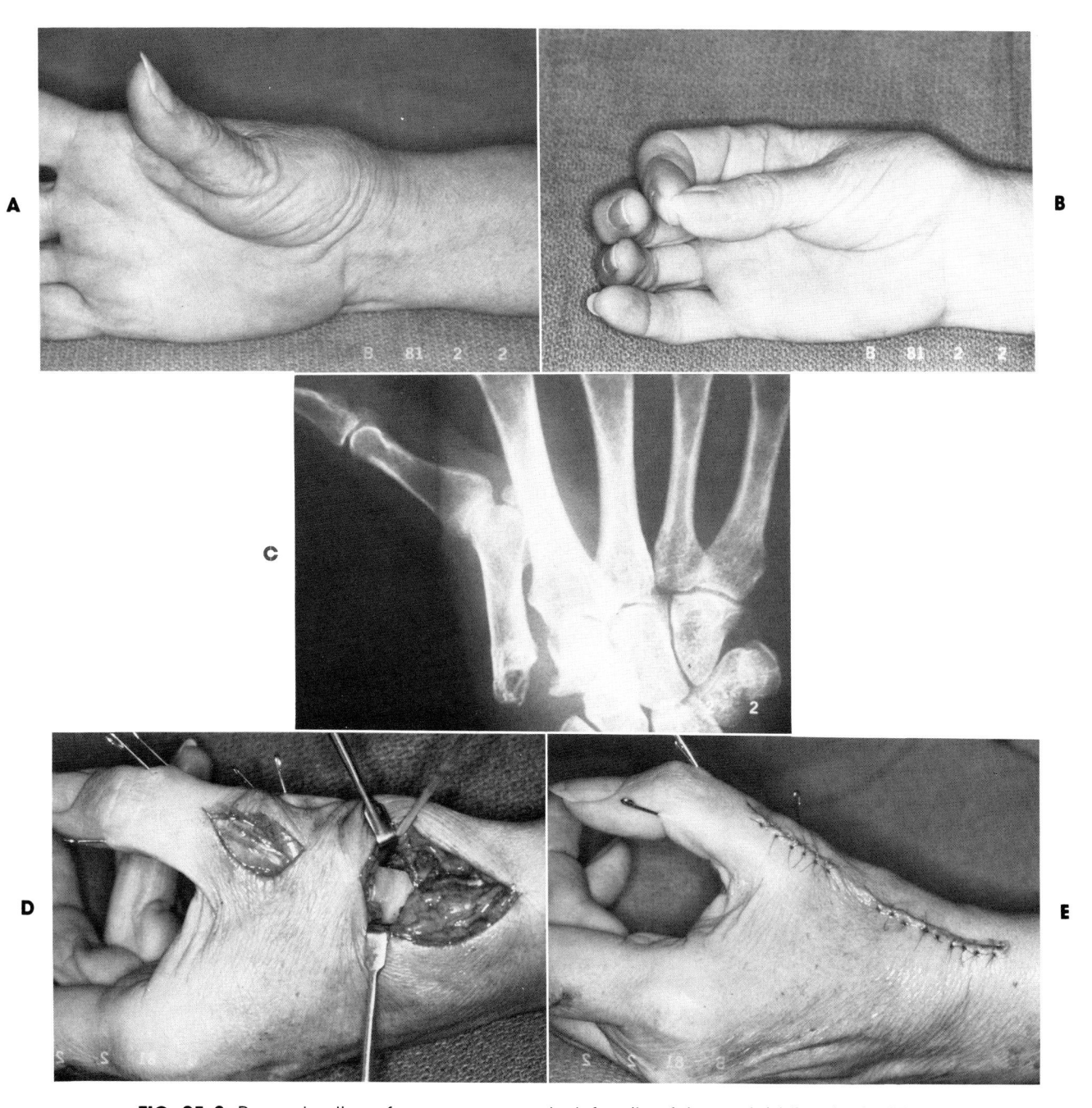

CHAPTER 25 COMPLEX ARTHRITIC DISABILITIES OF THE THUMB

FIG. 25-8. Reconstruction of severe swan-neck deformity of rheumatoid thumb. **A,** Clinical appearance of swan-neck deformity with adduction contracture of first metacarpal, hyperextension of MCP joint, but satisfactory position of IP joint. **B,** Inefficient pinch produced by basilar joint collapse and adducted posture of metacarpal in combination with unstable MCP joint. **C,** X-ray appearance of destroyed CMC joint, adducted first metacarpal, and hyperextension of MCP joint. **D,** Appearance of reconstructed thumb at time of surgery with implant arthroplasty of basilar joint and satisfactory mobilization of first metacarpal without webspace release. Transmetacarpal fixation was used to maintain thumb abduction-extension, and arthrodesis of MCP joint was carried out. **E,** Appearance of thumb at time of wound closure.

Continued.

SECTION 7 RHEUMATOID ARTHRITIS PROBLEMS

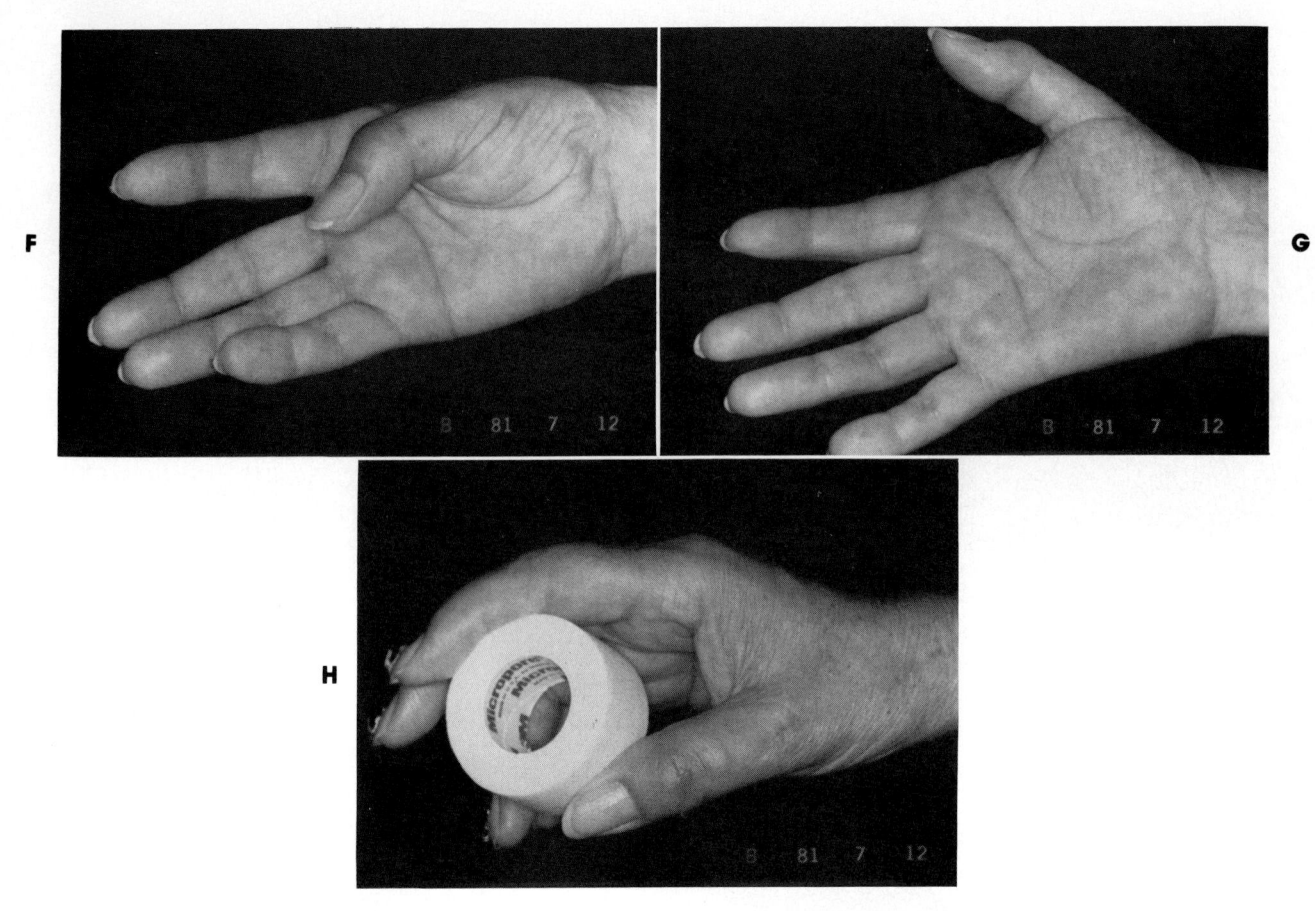

FIG. 25-8, cont'd. F, Appearance of reconstructed thumb at 6 months with satisfactory abduction. **G,** Stable adduction without collapse of CMC and MCP joints. **H,** Marked improvement in abduction mobility and pinch and grasp stability.

SUMMARY

This chapter has attempted to summarize the pathomechanics of complex deformities of the rheumatoid thumb and to offer management considerations for each deformity. If there is an appreciation of the underlying cause of each deformity, and if appropriate reconstructive procedures are carried out, the return of stable, pain-free thumb function may occur, which would be extremely gratifying to the patient.

REFERENCES

1. Ashworth, C.R., et al.: Silicone-rubber interposition arthroplasty of the carpometacarpal joint of the thumb, J. Hand Surg. **2:**345, 1977.
2. Brewerton, D.A.: Hand deformities in rheumatoid disease, Ann. Rheum. Dis. **16:**183, 1957.
3. Bunnell, S.: Surgery of the rheumatic hand, J. Bone Joint Surg. **37A:**759, 1955.
4. Clayton, M.L.: Surgery of the thumb in rheumatoid arthritis, J. Bone Joint Surg. **44A:**1376, 1962.
5. Dell, P.C., Brushart, T.N., and Smith, R.J.: Treatment of trapeziometacarpal arthritis: results of resection arthroplasty, J. Hand Surg. **3:**243, 1978.
6. Flatt, A.E.: The care of the rheumatoid hand, ed. 2, St. Louis, 1968, The C.V. Mosby Co.
7. Froimson, A.I.: Tendon arthroplasty of the trapeziometacarpal joint, Clin. Orthop. **70:**191, 1970.
8. Froimson, A.I.: Hand reconstruction in arthritis mutilans, J. Bone Joint Surg. **53A:**1377, 1971.
9. Gervis, W.H.: A review of excision of the trapezium for osteoarthritis of the trapeziometacarpal joint after 25 years, J. Bone Joint Surg. **55B:**56, 1973.
10. Goldner, J.L., and Clippinger, F.W.: Excision of the greater multiangular bone as an adjunct to mobilization of the thumb, J. Bone Joint Surg. **41A:**609, 1959.

11. Haffajee, D.: Endoprosthetic replacement of the trapezium for arthrosis in the carpometacarpal joint of the thumb, J. Hand Surg. **2**:141, 1977.
12. Inglis, A.E., et al.: Reconstruction of the metacarpophalangeal joint of the thumb in rheumatoid arthritis, J. Bone Joint Surg. **54A**:704, 1972.
13. Kessler, I.: Aetiology and management of adduction contracture of the thumb in rheumatoid arthritis, Hand **5**:170, 1973.
14. Mannerfelt, L.: Restoration of balance in the rheumatoid thumb. In Stack, H.G., and Bolton, H., editors: The Second Hand Club, London, 1975, British Society for Surgery of the Hand.
15. Marmor, L.: Surgery of rheumatoid arthritis, Philadelphia, 1967, Lea & Febiger.
16. Millender, L.H., and Nalebuff, E.A.: Reconstructive surgery in the rheumatoid hand, Orthop. Clin. North Am. **6**:709, 1975.
17. Millender, L.H., Nalebuff, E.A., Amadio, P., et al.: Interpositional arthroplasty for rheumatoid carpometacarpal joint disease, J. Hand Surg. **3**:533, 1978.
18. Murley, A.H.G.: Excision of the trapezium in osteoarthritis of the first carpometacarpal joint, J. Bone Joint Surg. **42B**:502, 1960.
19. Nalebuff, E.A.: Diagnosis, classification and management of rheumatoid thumb deformities, Bull. Hosp. Joint Dis. **29**:119, 1968.
20. Nalebuff, E.A.: Extensor pollicis longus re-routing in the rheumatoid thumb: a new operative approach, J. Bone Joint Surg. **51A**:790, 1969.
21. Nalebuff, E.A.: Restoration of balance in the rheumatoid thumb. In Stack, H.G., and Bolton, H., editors: The Second Hand Club, London, 1975, British Society for Surgery of the Hand.
22. Niebauer, J.J., and Landry, R.M.: Dacron-silicone prosthesis for the metacarpophalangeal and interphalangeal joints, Hand **3**:55, 1971.
23. Ratliff, A.H.C.: Deformities of the thumb in rheumatoid arthritis, Hand **3**:138, 1971.
24. Strickland, J.W.: Arthritis of the basal thumb joints: a technique for implant arthroplalsty. In Cowen, N.J., editor: Practical hand surgery, Chicago, 1980, Symposia Specialists.
25. Swanson, A.B.: Silicone rubber implants for replacement of arthritic or destroyed joints in the hand, Surg. Clin. North Am. **48**:1113, 1968.
26. Swanson, A.B.: Disabling arthritis at the base of the thumb: treatment by resection of the trapezium and flexible (silicone) implant arthroplasty, J. Bone Joint Surg. **54A**:456, 1972.
27. Swanson, A.B.: Disabilities of the thumb joints and their surgical treatment including flexible implant arthroplasty. In American Academy of Orthopaedic Surgeons: Instructional Course Lectures **22**:88, 1973.
28. Swanson, A.B.: Flexible implant resection arthroplasty in hand and extremities, St. Louis, 1973, The C.V. Mosby Co.
29. Swanson, A.B.: Reconstructive surgery in the arthritic hand and foot, Clin. Symp. **31**:1, 1979.
30. Swanson, A.B., and de Goot Swanson, G.: Thumb disabilities in rheumatoid arthritis: classification and treatment. In American Academy of Orthopaedic Surgeons: Symposium on Tendon Surgery in the Hand, St. Louis, 1975, The C.V. Mosby Co.
31. Swanson, A.B., de Goot Swanson, G., and Watermeier, J.J.: Trapezium implant arthroplasty, J. Hand Surg. **6**:125, 1981.
32. Swanson, A.B., and Herndon, J.H.: Flexible (silicone) implant arthroplasty of the metacaropphalangeal joint of the thumb, J. Bone Joint Surg. **59A**:362, 1977.
33. Vainio, K.: Indications and contra-indications for surgery in rheumatoid arthritis, Rheumatism **22**:10, 1966.

Chapter 26 Rheumatoid arthritis of the wrist

Julio Taleisnik

ANATOMIC CORRELATION OF EARLY RADIOGRAPHIC FINDINGS

The radiologic features of advanced rheumatoid involvement of the wrist are well known. Less emphasis has been placed on those early changes produced by synovitis at a stage when synovectomy could be most beneficial. These changes are not haphazard but develop in direct proportion to the concentration of synovium, the presence of synovial sacs and pouches in close relation to the supporting wrist ligaments, and the mechanical characteristics of the area involved.[2,10,12,13] Bywaters[2] described two sites where erosions are frequently seen: the ulnar styloid and head and the most lateral portion of the scaphotrapezial joint. Likewise, Martel, Hayes, and Duff[10] found that the ulnar styloid was most frequently involved and that the radial aspect of the scaphoid was the next most frequent location of rheumatoid involvement. Ranawat and associates,[12] in a report on arthrographic changes in the rheumatoid wrist, reviewed 76 wrist radiographs. The earliest bone lesions were marginal erosion of the ulnar styloid in 41, of the scaphoid and lunate in 40, and of the radial styloid in 28. Pseudocysts of the distal portion of the radius were present in 22 wrists. Abnormalities noted in arthrograms included, in addition, communications between the different wrist joint compartments; this correlated well with the surgical findings in 15 wrists, all of which showed, for instance, destruction of the scapholunate interosseous ligament. Resnick and Gmelich[13] also found predominant fragmentation at the level of the distal radioulnar joint and on the body of the scaphoid. In all these reports there is a recurrent pattern of involvement of the ulnar head and styloid and, less frequently, of the midportion of the scaphoid. A review of the anatomy of the wrist ligaments[7,16] suggests that synovitis of the prestyloid recess is the cause of ulnar styloid changes and that the scaphoid erosions occur deep to the radiocapitate, or "sling," ligament, which runs across the concavity of the scaphoid, spanning the distance between the radial styloid and the neck of the capitate. Other areas where a close anatomic correlation can be found for radiographic changes in the rheumatoid wrist are the radioscapholunate junction, the dorsal-ulnar corner of the radius, and the triquetrum.

Scaphoid "grooving": the sling (radiocapitate) ligament

In 1964 Martel[9] called attention to an area of erosion of the radial aspect of the scaphoid. In very early synovitis all that may be seen is a band of decreased bony density across the waist of the scaphoid (Fig. 26-1, B). This corresponds to the location of the radiocapitate ligament, one of three deep volar radiocarpal fascicles, best visualized after careful dissection of the overlying capsule (Fig. 26-1, A) or from within the joint.[7] (See Fig. 26-3, A). The concave volar waist of the scaphoid is weakly attached to this ligament, on which it rotates pretty much as a gymnast does on a horizontal bar while executing a hip circle. Synovitis in this area of continuous attrition is responsible for the appearance and progression of scaphoid grooving or notching (Fig. 26-1, C). It is one factor leading toward destabilization of the proximal pole of the scaphoid, eventual loss of radiocarpal height, and rotatory subluxation of the carpus.

Pseudocysts of the radius and scapholunate dissociation: the deep radioscapholunate ligament

Pseudocysts of the radius in rheumatoid wrists have been previously reported (Fig. 26-2).[4,6,8,12] The subchondral margin of the radius shows, in line with the scapholunate junction, a pseudocystic area of variable diameter. This corresponds to the origin of the deep radioscapholunate ligament,[16] the main stabilizing support of the proximal pole of the scaphoid. Distally this ligament attaches on both the scaphoid and the lunate and spreads to cover the scapholunate interosseous space. Corresponding to the pseudocyst of the radius, there are frequent erosions of the scaphoid and lunate and eventually a progressive scapholunate dissociation (Fig. 26-2, B), similar to that seen after traumatic ligament tears or avulsions. This, together with the detachment of the scaphoid from the radiocapitate ligament, completes the destabilization of the proximal pole of the

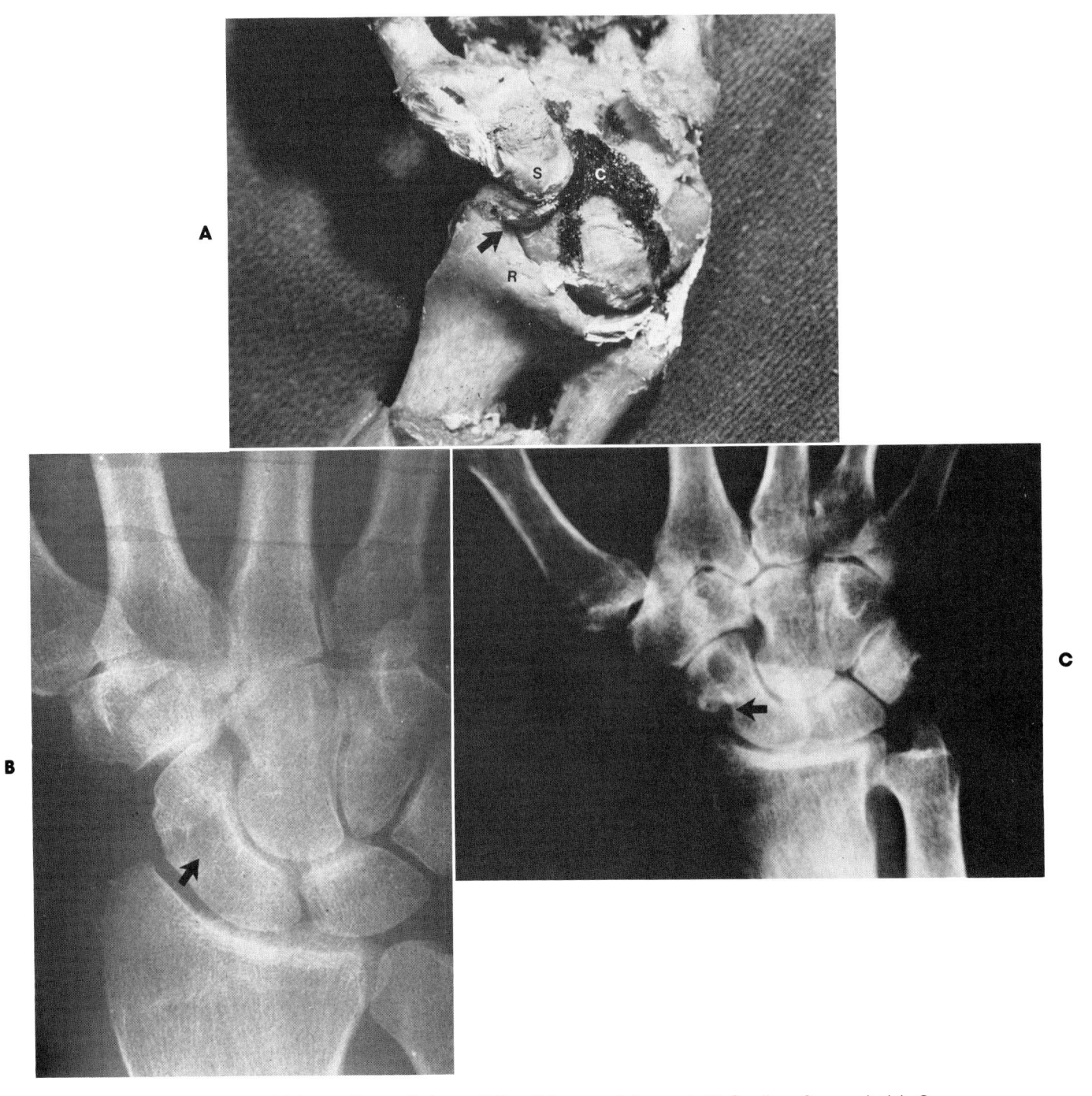

FIG. 26-1. A, Volar radiocapitate, or "sling," ligament *(arrow)*. *R,* Radius; *S,* scaphoid; *C,* capitate. **B,** Radiolucent band *(arrow)* across midscaphoid under radiocapitate ligament. **C,** Groove or notch *(arrow)* on midscaphoid. (**A** from Taleisnik, J.: J. Hand Surg. **1**:110, 1976.)

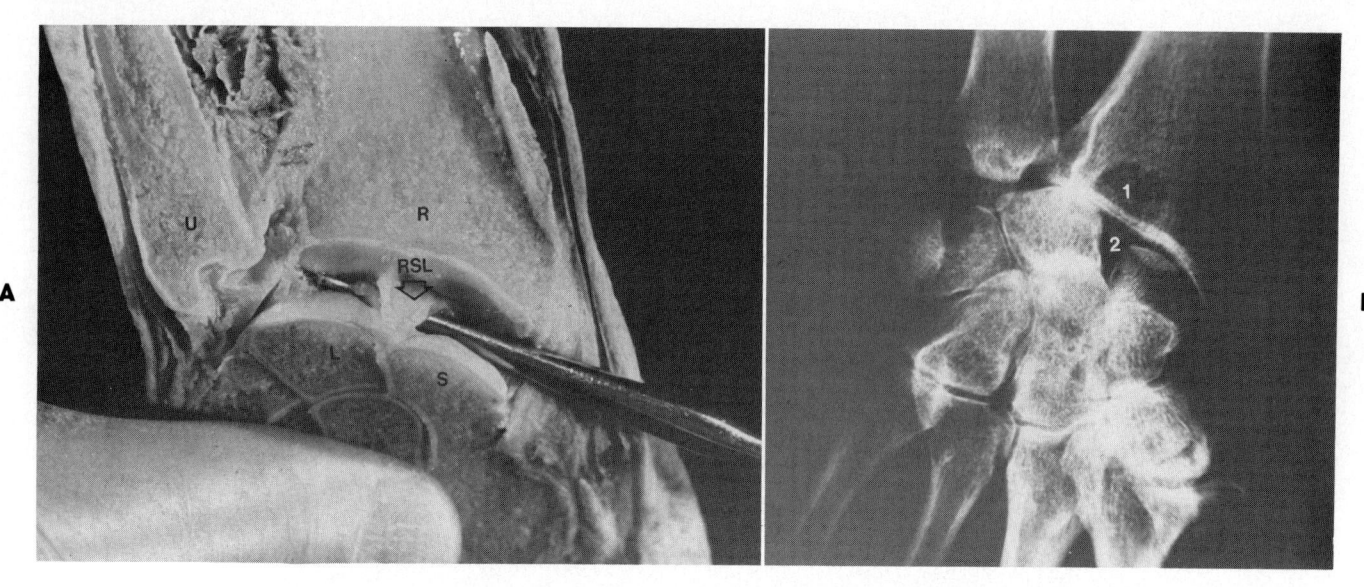

FIG. 26-2. A, Coronal section of wrist; volar half as seen from within joint. *U,* Ulna; *R,* radius; *RSL,* deep radioscapholunate ligament; *L,* lunate; *S,* scaphoid. **B,** Pseudocyst *(1)* and scaholunate dissociation *(2)* secondary to synovitis at origin and insertion of deep radioscapholunate ligament. Destabilized scaphoid is volar-flexed, seen from end in this anteroposterior x-ray view. (**A** from Taleisnik, J.: J. Hand Surg. **1:**110, 1976.)

scaphoid, allowing it to subluxate into a position perpendicular to the long axis of the radius.

Ulnar translocation: the radiolunate ligament

Ulnar migration of the carpus is a radiographic pattern seen in the rheumatoid wrist,[8] very likely related to a gradual loss of radiocarpal support, particularly the very strong volar radiolunate and dorsal radiocarpal ligaments. Because of their size and orientation, these structures are principally responsible for maintaining the lunate (and consequently the carpus) in its proper relationship to the radius. Both ligaments originate from the radius and progress in an almost horizontal direction medially and somewhat distally. They strongly tether the lunate laterally, preventing its ulnar migration. If this support is lost, the entire carpus may "slide" in an ulnar direction, creating the pattern seen in ulnar translocation (Fig. 26-3).

Erosions of the ulnar corner of the radius and the triquetrum: the ulnocarpal ligament complex

The ulnar half of the carpus is supported dorsally by a strong structure, the ulnocarpal meniscus homologue,[7] which originates primarily from the dorsal-ulnar corner of the radius and is not to be confused with the more familiar triangular fibrocartilage. Both these structures have a common origin, but, whereas the triangular fibrocartilage extends horizontally toward the head of the ulna, the meniscus homologue swings volarly and slightly distally in a semicircle around the ulnar border of the wrist to insert on the volar aspect of the triquetrum (Figs. 26-4, *A,* and 26-5). Proximal to these structures is the distal radioulnar joint. Erosive and cystic changes at the level of the origin and insertion of this ligament complex are frequent in rheumatoid wrists (Fig. 26-4, *B*). Loss of the dorsoradial support is a factor in the volar subluxation of the ulnar carpus seen in these patients. It also may be present in those wrists exhibiting ulnar translocation.

The ulnar styloid and prestyloid recess

As the triangular fibrocartilage and the ulnocarpal meniscus homologue diverge medially from their common origin at the radius, they enclose a triangular space filled with synovial villi (Fig. 26-4, *A*). This is the site of severe and early synovitis, a cause of erosive changes of the ulnar styloid (Fig. 26-4, *B*) and an additional factor of destabilization of the ulnar carpus.

FACTORS OF DEFORMITY

Loss of bone and joint stability and tissue laxity secondary to rheumatoid synovitis as well as to the elevation of the intraarticular pressures[3] are factors in rheumatoid wrist deformity. In 1968 Shapiro[14] called attention to

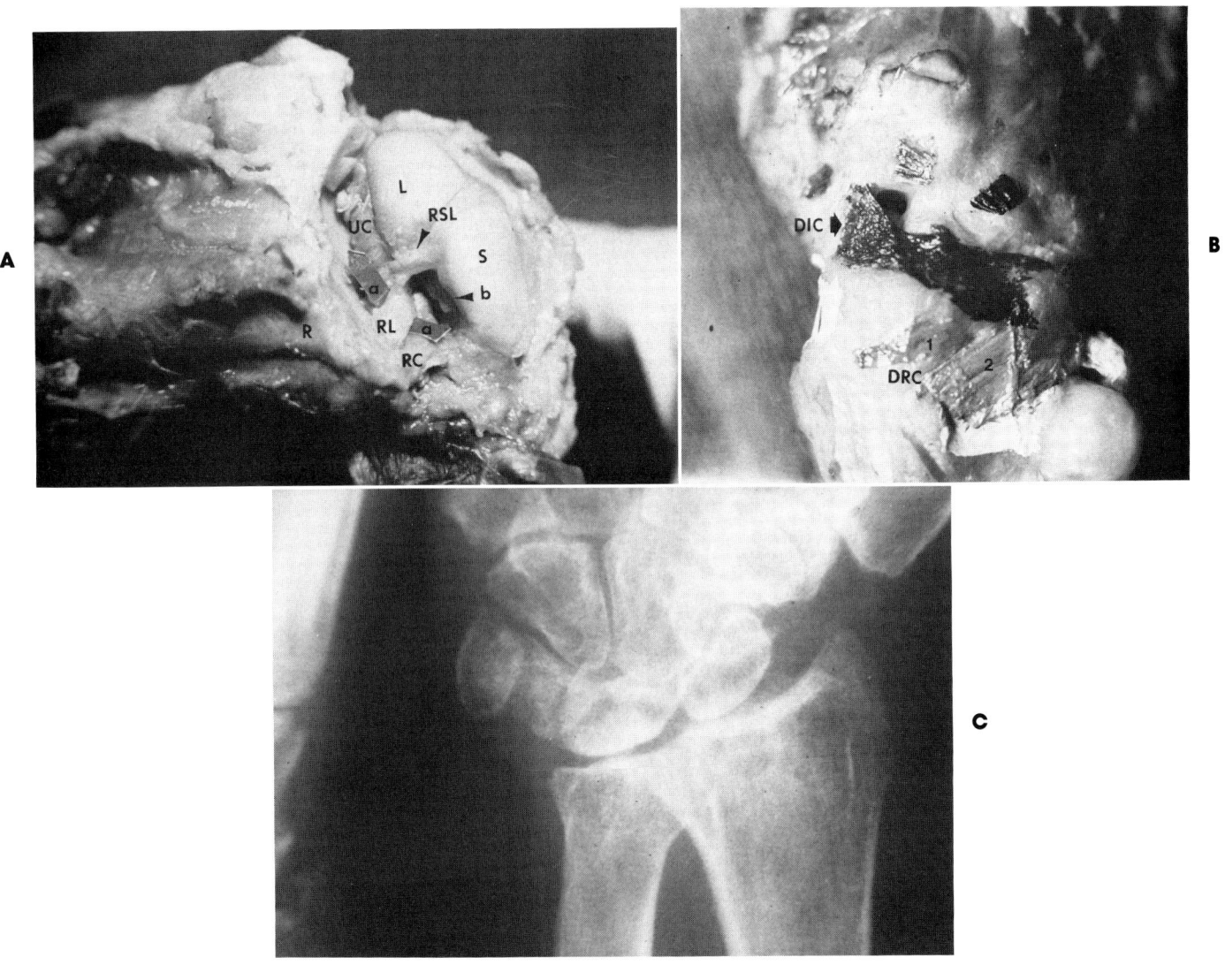

FIG. 26-3. A, Deep volar radiocarpal ligaments are visualized from within joint. Marker *(a)* is under deep radiolunate *(RL)* ligament. *R,* Radius; *S,* scaphoid; *L,* lunate; *RC,* radiocapitate ligament (weak scaphoid connection shown by *arrow, b*); *RSL,* deep radioscapholunate; *UC,* ulnocarpal ligament. **B,** *DRC,* Dorsal radiocarpal ligament; *1,* radiolunate; *2,* radiotriquetral fascicles; *DIC,* dorsal intercarpal ligament. **C,** Ulnar translocation of carpus. (**A** and **B** from Taleisnik, J.: J. Hand Surg. **1:**110, 1976.)

SECTION 7 RHEUMATOID ARTHRITIS PROBLEMS

FIG. 26-4. A, Coronal section of wrist; dorsal half is seen from within joint. *R,* Radius; *U,* ulna; *S,* scaphoid; *L,* lunate; *T,* triquetrum. Triangular fibrocartilage *(TF)* and ulnocarpal meniscus *(M)* share common origin from radius and enclose triangular space *(P),* prestyloid recess, filled with synovial villi. **B,** Erosive changes at distal radioulnar joint *(1),* ulnar styloid *(2),* and triquetrum *(3).* (**A** from Taleisnik, J.: J. Hand Surg. **1:**110, 1976.)

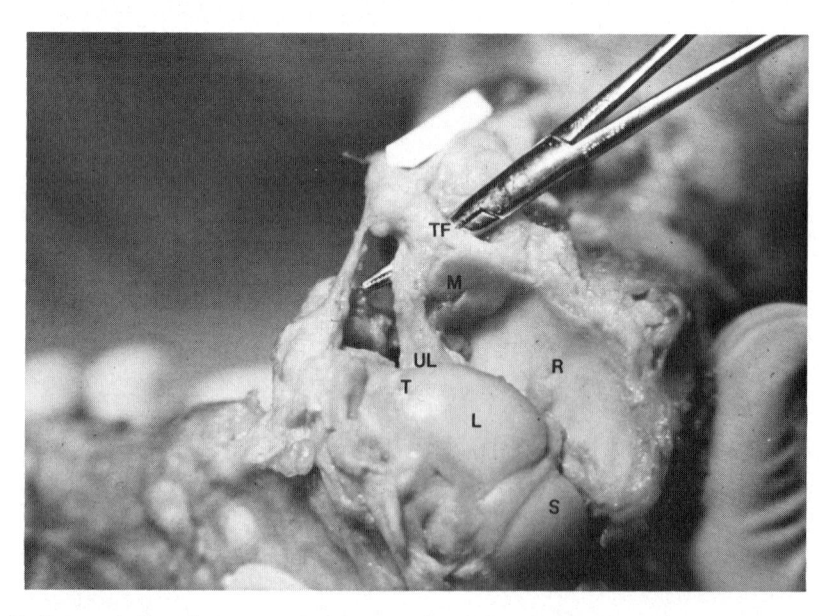

FIG. 26-5. Carpus is literally suspended from radius *(R)* on ligament sling originating from volar margin and dorsal-ulnar corner of radius. *S,* Scaphoid; *L,* lunate; *T,* triquetrum, *M,* ulnocarpal meniscus; *UL,* ulnolunate ligament; *TF,* triangular fibrocartilage.

radial deviation of the metacarpals, accompanied by radial rotation of the wrist, both deformities that are frequently associated with ulnar deviation of the fingers in rheumatoid patients. In 1971 he and his associates[15] further stated that "the individual who exhibits this set of variant findings (a normal tendency toward radial deviation during power grip) will be the one individual who may develop ulnar phalangeal drift should rheumatoid involvement occur."

The initial abnormality appeared to be a loss of the stabilizing influence of the extensor carpi ulnaris, a result of extensor carpi ulnaris tendon damage or rupture, subluxation, or muscle inhibition. The ulnar carpus thereafter would develop a progressive tendency toward volar subluxation. During power grip, radial rotation of the carpus would be increased, allowing the long digital flexors to exert an abnormal ulnar pull on already weakened finger joints. This inhibition of extensor carpi ulnaris activity was found, however, in rheumatoid patients with already established ulnar digital drift. Whether this inhibition was primary and preceded the onset of ulnar drift, as proposed by Shapiro and associates,[14] or secondary to an established ulnar drift was not clearly demonstrated. This correlation of wrist and finger deformities was further suggested by Pahle and Raunio's investigation[11] of wrist-hand alignment following wrist fusions. Their findings confirmed Shapiro's concept that radial metacarpal shift frequently would lead to ulnar digital drift. Conversely, ulnar metacarpal shift was conducive to radial deviation of the fingers. In these patients with wrists that had undergone arthrodesis, it was clearly the position of fusion that determined the phalangeal deviation and not the dynamic influence of the wrist motors, which were no long operative. Clinical experience further shows that patients deprived of the extensor carpi ulnaris through injury or transfer do not develop carpal malrotation provided all other supportive structures are intact. Therefore it must be assumed that in the wrist joint, just as in other rheumatoid joints, disorganization is initiated by intraarticular synovitis and the consequent loss of ligament support. Once articular malrotation and imbalance are present, then extensor carpi ulnaris inhibition or tearing becomes a factor of deformity, contributing to the development of the radial metacarpal shift.

Arkless[1] showed that changes in carpal function *do* occur in the early stages of rheumatoid involvement. Thirty-five of 55 wrists examined under cineradiography showed decreased or absent scaphoid rotation, and over half these had clear scapholunate joint widening. Linscheid[8] mentioned two predominant patterns of wrist involvement: ulnar translocation and radial metacarpal shift secondary to volar flexion of the scaphoid. In all instances an apparent collapse of the radial half of the carpus was shown. Hastings and Evans[6] confirmed this in measurements of normal and rheumatoid wrists. They attributed wrist collapse to loss of cartilage space, with or without bone erosions, to proximal migration of the capitate through an abnormal scapholunate separation, and to rotation of the scaphoid itself. They also showed that, even though volar flexion of the scaphoid was preserved, dorsiflexion was lost in the rheumatoid wrist. Similar abnormalities of wrist motion were previously noted in the cineradiographic studies of Arkless. In the ulnar half of the rheumatoid wrist, volar subluxation and relative supination of the carpus, together with distal radioulnar and extensor carpi ulnaris synovitis, allow the ulnar head to become prominent dorsally.

Anatomic and functional characteristics of the wrist

A review of the anatomic and functional characteristics of the wrist may assist the integration of all these different factors of deformity. The carpus is normally "suspended" from the radius by a ligamentous sling that originates predominantly from the volar radial and dorsal ulnar corners of the distal radius.[16] (See Fig. 26-5.) The radial half of this sling contributes to the stability of the lateral, or "mobile," carpal column (scaphoid) and the ulnar half to the stability of the medial, or "rotation," column (triquetrum). On the radial side attenuation or destruction of the deep radioscapholunate and radiocapitate ligaments effectively destabilizes the proximal pole of the scaphoid, which gradually assumes a volar-flexed position, its longitudinal axis perpendicular to that of the radius. (See Fig. 26-2, *B*.) The scaphoid appears foreshortened in the frontal roentgenogram, leading to a proportional loss of radiocarpal height.

On the ulnar side of the carpus the ulnar half of the radiocarpal sling is no longer capable of providing dorsal support. The entire medial column gradually sinks volarward, which appears clinically as an increased metacarpal descent angle (Fig. 26-6). This deformity, described by Zancolli,[18] therefore may be secondary to these more proximal radiocarpal changes rather than to synovitis of the fourth and fifth carpometacarpal joints alone, as he had suggested. The ulnar head becomes prominent dorsally, which is further accentuated by distal radioulnar joint synovitis, allowing dorsal ulnar subluxation. The combination of radiocarpal shortening, ulnar carpal volar subluxation, and dorsal subluxation of the ulnar head produces a relative carpal malrotation into supination, in relation to the distal aspects of the radius and ulna. Every time the patient makes a fist or attempts to grasp, this abnormal supination is dynamically accentuated, because the function of the extensor carpi radialis longus is facilitated, and also because on the opposite side the extensor carpi ulnaris fails to act as a dorsiflexor as it

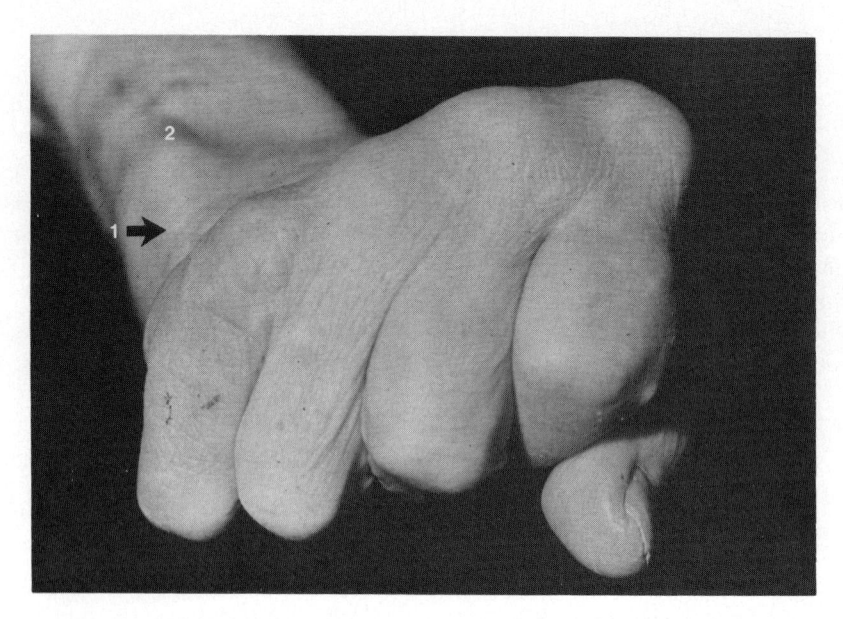

FIG. 26-6. Increased metacarpal descent typical of rheumatoid deformity. There is volar subluxation of ulnar carpus (1) and dorsally prominent ulnar head (2).

gradually subluxates volar to the prominent ulnar head. Further progression of destruction of the volar radiocarpal support leads to a frank dissociation of the scapholunate joint and a rapidly accelerating wrist collapse. It is clear that, although initial wrist involvement is not as frequent as early isolated involvement of the finger joints, once present, wrist collapse will facilitate the progression of digital deformity. Most important, it will interfere with the successful correction of ulnar drift of the fingers, unless the wrist itself is treated first.

Treatment plan

The treatment plan is based on the clinical and radiologic findings and may include the following:

1. Synovectomies of all involved compartments, including the volar radiocarpal and midcarpal joints when volar synovitis is suggested by x-ray changes (scaphoid notching, radial pseudocysts, scapholunate dissociation, and triquetral erosions)
2. Ligament repair or reconstruction for stabilization of the malrotated scaphoid and correction of the scapholunate dissociation
3. Relocation of the extensor carpi ulnaris dorsal to the ulnar head and transfer of the extensor carpi radialis longus to the extensor carpi ulnaris insertion to counteract radial rotation of the metacarpals[5]
4. Distal radioulnar joint synovectomy and reduction or excision of the subluxated ulnar head with transposition of the extensor retinaculum deep to the extensor tendons
5. Radiolunate fusion for ulnar translocation of the carpus, provided that the radioscaphoid and midcarpal joints are relatively well preserved[17]

A well-aligned, strong, and symptom-free wrist enormously facilitates the treatment and postoperative rehabilitation after surgery of the hand itself.

REFERENCES

1. Arkless, R.: Rheumatoid wrists: cineradiography, Radiology **88**:543, 1967.
2. Bywaters, E.G.L.: The early radiological signs of rheumatoid arthritis, Bull. Rheum. Dis. **11**:231, 1960.
3. Clark, L.P., James, D.F., and Colwill, J.C.: Intra-articular pressure as a factor in initiating ulnar drift, J. Bone Joint Surg. **60A**:325, 1978.
4. Collins, L.C., Lidsky, M.D., Sharp, J.T., and Moreland, J.: Malposition of carpal bones in rheumatoid arthritis, Radiology **103**:95, 1972.
5. Ferlic, D.C., and Clayton, M.L.: Tendon transfer for radial rotation in the rheumatoid wrist, J. Bone Joint Surg. **55A**:880, 1973.
6. Hastings, D.E., and Evans, J.A.: Rheumatoid wrist deformities and their relation to ulnar drift, J. Bone Joint Surg. **57A**:930, 1975.
7. Lewis, O.J., Hamshere, R.J., and Bucknill, T.M.: The anatomy of the wrist joint, J. Anat. **106**:539, 1970.
8. Linscheid, R.L.: Mechanical forces affecting the deformity of the rheumatoid wrist, Presented at meeting of the American Society for Surgery of the Hand, New York, 1969.
9. Martel, W.: The pattern of rheumatoid arthritis in the hand and wrist, Radiol. Clin. North Am. **2**:221, 1964.
10. Martel, W., Hayes, J.T., and Duff, I.F.: The pattern of

bone erosion in the hand and wrist in rheumatoid arthritis, Radiology **84:**204, 1965.
11. Pahle, J.A., and Raunio, P.: The influence of wrist position on finger deviation in the rheumatoid hand: a clinical and radiological study J. Bone Joint Surg. **51B:**664, 1969.
12. Ranawat, C.S., Freiberger, R.H., Jordan, L.R., and Straub, L.R.: Arthrography in the rheumatoid wrist joint, J. Bone Joint Surg. **51A:**1269, 1969.
13. Resnick, D., and Gmelich, J.R.: Bone fragmentation in the rheumatoid wrist: radiographic and pathologic considerations, Radiology **114:**315, 1975.
14. Shapiro, J.S.: Ulnar drift—report of a related finding, Acta Orthop. Scand. **39:**346, 1968.
15. Shapiro, J.S., Heijna, W., Nasatir, S., and Ray, R.D.: The relationship of wrist motion to ulnar phalangeal drift in the rheumatoid patient, Hand **3:**68, 1971.
16. Taleisnik, J.: The ligaments of the wrist, J. Hand Surg. **1:**110, 1976.
17. Watson, H.K., Johnson, T.R., Hempton R.F., and Jones, D.S.: Limited wrist arthrodesis, Presented at thirty-fourth meeting of the American Society for Surgery of the Hand, San Francisco, Feb. 20, 1979.
18. Zancolli, E.: Structural and dynamic bases of hand surgery, Philadelphia, 1968, J.B. Lippincott Co.

Chapter 27 The surgical management of multiple-level deformities of the rheumatoid hand: a practical approach

James W. Strickland

William B. LaSalle

In the zeal to reconstruct the severely deformed rheumatoid hand the surgeon must pause to carefully consider the overall condition of the patient and the patient's needs, expectations, and motivation.[21] It is equally important that the condition of the hand be assessed in its entirety rather than as a series of isolated considerations of specific levels of joint involvement.[19] Both the patient and the surgeon must realistically analyze the goals of any contemplated surgical procedures with regard to the correction of existing deformities, prevention of additional deformity, pain relief, and improvement of hand function.

Because of its chronicity and disabling sequelae, rheumatoid arthritis almost always has a severe economic impact on its victims. It is mandatory that the surgeon carefully plan and coordinate the reconstructive process to minimize the number of surgical procedures and hospitalizations and the postoperative rehabilitative costs.[16,20] To subject the patient to multiple procedures carried out on one or both hands over a protracted period may have a profoundly negative influence on the patient's health, financial status, and motivation. It is not unusual for such a patient to abruptly terminate the reconstructive effort after the completion of one of several planned stages on a hand or to choose not to have the opposite side done after successful reconstruction of one hand. A single-stage, well-planned, multiple-level reconstructive approach may prevent the deterioration of patient morale and cooperation without the sacrifice of rehabilitative goals.

GENERAL CONSIDERATIONS

The general indications for surgery of the rheumatoid hand have been enumerated by many authors; failure of medical treatment, persistent synovitis, pain, tendon rupture, joint instability, deformity, and nerve compression are the most frequently mentioned reasons for surgical intervention.* The contraindications to such reconstructive efforts also are well known and include inadequate medical control of arthritis, advanced age, satisfactory adaptation to deformity, poor general medical condition, arteritis, and patient apathy.*

The objectives of surgical correction in the rheumatoid hand consist of the preservation or restoration of stability and mobility, correction of deformity, relief of pain, increase of strength, and cosmetic improvement.† A useful classification of the stages of rheumatoid hand involvement, as a guide to the selection of appropriate operative procedures, has been provided by Savill.[19]

Souter[21] has emphasized that the mere existence of deformity is not necessarily an indication for surgery and that the specific program must be tailored to the individual rheumatoid patient. He stressed that surgical planning must be preceded by a careful clinical and radiologic examination of the hand and consideration of the demands placed on the upper limbs, particularly with regard to the use of walking aids in those patients with severe lower limb involvement. He emphasized that rheumatoid involvement of the elbow or shoulder may have a very substantial effect on the success of hand surgery.

In his own personal series of over 6500 surgical procedures on patients with rheumatoid arthritis, Vainio[29] reported that there was not a single flare of the disease as a result of surgery. Vainio also states that the patient must be well motivated and medically able to withstand the anesthesia and surgery but need not be in a complete remission from the rheumatoid disease.

It is not uncommon for patients to have additional joints of either the upper or lower extremities that also require reconstructive surgical efforts, and under apropriate circumstances it is possible to carry out a reconstructive procedure on a lower extremity concomitant with or shortly after surgery on the upper extremity. This multiple-extremity approach reduces the risk of repeated anesthesia, and, by decreasing the number of

---

*References 14, 17, 18, 20, and 29.

*References 5, 14, 18, 21, and 29.
†References 16-18, 20, 21, and 27.

CHAPTER 27 THE SURGICAL MANAGEMENT OF MULTIPLE-LEVEL DEFORMITIES OF THE RHEUMATOID HAND

surgical procedures and hospitalizations, patient motivation and morale can be sustained at a much higher level.

It has been emphasized that each rheumatoid hand has a different pattern of joint-tendon involvement, and operations must be selected that will provide the best return of function based on individual deformities.[21] The prerequisites for the return of useful function for both grasp and pinch activities include a good range of motion at the metacarpophalangeal (MCP) joints of the fingers and the carpometacarpal (CMC) joint of the thumb. It is generally agreed that, if this combination can be achieved, one can afford to fuse the wrist and distal two joints of the thumb and fingers.[7,17,18] This practice of achieving motion at one level while carrying out stabilizing procedures at adjacent joints has become a very practical approach for the restoration of the severe rheumatoid hand and has allowed the surgeon to proceed with single-stage total hand reconstruction in appropriate circumstances.[7]

The purpose of this chapter is to review the practical considerations for surgical reconstruction of the severely involved wrist and digital joints in the hands of patients afflicted with rheumatoid arthritis. Recommendations for surgical procedures at each level are followed by a discussion of how these procedures can be coordinated into a single reconstructive effort that will allow the maximal benefit for each hand. Early palliative procedures such as small joint synovectomy are controversial and beyond the scope of this discussion.

CONSIDERATION BY LEVEL
The wrist

By virtue of its position between the forearm and the hand, the wrist serves as the key joint for the proper functional performance of the hand. Although a number of procedures are available for reconstruction of the severely involved rheumatoid wrist, it is important to realize that many patients have wrists that are stable and essentially pain free. Even though radiographs of these patients may indicate substantial carpal destruction and coalition, no surgical efforts are indicated, and the surgeon can direct efforts to other areas that are more functionally disabling. On other occasions clinical examination of the rheumatoid wrist may indicate that the only pain is around the distal aspect of the ulna as a result of its subluxation in the *caput ulnae* syndrome, and a simple Darrach excision of the distal part of the ulna and local synovectomy may suffice despite rather marked changes in the carpus. Resurfacing of the distal ulnar stump following Darrach excision using the silicone rubber cap designed by Swanson[25,27] has given good results, although its role in preventing ulnar translocation or carpal collapse is questionable.

Occasionally patients with MCP joint destruction sufficient to require reconstructive surgery will also have chronic, minimally symptomatic synovitis of the dorsal aspect of the wrist. To lessen the chance of extensor tendon rupture, it is probably worthwhile to carry out at least a "limited" synovectomy of the dorsal portion of the wrist at the time of digital joint reconstruction. We have found no problems with concomitant wrist and MCP joint procedures.

Rebalancing the wrist using the Clayton[4] transfer of the extensor carpi radialis longus to the extensor carpi ulnaris may be indicated if there is early ulnar translocation of the carpus. Volar repositioning of the extensor retinaculum as recommended by Clayton also has proved effective in decompressing the extensor tendons and buffering them from possible carpal abrasion and rupture. Taleisnik has indicated that early reconstruction of the scapholunate ligament complex maybe beneficial in preventing the dissociation pattern that occurs frequently in that area of the rheumatoid wrist. (See Chapter 26.) The long-term benefits of this technique will have to be carefully monitored.

Procedures recommended for advanced destruction of the wrist in rheumatoid arthritis include intracarpal or total wrist arthrodesis (Fig. 27-1) using the methods described by Watson and Hempton,[30] Abbott, Saunders, and Bost,[1] Carroll and Dick,[3] or Millender and Nalebuff[15] (Fig. 27-2). Proximal row carpectomy occasionally has been advocated, and dorsal stabilization of the rheumatoid wrist has been described recently by Kulick and associates.[9] The use of various prosthetic devices for wrist arthroplasty has enjoyed some popularity, and the need to rebalance the deformed wrist following the use of such implants has been emphasized, although duplicating normal wrist mechanics may be difficult.[10,26,27]

In an effort to simplify the indications for various procedures in the badly deformed rheumatoid wrist, our recommendation has been that, if the wrist is stable and without substantial deformity at the time of surgery, the flexible silicone rubber implant of Swanson[22,24-26] will provide an excellent interpositional arthroplasty with the retention of approximately 50% of normal wrist motion with satisfactory stability and pain relief. The articulated prostheses of Volz[10] and others also can provide the same type of satisfactory rheumatoid wrist reconstruction, although there have been some problems achieving the proper rotational axis and preventing loosening. The use of the Swanson implant in the stable wrist eliminates the need for extensive revision and rebalancing of the capsule and tendons about the joint. The long-term performance of the implant appears to be more predictable without the stresses generated by an imbalanced situation. Using this rather strict indication for implantation, we have not had any fractures of the silicone rubber wrist implants and have found them to pro-

SECTION 7 RHEUMATOID ARTHRITIS PROBLEMS

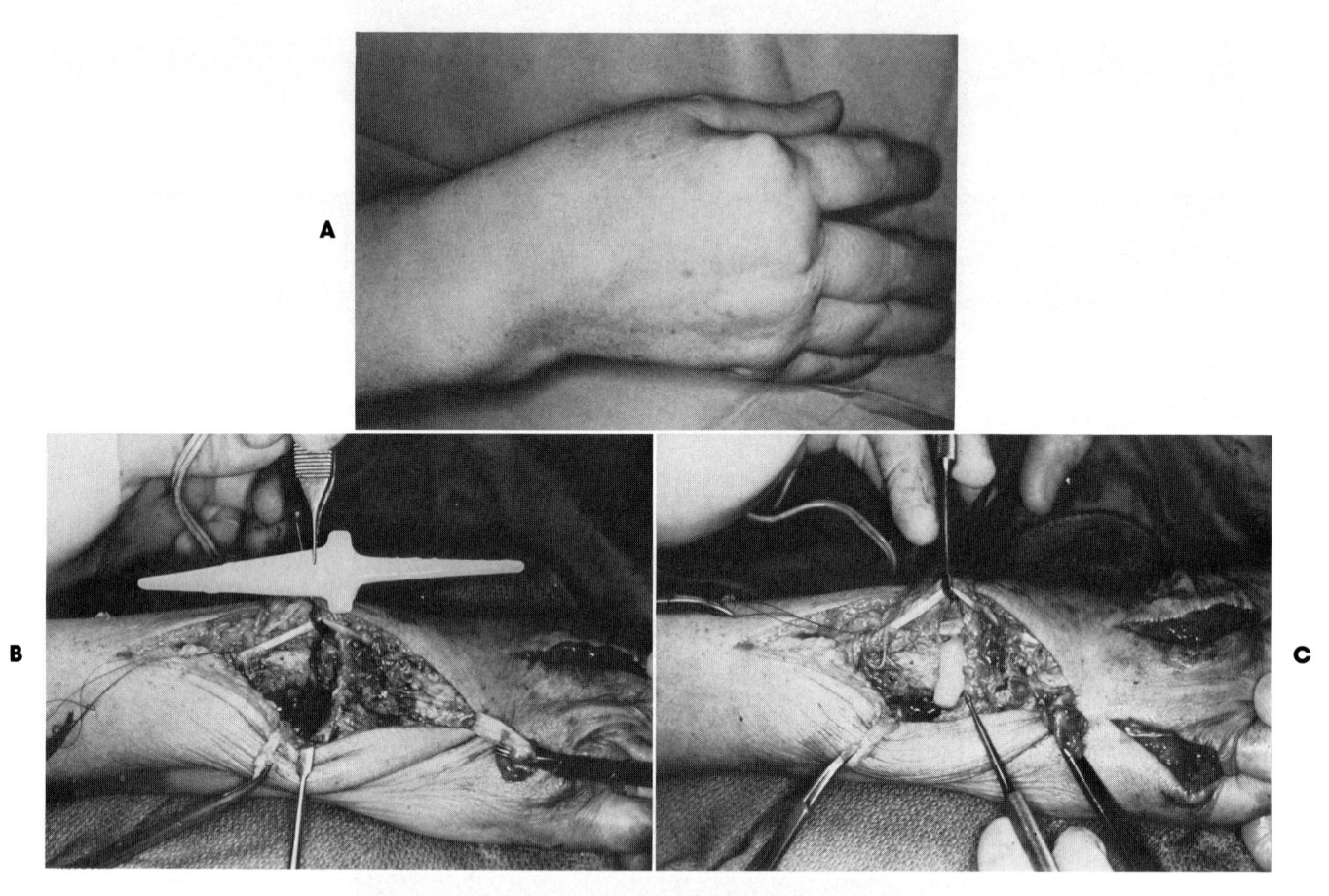

FIG. 27-3. Multiple-level involvement of rheumatoid wrist and hand, including painful but stable wrist, rupture of extensor tendons to long, ring, and small fingers, MCP joint subluxation, and painful instability of MCP joint of thumb. **A,** Preoperative appearance of hand and wrist. **B,** Carpal defect and preparation for implantation of silicone rubber interpositional implant. Note ruptured extensor tendons proximally and distally. **C,** Appearance of wrist following seating of silicone rubber implant prior to completion of MCP joint fusion of thumb, MCP joint arthroplasty of index, long, ring, and small fingers, and extensor tendon reconstruction using extensor carpi radialis brevis.

CHAPTER 27 THE SURGICAL MANAGEMENT OF MULTIPLE-LEVEL DEFORMITIES OF THE RHEUMATOID HAND

surgical procedures and hospitalizations, patient motivation and morale can be sustained at a much higher level.

It has been emphasized that each rheumatoid hand has a different pattern of joint-tendon involvement, and operations must be selected that will provide the best return of function based on individual deformities.[21] The prerequisites for the return of useful function for both grasp and pinch activities include a good range of motion at the metacarpophalangeal (MCP) joints of the fingers and the carpometacarpal (CMC) joint of the thumb. It is generally agreed that, if this combination can be achieved, one can afford to fuse the wrist and distal two joints of the thumb and fingers.[7,17,18] This practice of achieving motion at one level while carrying out stabilizing procedures at adjacent joints has become a very practical approach for the restoration of the severe rheumatoid hand and has allowed the surgeon to proceed with single-stage total hand reconstruction in appropriate circumstances.[7]

The purpose of this chapter is to review the practical considerations for surgical reconstruction of the severely involved wrist and digital joints in the hands of patients afflicted with rheumatoid arthritis. Recommendations for surgical procedures at each level are followed by a discussion of how these procedures can be coordinated into a single reconstructive effort that will allow the maximal benefit for each hand. Early palliative procedures such as small joint synovectomy are controversial and beyond the scope of this discussion.

CONSIDERATION BY LEVEL
The wrist

By virtue of its position between the forearm and the hand, the wrist serves as the key joint for the proper functional performance of the hand. Although a number of procedures are available for reconstruction of the severely involved rheumatoid wrist, it is important to realize that many patients have wrists that are stable and essentially pain free. Even though radiographs of these patients may indicate substantial carpal destruction and coalition, no surgical efforts are indicated, and the surgeon can direct efforts to other areas that are more functionally disabling. On other occasions clinical examination of the rheumatoid wrist may indicate that the only pain is around the distal aspect of the ulna as a result of its subluxation in the *caput ulnae* syndrome, and a simple Darrach excision of the distal part of the ulna and local synovectomy may suffice despite rather marked changes in the carpus. Resurfacing of the distal ulnar stump following Darrach excision using the silicone rubber cap designed by Swanson[25,27] has given good results, although its role in preventing ulnar translocation or carpal collapse is questionable.

Occasionally patients with MCP joint destruction sufficient to require reconstructive surgery will also have chronic, minimally symptomatic synovitis of the dorsal aspect of the wrist. To lessen the chance of extensor tendon rupture, it is probably worthwhile to carry out at least a "limited" synovectomy of the dorsal portion of the wrist at the time of digital joint reconstruction. We have found no problems with concomitant wrist and MCP joint procedures.

Rebalancing the wrist using the Clayton[4] transfer of the extensor carpi radialis longus to the extensor carpi ulnaris may be indicated if there is early ulnar translocation of the carpus. Volar repositioning of the extensor retinaculum as recommended by Clayton also has proved effective in decompressing the extensor tendons and buffering them from possible carpal abrasion and rupture. Taleisnik has indicated that early reconstruction of the scapholunate ligament complex maybe beneficial in preventing the dissociation pattern that occurs frequently in that area of the rheumatoid wrist. (See Chapter 26.) The long-term benefits of this technique will have to be carefully monitored.

Procedures recommended for advanced destruction of the wrist in rheumatoid arthritis include intracarpal or total wrist arthrodesis (Fig. 27-1) using the methods described by Watson and Hempton,[30] Abbott, Saunders, and Bost,[1] Carroll and Dick,[3] or Millender and Nalebuff[15] (Fig. 27-2). Proximal row carpectomy occasionally has been advocated, and dorsal stabilization of the rheumatoid wrist has been described recently by Kulick and associates.[9] The use of various prosthetic devices for wrist arthroplasty has enjoyed some popularity, and the need to rebalance the deformed wrist following the use of such implants has been emphasized, although duplicating normal wrist mechanics may be difficult.[10,26,27]

In an effort to simplify the indications for various procedures in the badly deformed rheumatoid wrist, our recommendation has been that, if the wrist is stable and without substantial deformity at the time of surgery, the flexible silicone rubber implant of Swanson[22,24-26] will provide an excellent interpositional arthroplasty with the retention of approximately 50% of normal wrist motion with satisfactory stability and pain relief. The articulated prostheses of Volz[10] and others also can provide the same type of satisfactory rheumatoid wrist reconstruction, although there have been some problems achieving the proper rotational axis and preventing loosening. The use of the Swanson implant in the stable wrist eliminates the need for extensive revision and rebalancing of the capsule and tendons about the joint. The long-term performance of the implant appears to be more predictable without the stresses generated by an imbalanced situation. Using this rather strict indication for implantation, we have not had any fractures of the silicone rubber wrist implants and have found them to pro-

SECTION 7 RHEUMATOID ARTHRITIS PROBLEMS

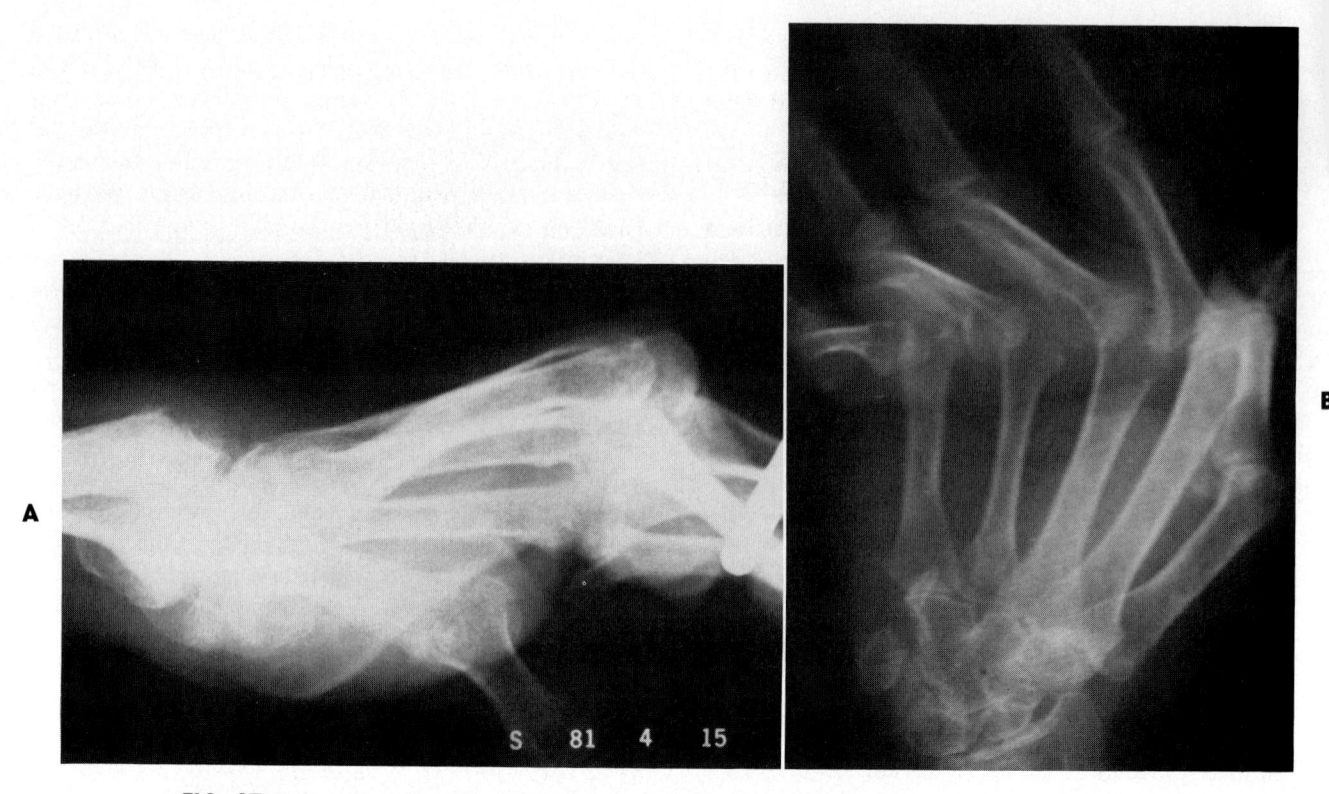

FIG. 27-1. Severe deformities of rheumatoid wrist. **A,** Carpal coalition and joint destruction with partial volar subluxation and dorsal dislocation of ulna. **B,** Ulnar translocation of carpus with radiocarpal and intracarpal destruction. In both cases dislocation has occurred at MCP joints.

vide predictable pain relief and stability while preserving adequate motion (Fig. 27-3).

In those instances where there has been marked collapse or deviation of the wrist secondary to volar subluxation of the carpus beneath the radius or severe ulnar translocation of the carpus, fusion procedures remain effective in regaining length and stability, relieving pain, restoring strength, and preserving forearm rotation.[15] Although simple dorsal stabilization of the rheumatoid wrist might be applicable in some instances,[9] it seems that the predictable stability provided by arthrodesis techniques would be preferable. A formal Abbott[1] or Carroll[3] arthrodesis of the wrist with the use of iliac crest bone is unfortunately a rather time-consuming procedure that may limit the option to proceed with additional reconstructive efforts at more distal levels.

Millender and Nalebuff[15,16] described a practical arthrodesis technique involving a limited preparation of the carpus and the use of a Steinmann pin driven down the web space between the second and third metacarpals and into the distal aspect of the radius. They[16] also have recommended a "closed wrist fusion," which consists of introducing a Steinmann pin down the third metacarpal and into the radius at the time of MCP joint arthroplasty. These techniques have provided excellent wrist stability despite the fact that complete bony coalition does not always occur. The procedure (open or closed) is relatively quick and easily combined with additional reconstruction of the digital joints (Fig. 27-4).

When restoration of carpal height is desired to achieve correct tendon balance in a severe collapsed wrist deformity, occasionally we have used the *instant wrist fusion* technique described by Heiple, Burstein, and Gradisar.[8] This procedure uses a rabbit-eared, perforated metal scaffolding, which is surrounded by methyl methacrylate after appropriate carpal excision and preparation. (See Fig. 27-2, *C*.) The technique is rapid and predictable and can be combined with additional reconstruction at the digital joint level (Fig. 27-5). Unfortunately the scaffolding device is no longer available, although an improvising surgeon should be able to create similar stability with the use of Kirschner wires or small Steinmann pins encompassed by methyl methacrylate.

In a departure from conventional advice we have not hesitated to carry out appropriate transfers for ruptured extensor tendons at the same time as wrist arthroplasty

Text continued on p. 232.

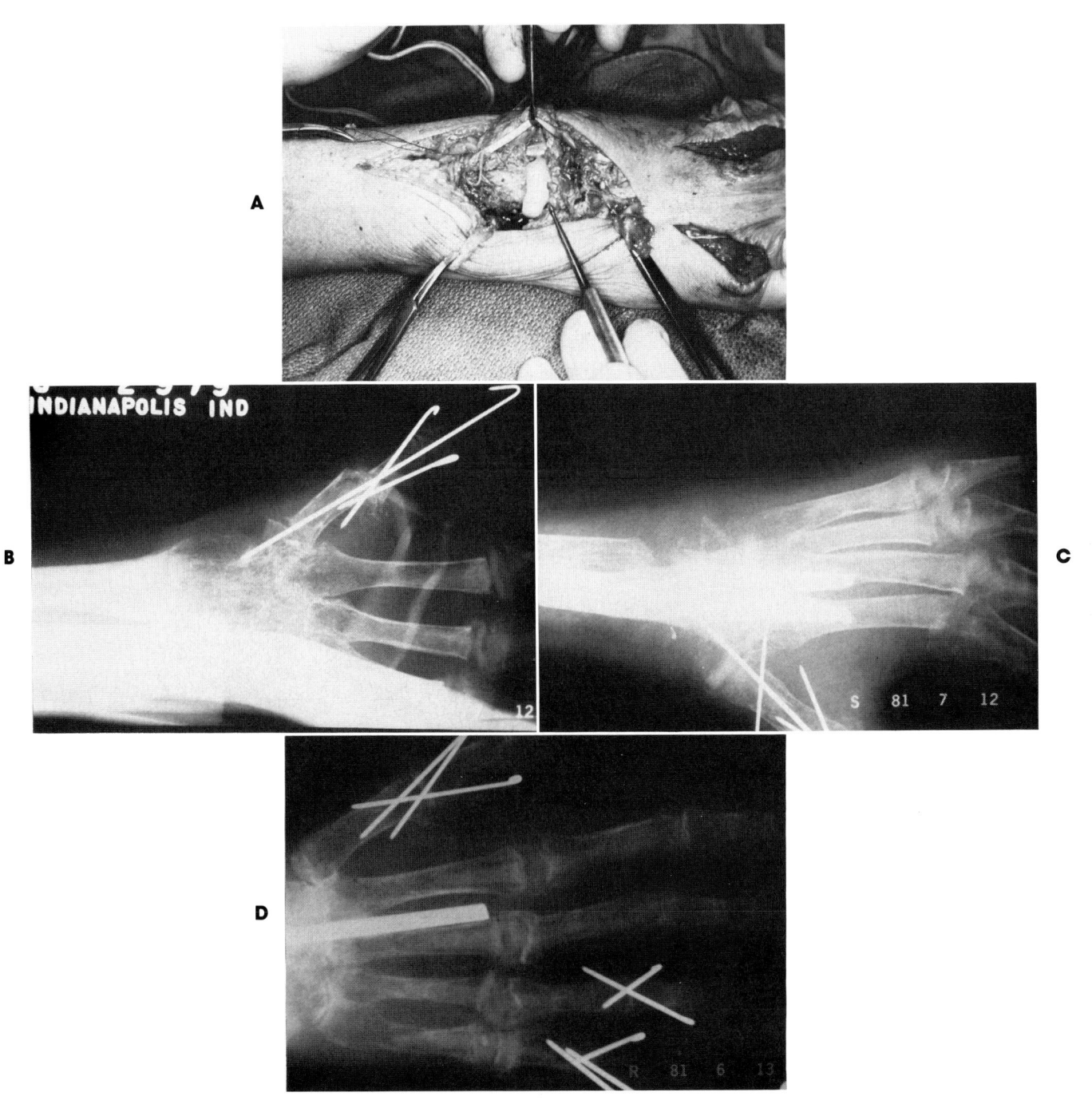

CHAPTER 27 THE SURGICAL MANAGEMENT OF MULTIPLE-LEVEL DEFORMITIES OF THE RHEUMATOID HAND

FIG. 27-2. Techniques for reconstruction of rheumatoid wrist. **A,** Implant arthroplasty combined with extensor tendon reconstruction and MCP joint arthroplasty. **B,** Previous formal wrist arthrodesis (Abbott) with MCP joint arthroplasties and thumb reconstruction at three levels. **C,** Wrist stabilization using metal scaffolding and methyl methacrylate. Note reconstruction of basilar thumb joint using great toe prosthesis and arthroplasties of MCP joints. **D,** Wrist stabilization with large Steinmann pin (Millender and Nalebuff[15]) combined with MCP joint arthroplasty and arthrodesis of MCP joint of thumb and proximal interphalangeal (PIP) joints of ring and small fingers.

SECTION 7 RHEUMATOID ARTHRITIS PROBLEMS

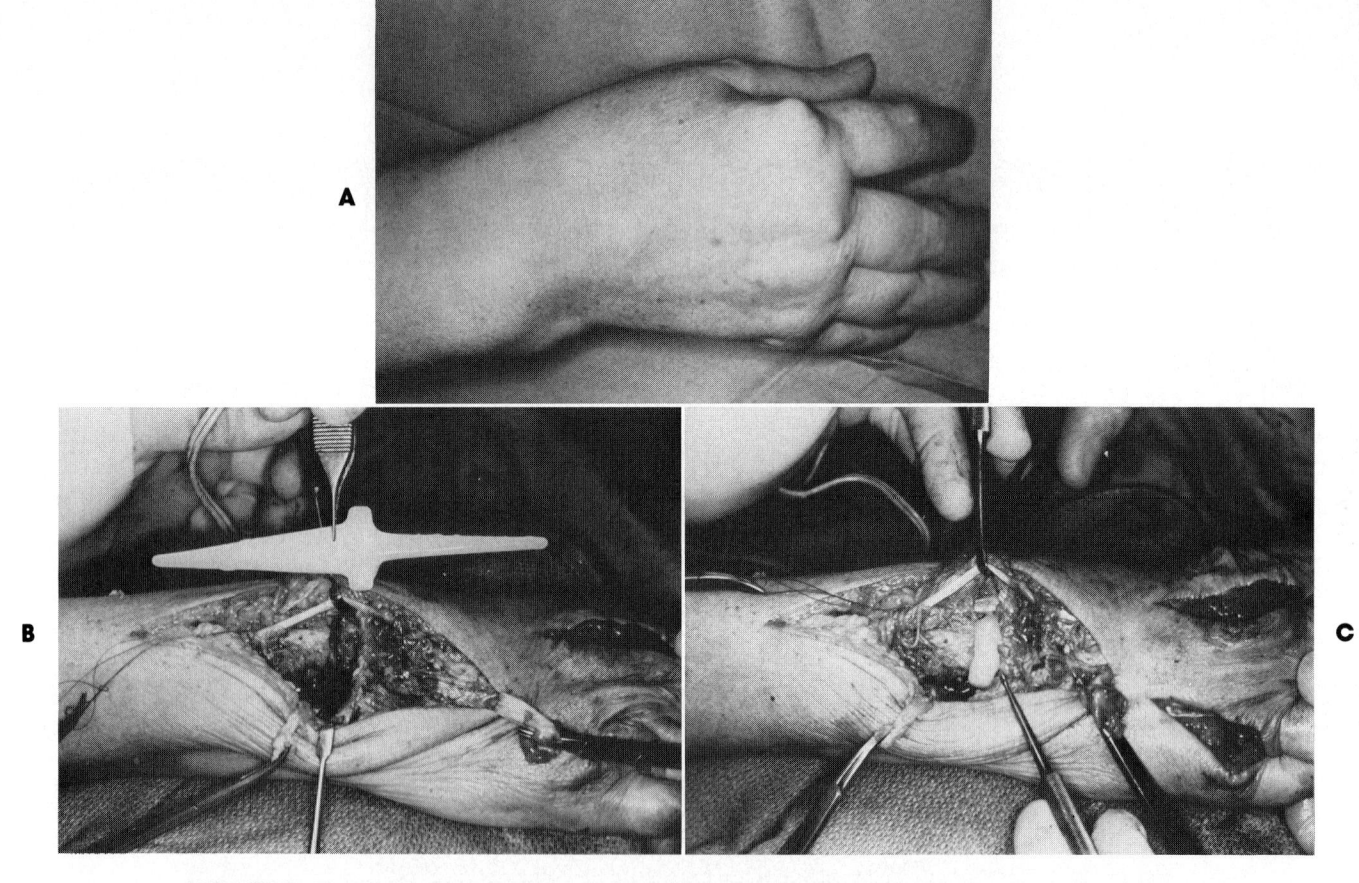

FIG. 27-3. Multiple-level involvement of rheumatoid wrist and hand, including painful but stable wrist, rupture of extensor tendons to long, ring, and small fingers, MCP joint subluxation, and painful instability of MCP joint of thumb. **A,** Preoperative appearance of hand and wrist. **B,** Carpal defect and preparation for implantation of silicone rubber interpositional implant. Note ruptured extensor tendons proximally and distally. **C,** Appearance of wrist following seating of silicone rubber implant prior to completion of MCP joint fusion of thumb, MCP joint arthroplasty of index, long, ring, and small fingers, and extensor tendon reconstruction using extensor carpi radialis brevis.

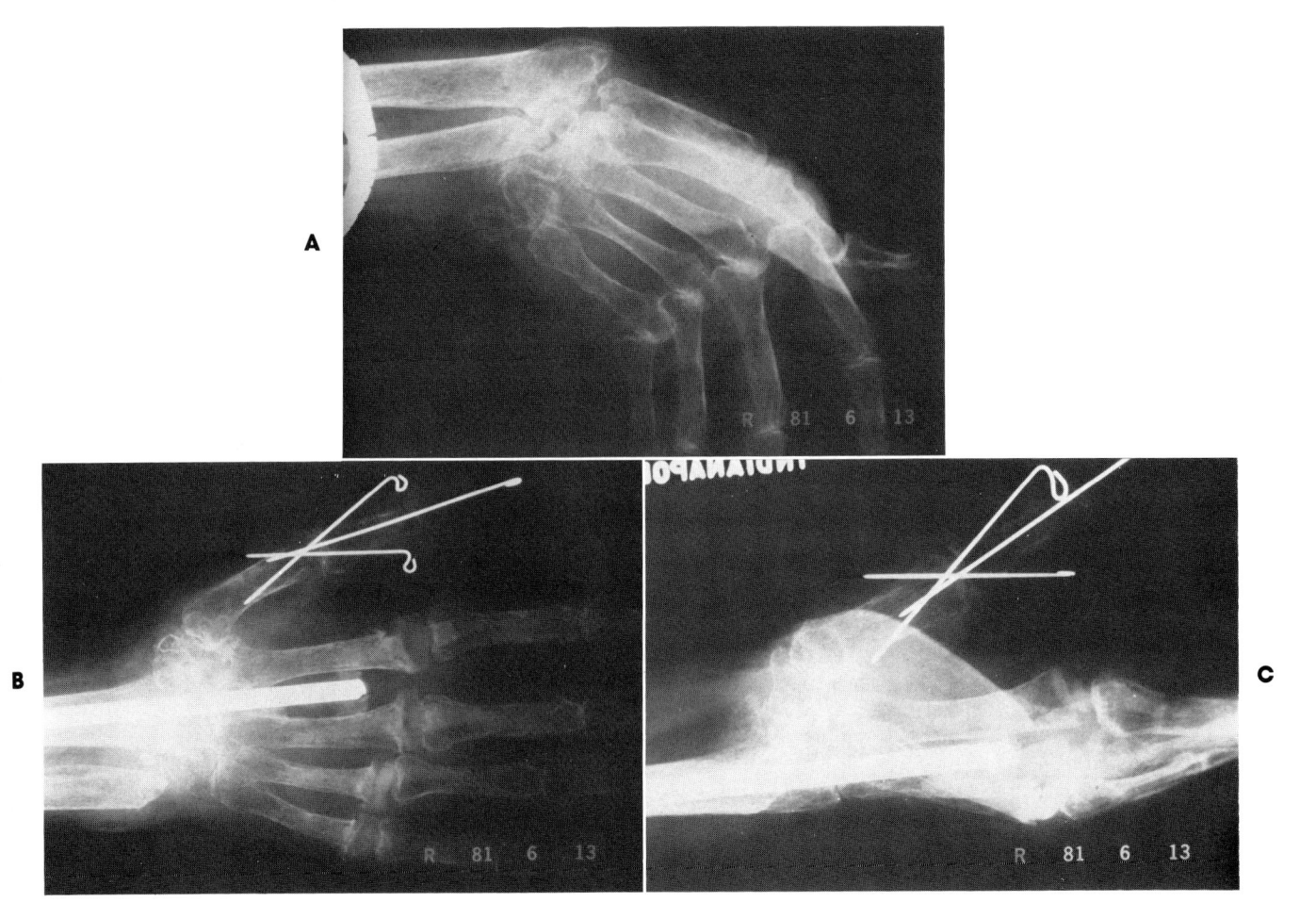

CHAPTER 27 THE SURGICAL MANAGEMENT OF MULTIPLE-LEVEL DEFORMITIES OF THE RHEUMATOID HAND

FIG. 27-4. Wrist stabilization using technique of Millender and Nalebuff.[16] **A,** Marked wrist destruction with ulnar-volar dislocation of carpus. Note concomitant dislocation of MCP joints. **B,** Anteroposterior view following repositioning of carpus and stabilization with large Steinmann pin driven between second and third metacarpals and into radius. **C,** Lateral view of wrist stabilization procedure. Note arthrodesis of MCP joint of thumb and silicone rubber implant arthroplasty of MCP joints of index, long, ring, and small fingers, carried out concomitant with wrist stabilization.

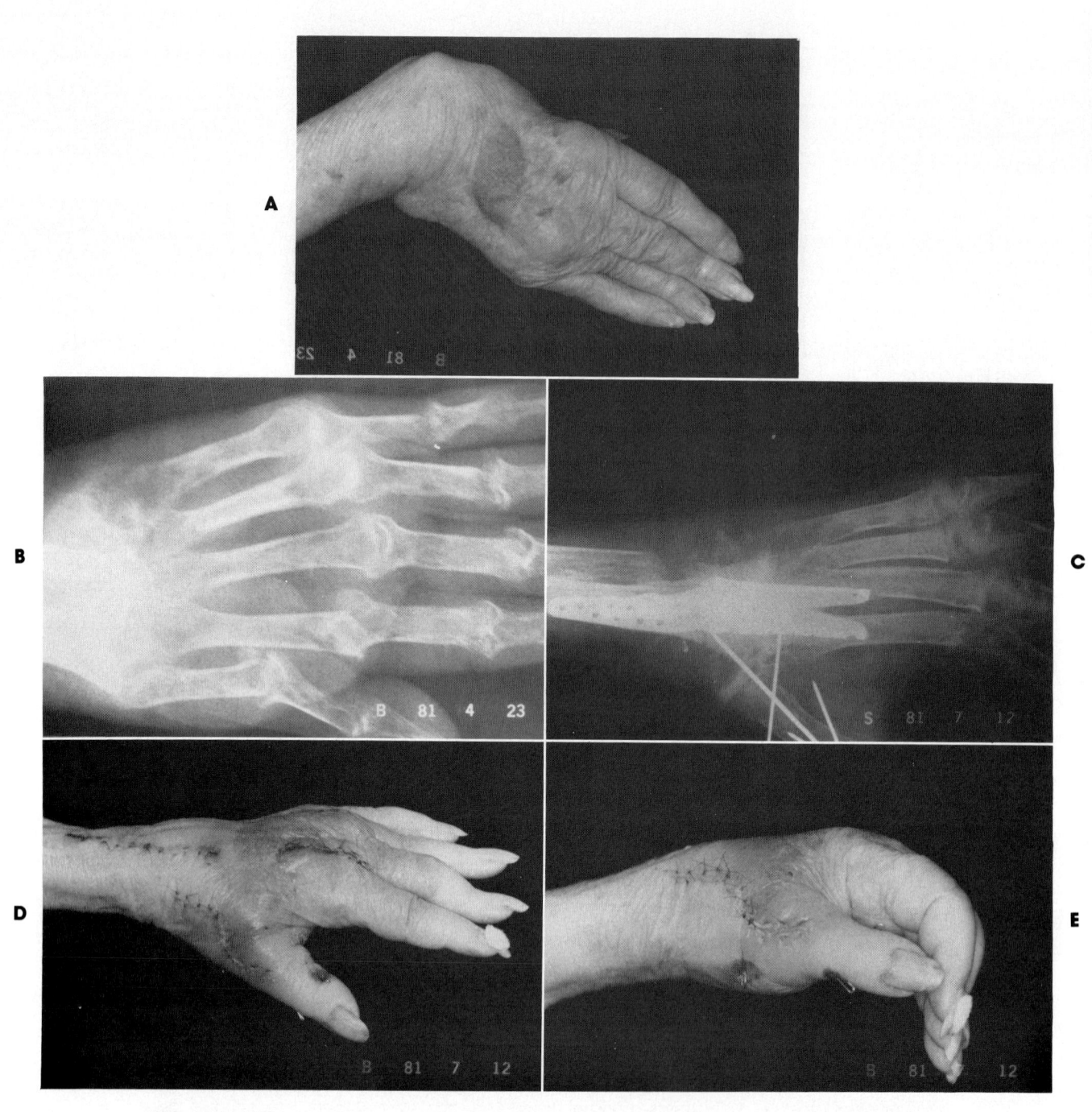

FIG. 27-5. Wrist stabilization and hand reconstruction using *instant wrist arthrodesis* devised by Heiple, Burstein, and Gradisar.[8] **A,** Markedly unstable and dislocated wrist in patient with severe rheumatoid arthritis involving all hand joints. **B,** Appearance of collapsed wrist and destroyed MCP and interphalangeal (IP) joints. **C,** X-ray appearance of wrist and hand following wrist stabilization using rabbit-eared, perforated metal scaffolding and methyl methacrylate. Concomitant MCP joint arthrodesis and basilar joint arthroplasty using toe prosthesis was carried out together with silicone rubber replacement arthroplasty of index, long, ring, and small fingers. **D** and **E,** Appearance of hand at 10 days with improved wrist, thumb, and digital positioning.

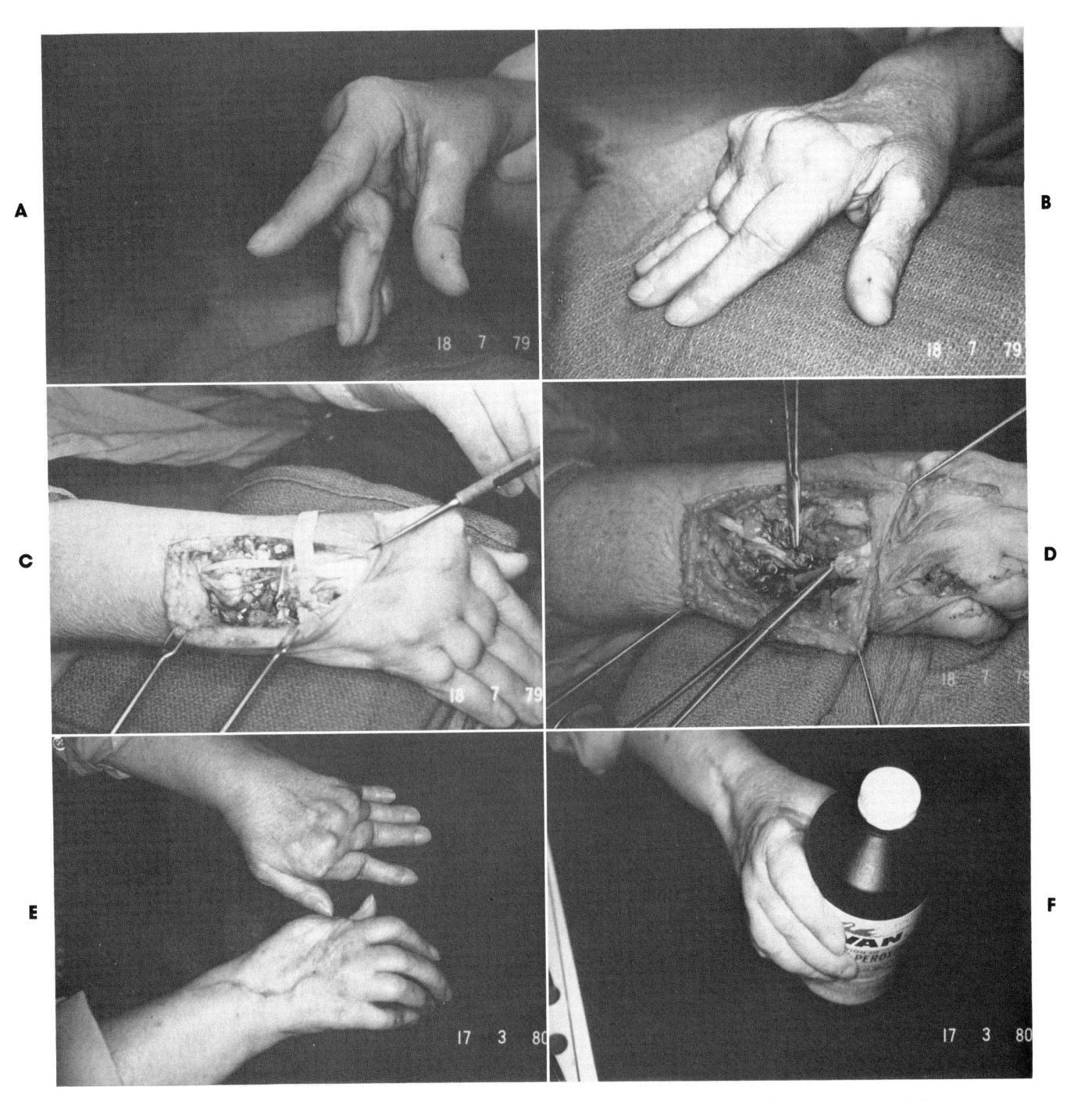

CHAPTER 27 THE SURGICAL MANAGEMENT OF MULTIPLE-LEVEL DEFORMITIES OF THE RHEUMATOID HAND

FIG. 27-6. Reconstruction of severely involved rheumatoid hand with simultaneous wrist stabilization, tendon transfer, MCP joint arthroplasty, and open capsulectomy of PIP joints. **A,** Inability to extend index, long, ring, or small fingers subsequent to extensor tendon rupture. **B,** Severe MCP joint flexion and PIP hyperextension deformities in digits. **C,** Appearance of wrist at time of stabilization. Note distal stumps of ruptured extensor tendons. **D,** Preparation for completion of superficialis transfers to extensor tendon stumps, with open capsulectomies of PIP joints and MCP joint arthroplasties having already been completed. A Darrach excision of distal ulna and wrist rebalancing (extensor carpi radialis brevis to extensor carpi ulnaris) also were carried out. **E,** Appearance of reconstructed hand at 8 months compared with similarly deformed opposite hand. **F,** Improved hand stability, motion, and function following this combined reconstruction.

or stabilization even in combination with MCP joint replacement arthroplasty (Fig. 27-6). It is difficult to understand how the digits can be "rebalanced" prior to wrist or digital reconstruction when one is not certain of the amount of bone that will be resected—a factor that will substantially influence the tension of the transfers at the time of tendon restoration. We have found no significant problems with simultaneous tendon reconstruction and implant arthroplasty, although the obligatory postoperative immobilization of the tendon repairs has been slightly prejudicial to the ultimate performance of the arthroplasties.

Carpal tunnel release can be carried out concomitant with procedures on the dorsal aspect of the wrist such as synovectomy, Darrach excision, arthroplasty, or arthrodesis. Despite varying combinations of additional procedures, surgical decompression of the median nerve has been performed routinely whenever indicated with no noticeable sequelae.

In summary, the indications for surgery on the rheumatoid wrist include unrelenting synovitis with nerve compression (carpal tunnel syndrome) or impending tendon rupture, caput ulnae syndrome, chronic pain, instability, and deformity, or the presence of one or more ruptured extrinsic tendons. The appropriate procedures for these conditions include synovectomy with dorsal retinacular transposition, median nerve decompression, Darrach excision of the distal portion of the ulna with or without ulnar head replacement, interpositional or replacement arthroplasty, wrist stabilization or fusion, and tendon transfer. Time-efficient surgical techniques such as the Swanson[22,24-26] silicone rubber interpositional arthroplasty for the stable rheumatoid wrist or the Millender-Nalebuff[15] arthrodesis technique in unstable situations may be carried out by experienced surgeons without limiting the option of simultaneously reconstructing more distal levels of digital joint disease.

MCP joints

The MCP joints will be involved in a large percentage of patients with complex deformities of the rheumatoid hand. The classic triad of MCP joint flexion, ulnar dislocation of the extensor tendons, and ulnar deviation of the digits continues to represent a restorative challenge for the hand surgeon. Secondary deformities at the proximal interphalangeal (PIP) joints resulting from MCP joint collapse will compound digital disability, and a prerequisite to their correction is reconstruction at the MCP joint level.

A classification of MCP joint deformities after long-standing synovial invasion has been suggested by Millender and Nalebuff[16] and is useful for making management decisions at the time of surgical correction. Although there is an occasional place for surgical synovectomy of the MCP joint in rheumatoid arthritis, the procedure should be reserved for those patients who have had unrelenting synovial activity for at least 6 months with the evolution of a boggy, chronically inflamed synovial membrane.[20] Procedures designed to prevent or correct ulnar deviation of the digits prior to cartilage destruction[31] have had disappointing long-term success.

MCP joint arthroplasty using a flexible silicone rubber implant has now reached the stage of predictability and reliability that makes it the procedure of choice for most advanced deformities at that level.* These prostheses, which have been in use since 1967 and currently are constructed out of high-performance silicone rubber, are well tolerated and appear to have a low fracture rate. The indications for MCP joint interpositional arthroplasty with concomitant realignment of the extensor tendons and collateral ligament reconstruction include fixed flexion deformities, joint subluxation, severe ulnar deviation, destruction of articular cartilage, protracted pain, and joint instability.[27] It is our opinion that the destruction of three or more of the digital MCP joints should be an indication for replacement of all four, because a single joint left unoperated will inevitably deteriorate and require later reconstruction. The so-called eggcup deformity created by long-standing erosion of the metacarpal head into the base of the proximal phalanx will often perform satisfactorily without surgical intervention, whereas in other instances chronic pain and instability will ultimately require replacement arthroplasty.

Millender and Nalebuff[16] have emphasized that any significant wrist deformity should be corrected prior to MCP joint arthroplasty or at the time of arthroplasty, which we feel is the preferable approach. They also have emphasized the need to assess the continuity and amplitude of both the flexor and extensor tendon systems prior to implant arthroplasty, and it has proved possible to carry out extensor tendon transfer or flexor tenolysis at the same time as MCP joint reconstruction.

Proximal and distal interphalangeal joints

Several patterns of deformity may exist at the PIP joint in rheumatoid arthritis and occur either independently or in combination with deformity at the MCP joint. The swan-neck hyperextension or boutonniere flexion deformities of the PIP joint may be flexible or rigid (Fig. 27-7). Interesting combinations of PIP joint flexion and extension deformities may occur in the same hand. It is important to develop a practical management plan for these deformities, particularly when they occur in combination with MCP joint destruction. One-stage

---

*References 16, 22-24, 26, and 27.

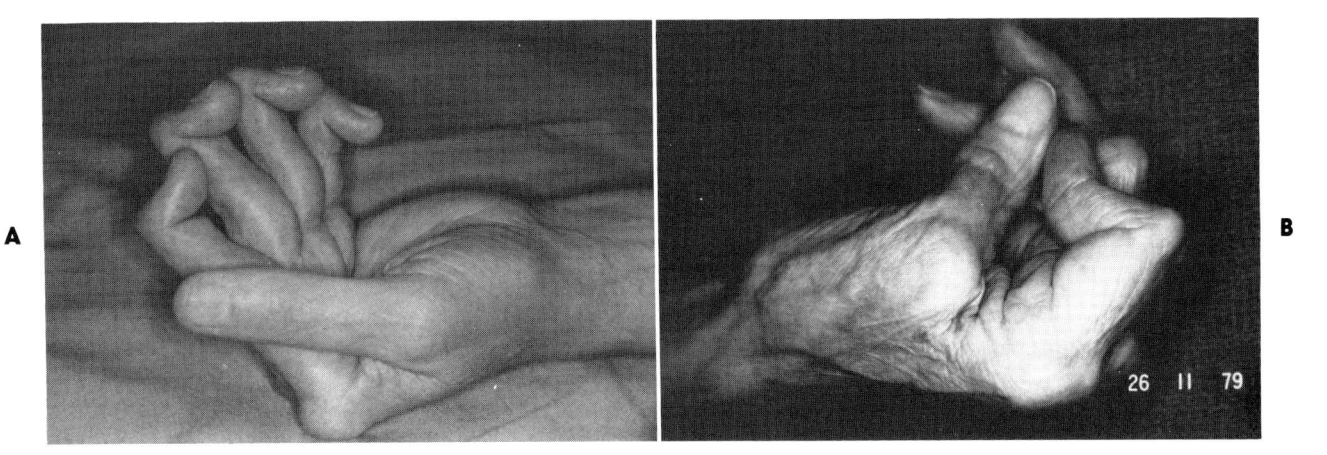

CHAPTER 27 THE SURGICAL MANAGEMENT OF MULTIPLE-LEVEL DEFORMITIES OF THE RHEUMATOID HAND

FIG. 27-7. Characteristic disabilities of PIP and DIP joints in rheumatoid arthritis. **A,** Severe fixed swan-neck deformities with hyperextension of PIP joints and flexion deformities of DIP joints. **B,** Severe boutonniere flexion deformities of PIP joints of index and long fingers with hyperextension at DIP level. Boutonniere lesion of thumb is also present.

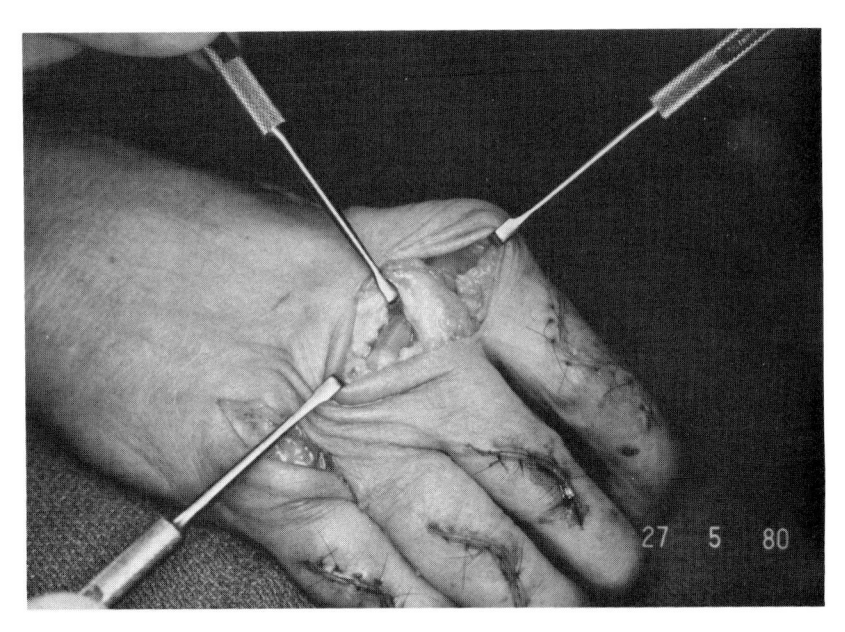

FIG. 27-8. Concomitant MCP joint arthroplasty and open dorsal capsulectomy of PIP joints to mobilize severe, fixed swan-neck deformities.

reconstruction at both levels is frequently possible, provided the surgeon is experienced and the goals of surgery are realistic.

The management of flexible swan-neck deformities of the PIP joint in rheumatoid arthritis may be accomplished by the procedure described by Littler[11] in which a single lateral band is detached proximally, transferred volar to the retaining skin ligaments (Cleland's ligaments), and attached proximally to either bone or the flexor tendon sheath to create a dynamic tenodesis similar in function to that of the oblique retinacular ligament.[6,28] When PIP joint hyperextension has become fixed but satisfactory articular surfaces remain, a longitudinal splitting of the lateral bands away from the central slip combined with dorsal capsulectomy and extensor tenolysis may be sufficient to restore flexion of that joint. The volar displacement of the lateral bands created by this procedure will augment joint flexion, and protective splinting in the postoperative period often will prevent the recurrence of the deformity, particularly when done in combination with MCP joint arthroplasty and intrinsic decompression (Fig. 27-8). We have rarely found it necessary to lengthen the central extensor tendon to achieve the restoration of PIP joint flexion. When significant cartilage destruction has occurred, prosthetic replacement arthroplasty may be considered. If implant arthroplasty has been carried out at the MCP joint, it is usually preferable to perform an arthrodesis of the PIP joint particularly when multiple digital deformities exist.[7,17,18]

When a boutonniere deformity is present with flexion at the PIP joint and hyperextension at the distal interphalangeal (DIP) joint, the condition of the articular surfaces and the passive mobility of the middle joint will be important considerations in determining the appropriate reconstructive procedure. A flexible boutonniere deformity in the presence of satisfactory articular cartilage should allow one to reconstruct the attenuated central extensor slip or use the technique of Matev[12,13] to augment PIP joint extension and improve DIP joint flexion. If the boutonniere deformity has become fixed, the reconstructive options are implant arthroplasty with extensor reconstruction or arthrodesis, a procedure that is particularly applicable when concomitant MCP joint arthroplasties are being carried out (Fig. 27-9). Arthrodesis of the DIP joint for long-standing fixed deformities, whether in extension or flexion, has proved to be a very satisfactory procedure and can be easily carried out in combination with more proximal reconstructive efforts.

For severe multiple-level joint deformities, arthroplasty of the MCP joints combined with PIP joint arthrodesis is an effective and reliable method of returning effective digital function.[7,17,18] In our experience replacement arthroplasty of both MCP and PIP joints of all digits may be performed (Fig. 27-10), but it is difficult to achieve a predictable long-term result at both levels. In many instances MCP joint flexion will remain satisfactory, but a slow loss of motion will occur at the more distal joint level. For that reason we usually have opted for PIP joint arthrodesis combined with MCP joint ar-

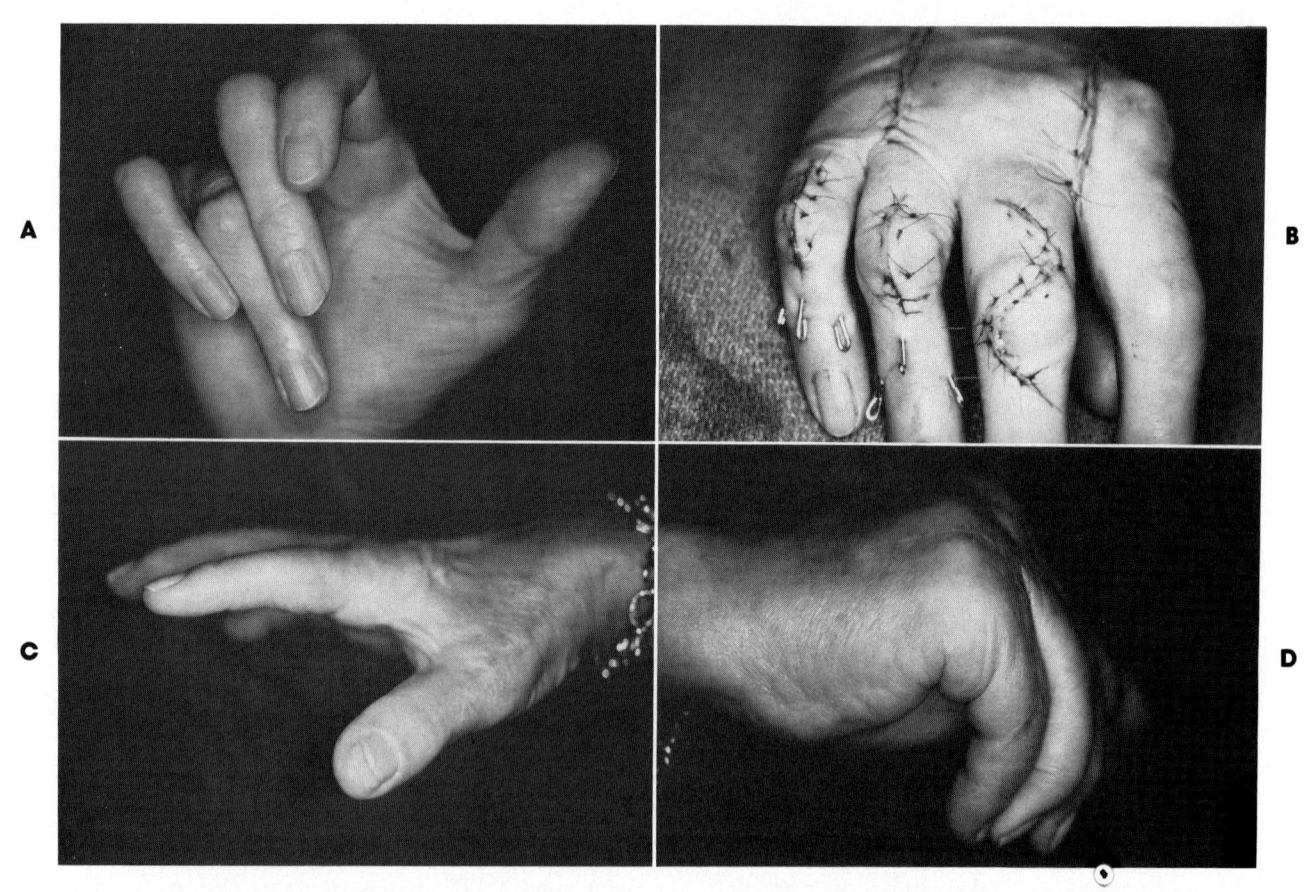

FIG. 27-9. Management of combined MCP joint destruction and boutonniere deformity of fingers. **A,** Fixed boutonniere flexion deformities of PIP joints of long, ring, and small fingers in excess of 70 degrees. **B,** Appearance of hand following completion of MCP joint arthroplasty of index, long, ring, and small fingers, arthrodesis of PIP joints of ring and small fingers, and reconstruction of extensor mechanism of long finger after capsulectomy. **C,** Improved digital extension at 6 months. **D,** Lateral view of flexion capability at 6 months.

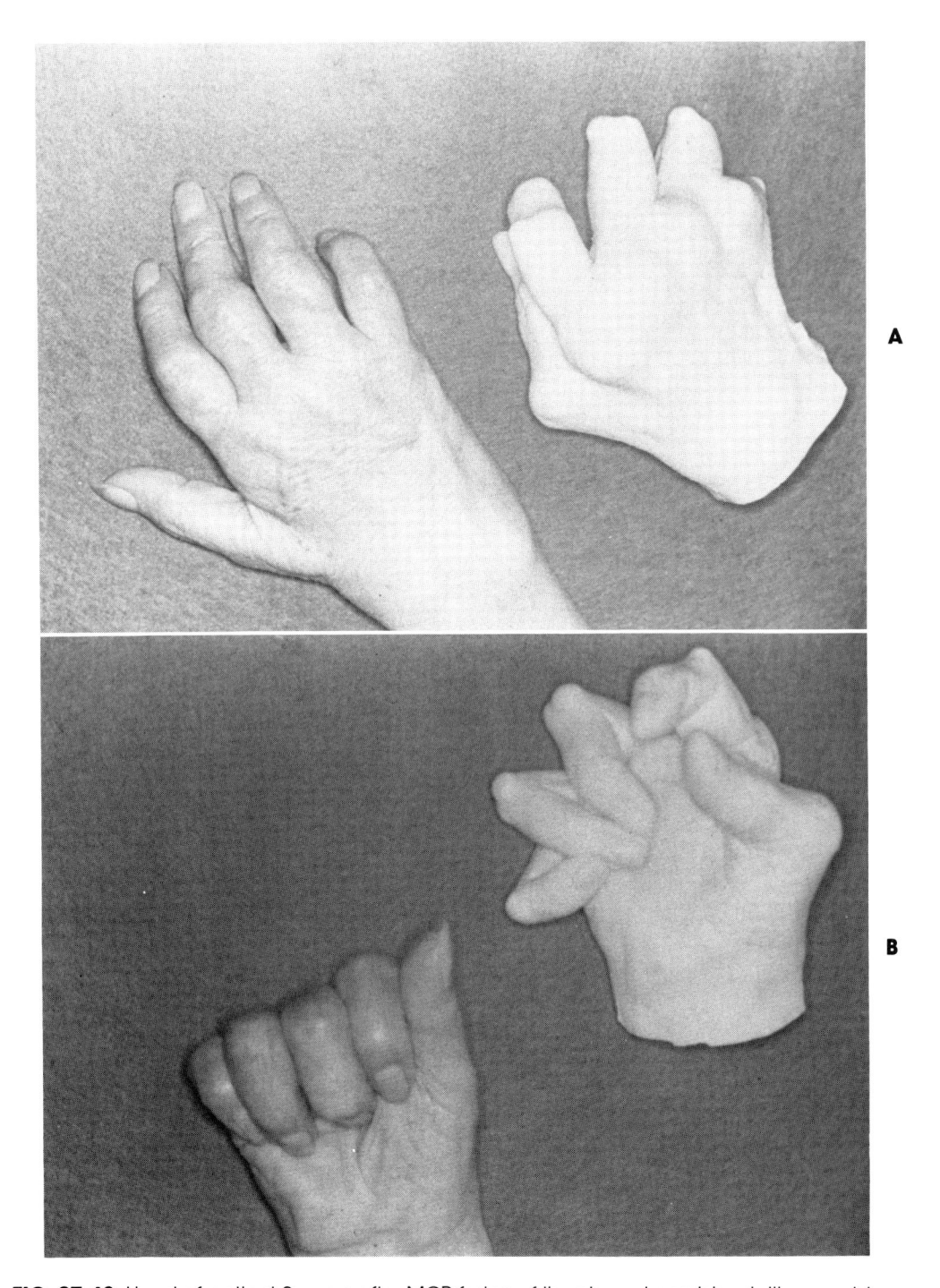

CHAPTER 27 THE SURGICAL MANAGEMENT OF MULTIPLE-LEVEL DEFORMITIES OF THE RHEUMATOID HAND

FIG. 27-10. Hand of patient 2 years after MCP fusion of thumb and combined silicone rubber replacement arthroplasty at both MCP and PIP joints of index, long, ring, and small fingers. **A** and **B,** Appearance of hand compared with model of hand made just prior to surgery: despite excellent early performance, there has been gradual deterioration in range of motion at PIP joint level.

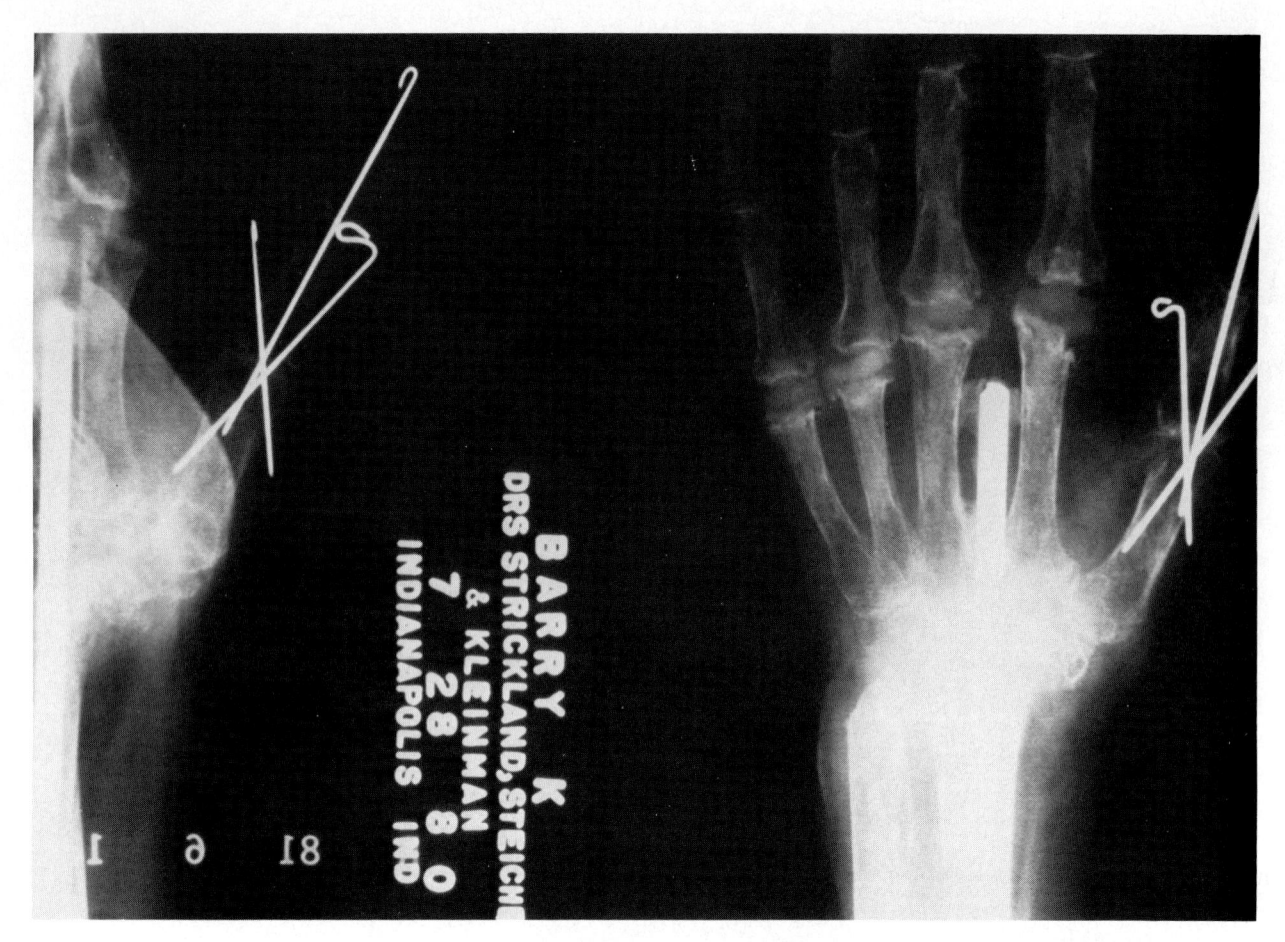

FIG. 27-11. X-ray appearance of hand following combined wrist stabilization (Millender-Nalebuff[16]), MCP arthrodesis of thumb, and MCP joint arthroplasties.

throplasty except when the indications for arthroplasty exist at only one or two PIP joints. It appears that the performance of MCP joint arthroplasty may be enhanced by stabilization of the PIP joints, thereby allowing the patient to use the full amplitude of the long flexor tendons at the MCP level.

The thumb

The management of complex deformities of the rheumatoid thumb is discussed in Chapter 25. The most common presentation is the boutonniere deformity with fixed flexion at the MCP joint and hyperextension at the interphalangeal (IP) joint. In many cases a simple arthrodesis of the MCP joint will tend to adequately rebalance the IP joint and restore satisfactory thumb stability and alignment. Arthrodesis of both MCP and IP joints will be necessary on rare occasions. In the more complex deformities involving collapse at the carpometacarpal (CMC) joint some type of interpositional arthroplasty of the basilar joint may prove beneficial.

When arthrodesis of the wrist has been carried out, it may be difficult to reconstruct the basilar thumb joint with a trapezial prosthesis, and in these instances we have relied on creating a small slot for the insertion of a great toe prosthesis[27] or an Ashworth-Blatt[2] type of prosthetic implant. There has been little difficulty in proceeding with thumb reconstruction concomitant with wrist arthroplasty or arthrodesis, tendon transfers, MCP joint prosthetic replacement, or procedures designed to reconstruct or stabilize the PIP and DIP joints of other digits (Fig. 27-11).

DISCUSSION

Numerous authors* recommend the staging of reconstructive procedures on the rheumatoid wrist and hand, with the implication that simultaneous major reconstructive surgery at multiple levels is prejudicial to final hand performance. These authors emphasize that maximal re-

---

*References 16, 18, 19, 21, and 27.

covery from each procedure should be achieved before the next procedure is undertaken.[19] Most agree that the treatment of the wrist should be completed before surgery is initiated on the thumb and digital joints.[16,19,21,27] It is widely held that synovectomy of the joints and tendon sheaths and rebalancing of the joints by tendon transfer should precede arthroplasty procedures.[18,27]

Possible combinations of hand reconstructive procedures have been proposed, with most authors[18,19,27] indicating that wrist and digital procedures usually should be done separately. It has been suggested that MCP joint arthroplasty may be carried out concomitant with thumb reconstructive procedures or, on occasion, with procedures designed to overcome swan-neck or boutonniere deformities at the PIP joint.[27] The MCP joints are usually given first priority with regard to the preservation of digital motion.[7,17,27]

In our experience in the surgical management of these deformities, however, it becomes apparent that simultaneous reconstruction of tendons and joints of the rheumatoid wrist and hand is not as contradictory as it might initially seem. Provided the indications for surgery at each level are carefully considered and procedures selected that will complement efforts at other levels, it is usually possible to carry out one-stage multiple-level reconstruction without the need to subject the patient to repeated operations over a prolonged period.

In an excellent evaluation of the practical value of various surgical procedures in the rheumatoid hands, Souter[21] indicates that fusion of the MCP joint of the thumb and extensor synovectomy with ulnar head resection are the most reliable and consistently useful operations. Flexor tendon synovectomy and MCP joint arthroplasty also are thought to produce excellent results, whereas PIP joint fusion and wrist stabilization are believed to be valuable, although their application is usually confined to the later stages of the disease in severely crippled hands, and their success depends on careful patient selection. Souter further grouped the correction of swan-neck deformity, MCP and IP joint synovectomy, and IP joint fusion of the thumb as procedures with a relatively limited field of application; he believed that, with the exception of thumb IP joint fusion, the reliability and value of these procedures were somewhat controversial. Finally, PIP joint arthroplasty and plastic procedures for the correction of boutonniere deformity achieved a poor rating and were not recommended for general use. He felt that these procedures demanded great technical expertise from the surgeon in handling hood tissues and should only be attempted by experienced surgeons.

Souter[21] favored a sequential, staged plan of operative reconstruction and emphasized that the program should be initiated with a procedure that was "guaranteed to be a winner" from the symptomatic and functional point of views and was likely to make the least demands on the patient. The procedures that he thought were most consistent with these goals were extensor synovectomy and excision of the head of the ulna. His recommendation with regard to the sequence of surgery was as follows:

1. Extensor tendon synovectomy and excision of the head of the ulna plus wrist stabilization, when necessary
2. Flexor tendon synovectomy
3. MCP joint surgery
4. PIP joint surgery and correction of finger deformities
5. Realignment of the thumb in the most useful position relative to the reconstructed fingers

It was Souter's opinion[21] that it was preferable to undertake several smaller operations at relatively frequent intervals rather than to carry out a "major onslaught" likely to result in massive edema and serious difficulties with mobilization. He emphasized that extensor and flexor tendon surgery should not be undertaken at the same sitting, nor should a major tenosynovectomy be coupled with major surgery.

Although we are essentially in agreement with Souter's rating[21] of the various surgical procedures for the rheumatoid hand, our own experience has been decidedly different with regard to the staging of procedures. We now feel strongly that, as long as procedures are not carried out that would prove contradictory in terms of postoperative therapy programs, a much more aggressive approach, with reconstructive efforts made at multiple levels in one sitting, has proved more effective.

Millender and Nalebuff[16] have emphasized the importance of a pain-free wrist with proper alignment and stability as a prerequisite for satisfactory MCP joint arthroplasty. They stated that closed wrist fusion in conjunction with MCP joint arthroplasty has produced pleasing results in selected cases. They thought the procedure could not be done if the wrist had been dislocated or if there were a severe flexion contracture and that it should not be done if inadequate bone stock were present. If the situation required opening the wrist to correct the deformity, it was felt that additional reconstruction at the MCP joint level; was precluded. In our experience of over thirty cases of wrist arthroplasty using the flexible implant of Swanson[22,24-27] or arthrodesis using either the technique of Millender and Nalebuff[15] or the metal implant with methyl methacrylate described (but not published) by Heiple,[8] there has been no reason to feel that these procedures cannot be effectively combined with MCP joint reconstruction in a single operative effort (Fig. 27-12).

Millender and Nalebuff[16] also state that flexor tenosynovectomy or single or double extensor tendon recon-

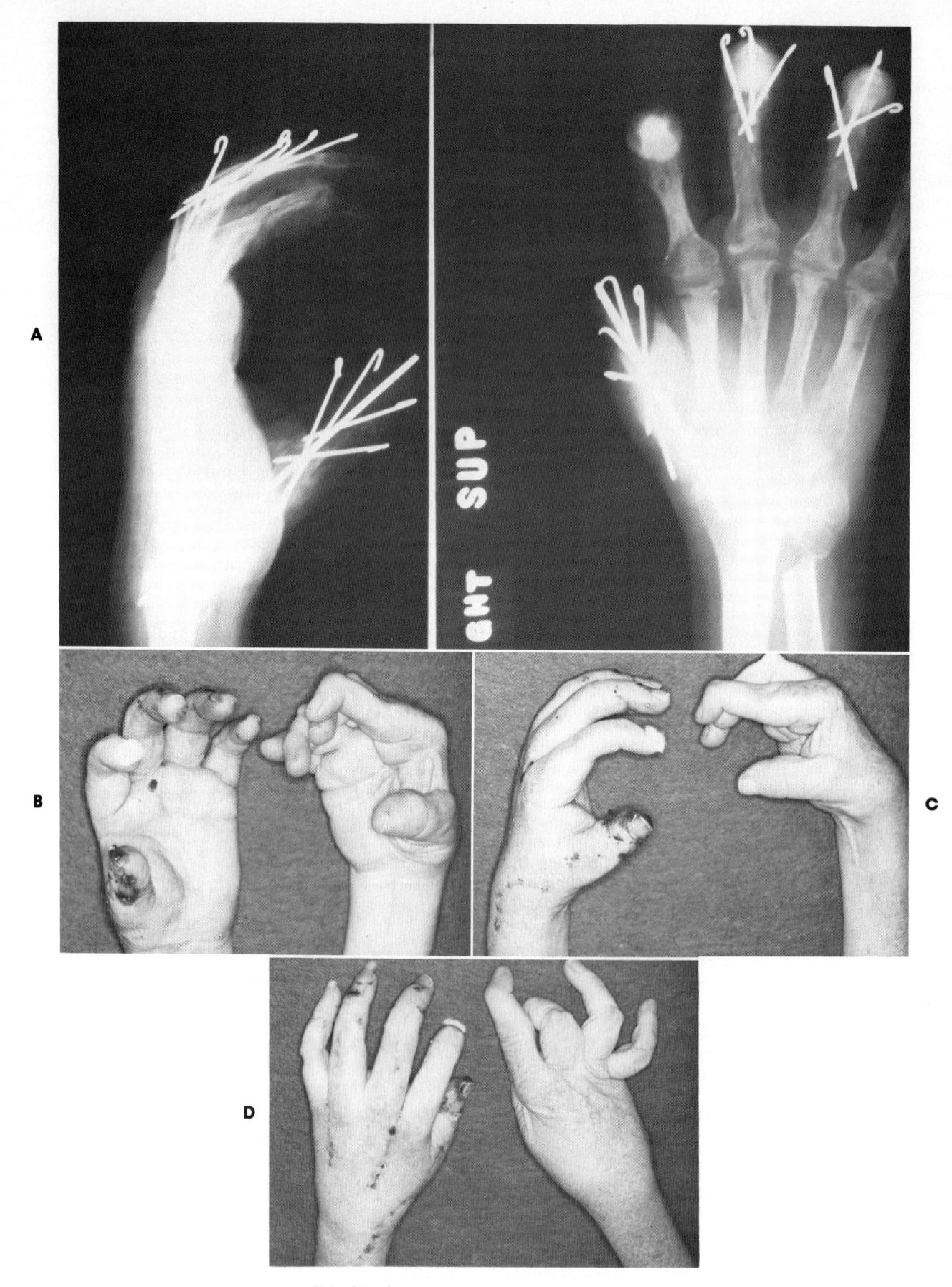

FIG. 27-12. For legend see opposite page.

struction can be combined with MCP joint arthroplasty. For more extensive tendon ruptures, however, their advice has been to withhold tendon reconstruction until MCP joint arthroplasties have been completed. Again, our experience would contradict this advice in that we have found that tendon transfers to all four digits can be effectively carried out at the same time as MCP joint arthroplasty, and, further, that wrist reconstruction and thumb stabilization also can be added to this restorative effort. There is no question that the obligatory 3 weeks of immobilization following tendon transfer can have a somewhat prejudicial effect on the ultimate performance of the MCP joint arthroplasties. However, in our experience a very satisfactory range of motion still has been achieved by a vigorous splinting program initiated 3 to 4 weeks postoperatively. It would seem that a rebalancing of the digits is best carried out at the same time as arthroplasty procedures so that one can more accurately assess the proper tension for tendon transfer suture and the effects of these transfers at each joint level.

Swanson[27] states that proper staging of reconstructive procedures is an important consideration and that tendon repair and synovectomy of the tendon sheaths must precede arthroplasty by 8 weeks. He further indicates that, in patients with involvement of both the MCP and PIP joints, MCP joint reconstruction has priority. When severe MCP joint and wrist involvement is present concomitantly, he suggests that the wrist be managed first. Swanson also indicates that it is unwise to carry out any surgical procedure on the rheumatoid patient that might exceed 2 hours. We would take issue with these statements in that we have found no significant problems with combining multiple-level reconstructive procedures.

The experienced reconstructive hand surgeon, adept at the procedures now available for the restoration or preservation of function in the rheumatoid hand, can expediently combine techniques such as wrist stabilization, MCP joint arthroplasty, thumb stabilization, and tendon reconstruction or lysis without causing undue hardship on the patient at the time of surgery and without affecting the performance of any of these procedures. When multiple-level disease is present within the digits, MCP joint arthroplasty combined with PIP joint mobilization or fusion also may be effectively carried out and can be further combined with wrist arthroplasty or arthrodesis under suitable circumstances.

Periodic release of the pneumatic tourniquet with appropriate external tissue compression and subsequent reinflation can allow one to proceed for three to four hours without any harmful effects. This is sufficient time for the performance of almost any combination of rheumatoid reconstructive procedures.

We would further question the acceptability of the staging of hand reconstruction in the severe rheumatoid patient with multiple-extremity involvement whose requirements include not only reconstruction of the wrist and hand but also of other joints, including elbows, hips, knees, ankles, or feet. The financial impact of multiple surgical procedures, hospitalizations, and rehabilitation may be so enormous as to negatively affect the patient's ability to carry through with the entire program. Perhaps most important, the motivational drive of the patient may be largely destroyed by the protracted sequence of surgery and rehabilitation necessitated by this approach.

SUMMARY

The surgeon undertaking the managemet of a rheumatoid arthritic patient with multiple-level hand involvement has an obligation to determine the realistic goals of reconstructive surgery and to thoroughly convey them to the patient. Consideration of the many physical, economic, or emotional problems that plague these patients must strongly enter into the decision as to which procedures will be most beneficial. Single-stage reconstructive efforts that involve complementary reconstructive procedures on the wrist, MCP joints, PIP joints, thumb, or tendons should be undertaken commensurate with operative efficiency, patient tolerance, and the skill of the surgeon. This seemingly aggressive approach has proved to be much more effective than the conventional staged approach with its inevitable deleterious effect on the patient's monetary and motivational resources.

FIG. 27-12. Combined procedures at three digital levels and thumb (three levels). **A,** X-ray appearance of hand shortly following wrist stabilization (Millender-Nalebuff[16]) with Steinmann pin driven down third metacarpal just prior to silicone replacement arthroplasty of MCP joint. Concomitant silicone rubber replacement arthroplasty of MCP joints of index, long, ring, and small fingers and arthrodesis of PIP joints of long and ring fingers were carried out together with combined arthrodesis at MCP and IP level of thumb and arthroplasty of basilar joint. **B, C,** and **D,** Three views of reconstructed left hand at 1 week compared with similar deformities of opposite hand. Note improved wrist and digital positioning at this early stage of motion.

SECTION 7 RHEUMATOID ARTHRITIS PROBLEMS

REFERENCES

1. Abbott, L.C., Saunders, J.B.De.C.M., and Bost, F.C.: Arthrodesis of the wrist with the use of grafts of cancellous bone, J. Bone Joint Surg. 24:883, 1942.
2. Ashworth, C.R., et al.: Silicone-rubber interposition arthroplasty of the carpometacarpal joint of the thumb, J. Hand Surg. 2:345, 1977.
3. Carroll, R.E., and Dick, H.M.: Arthrodesis of the wrist for rheumatoid arthritis, J. Bone Joint Surg. 53A:1365, 1971.
4. Clayton, M.L.: Surgical treatment at the wrist in rheumatoid arthritis: a review of 37 patients, J. Bone Joint Surg. 47A:741, 1965.
5. Cummings, J.K., and Taleisnik, J.: Peripheral gangrene as a complication of rheumatoid arthritis: report of a case and review of the literature, J. Bone Joint Surg. 53A:1001, 1971.
6. Flatt, A.E.: The care of the rheumatoid hand, ed. 2, St. Louis, 1974, The C.V. Mosby Co.
7. Froimson, A.I.: Hand reconstruction in arthritis mutilans: a case report, J. Bone Joint Surg. 53A:1377, 1971.
8. Heiple, K.G., Burstein, A.H., and Gradisar, I.: "Instant wrist fusion"—a preliminary report, J. Bone Joint Surg. 56A:1086, 1974.
9. Kulick, R.G., et al.: Long-term results of dorsal stabilization in the rheumatoid wrist, J. Hand Surg. 6:272, 1981.
10. Lamberta, F.L., Ferlic, D.C., and Clayton, M.L.: Volz total wrist arthroplasty in rheumatoid arthritis: a preliminary report, J. Hand Surg. 5:245, 1980.
11. Littler, J.W.: Restoration of the oblique retinacular ligament for reconstructing hyperextension deformity for the proximal interphalangeal joint. In Group d'Etude de la Main: La main rheumatismale, Paris, 1966, L'Expansion Scientifique Française.
12. Matev, I.: Transposition of the lateral slips of the aponeurosis in treatment of long-standing "boutonniere deformity" of the fingers, Br. J. Plast. Surg. 17:281, 1964.
13. Matev, I.: The boutonniere deformity, Hand 1:90, 1969.
14. McCollum, D.E., et al.: Surgery of the hand in rheumatoid arthritis—indications, contra-indications and expectations, J. Bone Joint Surg. 47A:1285, 1965.
15. Millender, L.H., and Nalebuff, E.A.: Arthrodesis of the rheumatoid wrist: an evaluation of 60 patients and a description of a different surgical technique, J. Bone Joint Surg. 55A:1026, 1973.
16. Millender, L.H., and Nalebuff, E.A.: Reconstructive surgery in the rheumatoid hand, Orthop. Clin. North Am. 6:709, 1975.
17. Nicolle, F.V.: Recent advances in the management of joint disease in the rheumatoid hand, Hand 5:91, 1973.
18. Nicolle, F.V., and Dickson, R.A.: Surgery of the rheumatoid hand: a practical manual, London, 1979, William Heinemann Medical Books, Ltd.
19. Savill, D.L.: Assessment of rheumatoid hand for reparative and reconstructive surgery, J. Bone Joint Surg. 46B:786, 1964.
20. Sones, D.A.: Surgery for rheumatoid arthritis—timing and techniques: general and medical aspects, J. Bone Joint Surg. 50A:576, 1968.
21. Souter, W.A.: Planning treatment of the rheumatoid hand, Hand 11:3, 1979.
22. Swanson, A.B.: Silicone rubber implants for replacement of arthritic or destroyed joints in the hand, Surg. Clin. North Am. 48:1113, 1968.
23. Swanson, A.B.: Finger joint replacement by silicone rubber implants and the concept of implant fixation by encapsulation: workshop on artificial finger joints, Ann. Rheum. Dis. (Suppl.) 28:47, 1969.
24. Swanson, A.B.: Flexible implant resection arthroplasty, Hand 4:119, 1972.
25. Swanson, A.B.: The ulnar head syndrome and its treatment by implant resection arthroplasty, J. Bone Joint Surg. 54A:906, 1972.
26. Swanson, A.B.: Flexible implant resection arthroplasty in the hand and extremities, St. Louis, 1973, The C.V. Mosby Co.
27. Swanson, A.B.: Reconstructive surgery in the arthritic hand and foot, Clin. Symp. 31(6):1, 1979.
28. Thompson, J.S., Littler, J.W., and Upton, J.: The spiral oblique retinacular ligament (SORL), J. Hand Surg. 3:482, 1978.
29. Vainio, K.: Indications and contra-indications for surgery in rheumatoid arthritis, Rheumatism 22:10, 1966.
30. Watson, H.K., and Hempton, R.F.: Limited wrist arthrodeses. I. The triscaphoid joint, J. Hand Surg. 5:320, 1980.
31. Zancolli, E.: Correction of the arthritic ulnar drift before cartilage destruction—an operation to rebalance the metacarpophalangeal forces. In Gramer, L.M., and Chase, R.A., editors: Symposium on the Hand, St. Louis, 1971, The C.V. Mosby Co.

SECTION EIGHT MICROVASCULAR PROBLEMS

Chapter 28 A rationale for digital salvage

James W. Strickland

The refinements in microsurgical techniques have made replantation of digits a clinical reality. Subsequent to the initial report by the replantation team at the Sixth People's Hospital in Shanghai,[14] numerous additional surveys[6,15-17] have indicated a success rate approaching 90% in both complete and incomplete amputations. Although some controversy exists, it is generally agreed that a replantation effort is worthwhile when there has been multiple finger amputation or thumb amputation.[8,11,15]

GENERAL CONSIDERATIONS FOR DIGITAL SALVAGE

In the midst of the sometimes unbridled enthusiasm for the heroics of digital salvage after severe multiple tissue injury, devascularization, or amputation, the hand surgeon must weigh the realistic potential for functional recovery before proceeding with an effort at finger preservation. Although the only absolute indication for primary amputation is an irreversible loss of blood supply to a digit, other important considerations include the nature of the injury, taking into account the tissues involved and the severity of damage, the digit involved, the functional prognosis, injury to other digits, and patient factors, including age, occupation, and sex. The minimal requirements for digital function include length sufficient to participate in pinch and grasp, the preservation of sensibility (with the radial side of the digits usually more important than the ulnar side), and satisfactory motion at either the metacarpophalangeal (MCP) joint or the proximal interphalangeal (PIP) joint. It is also important that the retained digit be minimally painful, or it will not participate in hand function.[16] Hand surgeons have long recognized the difficulty in restoring satisfactory digital function after severe phalangeal fractures, interruption of one or both flexor tendons, substantial extensor tendon injury, severance of one or both digital nerves, crushing, or severe avulsion of skin and soft tissue. Combinations of these injuries have been even more prejudicial to the final digital performance. This realization has resulted in valuable advice from experienced hand surgeons when writing about the management of digital injuries. Some examples of these admonitions are the following:

If too much is damaged to be worth reconstructing or the circumstances are such that expense and time of reconstruction would be impossible, amputation is a quick solution. This is preferable to long treatment . . . and having a stiff finger as the result *(Bunnell*[1]*)*.

Reparative surgery is wasteful and bad treatment without reasonable prospect of a worthwhile result *(Rank and Wakefield*[12]*)*.

Amputation should be considered whenever too much is wrong with important factors being: 1) Amount of bone and soft tissue loss, 2) amount of circulation of the part, 3) damage to the flexor and extensor tendons at the same level, 4) irreparable nerve damage, and 5) excessive crush of all tissues *(Howard*[7]*)*.

When three or more of the five tissue areas (skin, tendon, nerve, bone and joint) require special procedures . . . , amputation should be strongly considered *(Milford*[10]*)*.

[I]t must be made clear that if he elects to keep the finger he will be retaining a stiff and useless digit which might be a liability to him in his occupation *(Flatt*[4]*)*.

Not only is this advice still applicable when weighing the decision as to whether a digit should be salvaged, but also it should strongly enter into the microvascular surgeon's decision to attempt revascularization. Certainly the restoration of digital function following the severance of all or almost all major digital tissues in these injuries should be expected to have no better functional prognosis than the same multiple tissue injuries when vascularity is not a problem.

DIGITAL FUNCTION AFTER REPLANTATION

Long-term studies of digital function after replantation are now beginning to surface in the literature, and the merit of digital replantation particularly with single finger involvement will await the accumulated evidence of these studies. Gelberman and associates[5] reported that two-point discrimination was not as good in replanted digits as in digits with isolated nerve injuries. Matsuda, Shibahara, and Kato[9] reported 60% recovery of effective

SECTION 8 MICROVASCULAR PROBLEMS

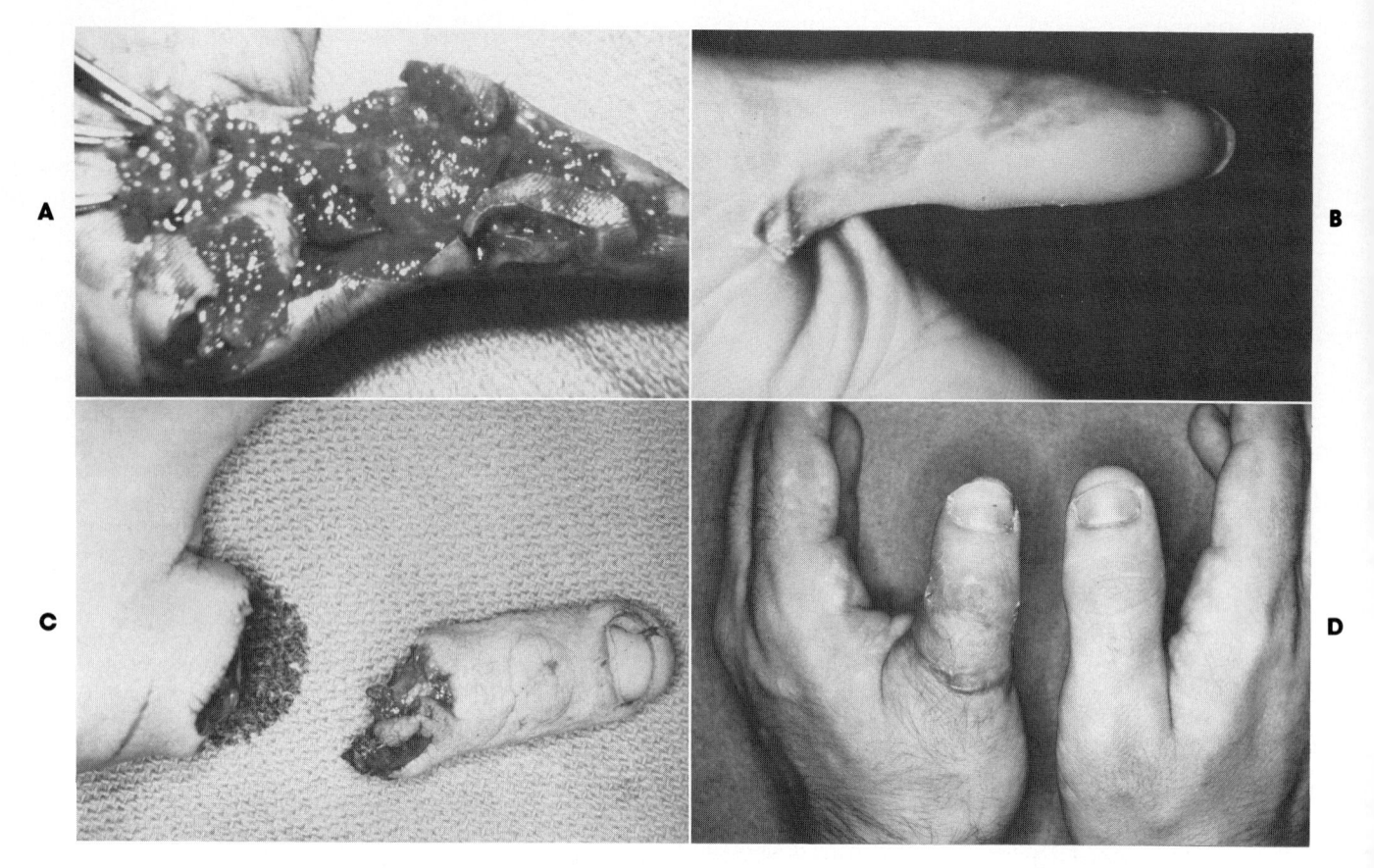

FIG. 28-1. Importance of thumb salvage can be seen in these two cases. **A,** A 24-year-old man (C.J.) with mutilation of volar aspect of thumb, including destruction of both MCP and IP joints and ulnar neurovascular structures: salvage was achieved by primary arthrodesis of both joints and coverage by means of local flap suture and split-thickness skin grafting. **B,** Appearance of thumb at 1 year with satisfactory sensation maintained on critical ulnar side of distal aspect of thumb and good function despite MCP and IP joint fusion. **C,** Amputation of thumb through midproximal phalanx. **D,** Satisfactory return of thumb function and sensibility 6 months after replantation.

pinch, grasp, and sensation, whereas Schlenker, Kleinert, and Tsai[13] reported that more than two thirds of 64 patients with thumb amputations returned to work when evaluated 2½ years after injury. Ch'en, Yun'Quing, and Zhong'Jia[3] have evaluated their results with respect to working ability, range of motion, sensation, and muscle power and found them to be disappointing.

THUMB SALVAGE

Bunnell[1] stated that "The thumb is so important that whatever the injury, we should salvage every portion rather than amputate." There is no question that this advice plus the well-known importance of the thumb to hand function has led to ultraconservatism with regard to the thumb. It is important to salvage all thumb length compatible with satisfactory function. The minimal requirements for thumb function include sufficient length to oppose other digits, adequate sensibility, minimal pain, and correct positioning with motion maintained at least at the basilar level. There is also universal agreement among replantation surgeons that thumb salvage has been consistently rewarding with excellent functional restoration usually achieved even if substantial MCP and interphalangeal (IP) motion is lost (Fig. 28-1).

MULTIPLE DIGIT INJURIES

Other areas of special consideration include multiple digit injuries when functional loss would be substantial, although this situation does not necessarily give one license to replant or salvage digits whose damage has been so great that they will remain painful, insensate, or of no functional value (Fig. 28-2). Temporary salvage may be indicated if parts of a digit may be useful in reconstructing other digits. This principle has been advocated by Chase,[2] who demonstrated the excellent reconstructive potential of tissues from otherwise nonfunc-

CHAPTER 28 A RATIONALE FOR DIGITAL SALVAGE

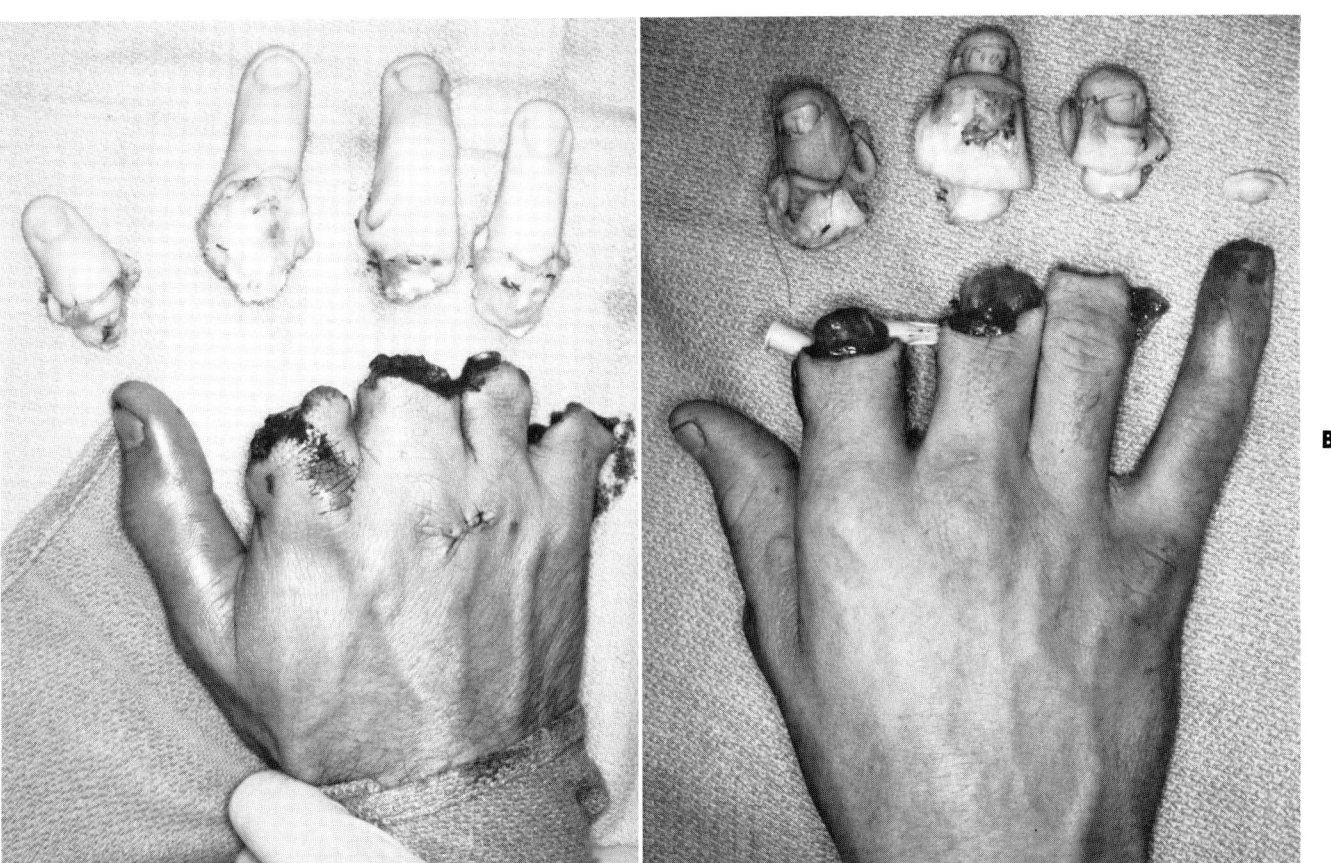

FIG. 28-2. Examples of multiple digit loss in young patients. Under appropriate circumstances efforts of replantation are indicated. **A,** Loss of all four fingers through proximal phalanges. **B,** Loss of index and long fingers through proximal phalanges, ring finger through middle phalanx, and tip of small finger.

SECTION 8 MICROVASCULAR PROBLEMS

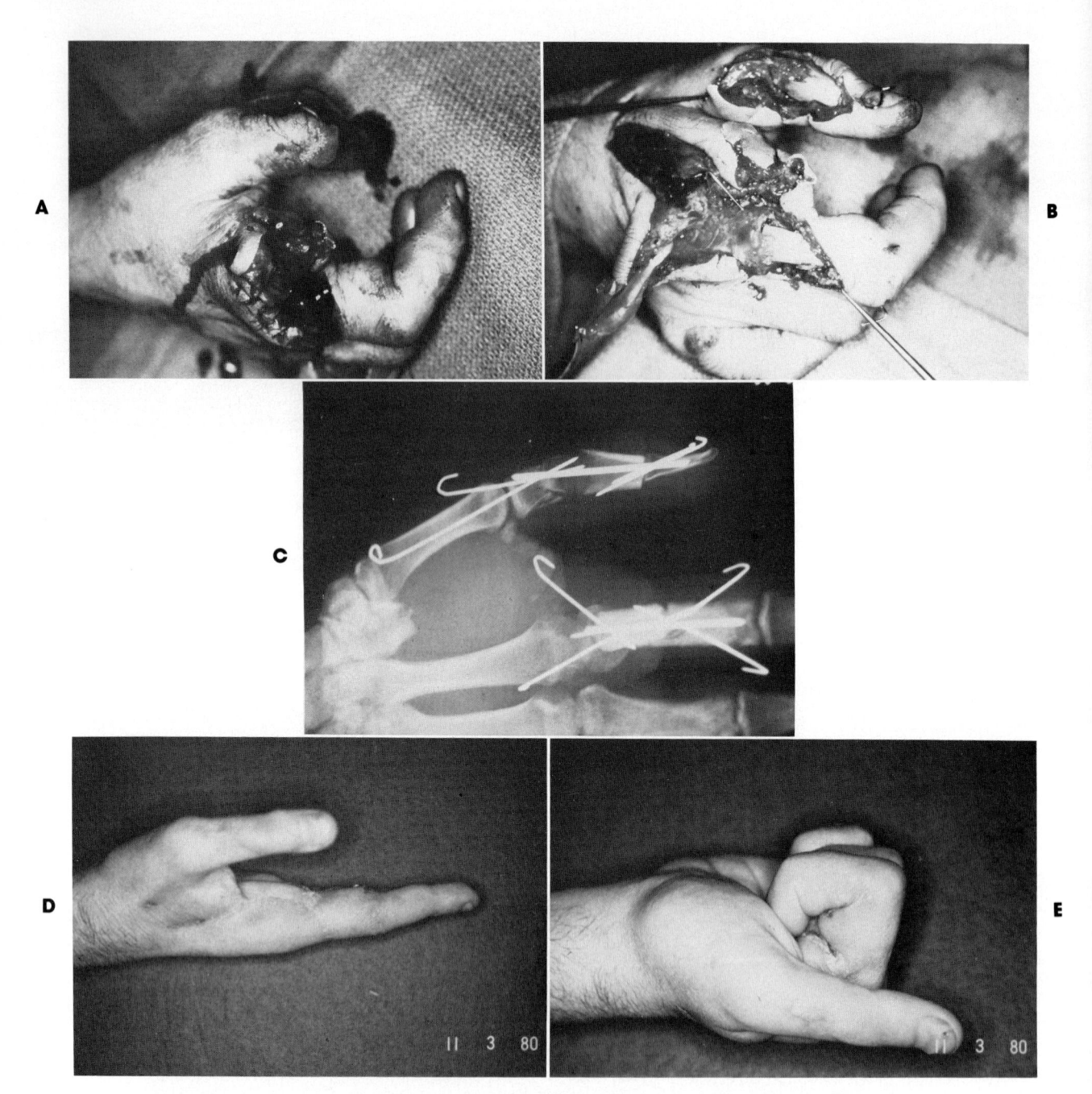

FIG. 28-3. Use of tissues from amputated digit to reconstruct adjacent digits is illustrated by this 24-year-old man, who suffered severe crushing injury involving thumb and index and long fingers, with index finger nonviable and unsalvageable. **A,** Appearance of hand at time of injury, indicating unsalvageable situation in index finger. There was comminution of almost entire proximal phalanges of thumb and long fingers, although those digits were viable. **B,** After excision of comminuted fragments of proximal phalanges of thumb and long finger and ray amputation of index finger, cylindric portions of second metacarpal were interposed between proximal and distal ends of proximal phalanges. In addition, extensor communis tendon from index finger was used to replace badly destroyed extensor to long finger. **C,** X-ray appearance of thumb and long finger following primary grafting from amputated index finger. Primary arthrodesis of IP joint of thumb was carried out. **D,** Following bony healing and extensor lysis, this patient demonstrated full digital extension. **E,** Full long finger flexion was achieved and satisfactory thumb function maintained at carpometacarpal (CMC) and MCP joints.

tional digits when skillfully used by imaginative surgeons (Fig. 28-3).

DIGITAL SCORING SYSTEM

We have employed on occasion a digital scoring system in which one assesses the degree of damage to each of six major digital tissues and provides a numeric rating for each tissue, which is then summated to provide an indicator of the degree of damage and functional potential of that digit. The specific scoring system used is listed below for each tissue:

Skin and subcutaneous tissue
No involvement	0
Simple laceration	1
Compound laceration or crush	2
Extensive involvement (requiring graft or flap)	3

Bone (stability)
No involvement	0
Simple undisplaced fracture	1
Displaced fracture without comminution	2
Displaced fracture with comminution	3

Joint (motion)
No involvement	0
Mild crush or adjacent undisplaced fracture	1
Moderate crush or adjacent displaced fracture	2
Severe crush or articular fracture	3

Tendon (motion)
No involvement	0
One tendon repairable	1
Two tendons, one or both repairable	2
Two tendons irreparable	3

Nerve (sensation)
No involvement	0
One nerve repairable	1
Both nerves repairable	2
One or both nerves irreparable	3

Vessel (circulation)
No involvement	0
Single artery	1
Both arteries, one or both repairable	2
Both arteries irreparable	3

An example of scoring for a particular digital injury is the following:

Skin	Bone	Joint	Tendon	Nerve	Vessel
1	3	3	0	1	2

TOTAL: 10

Additional examples are shown in illustrations of several digital injuries (Figs. 28-4 and 28-5). Clinical experience would indicate that a digit with a score of 10 or greater should be strongly considered for amputation rather than attempted salvage.

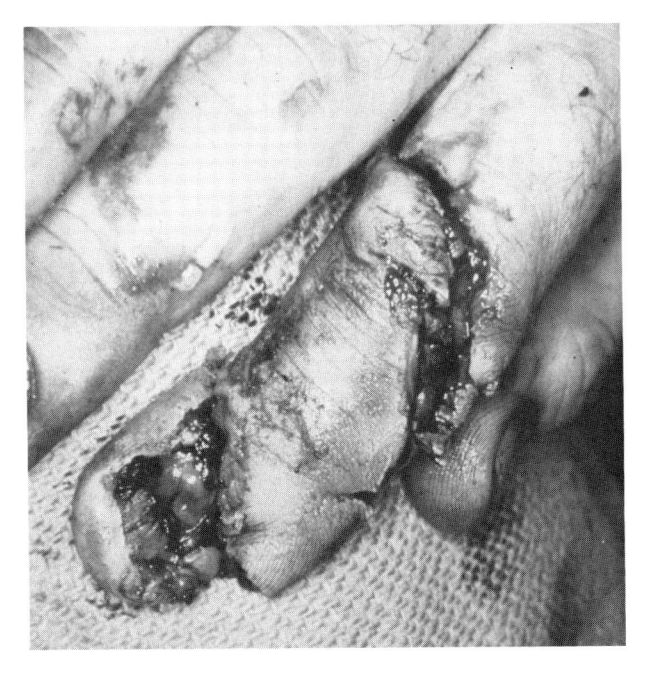

FIG. 28-4. Severe crushing of distal aspect of index finger in 22-year-old man. Numeric rating of that digit would be: vessel—3, skin—1, bone—2, joint—3, nerve—3, tendon—2; TOTAL—14. Although viable, this digit's prospects for useful function were extremely poor, and amputation was carried out.

SECTION 8 MICROVASCULAR PROBLEMS

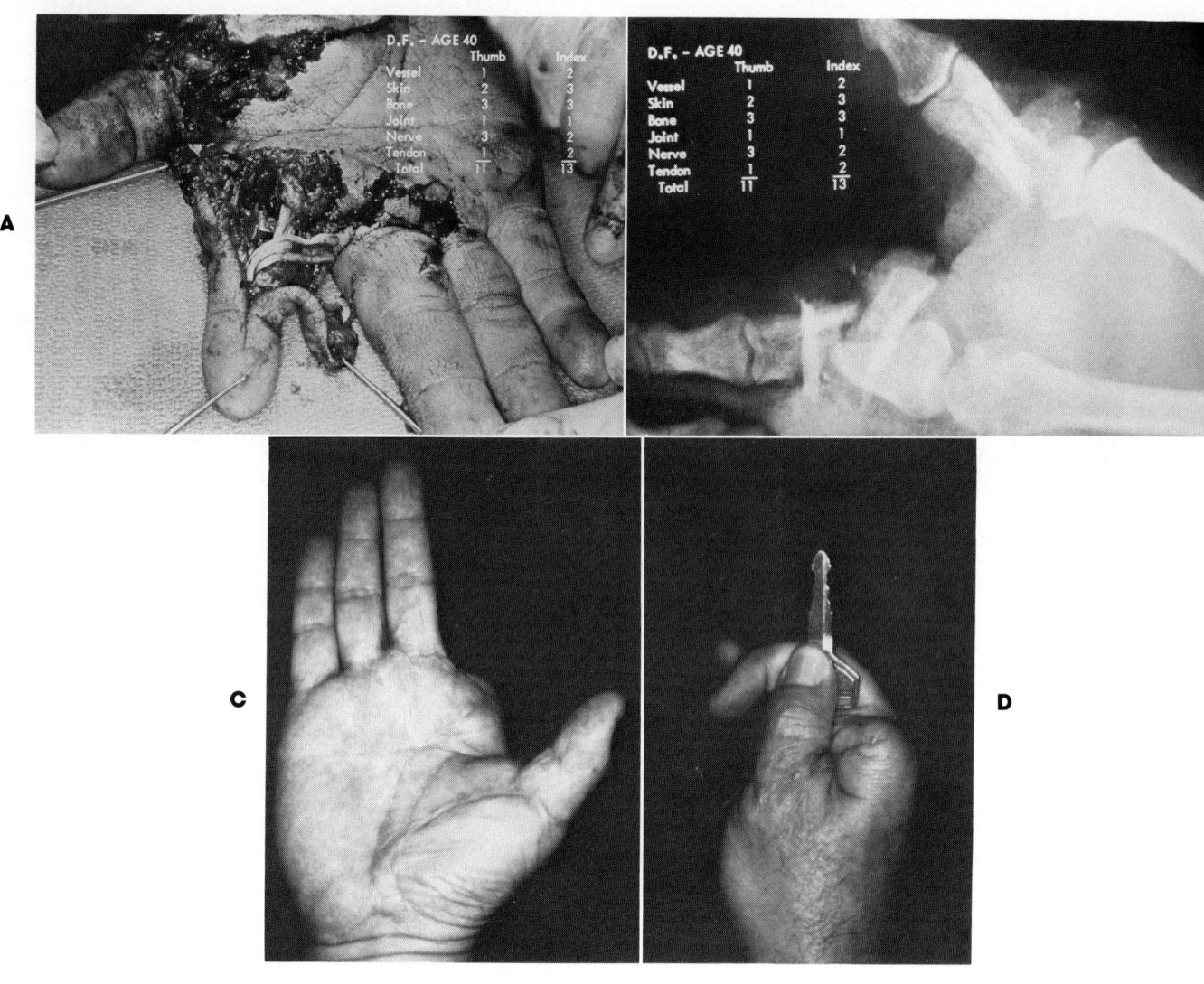

FIG. 28-5. Example of numeric rating as applied to badly damaged thumb and index finger of this 40-year-old man. Again, use of tissue parts from amputated digit is illustrated. **A,** Appearance of thumb and index finger after crushing by industrial machine. Severe involvement of almost all tissues resulted in score of 13 for index finger, and amputation was elected. Despite significant tissue destruction of thumb (score of 11), it was salvaged, and transfer of profundus tendon of index finger to flexor pollicis longus and radial digital nerve from index finger to ulnar digital nerve of thumb were of great value in functional restoration of this digit. **B,** X-ray appearance at time of initial injury, again with scoring system depicted. **C,** Appearance of patient's hand at 15 months after additional web space–deepening procedure, **D,** Maintenance of excellent thumb function at 15 months.

SINGLE DIGIT REPLANTATION

The rationale for single digit replantation has perhaps been the most severely questioned, although O'Brien[11] has indicated that any digit not severely crushed should be replanted in a child because of superior results following tendon and nerve repair in that age group. With that exception, single digit replantation is almost never indicated, although certain functional requirements should be kept in mind by the surgeon (Fig. 28-6). The radial aspects of the index and long fingers provide precision handling, and their sensory preservation is a paramount consideration. It is well known that the interruption of a single radial digital nerve to the index finger without other significant tissue damage may result in permanent disuse of that finger for fine pinch function regardless of the range of motion that is preserved in that digit (Fig. 28-7).[13] In an excellent essay entitled "Why I Hate the Index Finger," William White[18] documents the absurdity of overzealous attempts to salvage or restore that digit when it is so quickly bypassed after

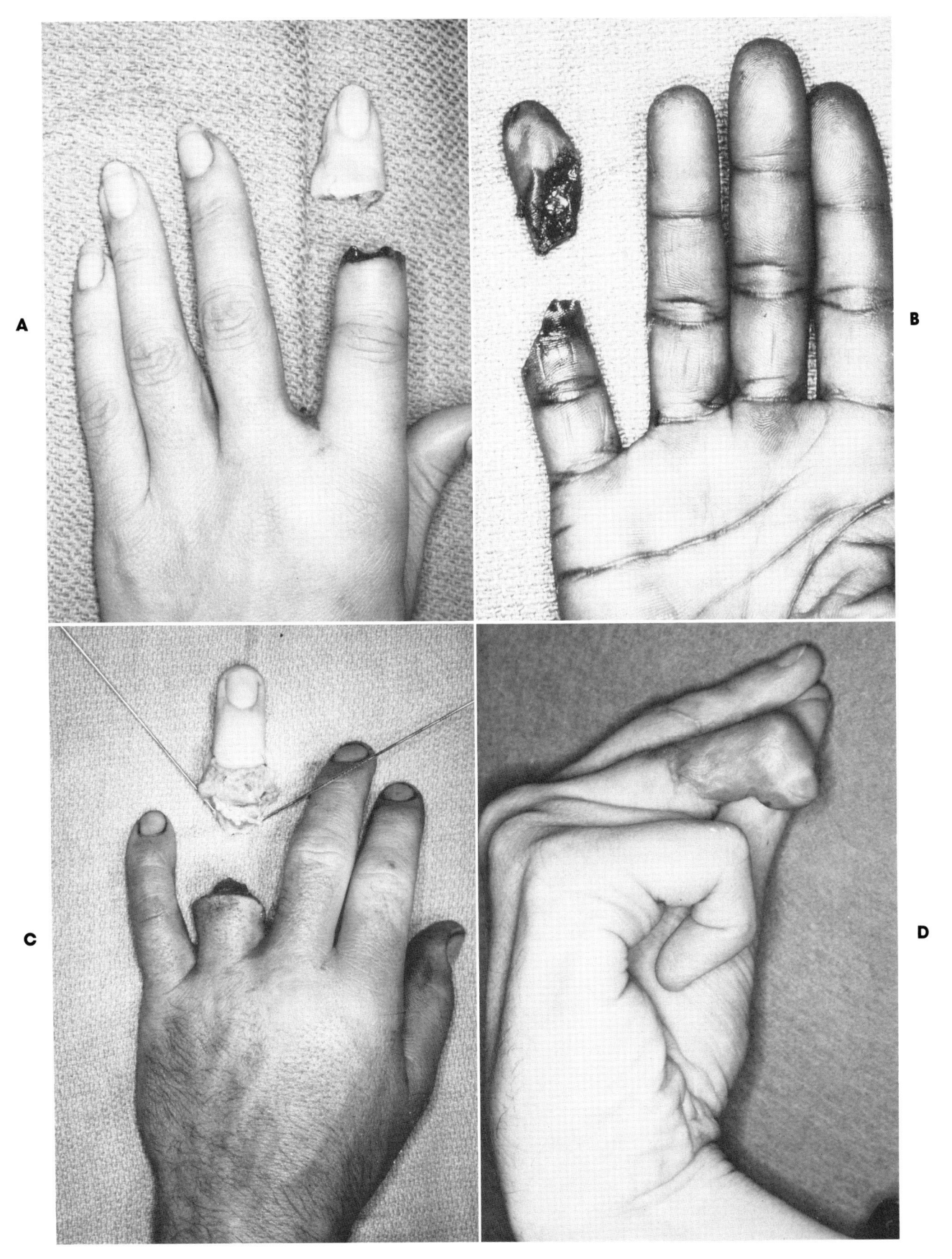

FIG. 28-6. Poor candidates for digital replantation. **A,** Amputation of index finger at level of distal interphalangeal joint. **B,** Amputation of small finger through middle phalanx. **C,** Isolated amputation of ring finger through proximal phalanx. **D,** Atrophic, insensate, unused distal aspect of long finger 6 months after replantation.

SECTION 8 MICROVASCULAR PROBLEMS

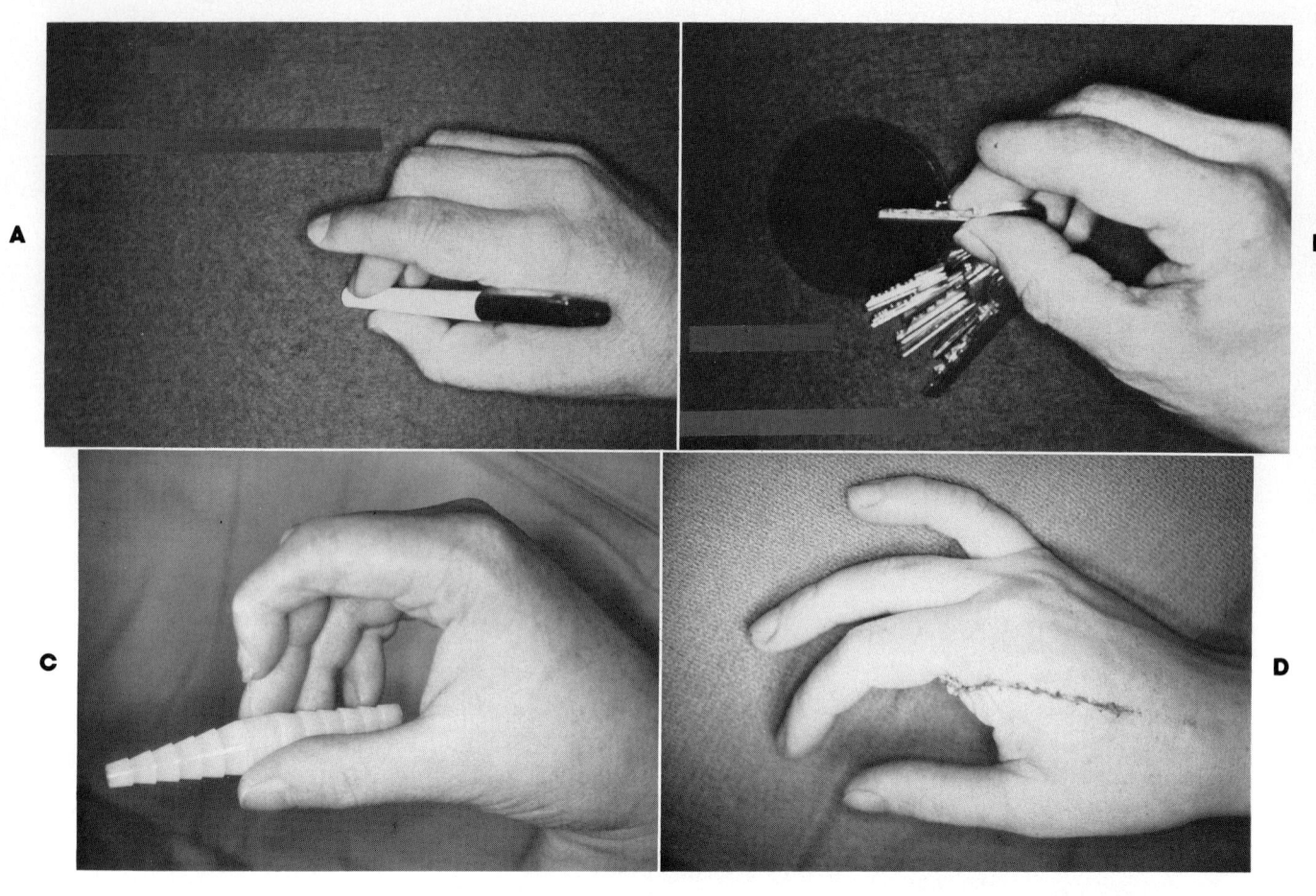

FIG. 28-7. Examples of disuse of index finger after injury. **A,** A 32-year-old woman who totally bypasses finger for fine pinch after severance and repair of radiodigital nerve index finger with adequate sensory return. **B,** Avoidance of sensitive stump of index finger following distal amputation. **C,** Functional avoidance of index following distal crush injury with partial sensory loss and joint contracture. **D,** Improved hand function following ray amputation of index finger.

injury and when hand function is so excellent after its deletion. The most ulnar digits consisting of the ring and small fingers constitute the basic unit of power grasp, and their sensory needs are considerably less. It is, however, necessary to preserve strong flexion at least at the MCP joint level with appropriate positioning of the distal joints in those digits if they are to continue to function in this capacity.

PATIENT CONSIDERATIONS

Before subjecting the patient to an attempt at digital preservation, the surgeon should recognize and relate to the patient the following considerations:
1. The initial surgical procedure may be quite long and involved.
2. Additional procedures may be necessary in the immediate postoperative period (e.g., reexploration, additional debridement, and skin grafts).
3. Expensive medications will be administered throughout the hospital course.
4. The patient may be hospitalized for a protracted period.
5. There will be an obligatory period of therapy.
6. Additional reconstructive procedures may be necessary (e.g., secondary nerve repair or grafting, tendon grafting or lysis, and bone grafting).
7. Most important, there will be a protracted time loss from work.

The total cost to the patient of such a salvage effort, both in terms of medical costs and income lost from the inability to work, may be staggering, particularly when compared with those same costs following primary digital amputation (Fig. 28-8). Failure to consider the economic impact of a digital injury on a patient's life and to weight it heavily in the decision-making process is inexcusable. It is not sufficient for the surgeon to attempt an

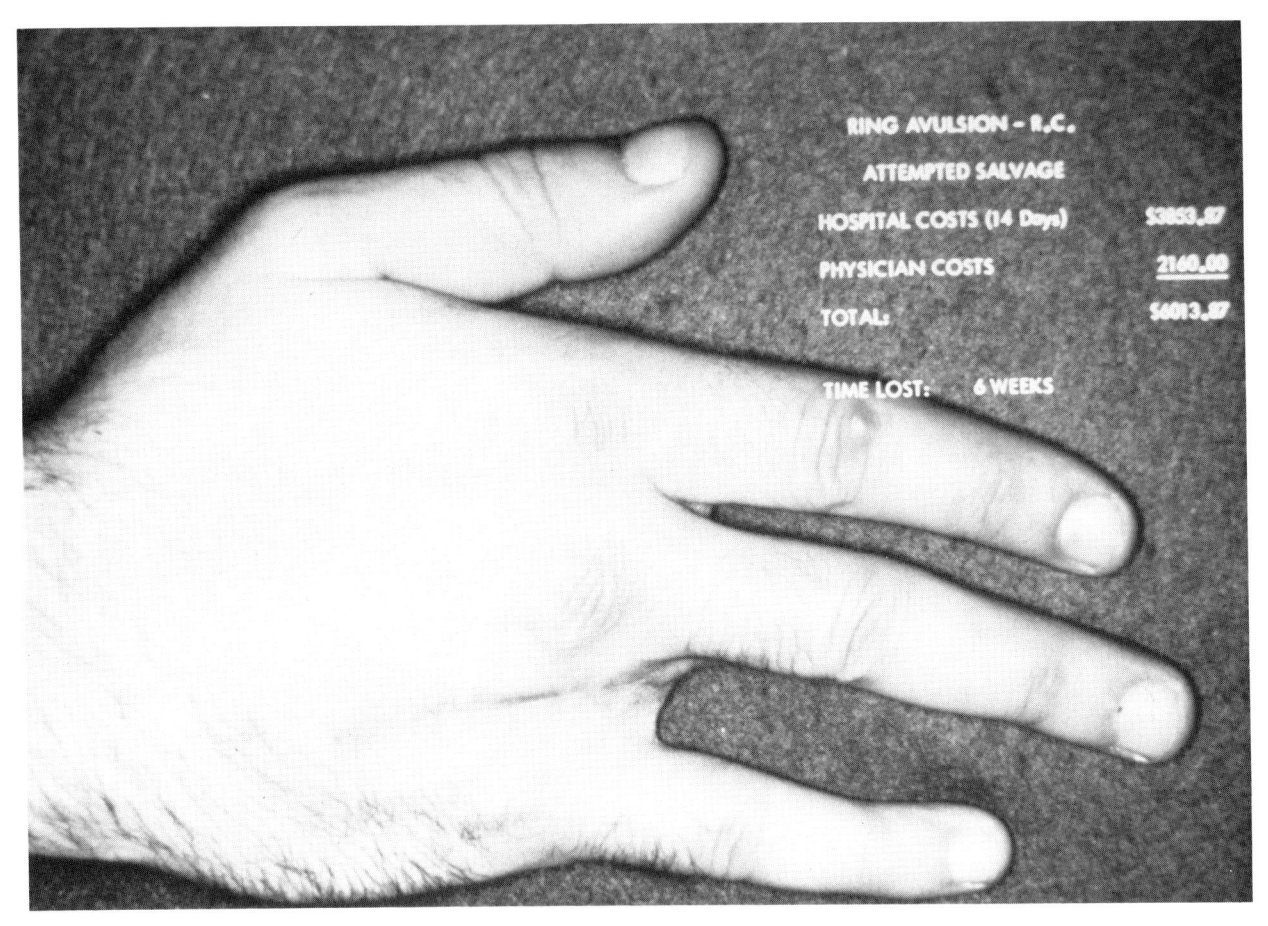

FIG. 28-8. Economic impact of attempted (but failed) effort at digital salvage following ring finger avulsion. In this case, hospital cost for 14 days, during which time vascularity of digit was precarious, was $3853.87. Physician costs, including initial revascularization effort and subsequent amputation, were $2160.00. Total cost to this patient was $6013.87, and time lost from work was 6 weeks.

ill-fated exercise in digital salvage based solely on the uninformed request of the patient. It should be recognized that the "desires of the patient" depend on the "advice of the surgeon." It is the absolute obligation of the surgeon to thoroughly inform the patient not only with regard to the intricacies of the surgery but more important as to the realistic likelihood of a return to function of the injured part. When appropriately informed, few patients will opt for a salvage procedure that will preserve a stiff, insensate, painful, or cosmetically unattractive digit.

SUMMARY

This chapter has attempted to dampen the current wave of enthusiasm for digital salvage brought on by technologic advances in microvascular restoration. The current state of the art does not yet permit any alteration of the previous concerns for the ultimate digital performance after severe multiple tissue digital injuries or amputation. The potential performance of a salvaged digit and moreover the performance of the hand of which that digit is a member must be the abiding concerns of the surgeon and must be accurately portrayed to the patient. Failure to do so is a breach of medical ethics and honesty. In our zeal to salvage the badly injured digit we should not forget the advice of Howard[7] in 1960 when he said "a good stump is a joy."

REFERENCES

1. Bunnell, S.: Surgery of the hand, ed. 1, Philadelphia, 1944, J.B. Lippincott Co.
2. Chase, R.A.: The damaged index digit: a source of components to restore the crippled hand, J. Bone Joint Surg. **50A:**1152, 1968.
3. Ch'en, C.W., Yun'Quing, Q., and Zhong'Jia, Y.: Extremity replantation, World J. Surg. **2:**513, 1978.

4. Flatt, A.E.: The care of minor hand injuries, ed. 2, St. Louis, 1963, The C.V. Mosby Co.
5. Gelberman, R.H., et al.: Digital sensibility following replantation, J. Hand Surg. 3:313, 1978.
6. Hamilton, R.B., et al.: Replantation and revascularization of digits, Surg. Gynecol. Obstet. 151:508, 1980.
7. Howard, L.D., Jr.: Fractures of the small bones of the hand, San Francisco, 1960, L.D. Howard, Jr.
8. Kleinert, H.E., Jablon, M., and Tsai, T.: An overview of replantation and results of 347 replants in 245 patients, J. Trauma 20:390, 1980.
9. Matsuda, M., Shibahara, H., and Kato, N.: Long-term results of replantation of 10 upper extremities, World J. Surg. 2:603, 1978.
10. Milford, L.: The hand, St. Louis, 1971, The C.V. Mosby Co.
11. O'Brien, B.M.: Microvascular reconstructive surgery, New York, 1977, Churchill Livingstone, Inc.
12. Rank, B.K., and Wakefield, A.R.: Surgery or repair as applied to hand injuries, ed. 1, Edinburgh, 1953, Churchill Livingstone.
13. Schlenker, J.P., Kleinert, H.E., and Tsai, T.: Methods and results of replantation following traumatic amputation of the thumb in 64 patients, J. Hand Surg. 5:63, 1980.
14. Shanghai Sixth People's Hospital, Research Laboratory for Replantation of Severed Limbs: Replantation of severed fingers: clinical experiences in 217 cases involving 373 severed fingers, Chin. Med. J. 1:184, 1975.
15. Tamai, S.: Digit replantation: analysis of 163 replantations in an 11 year period, Clin. Plast. Surg. 5:195, 1978.
16. Urbaniak, J.R.: Replantation of amputated parts—technique, results and indications. In Urbaniak, J.R., and Bright, D.S., editors: American Academy of Orthopaedic Surgeons: Symposium on Microsurgery, St. Louis, 1979, The C.V. Mosby Co.
17. Weiland, A.J., et al.: Replantation of digits and hands: analysis of surgical techniques and functional results in 71 patients with 86 replantations, J. Hand Surg. 2:1, 1977.
18. White, W.L.: Why I hate the index finger, Orthop. Rev. 9:23, 1980.

Chapter 29 Ulnar artery thrombosis: a rationale for management

James R. Urbaniak

L. Andrew Koman

Recent advances in microsurgical technique that have improved the technical ability to vein graft arterial defects reliably have added an additional modality to the management of thrombosis of the ulnar artery at the wrist. The restoration of arterial flow has obvious implications, but experienced microsurgical centers report failure rates approaching 50% with resection and vein grafting.[8,11,12] Alternative management techniques include surgical excision of the involved arterial segment and ligation,* local and regional sympathectomy,[4,5,12,13] and pharmacologic and psychologic palliation.[12] The purpose of this chapter is to present a patient-oriented treatment approach to this complex problem.

HISTORY

The first description of thrombosis of the ulnar artery at the wrist was by von Rosen[18] in 1934. In 1929 Allen[1] described a reliable bedside technique for the determination of patency of the ulnar and radial arteries at the wrist, providing the necessary methodology to confirm the clinical diagnosis. From 1937 until 1965 treatment was based on Leriche, Fontaine, and Dupertuis's principle[13] of surgical excision of the involved arterial segment and ligation of the artery. Resection of the involved segment and end-to-end repair was reported in 1964 by Trevaskis and associates,[17] and Kleinert and Volianitis[11] reported the first documented restoration of flow in 1965. Using microvascular technique, they reestablished ulnar artery flow by excision and direct repair or multiple arteriotomies and thrombectomies. The designation *hypothenar hammer syndrome* was applied to ulnar artery thrombosis in 1970 by Conn, Berigan, and Bell,[4] who proposed sympathectomy as the treatment of choice.

CLINICAL SYNDROME

Thrombosis of the ulnar artery at the wrist is typically unilateral and occurs in a man in the fifth decade of life with an occupational predisposition to trauma.[8,12,14] The dominant hand is usually involved, with nondominant-hand involvement generally explained on the basis of trauma or definable repetitive activity.[14] A history of either major trauma or repetitive minor trauma is usually elicitable.[12,14] In our series of 28 symptomatic and arteriogram-proven thrombosed ulnar arteries over 85% were men with dominant-hand involvement. Thirteen of 24 routinely used their hands as hammers or used pneumatic tools. The four patients who were younger than 35 years old at the onset of symptoms had significant trauma to the ulnar side of the hand or documented repetitive trauma. Our youngest patient was a baseball catcher at the time of diagnosis.

SYMPTOMS

All patients had pain, 80% had cold intolerance, and 80% had ulnar nerve distribution numbness or paresthesia (Fig. 29-1).

Pain

Prior to management all patients in our series complained of pain when using their hand or on direct contact with the hypothenar area. Pain generally was relieved by rest or splinting, increased with activity, and was exacerbated by cold weather. Pain was localized usually to the ulnar side of the hand and ulnar three

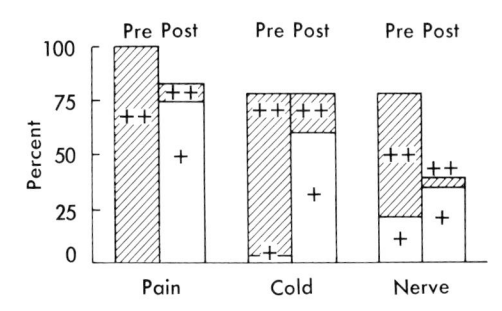

FIG. 29-1. Premanagement and postmanagement symptoms of 28 arteriogram-proven thrombosed ulnar arteries.

---
*References 6, 8, 10, 12, 13, 17, and 19.

digits but could involve the entire hand. Typical complaints were of "pain," further described as "tiredness," "cramping," or "discomfort." Night and rest pain was unusual and occurred only in patients with ulceration.

Cold intolerance

Eighty percent of our patients complained of significant discomfort secondary to exposure to a cold environment or on holding cold objects. This pain was different subjectively from the general pain just described.

Patients with cold intolerance were stress tested, comparing the digital temperature response and plethysmographic response of normal and involved digits while changing ambient temperature. Cold-intolerant digits showed a characteristic temperature response to cooling and rewarming over a 40-minute period (Fig. 29-2). When ambient temperature dropped below 10° C, there was a rapid drop in the temperature of symptomatic digits with temperatures approaching ambient temperature and the absence of periodic increases in temperature over the 20-minute cooling phase. "Normal" digital temperature remained above 24° C and showed characteristic transient elevations of temperature. Onset of pain occurred after 6 to 11 minutes of exposure in symptomatic patients. Symptomatic digits did not have the reactive hyperemia of the normal digits, and in most cases pulp temperatures did not equal or exceed ambient temperatures until 15 to 20 minutes into the rewarming phase. Three patients with arteriogram-proven ulnar artery thrombosis but without cold-related pain had essentially normal responses to isolated extremity temperature testing (Fig. 29-3).

Simultaneous digital plethysmography confirmed that pulsatile flow diminished when pulp temperature dropped. Fig. 29-4 represents the simultaneous plethysmography and temperature readings of a patient with arteriogram-proven ulnar artery thrombosis and cold intolerance. There was pain in the right little and ring fingers 10 minutes after exposure to ambient temperatures of less than 10° C. There was no discomfort on the left.

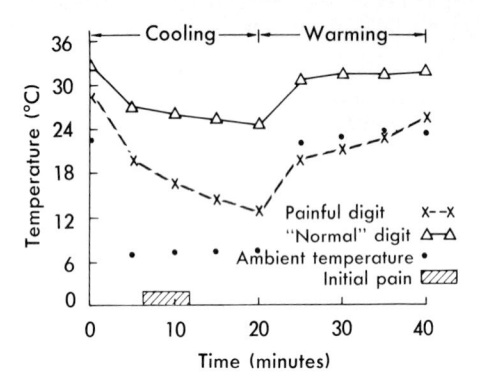

FIG. 29-2. Cold stress testing of isolated upper extremities of six patients with unilateral ulnar artery thrombosis: average pulp temperature from most painful digit of involved extremity is compared with contralateral digit over 40-minute period. There is significant statistical difference ($p < 0.0001$) in temperature response of painful digits and nonpainful digits during changing ambient temperature.

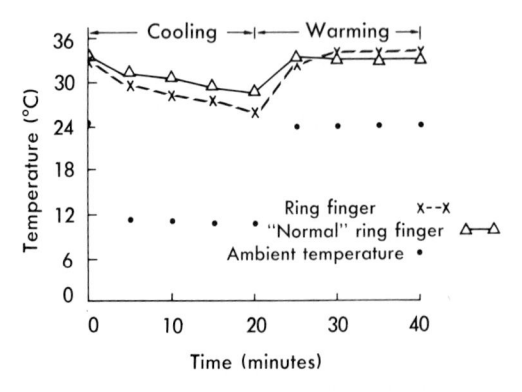

FIG. 29-3. Cold stress testing of isolated upper extremities of three patients with unilateral arteriogram-proven ulnar artery thrombosis but without symptoms of cold intolerance. Average pulp temperature of ring finger of hand with ulnar artery thrombosis is compared with digital temperature of "normal" ring finger of opposite hand while ambient temperature is decreased and increased over 40-minute period. There is no statistically significant difference in response.

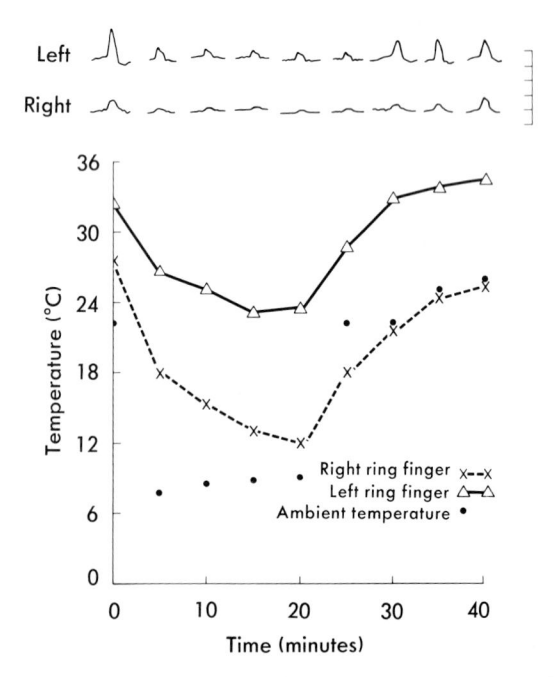

FIG. 29-4. Simultaneous digital plethysmography (above) and temperature monitoring (below) of patient with arteriogram-proven right ulnar artery thrombosis and cold intolerance.

In the normal patient, pulsatile flow diminishes with decreasing ambient temperature, falling to 70% to 80% of control values (Fig. 29-5). Patients with symptomatic ulnar artery thrombosis may have decreased flows to 10% of control values and do not exhibit the normal periodic flow increases seen at lower temperatures in normal fingers.

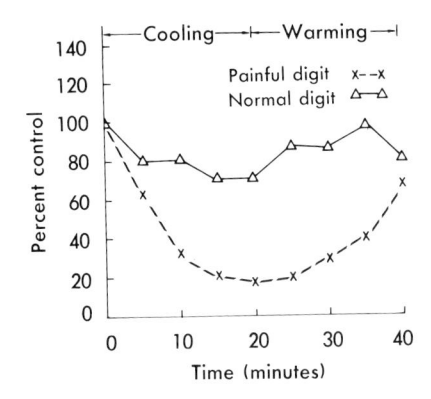

FIG. 29-5. Average percent of digital flow of six subjects with ulnar artery thrombosis as measured by digital plethysmography compared with time during 20-minute cooling period (ambient temperature 6° to 10° C) followed by rewarming period (ambient temperature 22° to 24° C). Percent flow is for individual finger compared with itself and is not reflection of absolute flow.

Numbness

Symptoms of ulnar nerve involvement occurred in over half the patients. (See Fig. 29-1.) Subjective sensibility changes ("numbness") and decreased sweating ("dryness") were the most common complaints. Triketohydrindene hydrate (Ninhydrin) testing confirmed the decreased sweating in two patients; two-point discrimination, electromyography, and conduction times were normal, although six patients with symptoms and a positive Tinel's sign responded to ulnar nerve decompression in association with other treatment.

SIGNS

Clinical signs seen in ulnar artery thrombosis are those of arterial insufficiency and nerve irritation. Inspection may reveal cyanosis or pallor, and ulceration or gangrene of the fingertips may exist. Palpable temperature differences and relative dryness in the ulnar distribution can be seen. Pressure over Guyon's canal usually is painful, and a mass may be present. A positive Tinel's sign may be elicited over the ulnar nerve. The Allen test will demonstrate diminished or absent arterial inflow through the ulnar artery (Fig. 29-6).

SPECIAL STUDIES
Electromyography/nerve conduction

Although a high percentage of patients with ulnar artery thrombosis have symptoms of ulnar nerve irritation,

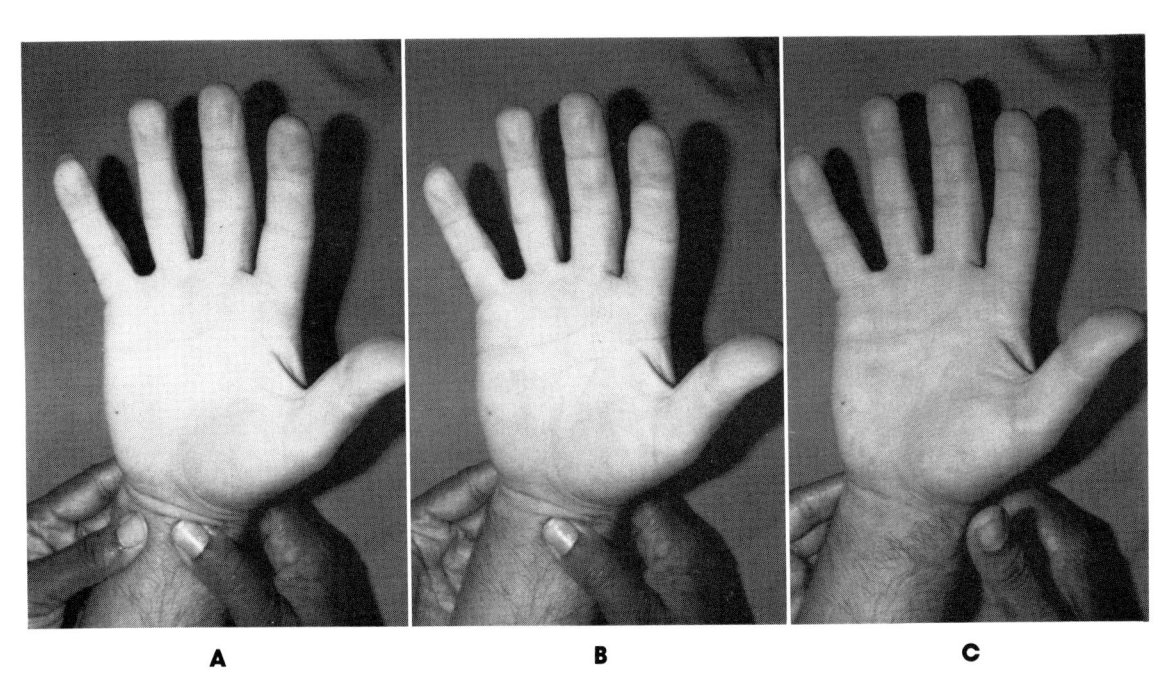

FIG. 29-6. Occlusion of radial and ulnar artery **(A)**. Positive Allen test showing absence of arterial inflow with release of ulnar artery but occlusion of radial artery **(B)**. Release of radial artery results in prompt capillary filling of the entire palm **(C)**. (From Koman, L.A., and Urbaniak, J.R.: Ulnar artery insufficiency—a guide to treatment, J. Hand Surg. **6:**16, 1981.)

SECTION 8 MICROVASCULAR PROBLEMS

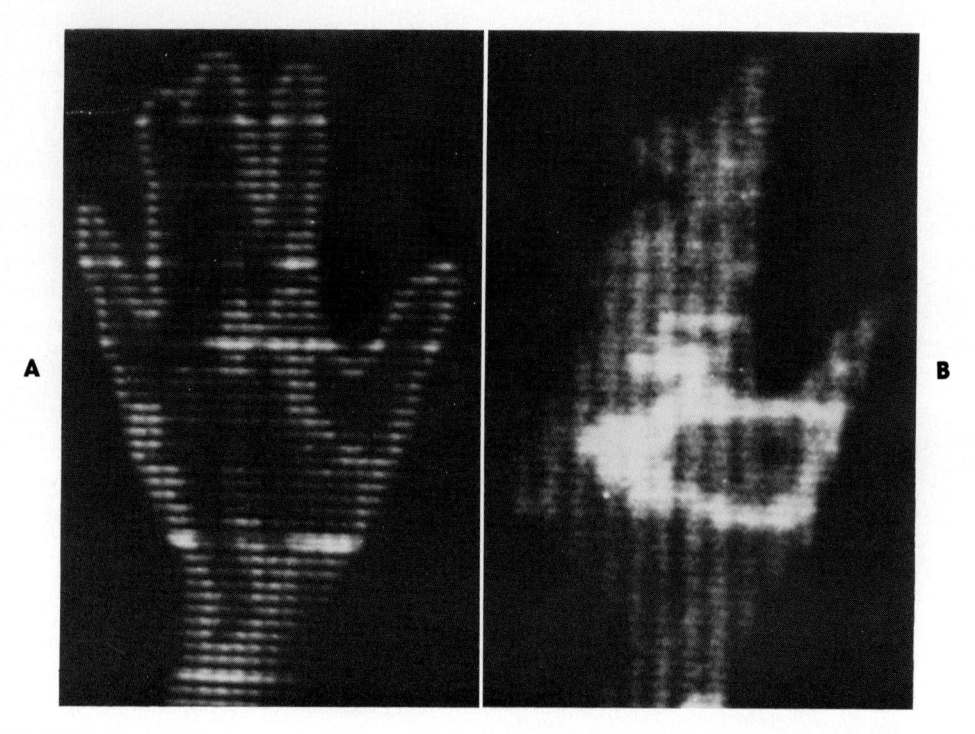

FIG. 29-7. Normal thermogram **(A)** and thermogram of hand with arteriogram-proven ulnar artery thrombosis **(B)**. (From Koman, L.A., and Urbaniak, J.R.: Thrombosis of ulnar artery at the wrist. In American Academy of Orthopaedic Surgeons: Symposium on Microsurgery: Practical Use in Orthopaedics, St. Louis, 1979, The C.V. Mosby Co.)

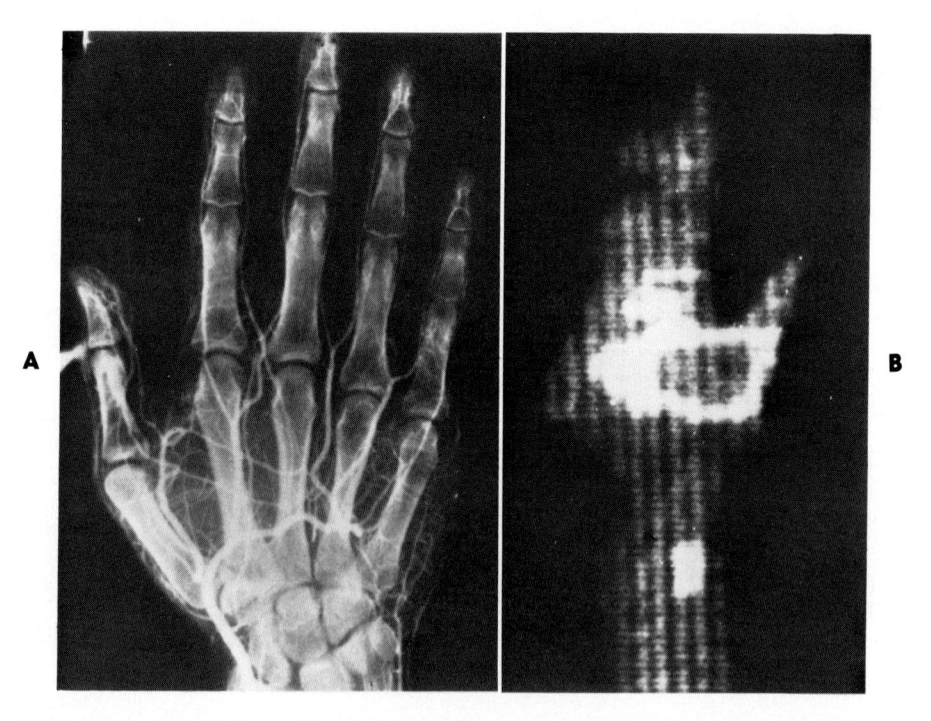

FIG. 29-8. Arteriogram **(A)** and thermogram **(B)** of hand with symptomatic ulnar artery thrombosis. (From Koman, L.A., and Urbaniak, J.R.: Thrombosis of ulnar artery at the wrist. In American Academy of Orthopaedic Surgeons: Symposium on Microsurgery: Practical Use in Orthopaedics, St. Louis, 1979, The C.V. Mosby Co.)

few will have abnormal electromyograms or conduction velocities. Tests of sensory conduction times were not done on any of our patients but potentially would be more sensitive. At exploration several patients had evidence of ulnar nerve compression and demonstrated symptom relief after surgical decompression.

Thermography/temperature probes

Differential temperature is a valuable noninvasive method to assess blood flow. Thermography and temperature probes provide similar information. The normal thermogram of the hand shows the mirror image of the uniform heat pattern of the hand (Fig. 29-7). The patient with ulnar artery thrombosis shows decreased heat over the ulnar distribution of the hand in the area of deficient arterial flow (Fig. 29-8). Multiple small temperature probes provide similar information. Both methods are most useful in assessing quantitatively the response to cold stress. Thermograms before and after immersion in ice baths provide excellent information about heat regulation and blood-flow characteristics. Stress testing of isolated upper extremities in a modified refrigeration unit with continuous monitoring of pulp pressure and plethysmographic response eliminates the problem of wet immersion and periodic measurements. (See discussion on cold intolerance.)

Digital plethysmography

The presence of pulsatile flow correlated with cold intolerance in our replanted digits.[7] We have had similar findings in patients with ulnar artery insufficiency. The absence of recordable pulsatile flow reflects inadequate collateral circulation and/or vasospasm. Without exception in our patients the absence of pulsatile flow was associated with severe symptoms. The pulse volume recordings and arteriogram in Fig. 29-9 are those of a 38-year-old male right-handed automobile mechanic. The patient used a pneumatic hammer and, when initially examined, had acute numbness, pain, and cyanosis of his right little and ring fingers. Serial plethysmography showed no recordable pulsatile flow in the ring or little fingers, after brachial block, after arteriography under brachial block and intraarterial tolazoline HCl, and after resection of the thrombosed segment. Because of the

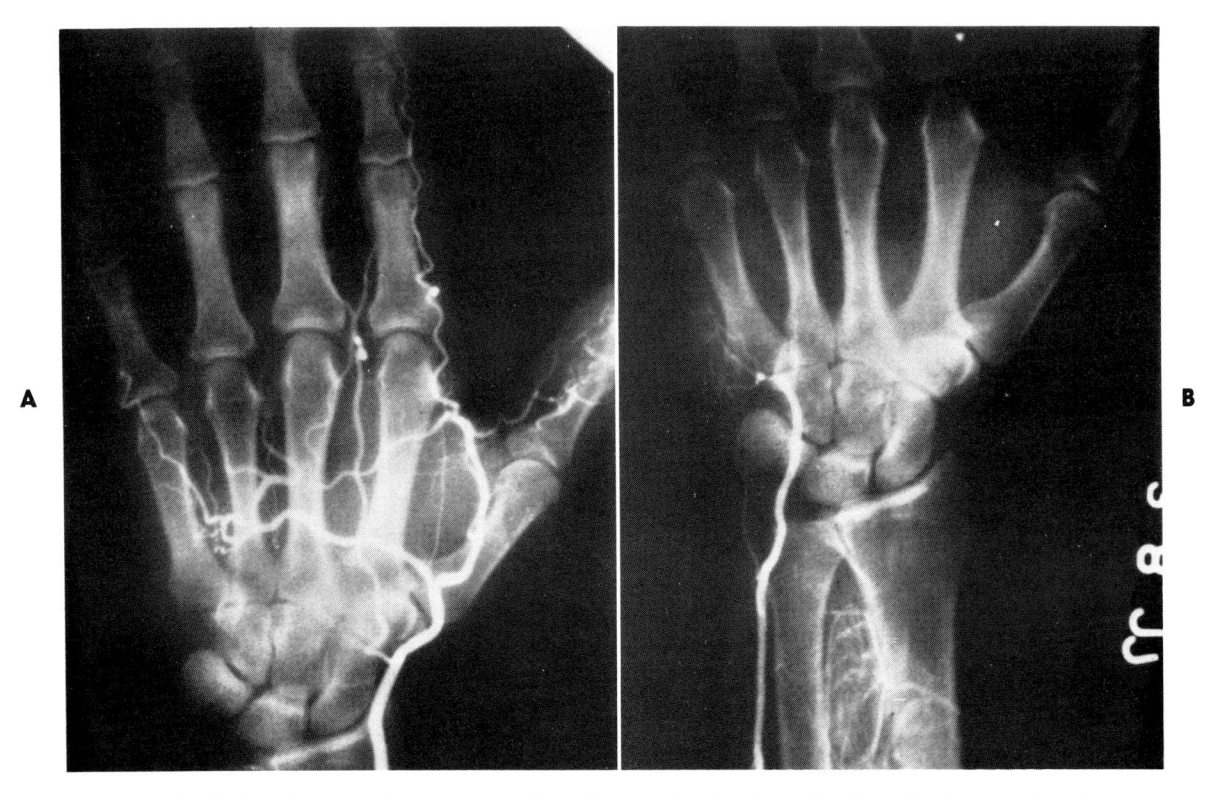

FIG. 29-9. Arteriogram of ulnar artery thrombosis. Injection into distal brachial artery showing filling of deep arch and partial filling of superficial arch from radial artery **(A)**. Selective injection of ulnar artery originating 12.5 cm above elbow **(B)** shows complete block in Guyon's canal. (From Koman, L.A., and Urbaniak, J.R. Thrombosis of ulnar artery at the wrist. In American Academy of Orthopaedic Surgeons: Symposium on Microsurgery: Practical Use in Orthopaedics, St. Louis, 1979, The C.V. Mosby Co.)

SECTION 8 MICROVASCULAR PROBLEMS

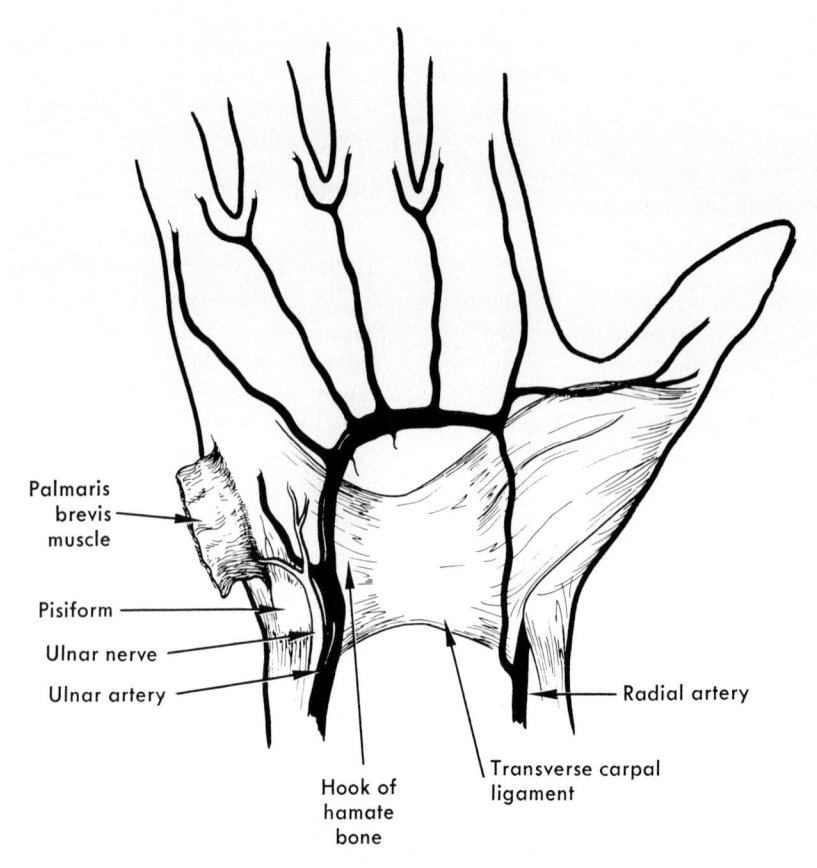

FIG. 29-10. Anatomy of Guyon's canal and superficial palmar arch. (From Koman, L.A., and Urbaniak, J.R.: Thrombosis of ulnar artery at the wrist. In American Academy of Orthopaedic Surgeons: Symposium on Microsurgery: Practical Use in Orthopaedics, St. Louis, 1979, The C.V. Mosby Co.)

persistent arterial insufficiency and lack of pulsatile flow, vein grafting was done.

Doppler mapping

Hand-held ultrasonic Doppler mapping of our patients prior to arteriography was performed. It allowed accurate mapping of arterial flow patterns in the palm and digits and correlated with arteriography.

Arteriography

Arteriography is the definitive study, permitting absolute confirmation of the clinical situation, accurate estimation of the extent of intimal damage or arteriosclerotic changes, and determination of the competence of the collateral circulation. During the arteriogram, intraarterial medications can be given, which may eliminate or postpone the necessity for further intervention.

Ideal studies are best obtained if potential spasm is eliminated by brachial or axillary block. Use of a femoral approach with selective catheterization of the brachial artery and test injections eliminates failure to detect a superficial radial or ulnar artery. (See Fig. 29-9.)

Anatomy/pathophysiology

Thrombosis of the ulnar artery usually occurs in Guyon's canal. Within the confines of "la loge de Guyon" the ulnar artery, with its paired veins, and the ulnar nerve are surrounded by the pisohamate ligament and respective carpal bones dorsoulnarly, the dorsal fascia of the palmaris brevis muscle and volar carpal ligament volarly, and the flexor retinaculum and transverse carpal ligament dorsoulnarly. In the classic description the superficial palmar arch is completed by the superficial palmar branch of the radial artery (Fig. 29-10). The superficial arch is defined as complete if there is direct anastomosis with the deep palmar arch, radial artery, or median artery. Based on studies of 650 specimens, Coleman and Anson[3] estimated that the arch was complete in 78.5% of hands and incomplete in the remaining 21.5% (Fig. 29-11). The clinical significance of an incomplete arch in the presence of acute ulnar artery thrombosis is obvious. Without adequate collateral circulation to allow pulsatile flow, symptoms and potentially nonviable digits would occur.

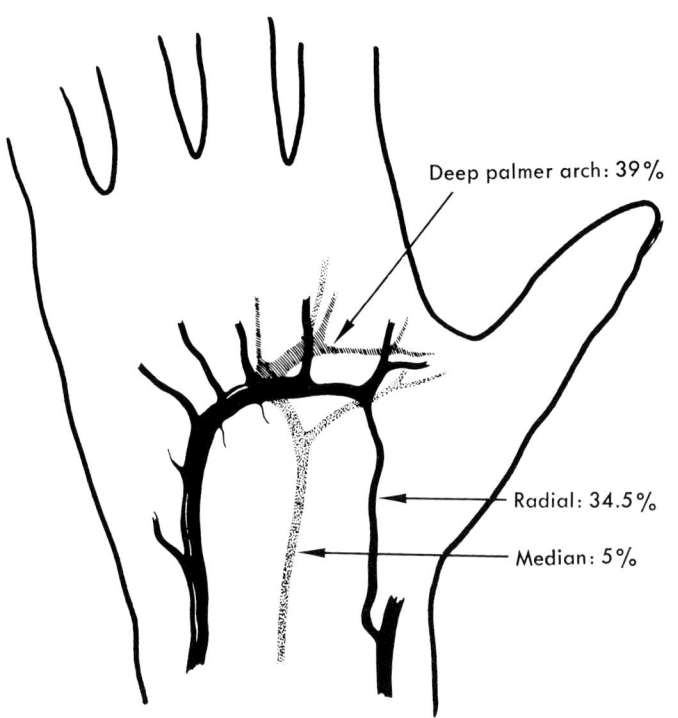

FIG. 29-11. Diagram of anatomic variations of superficial palmar arch, summarized from work of Coleman and Anson.[4] In 650 dissections, arch was found to be complete in 78.5%—39% from deep arch or princeps pollicis, 34.5% from superficial radial artery, and 5% from median artery—and incomplete in 21.5% of specimens. (From Koman, L.A., and Urbaniak, J.R.: Thrombosis of ulnar artery at the wrist. In American Academy of Orthopaedic Surgeons: Symposium on Microsurgery: Practical Use in Orthopaedics, St. Louis, 1979, The C.V. Mosby Co.)

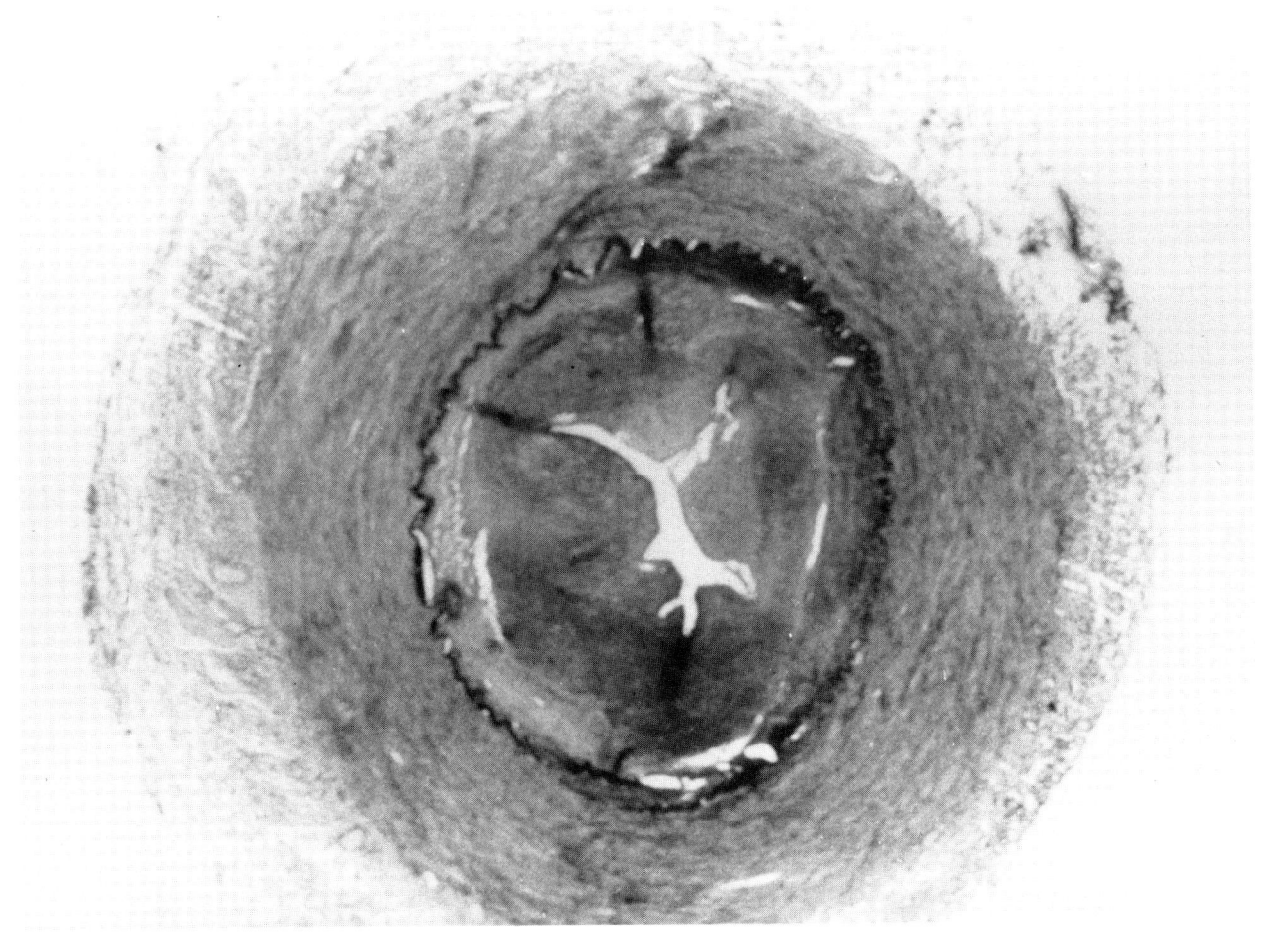

FIG. 29-12. Photomicrograph of cross-section of excised ulnar artery in patient with ulnar artery thrombosis. There is intimal hypertrophy and organized thrombus with partial recanalization. Internal elastic membrane is disrupted partially (Verhoeff's stain × 10).

The relative confinement of the ulnar artery by Guyon's canal predisposes the artery to damage secondary to blunt trauma. In spite of the protective value of the palmaris brevis muscle,[15] repeated trauma to the ulnar artery may result in intimal damage, subintimal hematoma, disruption of the internal elastic membrane, and thrombus formation (Fig. 29-12).

Differential diagnosis

In our series of patients with ulnar artery thrombosis the initial diagnosis was incorrect over 50% of the time. The differential diagnosis should include both systemic diseases and mechanical or other problems, including the following:

A. Systemic diseases
1. Arteriosclerosis
2. Thromboangiitis obliterans
3. Giant cell arteritis
4. Scleroderma
5. Raynaud's disease
6. Polycythemia

B. Mechanical and other problems
1. Thoracic outlet
2. Direct trauma
3. Embolic occlusion
4. Thrombotic occlusion
5. Median or ulnar nerve compression
6. Ergot poisoning

TREATMENT

Several modalities have been advocated for the treatment of ulnar artery thrombosis, and all provide some palliation. The ideal treatment would restore normal blood flow and eliminate predisposing or causative factors. Excision of the involved segment and vein grafting could potentially restore flow to close to normal. Unfortunately even experienced microsurgical centers have a high failure rate with thrombosis of the vein graft.[8,11,12] Since these same centers report 80% or greater patency rates in much smaller vessels, we must assume that intraoperative technique is not the limiting factor. Excision of the involved segment and end-to-end repair has an even higher failure rate, presumably secondary to the retention of damaged intima and tension at the site of repair. Furthermore surgical repair does not eliminate the reason for the initial thrombosis or the presence of erythrocytosis, which makes successful arterial reconstruction more difficult.

Our patients were treated by multiple regimens, including intraarterial reserpine or tolazoline HCl, fifteen; stellate blocks, eleven; sympathectomy, four; resection and ligation, eight; resection and vein grafting, four; and biofeedback plus additional modalities, one. A review of our results allows the following observations. All management programs decreased symptoms, and patients were able to return to work. (See Fig. 29-1.) There was no treatment, including patent vein grafting, that eliminated all symptoms. The presence or absence of pulsatile flow was the most important single factor correlating with ultimate symptoms.

The management of ulnar artery thrombosis remains a complex problem that requires individualized management. Our approach is presented in algorithmic form (Fig. 29-13).

Initial symptoms are those of arterial insufficiency or ulnar nerve irritation, and clinical suspicion of ulnar artery thrombosis can be confirmed by an Allen test. If the Allen test is negative (normal flow through the ulnar artery), then the diagnosis is in doubt, and other entities in the differential diagnosis must be investigated. If the Allen test is positive (no flow through the ulnar artery), additional confirmatory studies—thermography, temperature probes, Doppler mapping, or plethysmography—should be done. In the acute situation a stellate ganglion or brachial block should be done to diminish reflex vasospasm. The sympathetic block helps clarify the adequacy of the existing collateral circulation. If symptomatic relief is obtained, the patient may be observed. Two patients with acute ulnar artery thrombosis, later confirmed by arteriography, had potentially nonviable digits when first examined. Stellate ganglion blocks, followed by axillary blocks, were given in the emergency department, and symptoms were reduced with adequate blood flow to allow elective definitive treatment.

If the sympathetic blockade from a stellate ganglion block or an axillary block does not relieve symptoms, then arteriography should be performed. At the time of arteriography intraarterial medications may be given. Arteriography provides the definitive diagnosis and determines the extent of thrombus formation and the potential for operative intervention.

If the symptoms are decreased after the arteriogram, the patient may be observed. If after intraarterial medication there is no relief but the patient is a poor operative candidate for revascularization because of diffuse arteriosclerotic disease or inadequate distal runoff, other treatment modalities can be employed.

If symptoms persist and digital survival is questionable, then surgical intervention should take place immediately. At surgery the thrombosed area of ulnar artery and superficial arch are exposed and the thrombosed segment resected. After clamping the proximal segment, distal adequacy may be judged by the amount of back flow (Fig. 29-14). The amount and quality of back flow from the distal arch are important. The presence of pulsatile back flow through the superficial arch indicates excellent collateral circulation and is good evidence that

FIG. 29-13. Treatment algorithm.

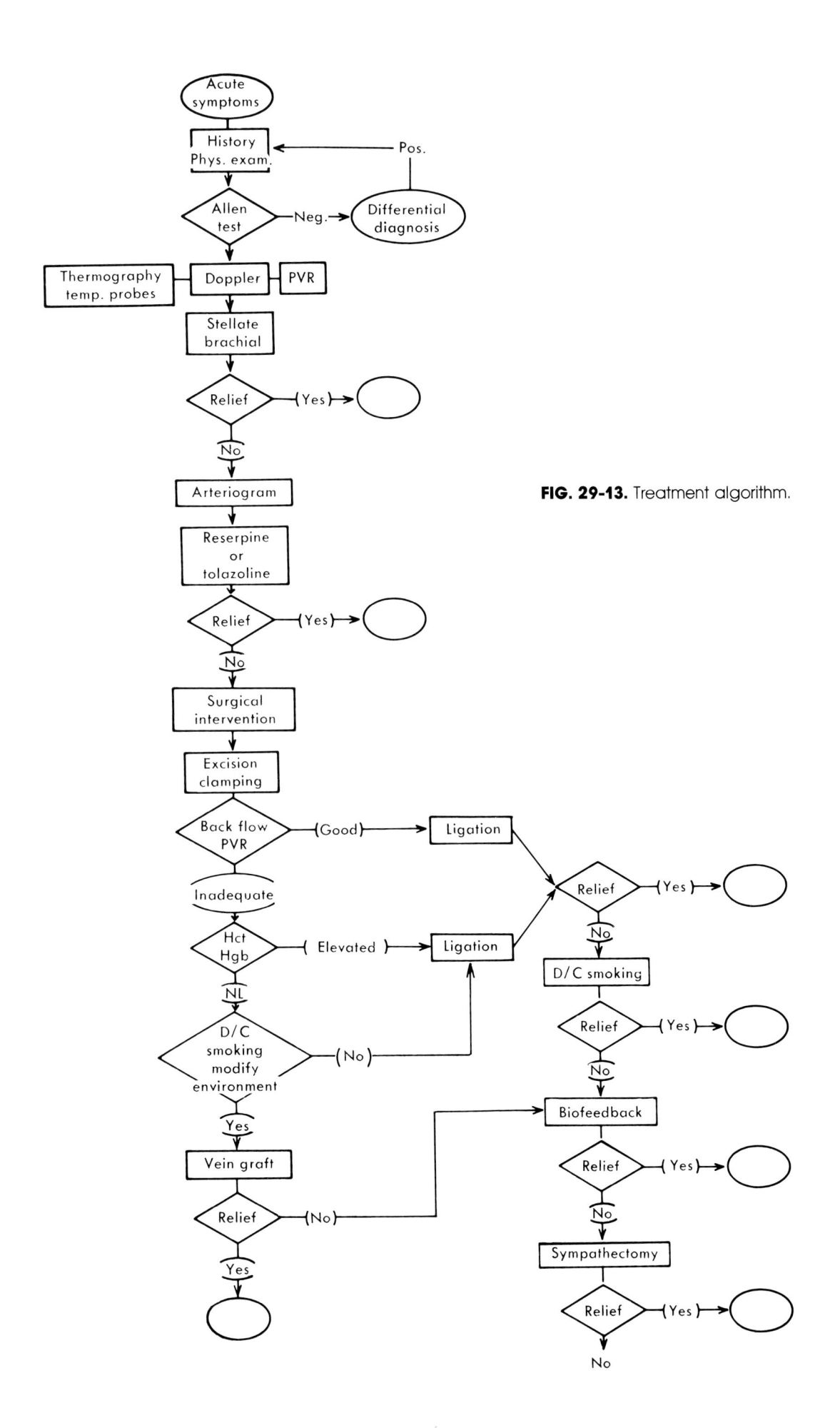

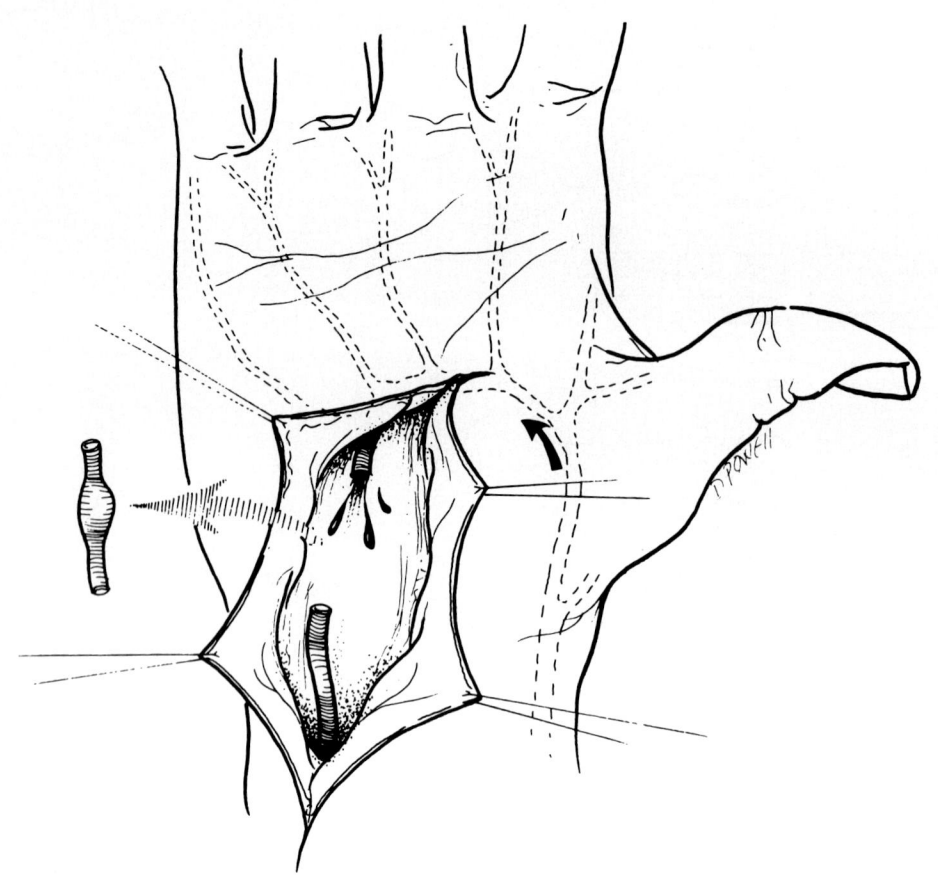

FIG. 29-14. Thrombosed segment of ulnar artery has been excised (left of *light arrow*) and tourniquet released. Pulsatile back flow through complete arch with clinical and plethysmographic evidence of adequate pulsatile flow is indication for ligation. Absence of back flow is contraindication to vein grafting, indicating probable distal obstruction. Back flow without pulsatile component in absence of other contraindications is indication for vein grafting.

revascularization is not necessary. Digital plethysmography may be done in the operating room to confirm the presence of digital pulsatile flow. The presence of digital and superficial arch pulsatile flow is an indication for ligation after suitable resection of the thrombosed arterial segment. Persistent postoperative symptoms, after resection and ligation in the presence of pulsatile flow, can usually be controlled by conservative measures. These include cessation of smoking, biofeedback techniques, and intermittent intraarterial medications. Sympathectomy can be used as a last resort but should not be necessary if good pulsatile flow exists.

If there is no back flow from the superficial arch after excision of the involved segment, this indicates probable distal obstruction and is a contraindication to vein grafting. Back flow without a pulsatile component or poor back flow without pulsatile digital flow is an indication for vein grafting. Contraindications to vein grafting are erythrocytosis, inability or refusal by the patient to modify the environment, or the continuation of smoking. If contraindications are present, then we feel that ligation should be done and other nonoperative management regimens used to control symptoms. If there are no contraindications, then vein grafting should be performed.

The involved artery is resected using the operating microscope until normal intima under high-power magnification is observed. A reversed vein graft from the forearm is then placed using microvascular techniques.

Persistent symptoms after management may be modified, as previously discussed. Sympathectomy can be used as a last resort but does have potential morbidity and may provide only temporary relief.

CONCLUSION

Thrombosis of the ulnar artery at the wrist occurs most frequently in men in the fifth decade of life. Symptoms are pain, cold intolerance, and numbness, and the degree of symptoms is related to the vascular anatomy of the superficial palmar arch and the presence of pulsatile blood flow. Diagnosis is confirmed by a positive Allen test and arteriography in conjunction with other specialized studies. Treatment should be patient oriented and aimed at the reconstitution of pulsatile digital blood flow. Management of ulnar artery insufficiency is a complex problem that often requires multiple treatment regimens.

REFERENCES

1. Allen, E.V.: Thromboangiitis obliterans: methods of diagnosis of chronic occlusive arterial lesions distal to the wrist with illustrative cases, Am. J. Med. Sci. **178**:237, 1929.
2. Benedict, K.T., Chang, W., and McCready, F.J.: The hypothenar hammer syndrome, Radiology **3**:57, 1974.
3. Coleman, S.S., and Anson, B.J.: Arterial patterns in the hand based upon a study of 650 specimens, Surg. Gynecol. Obstet. **113**:409, 1961.
4. Conn, J., Jr., Berigan, J.J., and Bell, J.L.: Hypothenar hammer syndrome, Surgery **68**:1122, 1970.
5. Dale, W.A.: Management of ischemia of the hand and fingers, Surgery **67**:62, 1970.
6. Eguro, H., and Goldner, J.L.: Bilateral thrombosis of the ulnar arteries in the hands, Plast. Reconstr. Surg. **52**:573, 1973.
7. Gelberman, R., Urbaniak, J.R., Bright, D.S., and Levin, L.S.: Digital sensibility following replantation, J. Hand Surg. **3**:313, 1978.
8. Given, K.G., Puckett, C.L., and Kleinert, H.E.: Ulnar artery thrombosis, Plast. Reconstr. Surg. **61**:405, 1978.
9. Guyon, F.: Note sur une disposition anatomique propre à la face antérieure de la région du poignet et non encore d'écorte, Bull. Soc. Anat. Paris **6**:184, 1861.
10. Herndon, W.A., Hershey, S.L., and Lambdin, C.S: Thrombosis of the ulnar artery in the hand, J. Bone Joint Surg. **57A**:994, 1975.
11. Kleinert, H.E., and Volianitis, G.J.: Thrombosis of the palmar arterial arch and its tributaries: etiology and newer concepts in treatment, J. Trauma **5**:447, 1965.
12. Koman, L.A., and Urbaniak, J.R.: Thrombosis of ulnar artery at the wrist. In American Academy of Orthopaedic Surgeons: Symposium on Microsurgery: Practical Use in Orthopaedics, St. Louis, 1979, The C.V. Mosby Co.
13. Leriche, R., Fontaine, R., and Dupertuis, S.M.: Arterectomy: with follow-up studies on 78 operations, Surg. Gynecol. Obstet. **64**:149, 1937.
14. Little, J.M., and Ferguson, D.A.: The incidence of the hypothenar hammer syndrome, Arch. Surg. **105**:684, 1972.
15. Shrewsbury, M.M.: The palmaris brevis: a reconsideration of its anatomy and possible function, J. Bone Joint Surg. **54A**:334, 1976.
16. Stirrat, C.R., Seaber, A.V., Urbaniak, J.R., and Bright, D.S.: Temperature monitoring in digital replantation, J. Hand Surg. **3**:352, 1978.
17. Trevaskis, A.E., Marcks, K.M., Pennisi, V.M., and Berg, E.M.: Thrombosis of the ulnar artery in the hand, Plast. Reconstr. Surg. **33**:73, 1964.
18. Von Rosen, S.: Ein fall von thrombose in der arteria ulnaris nach einwirkung von stumpfer gewalt, Acta Chir. Scand. **73**:500, 1934.
19. Zweig, J., Lie, K.K., Posch, J.L., and Larsen, R.D.: Thrombosis of the ulnar artery following blunt trauma to the hand, J. Bone Joint Surg. **51A**:1191, 1969.

Chapter 30 Traction avulsion amputations of the upper extremity replanted by microvascular anastomosis*

Harry J. Buncke

Elliott H. Rose

True traction avulsion amputations of the upper extremity are distinguished both clinically and prognostically from *shearing* (sharp) amputation. Salient clinical features of true traction avulsion amputations include the following:
1. Extensive soft tissue destruction at the wound margins
2. Disarticulation of the joint rather than fracture of the bony shaft
3. Extensive vascular and nerve injury proximal and distal to the point of division
4. Vessels more commonly avulsed from the distal part
5. Nerves more commonly avulsed from the proximal stump
6. Tendinous disruption at the musculotendinous aponeurosis

Suggestions for management to produce optimal results include the following:
1. Stabilization of the joint with minimal internal appliances and meticulous capsular reconstruction
2. Generous resection of damaged vessels beyond gross and microscopic injury (e.g., adventitial edema, dilated vasovasorum, intimal separation, and adherent clot
3. Tension-free anastomoses using long interpositional vein grafts
4. Early perfusion of the limb after arterial anastomosis to minimize ischemic time
5. Tendon resection with subsequent secondary tendon grafting
6. Nerve resection followed by secondary suralis nerve graft
7. Extensive soft tissue debridement of the wound margins and split-thickness skin graft to close the defect, even if necessary to do so over microvascular repairs or vein grafts

---

*Supported in part by the Microsurgical Fund of the Ralph K. Davies Medical Center, San Francisco.

TRACTION AVULSION AMPUTATIONS OF THE UPPER EXTREMITY

Survival rates of upper extremity replants are approaching 90% of selected cases in major replant centers.[3,5] Best results are reported in "guillotine and locally crushed digits," whereas survival rates of "diffusely crushed and avulsed" digits are dismal.[7] This latter category constitues a broad spectrum of mutilating injuries; however, no differentiation clinically or prognostically has been made between *true traction avulsion* (i.e., pulling) and *shearing avulsion* (cutting) amputation. This chapter presents five cases of true traction avulsion injuries that have been replanted by microvascular anastomosis.

CASE HISTORIES
Case 1

This 10-year-old girl (C.S.) caught her right thumb in a loop of rope during a tug-of-war game on May 18, 1977, sustaining a traction avulsion amputation at the metacarpophalangeal (MCP) joint level (Fig. 30-1). Transport time to the hospital was approximately 4 hours. On examination the soft tissue at the MCP joint was circumferentially transected with the exception of a small fibrous attachment of the flexor pollicis longus and extensor pollicis longus tendons. On the ulnar side the digital artery and digital nerve were separated at the wound level; on the radial side a lengthy segment of digital nerve was carried with the amputated specimen. Radiographically it was seen that the proximal phalanx was transected at the base of the shaft.

The surgical procedure consisted of slight bone shortening and longitudinal fixation with a single Kirschner wire. The long incision was carried midlaterally over the neurovascular bundles proximally and distally for exposure. The digital arteries and veins were extensively resected proximally and distally, resulting in a 6.0-cm gap between the two ends. This defect was bridged with an interpositional vein graft from the radiodigital artery proximally to the ulnar digital artery distally. Venous repair was by direct anastomosis of the dorsal vein on the radial side and a 2.0-cm vein graft to bridge the gap on the ulnar side. The tourniquet was released after the arterial repair to allow early perfusion of the digit. Total ischemic time prior to release was approximately 8 hours. The elongated distal segment of the radial nerve was repaired and sutured to the proximal ulnar segment with 9-0 nylon. The flexor pollicis longus was threaded through the flexor sheath and, through a counterincision on the volar aspect of the wrist,

CHAPTER 30 TRACTION AVULSION AMPUTATIONS OF THE UPPER EXTREMITY

anastomosed to a slip of the palmaris longus. The extensor pollicis longus was sutured to the transferred extensor indicis proprius on the dorsum of the wrist. Total operative time was 9 hours. Postoperatively a regimen of heparin, aspirin, dipyridamole (Persantin), and low-molecular weight dextran was maintained. Late on the second day the thumb was noted to be edematous and dusky.

Administration of intravenous dexamethasone (Decadron) was begun. On the third day an axillary block was performed, with no improvement. A technetium scan revealed the radiodigital artery to be clotted proximal to the proximal anastomosis. The graft itself was unclotted. On June 2, 1977, the left thumb was debrided, and the amputation stump was closed primarily.

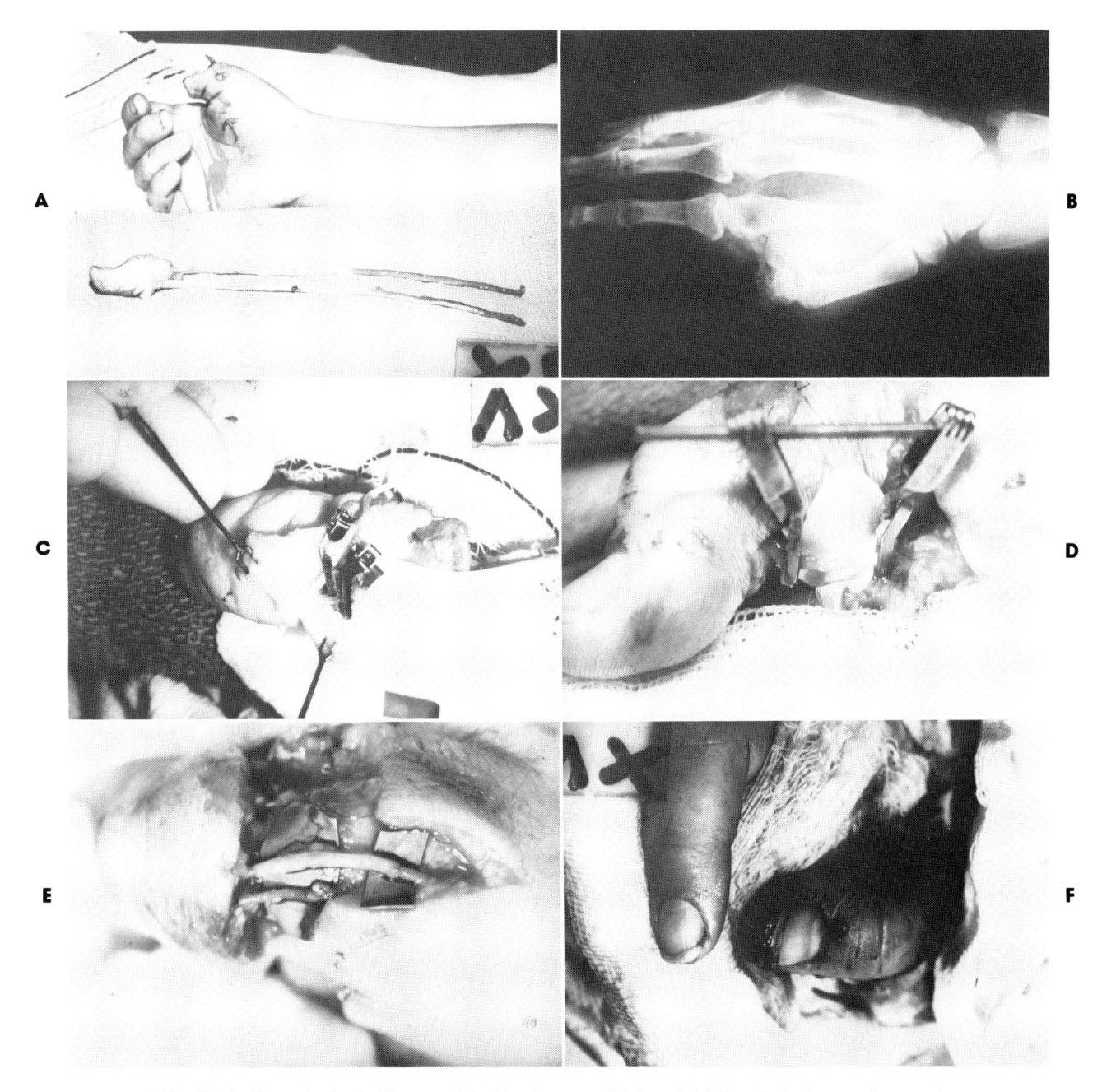

FIG. 30-1. Case 1. **A,** A 10-year-old-girl who caught her right thumb in loop of rope during tug-of-war. Note division of flexor pollicis longus and extensor pollicis longus at musculotendinous junction. **B,** X-ray demonstrating transection at metaphysis of proximal phalanx. Base is restrained by insertion of thenar intrinsics. **C,** Ulnar digital artery is identified at interphalangeal (IP) joint level (lower clamp). Ulnar digital nerve (upper clamp) is avulsed several centimeters proximally from stump. **D,** Length vein graft used in arterial reconstruction. **E,** Dorsal vein graft used for superficial venous drainage. **F,** Failed replant at 3 days.

SECTION 8 MICROVASCULAR PROBLEMS

Case 2

This 18-year-old man (J.F.) caught his left hand in an insulating packaging machine on May 21, 1977, sustaining a total avulsion of the left hand at the wrist level (Fig. 30-2). Transfer time to Ralph K. Davies Medical Center was 4½ hours.

On examination a circumferential soft tissue avulsion at the wrist level and disarticulation at the radiocarpal joint were found. All the flexors and extensors were avulsed with the amputated specimen from the full length of the forearm (i.e., the junction of the musculotendinous aponeurosis). Both proximal and distal segments of the ulnar and radial arteries were severely contused. A long stump of the median nerve was attached to the specimen.

In the operating room the soft tissue was radically debrided and the flexor and extensor tendons resected. The stabilization was with a proximal row carpectomy and two large Kirschner wires passed through the second and third metacarpal bones into the distal aspect of the radius. Both the radial and ulnar arteries as well as three dorsal veins were extensively debrided and reconstructed with lengthy interpositional vein grafts. The lengths of the vein grafts were 8.0 cm and 10.0 cm for the arterial and venous repairs, respectively. The tourniquet was released after the initial radial artery repair to allow perfusion. Total ischemic time was approximately 7 hours. The stump of the median nerve was debrided, and no nerve repair was attempted primarily. The split-thickness skin graft was placed directly over the arterial anastomosis on the volar side of the wrist for soft tissue coverage. Total operative time was 10 hours. Postoperative medications included dexamethasone from the second to sixth day, aspirin and dipyridamole for 8 days, low-molecular weight dextran for 4 days, and two units of whole blood. Good capillary fill color persisted, and the hand survived in its entirety. Secondary reconstruction of a 20.0-cm deficit in the median nerve and a 30.0-cm deficit in the ulnar nerve with suralis nerve grafts was carried out on December 5, 1977. Notably, the nerve injuries appeared to extend proximal to the points of major attachment, i.e., the median nerve at the pronator tunnel and the ulnar nerve at the cubital fossa.

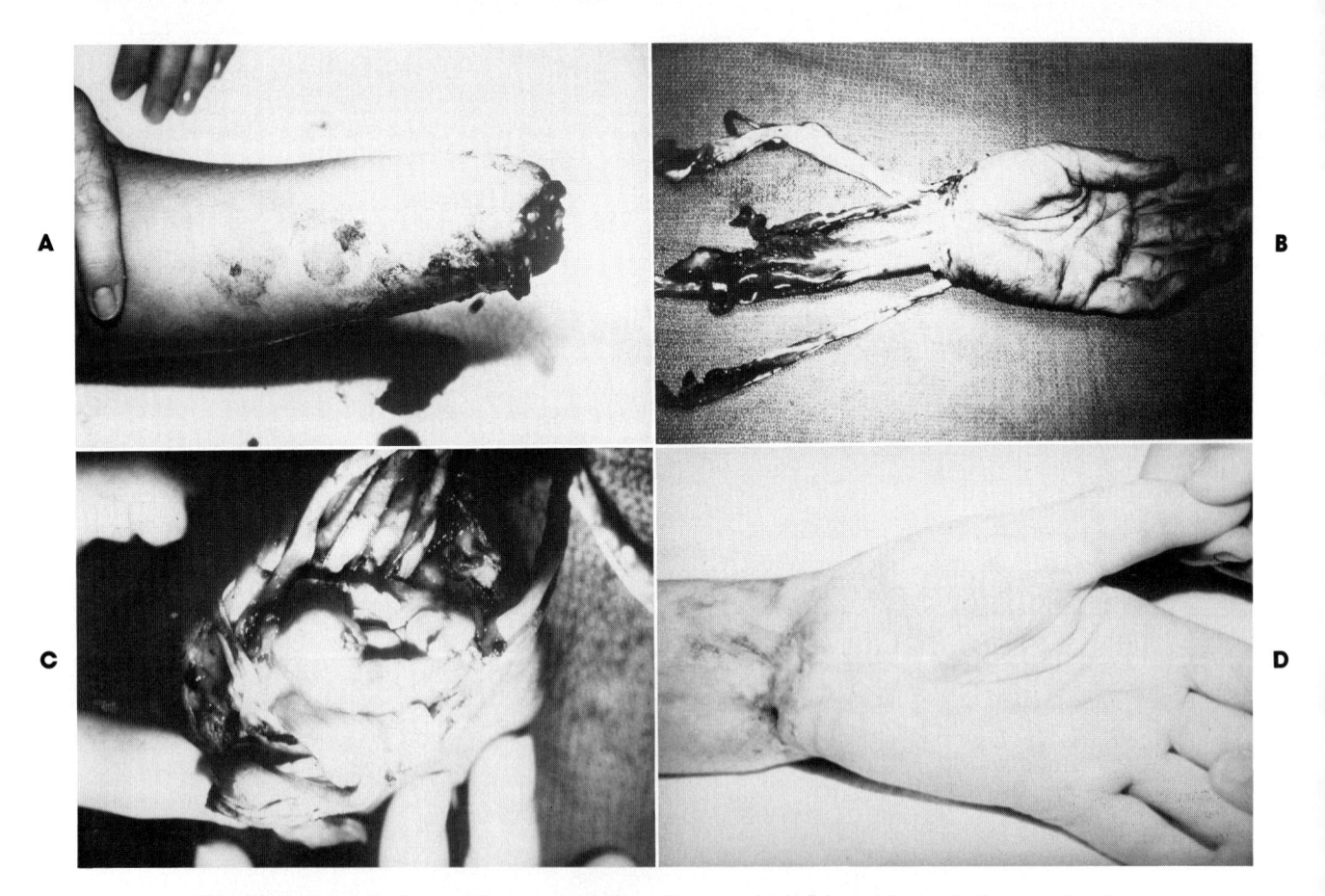

FIG. 30-2. Case 2. **A,** An 18-year-old man who caught left hand in insulating packaging machine. **B,** Flexor, extensors, and median nerve avulsed from forearm. **C,** Disarticulation at wrist level. **D,** Replanted hand at 6 months.

Case 3

This 34-year-old woman (F.S.) traumatically amputated the left forearm at the elbow level in an industrial machine on August 13, 1977 (Fig. 30-3). The amputated specimen was placed on ice at the local emergency room 30 minutes after amputation. The duration of the ambulance transport to Ralph K. Davies was 3 hours and 50 minutes. On examination the circumferential soft tissue severance was 3.0 cm distal to the elbow. The elbow joint was disarticulated without fracture. Severe vascular contusion extended 5.0 cm proximally and 10.0 cm distally. Operatively the elbow joint was fixed with a single large Kirschner wire through the trochlea and olecranon. The joint capsule was approximated with interrupted 3-0 Dexon sutures. The brachial artery and two large venae commitantes were repaired with lengthy 15.0-cm interpositional saphenous vein grafts with 8-0 nylon. Arterial repair was opened at 7½ hours. The traumatized ischemic muscle was extensively debrided and loosely approximated. The skin was closed dorsally, and a split-thickness skin graft was placed on the volar surface. Total operative time was 7 hours. Postoperatively the regimen consisted of low–molecular weight dextran, aspirin, cephalothin (Keflin), and dexamethasone in tapering doses for 3 days. On the first day marked forearm and hand congestion necessitated longitudinal "escharotomies" from above the elbow distal to the hand. Extensive hemorrhage from the incision sites prompted administration of a total of 21 units of whole blood, two units of fresh frozen plasma, and platelet concentrates. On the third through fifth days she became febrile to 38° C with progressive cyanosis and poor capillary refill. A serosanguineous drainage from the forearm grew heavy *Serratia marcescens* and enterococci; no clostridia were noted. On the sixth postoperative day the replanted arm was debrided at the elbow. Closure of the skin flaps was accomplished secondarily. The remainder of the course after amputation was uneventful.

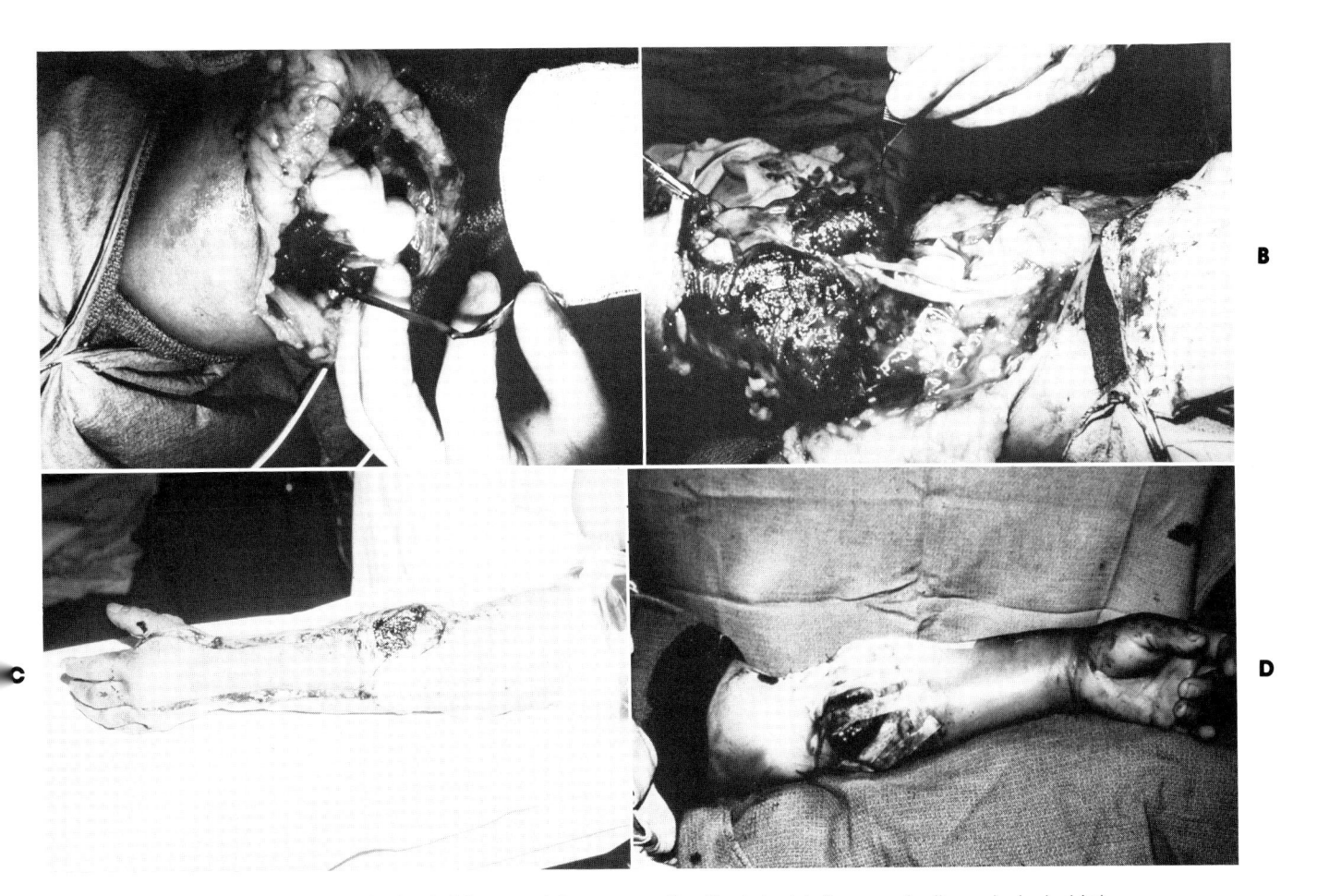

FIG. 30-3. Case 3. **A,** A 34-year-old woman disarticulated left arm at elbow in industrial machine. **B,** Saphenous vein grafts of 15.0 cm used for arterial and venous repairs. **C,** Skin and fascial releases for decompression at 3 days. **D,** Sepsis secondary to ischemic necrosis requiring amputation at 5 days.

SECTION 8 MICROVASCULAR PROBLEMS

Case 4

This 15-year-old girl (C.S.) caught her right little finger on a gatepost on October 7, 1977, sustaining a ring avulsion injury at the level of the proximal segment (Fig. 30-4). Warm ischemic time was 30 minutes. The time of transfer to Ralph K. Davies was 4 hours.

On examination the circumferential soft tissue laceration was found to be at the proximal interphalangeal (PIP) joint level, and the distal phalanx was disarticulated at the distal interphalangeal (DIP) joint. The flexor digitorum profundus was avulsed with the amputated specimen and measured 20.3 cm in length. On the proximal stump the proximal and middle phalanges were entirely skeletonized. The flexor digitorum superficialis insertion at the base of the middle phalanx was intact with good joint motion.

Surgically, the amputated specimen was replaced with a longitudinal Kirschner wire through the DIP joint at 30 degrees flexion. The neurovascular bundles were identified proximally and distally and extensively debrided. The ulnar digital artery and a volar digital vein was repaired with 5.0 cm interpositional vein grafts. A dorsal superficial vein was repaired directly. Nerve repairs were not carried out because of extensive avulsion injuries. The tourniquet was released after the arterial repair with a total ischemic time of approximately 6 hours. Total operative time was 5 hours. Postoperatively the regimen consisted of dexamethasone for 3 days, aspirin, heparin, and low–molecular weight dextran. Good capillary fill and turgor persisted throughout the postoperative course, and the finger survived in its entirety.

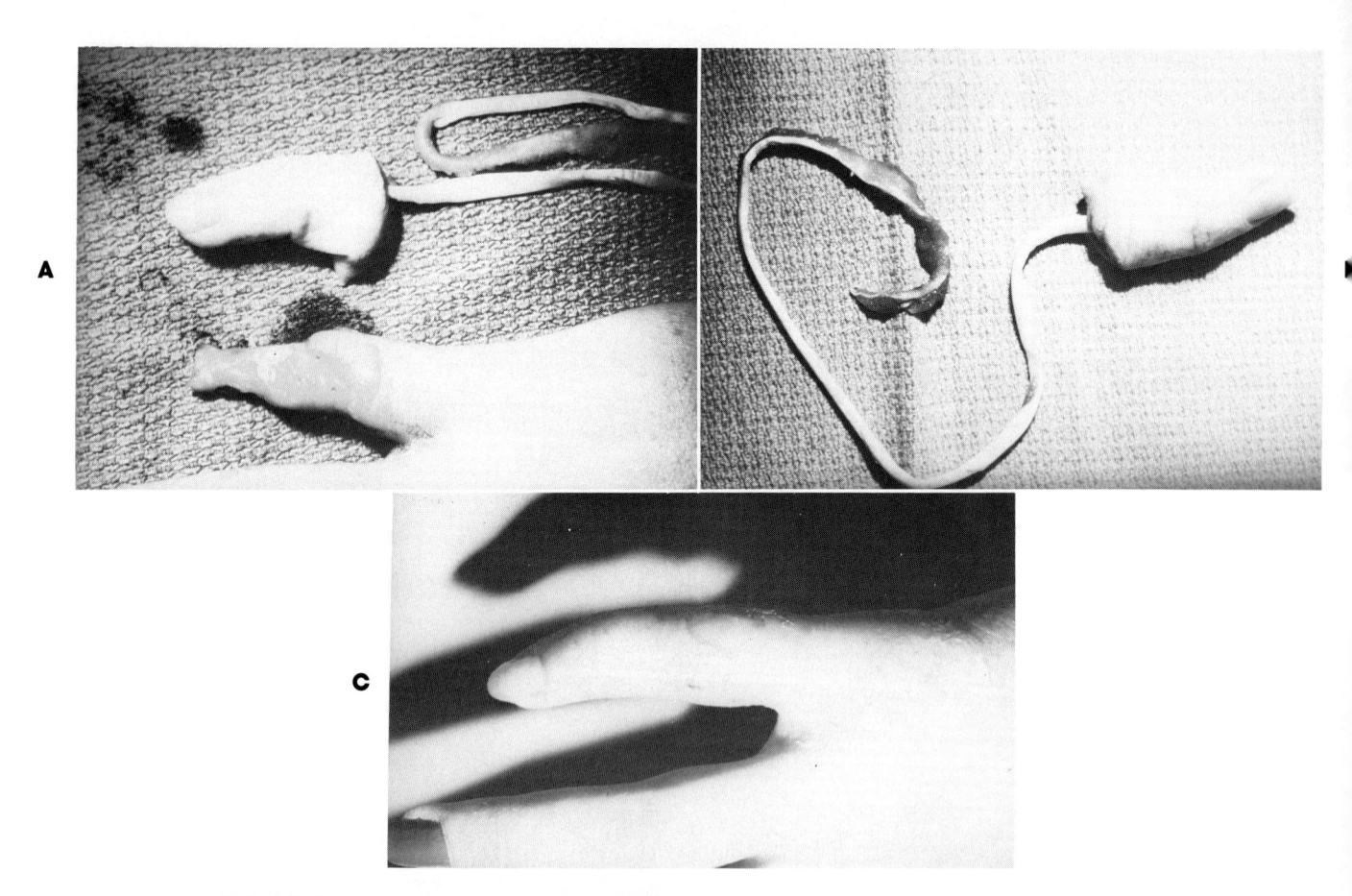

FIG. 30-4. Case 4. **A,** A 15-year-old girl with ring avulsion injury at base of right little finger. **B,** Disarticulation at DIP joint. Flexor digitorum superficialis is intact. **C,** Replanted finger at 3 months.

CHAPTER 30 TRACTION AVULSION AMPUTATIONS OF THE UPPER EXTREMITY

Case 5

This 21-year-old man (J.D.) caught his left thumb in a ditch jack, sustaining a traction avulsion amputation at the MCP joint level (Fig. 30-5). Radiographically the proximal phalanx was transected at its base just distal to the insertion of the thenar intrinsics. Both digital nerves were avulsed proximally at the midmetacarpal level and carried with the amputated specimen. Both digital arteries were avulsed distal to the interphalangeal (IP) joint. The flexor pollicis longus tendon was avulsed at its musculotendinous aponeurosis. Warm ischemic time was 5 minutes. Total time of transfer to Ralph K. Davies was 4 hours.

Operatively, after the proximal phalanx was stabilized with a single longitudinal Kirschner wire, the radiodigital artery distal to the IP joint was anastomosed proximally into the ulnar digital vessel via two 4.0-cm interpositional vein grafts crossed volarly over the proximal segment. Two dorsal superficial veins were directly anastomosed. Total ischemic time prior to repair of the arterial anastomosis was approximately 7 hours. Postoperatively aspirin and low–molecular weight dextran were used. Good capillary refill, color, and turgor were present until the fifth day when the finger abruptly became mottled and cyanotic after the patient had voluntarily moved the other digits. The Doppler tone was muffled at the level of the bony fixation. On reexploration it was found that the interpositional vein graft had fallen into the fracture site and abruptly occluded at that point. A second vein graft was interposed between the proximal ulnar arterial segment and the distal radial vessel. There was early capillary refill; however, the thumb went on to the progressive congestion and duskiness. Six weeks later the mummified necrotic skin of the distal segment and the volar proximal segment was debrided. The entire proximal phalanx and skin on the dorsal surface of the proximal segment were salvaged to the level of the IP joint. A temporary split-thickness skin graft has been applied in anticipation of secondary reconstruction with a neurovascular island pedicle flap with an incorporated distal phalanx of the great toe.

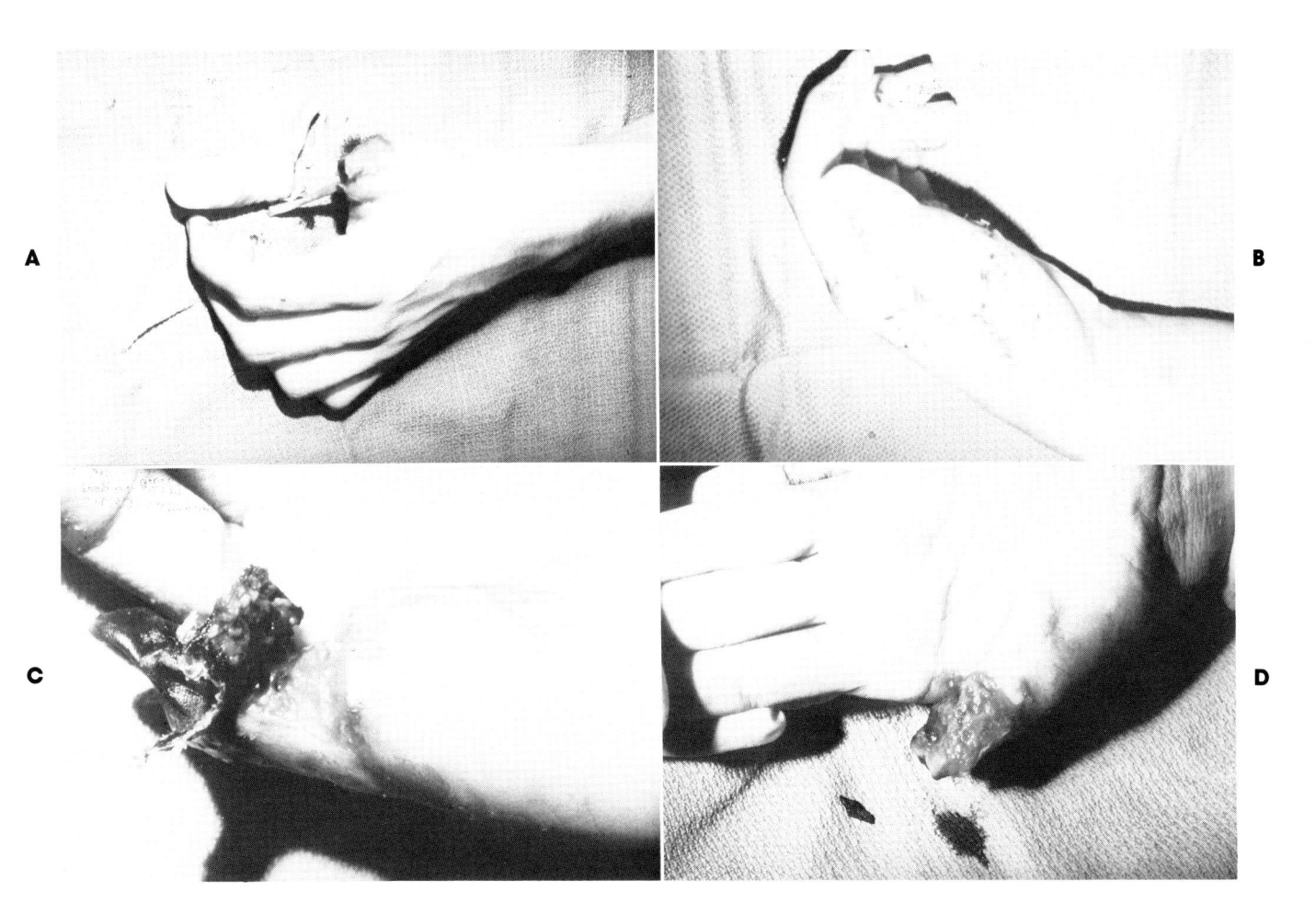

FIG. 30-5. Case 5. **A,** A 21-year-old man avulsed left thumb in ditch jack. Note extensive vascular pedicle on proximal stump. **B,** Replanted by cross-volar vein graft from ulnar to radiodigital artery. **C,** Partial loss debrided. **D,** Bony survival to IP joint.

CLINICAL FEATURES

Observations of clinical findings of true traction avulsion injuries include the following:

1. Extensive soft tissue destruction at the wound margins: linear lines of ecchymosis on both sides of the digit denote rupture of the localized bed.[4]
2. Disarticulation of the joint with disruption of the capsular attachments: the exception to this seems to be in the thumb where the strong tendinous insertion of the thenar intrinsics at the base of the proximal phalanx results in a shaft fracture.
3. Extensive vascular injury proximal and distal to the point of division: grossly, the adventitia is edematous, and the vasovasorum are dilated. At high-power magnification through the operating microscope there may be seen intimal separation, endothelial swelling, or adherent clot.
4. Vessels are more commonly avulsed at the site of the soft tissue injury or distally.
5. The nerves are more commonly avulsed quite proximally and carried with the amputation stump.
6. Tendinous disruption occurs at the musculotendinous aponeurosis.

RESULTS

Of the five cases of replantation of true traction avulsion amputations, two survived completely, two failed, and one partially survived (Table 30-1). The average ischemic time was 7.0 hours prior to vascular perfusion because of the long delays in transportation from remote parts of California, averaging 4 to 5 hours.

The average age was 19.6 years. The youngest in the series was 10 years old, and the oldest was 34 years old. The average length of interpositional vein grafts for arterial repairs was 7.6 cm. The average graft length for veins, when used, was 6.0 cm. Vein grafts were not used in repair of four superficial veins.

Sepsis secondary to myonecrosis developed in one case (forearm replant with 7½ hours of ischemic time). Thrombosis proximal to the anastomosis occurred in one case. Mechanical occlusion secondary to entrapment of the vein graft in a fracture site was responsible for partial loss in one case.

DISCUSSION

Although not optimal, the success rates of this series (50%) compare favorably with Morrison, O'Brien, and MacLeod's survival rates[5] in "diffusely crushed and avulsed digits." Long ischemic time predisposing the muscle to necrosis was probably the cause of loss of the most proximal amputation (case 3). Poor stabilization of the fracture site in case 5 allowed the vein graft to fall into the crevice with motion. In only one case did the loss appear to be caused by inadequate proximal resection of the artery, predisposing the vessel to thrombosis (case 1).

In traction injuries longitudinal trauma to vessels causes intimal damage that predisposes the vessel to thrombi.[7,8] Histologically this appears as intimal disruption and intramural ecchymosis.[2] Exposure of collagen-bearing tissue (media and adventitia) is thrombogenic, causing platelet adhesiveness.[6] Solid clots in the end of the vessel leave small bits of fibrin attached to the endothelial lining and act as stimuli for clot recurrence.

Extensive resection of the vessel with damaged intima and media some distance from the site of the amputation in both directions is mandatory.[7,9]

Table 30-1. Traction avulsion amputations of the upper extremity

Case	Age (years)	Level of amputation	Veins grafts (length in centimeters)		Ischemic time		Survival	Complications
			Arterial	Venous	Warm	Cold		
1	10	Right thumb MCP joint	Digital (6)	Two superficial (2, none)	Unknown	8 hours	No	Radiodigital artery clogged proximal to anastomosis
2	18	Left wrist	Ulnar (8)	Two superficial (10)	Unknown	7 hours	Yes	
3	34	Left elbow	Radial (8) Brachial (15)	Superficial (10) Deep (15)	30 minutes	7½ hours	No	Sepsis secondary to postoperative myonecrosis
4	15	Right little finger PIP joint	Digital (5)	Two superficial (5, none)	Unknown	6 hours	Yes	
5	21	Left thumb MCP joint	Digital (4)	Two superficial (none)	5 minutes	7 hours	Partial	Vein graft mechanically occluded in fracture site

Long interpositional vein grafts offer several advantages. Damaged vessels may be generously resected, and reconstruction may be accomplished with *tension-free* anastomoses. If shortened vessels are stretched for direct approximation, the intraluminal diameter is narrowed. As the diameter decreases, flow decreases to the fourth power of the decreased diameter (Poiseuille's law).

REFERENCES

1. Buncke, H.J., Rose, E.H., Brownsteing, M.D., and Chater, N.L.: Successful replantation of avulsed scalps by microvascular anastomosis, Plast. Reconstr. Surg. **61:**666, 1978.
2. Hayhurst, J.W.: Factors influencing patency rates. In Daniller, A.I., and Strauch, B., editors: Symposium of microsurgery, St. Louis, 1976, The C.V. Mosby Co.
3. Kleinert, H.E., Juhala, C.A., Tsai, T.M., and Van Beck, A.: Digital replantation—selection, technique and results, Orthop. Clin. North Am. **8:**309, 1977.
4. Kutz, J.E.: Preparation for replantation. In Daniller, A.I., and Strauch, B., editors: Symposium on microsurgery, St. Louis, 1976, The C.V. Mosby Co.
5. Morrison, W.A., O'Brien, B.M., and MacLeod, A.M.: Evaluation of digital replantation—a review of 100 cases, Orthop. Clin. North Am. **8:**925, 1977.
6. Mustard, J., and Packham, M.: Factors influencing platelet function, Pharmacol. Rev. **22:**97, 1970.
7. O'Brien, B.M., and MacLeod, A.M.: Digital replantation. In Daniller, A.I., and Strauch, B., editors: Symposium on microsurgery, St. Louis, 1976, The C.V. Mosby Co.
8. Wood, N.E., and Stutzman, F.L.: Initimal separation in arterial injuries, Angiology **14:**265, 1963.
9. Worman, L.W., Darin, J.C., and Kritter, A.E.: The anatomy of a limb replantation failure, Arch. Surg. **91:**211, 1965.

SECTION NINE TENDON TRANSFER PROBLEMS

Chapter 31 Restoration of lateral pinch in quadriplegia secondary to spinal cord injury: surgery selection by functional level

James H. House

Quadriplegia as the result of a spinal cord injury is a profound disability. The patient's entire life-style is radically changed, and the patient must be involved in a broadly based rehabilitation program to achieve the maximal function consistent with the level of injury. Selected patients with quadriplegia may derive significant benefit from surgical restoration of basic hand functions. The most useful function that can be restored in the majority of patients is lateral pinch. This chapter discusses several methods that have been described for restoring control of the thumb and relates the selection of each procedure to allow the maximal function consistent with the needs and the potential of each patient. Where appropriate, certain other procedures used to restore grasp and release are briefly presented for those patients with a lower level of injury and more retained function.

Before proposing surgery, it is important that ample time be allowed for the patient to learn to accept the handicap and through the rehabilitation process to become as skilled as possible with his or her retained function. Optimally the surgeon should be working closely with a rehabilitation team in the selection of patients for surgery and establishing realistic goals for self-care and vocational activities. Joint meetings with the surgeon, rehabilitation personnel who have been working with the patient, and other patients who have had surgery facilitate the evaluation procedure and often bring out significant functional needs of this similar but unique individual.

The preoperative evaluation must provide an exact characterization of each patient and includes a complete muscle test of the upper extremity and a careful sensory assessment identifying the quality and location of epicritic sensibility, as well as protective sensation. The presence of contractures and spasticity of distal muscles should be assessed, and a program to strengthen remaining functional muscles is useful. Through occupational therapy the patient is taught to become as independent as possible in the activities of daily living, using adaptive equipment and functional orthoses. Special self-care needs such as transfers, wheelchair propulsion, and the care of urinary collecting devices also must be learned. In addition, the patient may need the help of psychologic and social counseling to adjust to the emotional and dependency aspects of this severe disability prior to considering surgical reconstruction.

CLASSIFICATION BY FUNCTIONAL LEVEL

Quadriplegic patients are most usefully classified by identifying the lowest level of motor function retained. Fig. 31-1 shows the segmental innervation of muscles of the elbow, forearm, and hand with slight modifications after the observations of Zancolli.[11] Each of the cervical cord levels can be roughly identified through a brief examination of clinical function. The C5 functional group has elbow flexion, the C6 group has wrist extension, the C7 group has finger extension, the C8 group has finger flexion, and the T1 group has complete intrinsic function. This is somewhat oversimplified, but by relating the neurologic deficit to function rather than to the level of skeletal injury, each patient can be more accurately characterized. After a detailed motor and sensory examination a more specific subgroup of each limb can be identified. The classification of Zancolli,[11] as outlined in Fig. 31-2, facilitates communication and clarifies the rationale for selecting various surgical procedures. Moberg[8] also has developed a method of functional classification with appropriate emphasis on the sensory aspects of the disability.

Sensory function must be considered, particularly when contemplating surgery for patients with a C5 functional level. When function is preserved in the C6 root, there is usually two-point discrimination of less than 10 mm present in the thumb and often useful sensation in the index and middle fingers.

SURGICAL CONSIDERATION BY FUNCTIONAL LEVEL

Lesions of the upper cervical spinal cord, if not fatal, are associated with such profound deficits that surgical procedures are not indicated for those above C5. Below the C8 level, procedures for median and ulnar intrinsic paralysis can be readily performed if the patient requires

SECTION 9 TENDON TRANSFER PROBLEMS

CERVICAL				DORSAL
5	6	7	8	1

Muscle	C5	C6	C7	C8	D1
Biceps	■	■			
Brachialis	■	■			
Brachioradialis		■			
Supinator		■			
Extensor carpi radialis longus		■	■		
Extensor carpi radialis brevis			■		
Pronator teres			■		
Flexor carpi radialis			■		
Triceps			■	■	
Extensor digitorum communis				■	
Extensor digiti quinti				■	
Extensor carpi ulnaris				■	
Extensor indicis propius				■	
Extensor pollicis longus				■	
Pronator quadratus				■	
Flexor digitorum profundus				■	■
Flexor pollicis longus				■	■
Flexor carpi ulnaris				■	■
Lumbricalis				■	■
Flexor digitorum sublimis				■	■
Thenar muscles				■	■
Adductor pollicis				■	■
Interossei					■
Hypothenar muscles					■

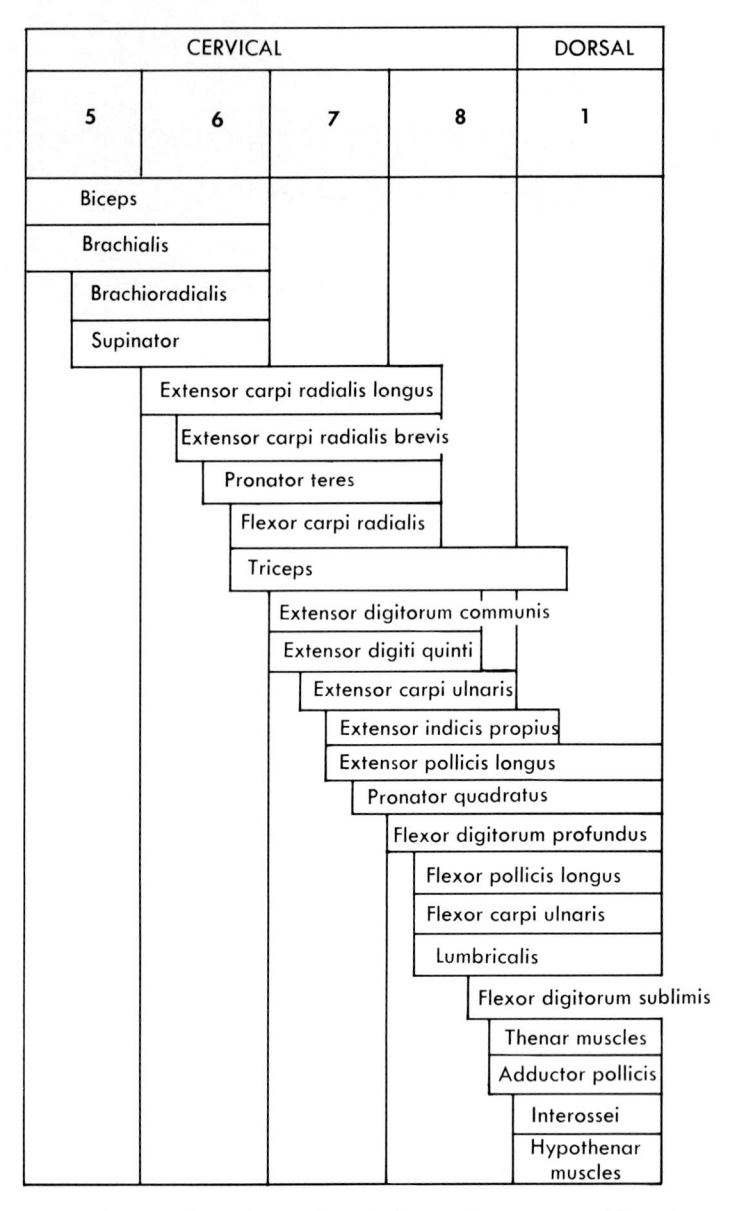

FIG. 31-1. Segmental innervation of muscles of elbow, forearm, and hand, as modified by Zancolli,[11] according to our clinical observations of traumatic quadriplegia. (Modified from Zancolli, E.: Clin. Orthop. **112:**101, 1975.)

more strength of finger flexion, better opposition, or control of clawing.

At the C5 level there is often sufficient function of the brachioradialis to allow transfer to the extensor carpi radialis brevis to provide some power of wrist extension so that the natural tenodesis of the extrinsic flexors and extensors can provide useful, although weak, gross grasp and enable the patient to use a wrist-driven orthosis such as those developed at Rancho Los Amigos or Northwestern University. Surgical tenodesis for extrinsic finger flexion and extension and thumb opposition can be performed; however, the sensory function is poor, and complex reconstructive procedures and multiple-joint fusions may result in a stiff hand that is not satisfying to either the surgeon or the patient.

Patients at the "weak" C6 functional level (subgroup II B1) with good wrist extension may be candidates for surgery to improve function. Limited improvement in function can be achieved by the procedure described by Moberg[7,8] (Fig. 31-3). The basic procedure involves tenodesis of the flexor pollicis longus tendon to the volar surface of the radius to provide thumb flexion as the

CHAPTER 31 RESTORATION OF LATERAL PINCH IN QUADRIPLEGIA SECONDARY TO SPINAL CORD INJURY

CLINICAL GROUP	LOWEST FUNCTIONING CORD SEGMENT	BASIC FUNCTIONING MUSCLES	SUBGROUPS			
I Flexor of the elbow —13%	5	Biceps, brachialis	A	Without brachioradialis		
			B	With brachioradialis		
II Extensor of the wrist —74%	6	Extensor carpi radialis longus and brevis	A	Weak wrist extension		
			B	Strong wrist extension —82%	1	Without pronator teres and flexor carpi radialis —76%
					2	With pronator teres and without flexor carpi radialis —16%
					3	With pronator teres, flexor carpi radialis, and triceps —8%
III Extrinsic extensor of the fingers —6.8%	7	Extensor digitorum communis, extensor digiti quinti, extensor carpi ulnaris	A	Complete extension of ulnar fingers and paralysis of radial fingers and thumb		
			B	Complete extension of all fingers and weak thumb extension		
IV Extrinsic flexor of the fingers and thumb extensor —6.2%	8	Flexor digitorum profundus, extensor indicis proprius, extensor pollicis longus, flexor carpi ulnaris	A	Complete flexion of ulnar fingers and paralysis of flexion of radial fingers and thumb; complete thumb extension		
			B	Complete flexion of all fingers and weak thumb flexion; weak thenar muscles; paralysis of the intrinsic muscles of the fingers without or with flexor superficialis		

FIG. 31-2. Clinical classification of quadriplegic hand: observations of 97 patients. (From Zancolli, E.: Clin. Orthop. **112**:101, 1975.)

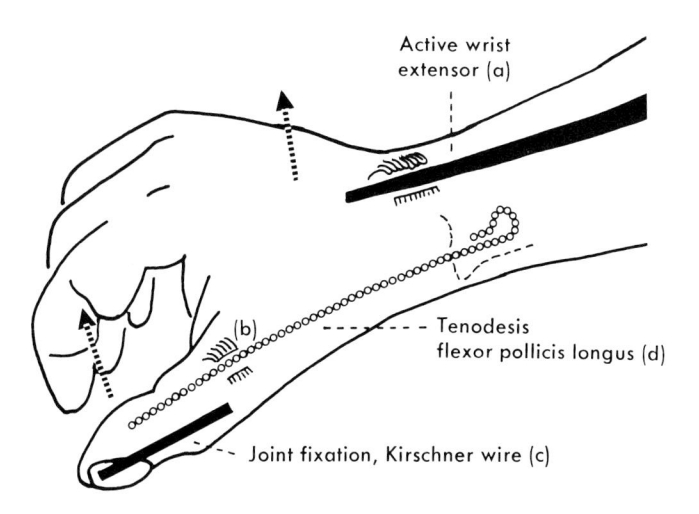

FIG. 31-3. Basic steps in procedure to provide key grip. Brachioradialis (a) is used as wrist extensor; b and d, flexor pollicis longus is tenodesed to volar surface of radius, and annular ligament at MCP joint is resected to permit tendon to bowstring and increase strength of key grip; c, arthrodesis is done of thumb IP joint with Kirschner wire to prevent flexion (Froment's sign) and to maintain broad contact surfaces. (From Moberg, E.: J. Bone Joint Surg. **57A**:200, 1975.)

wrist is extended. When necessary, the brachioradialis is transferred to augment wrist extension. Moberg has discovered that it is desirable to release the flexor pollicis longus tendon from the annular ligament at the metacarpophalangeal (MCP) joint to increase the mechanical advantage of the weak flexor system. The distal joint of the thumb is stabilized with a longitudinally inserted buried Kirschner wire to prevent hyperflexion. Three or more procedures are performed at one or more sittings to create an active wrist extensor and a thumb flexor grip to provide lateral pinch. He emphasizes that simplicity is a "must" in these severely involved patients and recommends that only one hand be reconstructed when the sensory function is poor. He does not perform finger flexor tenodesis, preferring to allow the fingers to remain supple for "human contact."

Satisfactory balance of the thumb by tenodesis of the flexor pollicis longus alone is difficult to achieve because of carpometacarpal (CMC) joint instability. An alternative method employing arthrodesis of the CMC joint in a position to allow lateral pinch can be combined with the tenodesis or a transfer to the flexor pollicis longus to assist in attaining the limited functional goal of voluntary lateral pinch in selected, well-motivated patients with adequate thumb sensibility and a weak C6 motor level.

There is more to offer the "strong" C6 group (subgroup II B2 or B3) with four or five functional muscles in the forearm. Those patients with function of the pronator teres and flexor carpi radialis, in addition to both radial wrist extensors and the brachioradialis, are good candidates for surgery. Active wrist extension is essential and is maintained by the extensor carpi radialis brevis, which is usually strong and is located centrally. If present, the flexor carpi radialis is preserved, since this muscle will increase power for wheelchair propulsion, assist in transfers, and augment the function of any extensor tenode-

Table 31-1. Plan for reconstruction (part I): transfers for "strong" C6 quadriplegia

Muscle or tendon	Procedure	Provides
Extensor carpi radialis brevis	Retained	Wrist extension
Flexor carpi radialis	Retained	Wrist flexion
Extensor carpi radialis longus	Transfer to flexor digitorum profundus	Finger flexion
Pronator teres	Transfer to flexor pollicis longus	Thumb flexion
Brachioradialis	Transfer via flexor digitorum superficialis graft	Thumb adduction-opposition
Extensor digitorum communis	Tenodesis to distal aspect of radius	Finger extension
Extensor pollicis longus and abductor pollicis longus (rerouted)	Tenodesis to distal aspect of radius	Thumb extension
Free-tendon graft	Tenodesis of index and middle fingers to second metacarpal through lumbrical canals	Intrinsic balance

Modified from Zancolli, E.: Clin. Orthop. **112**:101, 1975.

Table 31-2. Plan for reconstruction (part II)

Muscle or tendon	Procedure	Provides
Extensor carpi radialis brevis	Retained	Wrist extension
Flexor carpi radialis	Retained	Wrist flexion
Extensor carpi radialis longus	Transfer to flexor digitorum profundus	Finger flexion
Pronator teres	Transfer to flexor pollicis longus	Thumb flexion
	Transfer of paralyzed flexor digitorum superficialis (lasso procedure)	Intrinsic balance
Brachioradialis	Transfer to extensor digitorum communis and extensor pollicis longus	Finger and thumb extension
	CMC arthrodesis	Thumb alignment stability

From Zancolli, E.: Clin. Orthop. **112**:101, 1975.

sis. These patients usually retain good sensibility in the thumb and adequate sensation of the index finger for satisfactory function.

There are several methods[1-3,5-7] that have been used to restore grasp and lateral pinch in these patients, but two alternative methods are discussed in some detail (Tables 31-1 and 31-2).

Zancolli[10] in 1968 presented his concept of reconstruction for these patients. He performs a tenodesis of the extensor digitorum communis into the radius, providing finger extension as the wrist is flexed. The abductor pollicis longus is rerouted through the third dorsal compartment and joined with the extensor pollicis longus before tenodesis to the dorsum of the distal aspect of the radius, providing balanced thumb extension when the wrist is flexed. An intrinsic tenodesis likewise inserted into the radius was used to prevent clawing. Reconstruction of the flexor plane of the hand was accomplished through transfer of the extensor carpi radialis longus to the flexor digitorum profundus, transfer of the brachioradialis to the flexor pollicis longus, and abduction of the thumb through a tenodesis using the extensor pollicis brevis.

This technique was modified by House and associates[4] using a similar concept of extrinsic tenodesis in the extensor phase but incorporating an intrinsic tenodesis for only the index and middle fingers (Figs. 31-4 and 31-5).

Digital flexion is restored by transfer of the extensor carpi radialis longus to the flexor digitorum profundus, leaving the brachioradialis and pronator teres for use as active transfers to the thumb to restore adduction-opposition and flexion (Figs. 31-6 and 31-7). The pronator teres becomes a useful motor when extended by a strip of periosteum from the radius reinforced with nonabsorbable suture. By employing the paralyzed flexor digitorum superficialis as an in situ tendon graft and using a subcutaneous pulley at the ulnar border of the palmar fascia, the vector of force transmitted to the thumb provides a good position for lateral pinch, the strength of which is further augmented by active transfer of the other available motor to the flexor pollicis longus. A significant problem with this procedure is the development of a flexion deformity at the interphalangeal (IP) joint of the thumb because the thumb extensor tenodesis relaxes as soon as the wrist begins to extend, and the unopposed flexor pollicis longus transfer often will flex the IP joint prematurely. Arthrodesis of the IP joint or tenodesis of the IP joint with a distal slip of the extensor pollicis

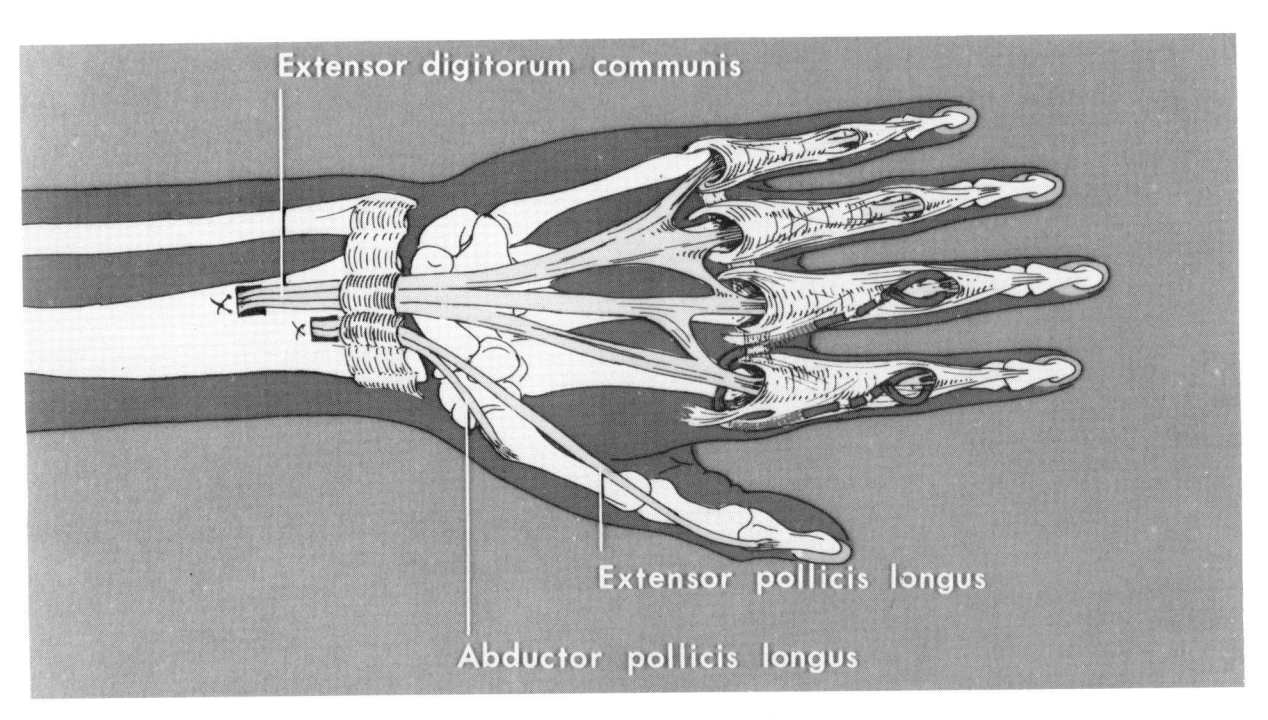

FIG. 31-4. Extensor phase (dorsal view) with tenodesis of extensor digitorum communis, extensor pollicis longus, and rerouted abductor pollicis longus to distal aspect of radius. Free-tendon grafts are routed through lumbrical canals of index and middle fingers, fixed proximally by subperiosteal loop placed dorsally around second metacarpal and sutured distally to extensor hood to produce intrinsic tenodesis. (From House, J.H., Gwathmey, F.W., and Lundsgaard, D.K.: J. Hand Surg. **1**(2):154, 1976.)

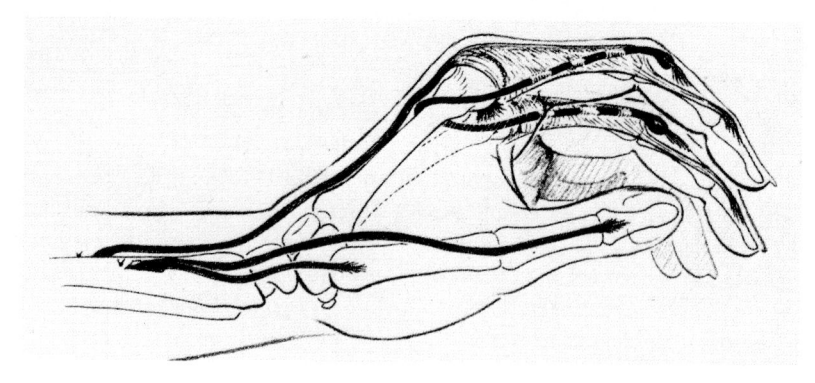

FIG. 31-5. Extensor phase (lateral view). Extrinsic tenodesis produces finger and thumb extension, and intrinsic tenodesis prevents MCP hyperextension and facilitates IP extension when wrist is flexed. (From House, J.H., Gwathmey, F.W., and Lundsgaard, D.K.: J. Hand Surg. **1**(2):154, 1976.)

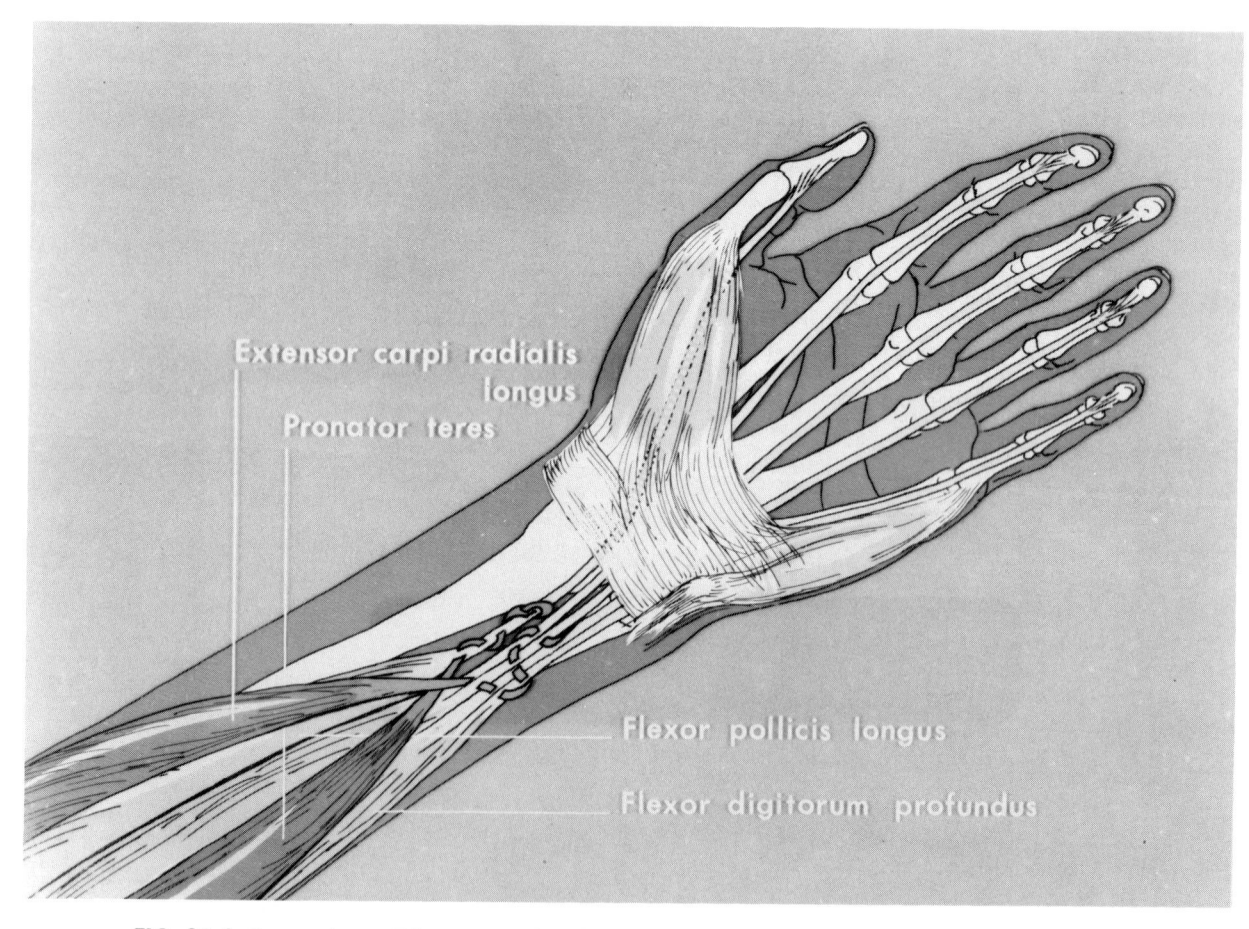

FIG. 31-6. Flexor phase. Extensor carpi radialis longus has been transferred to flexor digitorum profundus and pronator teres to flexor pollicis longus. (From House, J.H., Gwathmey, F.W., and Lundsgaard, D.K.: J. Hand Surg. **1**(2):154, 1976.)

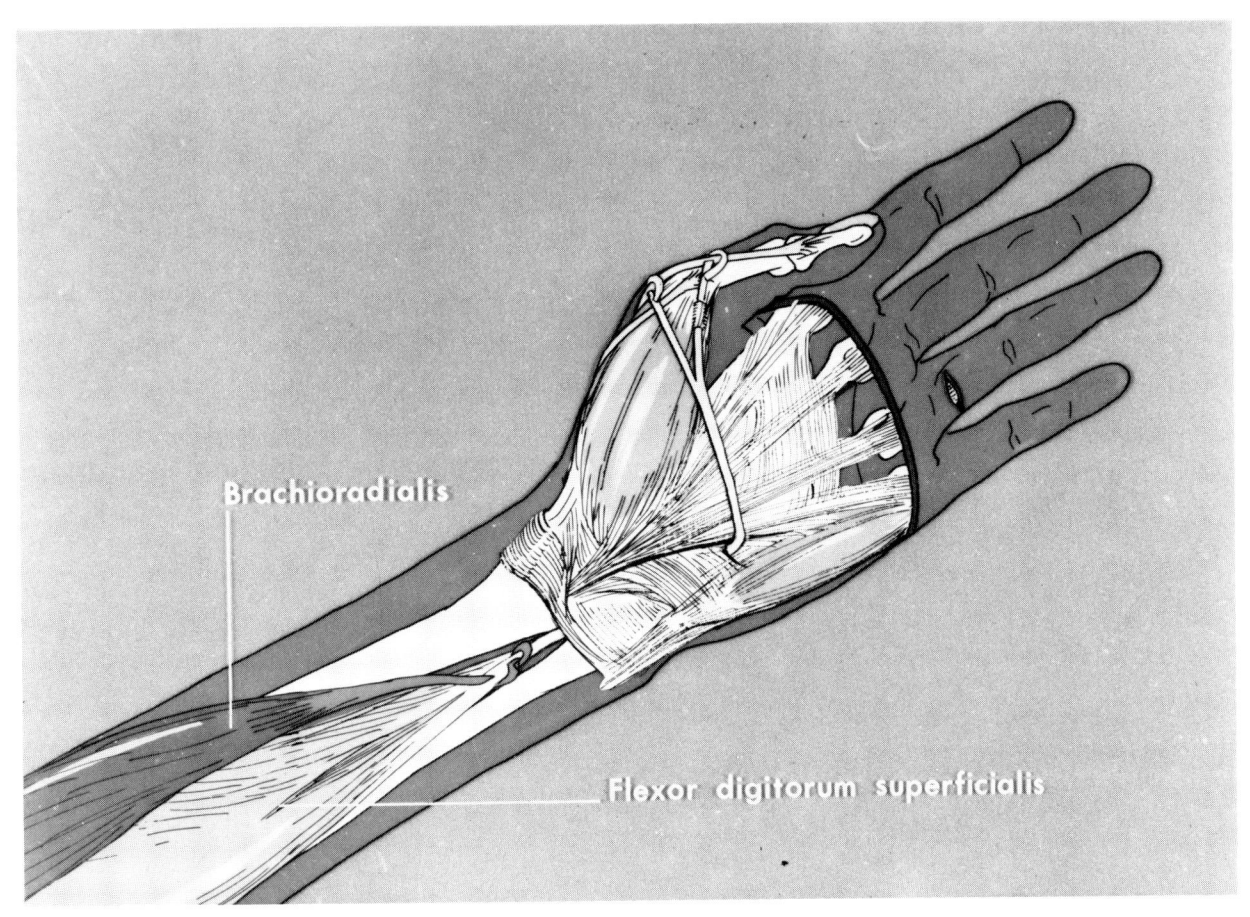

FIG. 31-7. Adduction-opponensplasty. Brachioradialis has been transferred to paralyzed flexor superficialis of ring finger as in situ tendon graft rerouted around palmar fascial pulley to split thumb insertion. (From House, J.H., Gwathmey, F.W., and Lundsgaard, D.K.: J. Hand Surg. **1**(2):154, 1976.)

longus has been used in several patients; however, most patients have adapted to this problem and have learned ways to minimize its functional interference, preferring to maintain their full range of IP flexion.

Zancolli[1] in 1975 introduced the concept of arthrodesis of the CMC joint of the thumb in a position to facilitate lateral pinch, a technique that simplified control of the thumb (Fig. 31-8). Arthrodesis in approximately 45 degrees of palmar abduction and 20 degrees of extension, as measured between the first and second metacarpals, provides a suitable thumb position and prevents the problems of rigidity of the hand associated with the "opponens bone block" procedure that was designed for three-point chuck function described by Nickel and Perry.[9] With the CMC joint fused in the proper position, the thumb still retains sufficient mobility at the adjacent joints to allow the hand to be used in a palm-down position for bed-to-wheelchair transfer. In conjunction with a CMC arthrodesis the brachioradialis can be transferred to the extensor digitorum communis and extensor pollicis longus to provides active digital extension in addition to the tenodesis effect. Transfer of the extensor carpi radialis longus and pronator teres to restore finger and thumb flexion will then provide grasp and lateral pinch. The active thumb extension provided by this method precludes the problem of premature flexion of the thumb that is observed in methods employing only a tenodesis for thumb extension.

The goals of surgery are even more optimistic in the C7 functional group, since the patient retains extrinsic finger extension and often has function of the extensor carpi ulnaris in addition to the muscles present in the strong C6 group. Sensory function of the thumb, index, and middle fingers is usually good. In these patients a "flexor phase," as described in the strong C6 group, is performed. There are usually enough motors present to allow tendon transfers for finger flexion, thumb flexion, and adduction-opposition. The thumb extensor may re-

SECTION 9 TENDON TRANSFER PROBLEMS

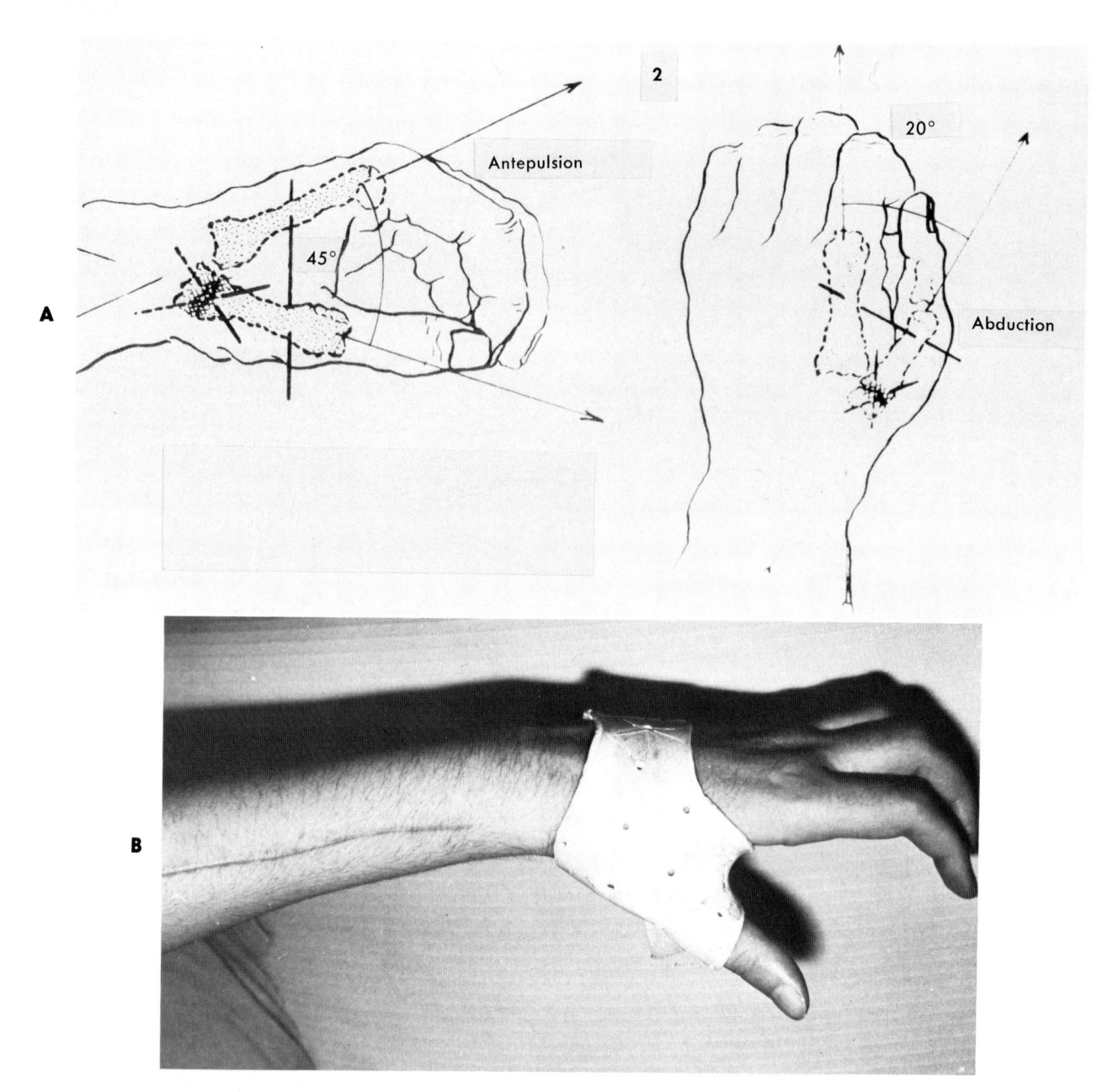

FIG. 31-8. A, Arthrodesis of CMC joint of thumb in this position enables thumb to develop effective lateral pinch with minimum of tendon transfers. **B,** Orthosis is worn to protect CMC joint while active motion of wrist and fingers is begun 4 weeks after surgery. (**A** from Zancolli, E.: Clin. Orthop. **112:**108, 1975.)

quire augmentation through transfer or by suturing it to the extensor digitorum communis. Intrinsic balance may be restored by free grafts from an available motor or by way of an intrinsic tenodesis.

Patients with C8 function usually have fairly good hand function, but tendon transfers to improve the strength of digital flexion, thumb opposition, or intrinsic function may be indicated. In these patients several "motors" are available for transfer to restore active intrinsic functions by "conventional" techniques.

CONCLUSION

There are many procedures that can be done to "change" a quadriplegic patient's function, but it is important that any irreversible procedure be selected only after careful consideration with the patient about how this change will affect the total function. Allowing a prospective patient to meet and talk in detail with a similarly involved patient who has had surgery is particularly valuable in the selection of specific surgical procedures and in establishing realistic goals.

CHAPTER 31 RESTORATION OF LATERAL PINCH IN QUADRIPLEGIA SECONDARY TO SPINAL CORD INJURY

CASE HISTORY

J.D. sustained a cervical spinal cord injury at age 19 in a skiing accident. He retained strong C6 function on the right and C7 function on the left. Fig. 31-9, *A*, demonstrates active extension and Fig. 31-9, *B*, active flexion 1 year after injury.

On the right hand an extensor and intrinsic tenodesis of all five digits was followed in 3 months by transfer of the extensor carpi radialis to the flexor digitorum profundus, the pronator teres to the flexor pollicis longus, and the brachioradialis by way of the ring finger flexor digitorum superficialis to the thumb for adduction-opposition.

Adequate extensor function was present in the left hand, so flexion was restored by transfer of the extensor carpi radialis longus to the flexor digitorum profundus, brachioradialis to the flexor pollicis longus, and flexor carpi ulnaris by way of the ring finger flexor digitorum superficialis to the thumb for adduction-opposition. Five years later the patient exhibited active flexion, extension, and lateral pinch (Fig. 31-9, *C* to *E*). In Fig. 31-9, *D*, note

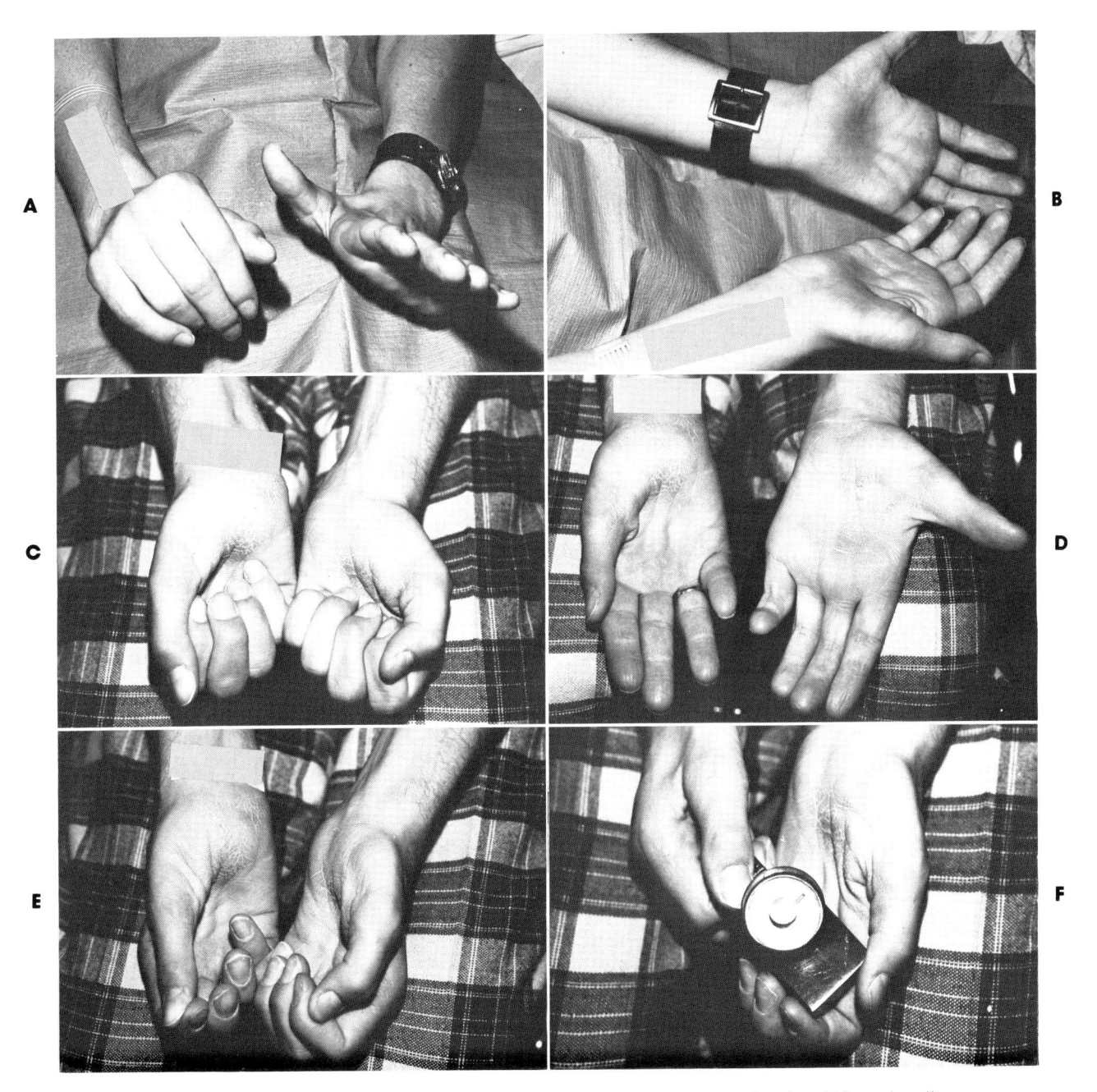

FIG. 31-9. Patient with cervical spinal cord injury displays active extension **(A)** and active flexion **(B)** 1 year after injury. Five years after surgical reconstruction he exhibited active flexion **(C)**, extension **(D)**, and lateral pinch **(E)**. **F,** Patient's key pinch.

Continued.

SECTION 9 TENDON TRANSFER PROBLEMS

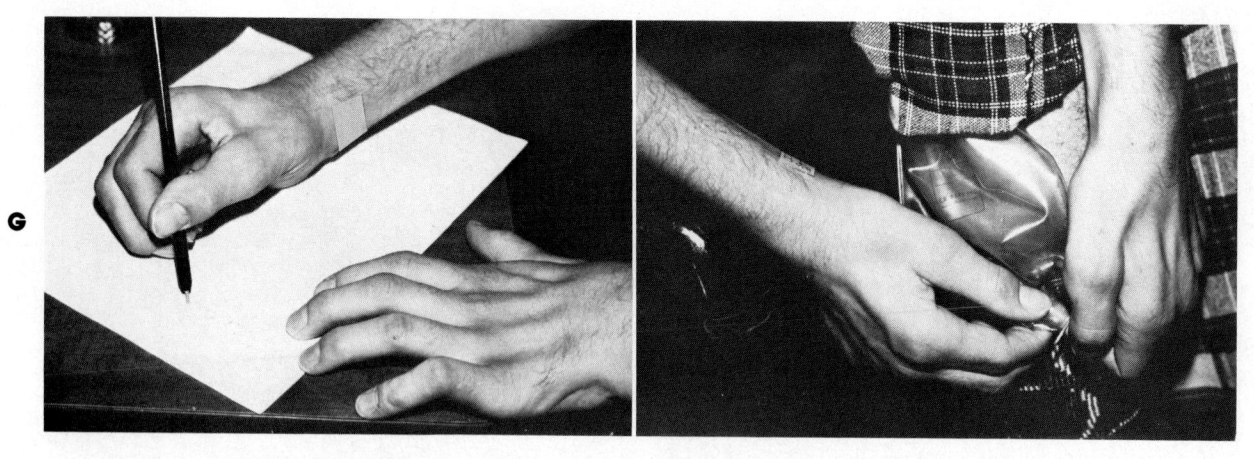

FIG. 31-9, cont'd. G, Patient writing and, **H,** emptying urinary collection bag.

the mild intrinsic-plus deformity on the right and intrinsic-minus deformity on the left, neither of which significantly interferes with function. He has 9.1 kg of grip bilaterally and key pinch of 5.5 kg on the right and 6.8 kg on the left. Fig. 31-9, *F* to *H*, shows the patient's key pinch and his ability to write and empty a urinary collection bag. He is totally independent, drives a car equipped for a paraplegic, and works as a counselor in a rehabilitation institution.

REFERENCES

1. Curtis, R.M.: Tendon transfers in the patient with spinal cord injury, Orthop. Clin. North Am. **5**:414, 1974.
2. Freehafer, A.A.: Tendon transfers to improve grasp after injuries of the cervical spine, J. Bone Joint. Surg. **56A**:951, 1974.
3. Henderson, E.D.: Transfer of wrist extensors and brachioradialis to restore opposition of the thumb, J. Bone Joint Surg. **44A**:513, 1962.
4. House, J., Gwathmay, F.W., and Lundsgaard, D.K.: Restoration of strong grasp and lateral pinch in tetraplegia, J. Hand Surg. **1**(2):154, 1976.
5. Lamb, D.W.: The hand in quadriplegia, Hand **3**:31, 1971.
6. Lipscomb, L.R.: Tendon transfers to restore function of hands in tetraplegia, especially after fracture dislocation of the sixth cervical vertebra in the seventh, J. Bone Joint Surg. **40A**:1061, 1958.
7. Maury, M.: Our experience of upper limb transfers in cases of tetraplegia, J. Paraplegia **11**:245, 1973.
8. Moberg, E.: Surgical treatment for absent simple hand grip and elbow extension in quadriplegia, J. Bone Joint Surg. **57A**:146, 1975.
9. Nickel, V.L.: Development of useful functions in the severely paralyzed hand, J. Bone Joint Surg. **45A**:933, 1963.
10. Zancolli, E.: Structural and dynamic bases of hand surgery, Philadelphia, 1968, J.B. Lippincott Co.
11. Zancolli, E.: Surgery for the quadriplegic hand with active strong wrist extension retained—a study of 97 cases, Clin. Orthop. **112**:101, 1975.

Chapter 32 Low ulnar nerve palsy: evaluation and treatment considerations

Hill Hastings II

Paralysis of the ulnar innervated intrinsic muscles of the hand presents a pattern of muscular imbalance and weakness that is often very disabling. The pattern of deficit may vary according to the patient's age and sex, relative laxity of the articular structures, time elapsed since onset of the palsy, and other associated injuries. Accordingly treatment will vary from one patient to another and depend on a thorough understanding of each patient's deficits, needs, and treatment options.

PATTERN OF INVOLVEMENT AND DEFICIT

The causes of low ulnar nerve palsy vary widely from spinal-muscular disease (e.g., Charcot-Marie-Tooth disease) and infections (e.g., leprosy) to compressive and traumatic injury. Accordingly the extent,stability, or progression of involvement and the prognosis for recovery will vary. The level and mechanism of nerve injury will affect the likelihood for success of later treatment.[40] Patients with intrinsic paralysis from a proximal injury at or above the elbow rarely recover following surgical treatment, except for children. On the other hand, surgical treatment of ulnar nerve injury at the wrist level in many situations may give intrinsic motor return and obviate the need for further reconstructive procedures.

Occasionally complete ulnar nerve lesions may unexpectedly cause little deficit because of anomalous muscle innervations or median nerve branches contributing to the ulnar nerve in the forearm or palm. The forearm median-ulnar nerve communication, described by Martin[31] in 1763 and Gruber[27] in 1870, is relatively common with 15% to 44% incidence.[30,39,45] The communication is more common on the left side and in 26% of cases is bilateral. Although cases have been reported of ulnar to median nerve conveyance of innervation, usually the communication is from median to ulnar.[45] Communication can exist in the palm, as reported by Riche[37] and Cannieu[17] in 1897, but is less common (10% to 15%) and is of less certain significance.[30] Rarely the first dorsal interosseous muscle may have double median and ulnar innervation (2% to 4%).[9,39] Similar double innervation has been reported in the third and fourth lumbricals and in the adductor pollicis.[9,30] Thus the pattern of deformity and functional deficit may vary not only with the cause and time elapsed since injury but also with anomalous innervations and the presence or absence of median-ulnar communications.

INITIAL EVALUATION AND TREATMENT

After initial surgical treatment of the injured nerve a careful, complete examination is made and findings recorded. This should include a careful history and physical examination to determine how well the hand functions and what deficits, if any, are present. Disabilities and symptoms to note include the following:
  A. Impaired strength of grasp
    1. Easy fatigue
    2. Weakness holding hammers and other tools
    3. Difficulty opening jar lids
  B. Impaired strength of pinch
    1. Difficulty opening push-button car doors
    2. Difficulty pinching to turn door keys
    3. Difficulty opening tabs on cans
  C. Impaired sensation: accidental burns to ulnar side of hand and little finger
  D. Inability to assume intrinsic-plus position
    1. Trouble buttoning and unbuttoning shirts
    2. Difficulty picking up coins and other small objects

Active and passive range of motion, grip strength, chuck pinch, and key pinch measurements are made. Record is made of muscles paralyzed, and those still functioning are graded as to their relative strengths. The relative amount of joint ligamentous laxity is noted. Initially metacarpophalangeal (MCP) volar plate tightness may limit hyperextension at this joint and prevent clawing. With time, particularly in patients with ligamentous laxity, the volar plate will become stretched and the MCP joint hyperextended. The common digital extensors will become less effective in extending the interphalangeal (IP) joints, and clawing deformity will become more pronounced. Clawing will be particularly pronounced in low ulnar nerve palsy where still functioning flexor digitorum profundi contribute to IP joint

SECTION 9 TENDON TRANSFER PROBLEMS

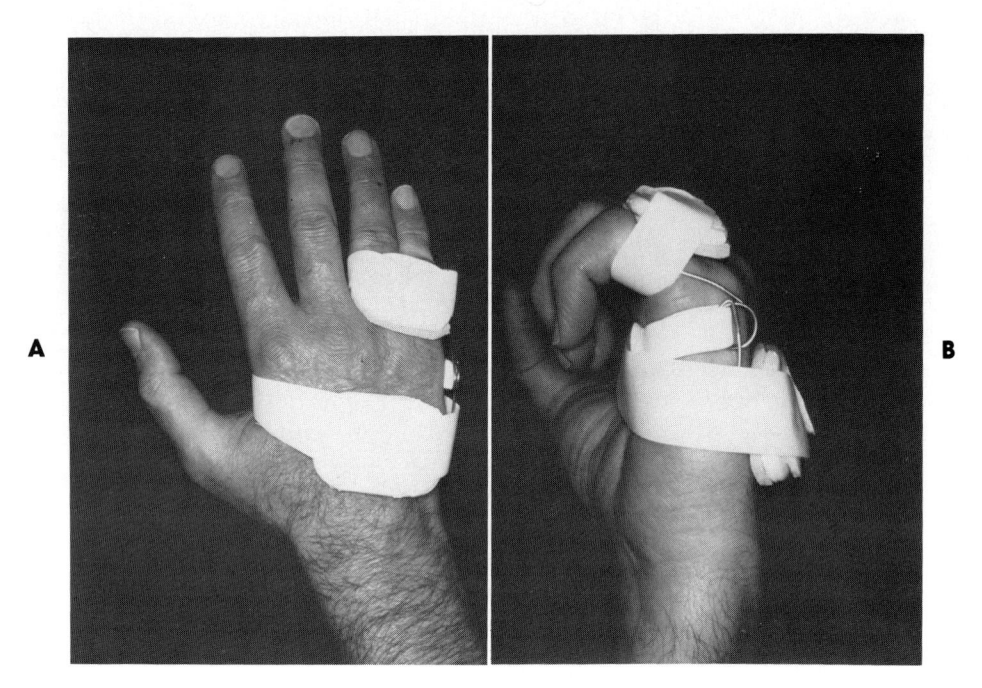

FIG. 32-1. Modified Wynn Parry[21] splint. **A,** This splint prevents hyperextension of ring and little finger MCP joints. **B,** Coil allows active flexion and functional use of splinted hand.

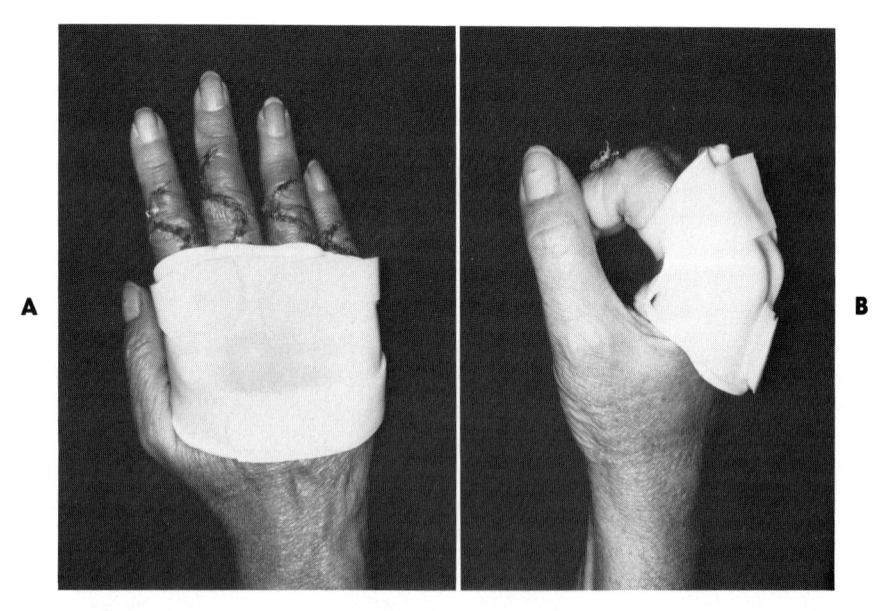

FIG. 32-2. Lumbrical bar splint. **A,** This splint prevents hyperextension at the MCP joints. **B,** Although it is easy to fabricate and allows active MCP joint flexion, this splint is cumbersome to wear.

flexion. Presence or absence of joint contracture is noted. The integrity of the extensor apparatus and the ability of the extensor digitorum communis to extend the IP joints is evaluated while joint hyperextension is prevented.[2]

Splinting therapy

While awaiting return of ulnar intrinsic function or surgical reconstruction, the patient should be fitted with a splint to prevent MCP joint hyperextension. This will allow the pull of the extensor digitorum communis to exert itself more distally to extend the IP joints. Dynamic splints such as the Wynn Parry[21,50] will not only prevent MCP joint hyperextension but also, to some extent, initiate MCP joint flexion (Fig. 32-1). Static splints such as the lumbrical bar[21] act only to prevent MCP joint hyperextension (Fig. 32-2). Only a few patients with stiff joints will successfully avoid hyperextension at the MCP joint and the need for splinting. Most patients should be placed in splints early to prevent deformity, and splinting should be continued until ulnar intrinsic function has returned or has been replaced by surgical reconstruction. No matter how comfortably and well the splint fits, almost all patients will find their total hand function somewhat compromised by the splint. Eventually most will discontinue splint use, and many will require surgical reconstruction.

Patients should be monitored and taught active and passive range of motion exercises to keep their hands supple and free from contracture. If contracture does exist, appropriate corrective splinting and range of motion exercises are carried out to achieve a contracture-free, supple state before surgical reconstructive procedures are undertaken (Figs. 32-3 to 32-5).

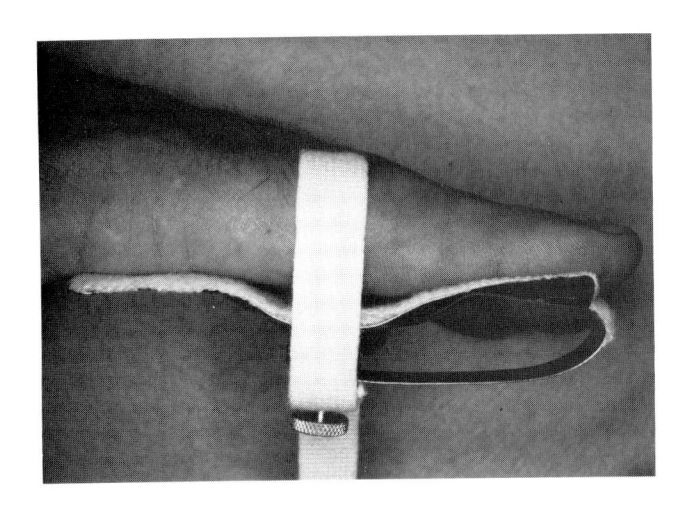

FIG. 32-3. Joint jack splint applies three-point correctional force to this proximal interphalangeal (PIP) joint flexion contracture.

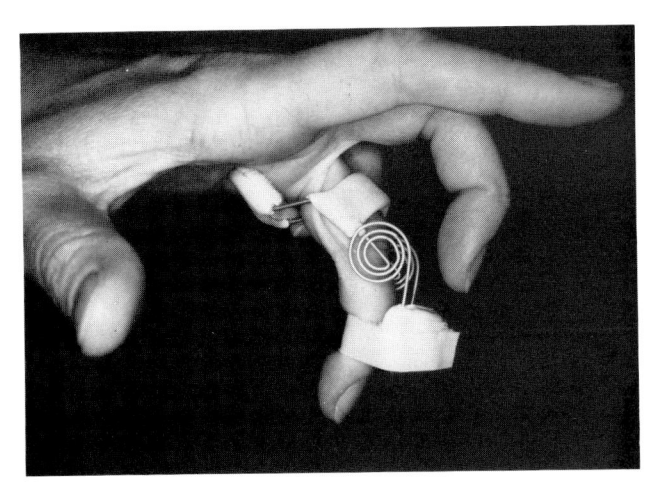

FIG. 32-4. Capener[18] splint dynamically assists extension of PIP joint through its bilateral coil springs.

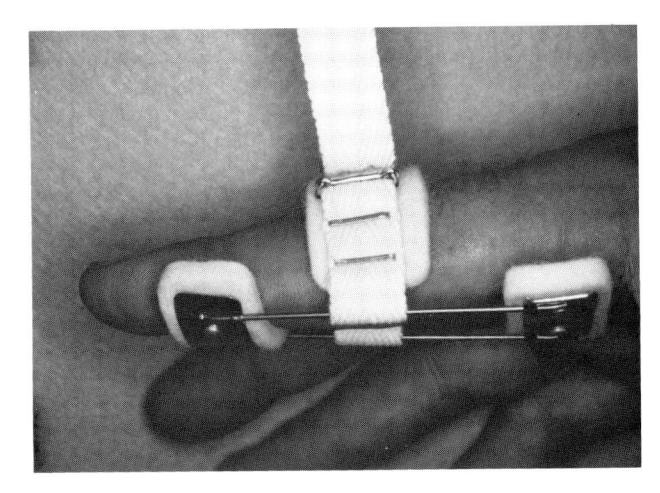

FIG. 32-5. Safety pin splint applies continuous three-point correctional force to this PIP joint flexion contracture.

SECTION 9 TENDON TRANSFER PROBLEMS

SURGICAL TREATMENT

Functional loss and disability in ulnar nerve palsy arises from the following:
1. Loss of sensation
2. Loss of digital abduction and adduction
3. Deformity
4. Weakness of pinch and grasp
5. Asynchronous finger flexion

Loss of sensation

In cases of laceration or other injury to the ulnar nerve current techniques of nerve repair should give at least protective or, it is hoped, close to normal sensory return. Although median nerve sensation is more crucial to hand function, obtaining at least protective ulnar sensation is important. An insensate digit will be used poorly and is prone to burns and other injuries.

Although classic textbooks often report contribution by the ulnar nerve to the dorsal-ulnar half of the middle finger,[34,48] this is rare (3% to 4%).[44] Likewise, contribution to the dorsoradial side of the ring finger is uncommon (16%).[44] On the volar side, ulnar nerve contribution to the middle finger is extremely rare, and contribution to the volar-radial side of the ring finger is present less than 16% of the time.[44] Return of ulnar nerve sensation is important but certainly does not preclude consideration of further reconstructive surgical procedures.

Loss of digital abduction and adduction

Compared with the other functional deficits and deformities of ulnar nerve palsy, loss of the ability to abduct and adduct the digit is usually of little consequence. The most common instances where treatment is considered are (1) a persistently abducted little finger (Wartenberg's sign),[49] (2) partial intrinsic paralysis resulting in imbalance and deviation of a single digit, and (3) weakness of pinch where inability to radially deviate the index and middle fingers contributes to the weakness.

Abducted little finger. An abducted little finger can annoyingly catch while putting one's hand into a pocket,

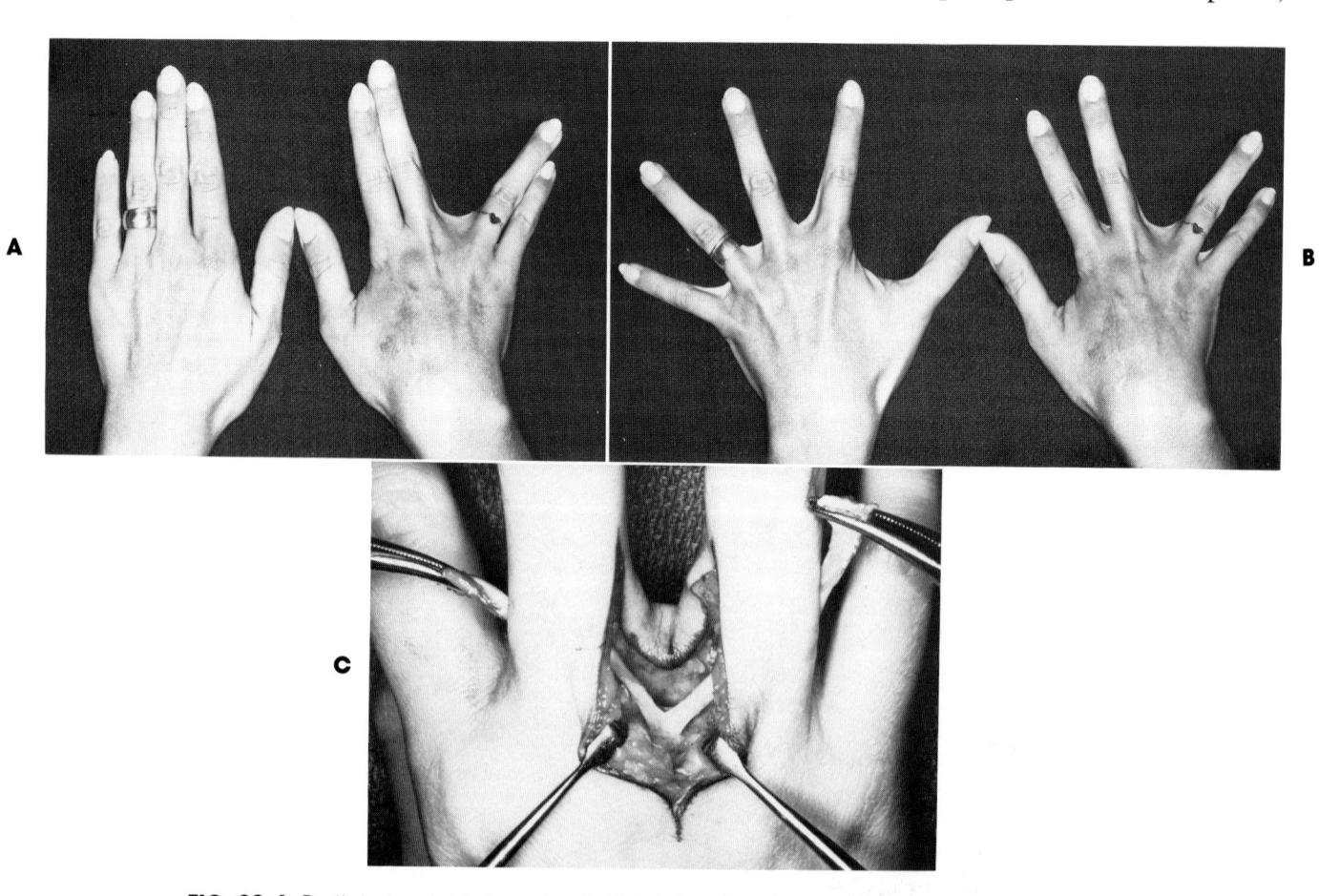

FIG. 32-6. Partial ulnar intrinsic palsy. **A,** Third dorsal and second volar interossei are paralyzed. Patient cannot actively adduct middle and ring fingers. **B,** On attempt to abduct fingers, intrinsic imbalance is still evident. **C,** Tendon transfer of middle finger flexor digitorum superficialis to ulnar side of middle finger and radial side of ring finger. (Courtesy James B. Steichen, M.D.)

shirt sleeve, or any confining space. Depending on how far ulnar to the longitudinal MCP joint axis the extensor digiti minimi tendon inserts, the patient will show varying attitudes of little finger abduction.[1] Corrective procedures depend on the severity of deformity and whether clawing deformity is present. When clawing deformity is present, the extensor digiti minimi tendon is transferred deep to the transverse metacarpal ligament to insert into the radial rim of the flexor tendon sheath over the proximal phalanx.[1,8,22] The deforming abduction force is removed and converted into a correcting adduction and flexion force. When hyperextension of the MCP joint is not significant, simple dorsal tendinous reinsertion of the extensor digiti minimi radial to the longitudinal axis of the MCP joint motion is all that is needed.[1]

Partial ulnar intrinsic palsy. Occasionally partial ulnar intrinsic palsy will affect certain dorsal or volar interossei while sparing others. For example, isolated paralysis of the third dorsal and second volar interossei will cause splaying deformity of the middle and ring fingers on extension (Fig. 32-6, A and B). This can be an annoying and difficult problem to treat. The middle finger flexor digitorum superficialis is transferred dorsal to the transverse intermetacarpal ligament to insert into the ulnar side of the middle finger proximal phalanx and radial side of the ring finger proximal phalanx (Fig. 32-6, C). Correction in these cases eventually may necessitate surgical release of the contracted, scarred, deforming intrinsics as well.

Flexion and radial deviation. Flexion and radial deviation of the index and middle fingers are important components of power pinch (Fig. 32-7). Bunnell's original intrinsic tendon transfer[14] was intended to restore this movement and also that of ulnar deviation. The original Stiles-Bunnell[42] transfer has not been successful. It has subsequently been modified to only correct flexion and radial deviation. Brand[4-6] has recommended insertion of the transfer into the ulnar side of the index finger to better stabilize the index and middle fingers together for chuck pinch. Passing the transfer volar to the intermetacarpal ligament (which is nonexistent on the radial side of the index figer) ensures that the transfer will stay volar to the index finger MCP joint axis. If the Brand transfer is passed through a volar route, such as the carpal canal, it may be inserted safely into the radial lateral band of the index finger as characteristically is done in the remaining digits. Zancolli[52] describes a similar transfer of the flexor digitorum superficialis of the middle finger with split insertions into the first dorsal interosseous and deep fascicle of the second dorsal interosseous muscles. If motors are available, tendon transfer to restore index and middle finger abduction can be done to better restore power pinch. Isolated tendon transfer to replace the first dorsal interosseous,* however, rarely is indicated. If the transfer is done with sufficient power to be effective, an annoying, radially deviated index finger will often result, which also impairs chuck pinch.

---

*References 11, 12, 25, 29, and 53.

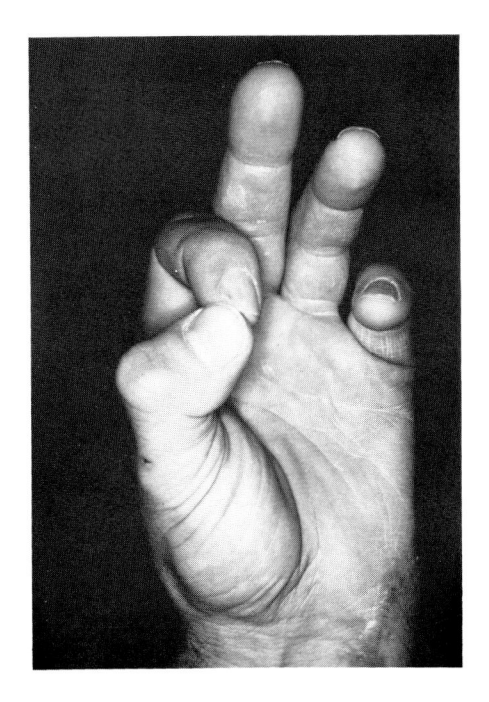

FIG. 32-7. Thumb to index finger pinch is awkward. Longitudinal instability of thumb results in MCP joint extension (Jeanne's sign[28]) and IP joint hyperflexion (Froment's sign[24]).

Deformity

The more significant deformities requiring treatment of low ulnar nerve palsy and their signs are the following:

1. Hyperflexion of thumb IP joint on powerful pinch (Froment's sign[24])
2. Hyperextension of thumb MCP joint on powerful pinch (Jeanne's sign[28])
3. Clawing of ring and little fingers (Duchenne's sign[19,20]) (Fig. 32-10)
4. Inability to actively adduct little finger (Wartenberg's sign[49])
5. Flattened metacarpal arch (Masse's sign[32])

Thirty-two percent of the time the entire flexor pollicis brevis is denervated.[39] Paralysis of the adductor pollicis and all or part of the flexor pollicis brevis severely weakens thumb MCP joint flexion and IP joint extension. Longitudinal stability of the first ray is lost, resulting in the characteristic hyperflexion of the IP joint (Froment's sign[24]) and hyprextension of the MCP joint (Jeanne's sign[28]) on power pinch. (See Fig. 32-7.) The resulting pinch is not only very weak but also awkward. Correction of this deformity will require restoration of powerful pinch, as discussed later. The transverse metacarpal arch of the hand is especially flattened when low median nerve palsy is present along with low ulnar nerve palsy (Masse's sign[32]) (Fig. 32-8). When there is combined low median nerve palsy and low ulnar nerve palsy, a hyperflexion deformity of the index IP joints also will occur, which may require intrinsic tendon transfer to augment the power of IP joint extension (Fig. 32-9).

With low ulnar nerve palsy of recent onset the relative tightness of the MCP joint volar plate may limit the amount of MCP joint extension, and clawing may be absent or very mild. With time the volar plates of the MCP joints will stretch, leading to MCP hyperextension and greater clawing (Fig. 32-10). If this situation persists, the MCP joints may become stiff in extension and the IP joints stiff in flexion. Eventually the extensor digitorum communis central slip over the proximal interphalangeal (PIP) joint will attenuate, and the lateral bands will migrate volar to the axis of joint motion. A permanent contracture at the PIP joint results, eventually leading to skin contracture as well. In an attempt to further augment the force of digital extension, many patients will assume a flexion pattern to their wrist

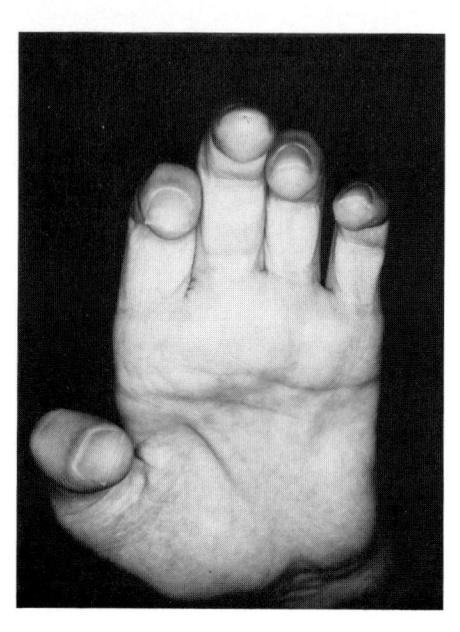

FIG. 32-8. Ulnar nerve palsy when combined with median nerve palsy causes flattening of transverse metacarpal arch (Masse's sign[32]).

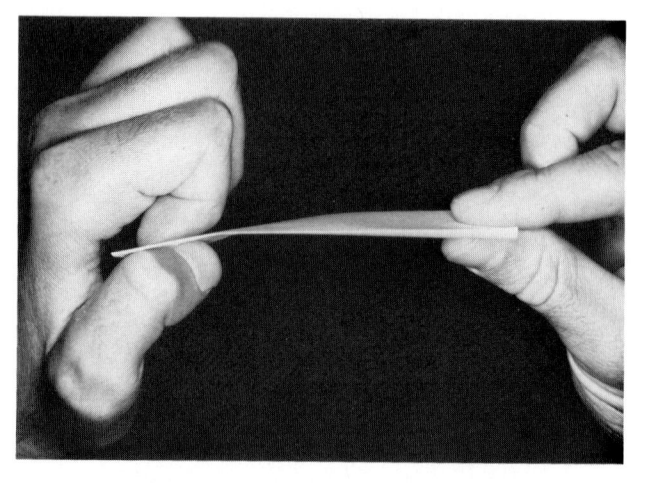

FIG. 32-9. Normal pinch on right compared with that in low median and ulnar nerve paralysis on left.

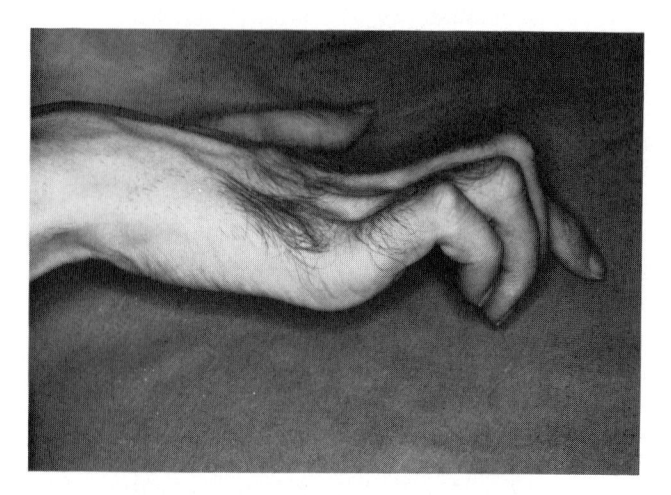

FIG. 32-10. Clawing deformity with marked MCP joint hyperextension and inability to actively extend IP joints.

on extending their fingers. Tendon transfer by the dorsal route to correct clawing deformity in these patients may contribute to the persistence of the wrist volar flexion pattern.

Extension contracture of the MCP joints, when mild, often will respond to dynamic flexion splinting (Fig. 32-11). When contracture is more established, dorsal MCP joint capsulectomy will be required. Dynamic extension splints with a lumbrical bar (Fig. 32-12) often will convert a moderate flexion contracture of the PIP joint to a milder contracture that will respond to safety pin, Capener,[18] or other extension splints. (See Figs. 32-3 to 32-5.) If progress of the spinting program plateaus, then surgical release of the PIP joint volar plate will be necessary. Mild distension of the PIP joint extensor apparatus usually responds to extension splinting. If, however, the distension is severe, then extensor reconstruction plus intrinsic tendon transfer to augment the power of IP joint extension through the lateral bands will be needed. Occasionally flexor tendon contractures or adhesions may be involved, which require tenolysis. *Only once these "complications" or sequelae of claw hand deformity are eliminated can surgical reconstruction for deformity, weakness, and asynchronous finger flexion be performed.*

Weakness of pinch

Procedures to restore power pinch have gained less attention than those for restoration of power grasp. Pinch in ulnar nerve palsy is reduced by over 80% in most patients and is one of the most disabling complaints. Palmar adduction of the thumb is weakened by 75%.[30] Only the extensor pollicis longus serves as a remaining secondary adductor. Even its contribution is lost when the wrist is flexed past 50 degrees, since in this position the extensor pollicis longus shifts radial to the longitudinal axis of the MCP joint.[30] There is little disability in light pinch, since substitution motors are effective. The abductor pollicis brevis and what portion of the flexor pollicis brevis is still innervated both act to flex the MCP joint and extend the IP joint of the thumb. The extensor pollicis longus will adduct and supinate the thumb for light pinch; but with strong pinch the characteristic collapse pattern occurs. The IP joint of the thumb hyperflexes, and at times the MCP joint of the thumb will hyperextend. Some strength of key pinch is preserved through the still functioning flexor pollicis longus; but because of the collapse pattern, the pinch is weak and awkward.

Surgical procedures to restore powerful pinch are indicated only if the adductor pollicis is irreversibly paralyzed and subjectively the patient considers the weakness of pinch to be a functional disability. There should be a supple, adequate first web space and a functioning thumb abductor of good strength. Tendon transfer for restoration of pinch should follow a direct route, have an adequate angle of approach to its insertion, and use a smooth, unyielding pulley.

Procedures that attempt to restore powerful pinch can be divided into those which (1) merely supplement power to the extensor pollicis longus (Table 32-1), (2) replace the transverse head of the adductor pollicis (Table 32-2), or (3) replace the deep head of the flexor pollicis brevis and oblique head of the adductor pollicis (Table 32-3). Tendon transfers that supplement the power of the extensor pollicis longus are the least effective. They have a very oblique, poor angle of approach and transmit very little of their amplitude and force to actual palmar adduction. They add little or no flexion force at the MCP joint of the thumb. A double insertion into the adductor pollicis and first dorsal interosseous slip may

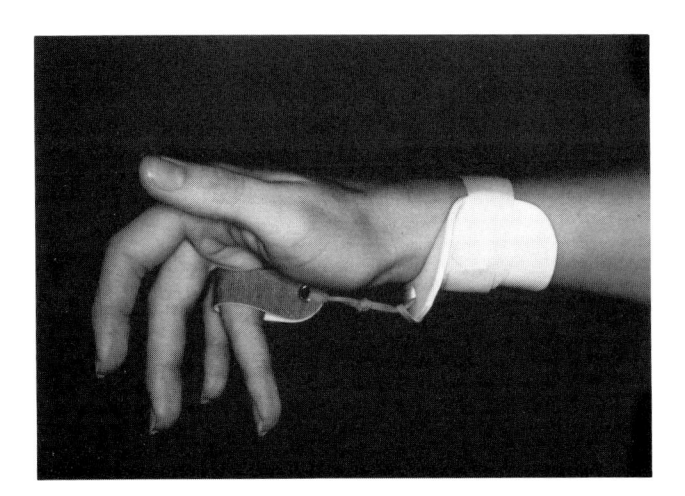

FIG. 32-11. Dynamic MCP joint flexion sling with wrist cuff.

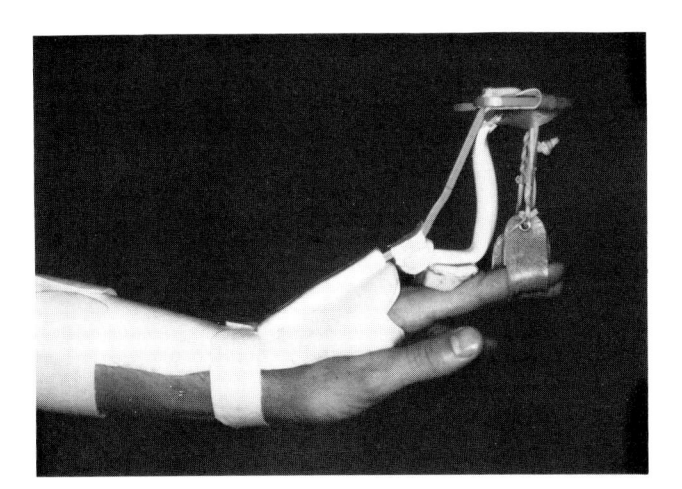

FIG. 32-12. Dynamic extension splint with lumbrical bar. Lumbrical bar prevents MCP joint hyperextension, allowing outriggers to better apply dynamic extension to PIP joints.

SECTION 9 TENDON TRANSFER PROBLEMS

Table 32-1. Tendon transfers for power pinch: supplement to extensor pollicis longus

Motor	Route	Insertion
Dorsal motors		
Extensor digiti minimi[53]	Dorsal aspect of hand	Adductor pollicis and first dorsal interosseous
Extensor digiti minimi[29]	Dorsal aspect of hand	Adductor pollicis
Extensor indicis proprius[35]	Dorsal aspect of hand	Adductor pollicis and first dorsal interosseous
Volar motors		
Flexor digitorum superficialis[26]	Between radius and ulna around extensor carpi ulnaris pulley	Thumb proximal phalanx
Flexor digitorum superficialis[29]	Around radial border of forearm and extensor carpi radialis longus pulley	Adductor pollicis and first dorsal interosseous

Table 32-2. Tendon transfers for power pinch: replacement of transverse head of adductor pollicis

Dorsal motor	Route	Insertion
Extensor carpi radialis brevis with graft[41,43]	Between second and third metacarpals	Adductor pollicis
Brachioradialis or extensor carpi radialis longus with graft[3]	Between third and fourth metacarpals	Adductor pollicis
Extensor indicis proprius[7]	Between second and third metacarpals	Adductor pollicis
Extensor indicis proprius[11,35]	Between third and fourth metacarpals	Adductor pollicis

Table 32-3. Tendon transfers for power pinch: replacement of deep head of flexor pollicis brevis and oblique head of adductor pollicis

Motor	Route	Insertion
Dorsal motors		
Extensor digitorum communis (index finger) with graft[3,14]	Around ulnar border of hand	Adductor pollicis
Extensor pollicis brevis[52]	Through carpal canal	Adductor pollicis
Extensor indicis proprius[52]	1. Around radial wrist, through carpal canal 2. Through interosseous membrane in forearm, through carpal canal 3. Around ulnar wrist	Radial side of thumb extensor apparatus
Volar motors		
Flexor digitorum superficialis[46]	Across palm	Adductor pollicis
Flexor digitorum superficialis[47]	Across palm	Adductor pollicis and extensor pollicis longus
Flexor digitorum superficialis[3,14]	Through carpal canal	Graft between first and fifth metacarpals
Flexor digitorum superficialis (little finger)[52]	Across palm	Adductor pollicis

severely limit the required excursion for adduction of the thumb.

The most effective surgical procedures are those which parallel either the transverse head of the adductor pollicis or oblique head of the adductor pollicis and deep head of the flexor pollicis brevis. Although those transfers which replace the transverse head of the adductor pollicis have the most advantageous angle of approach to restore strength of palmar adduction, they are less effective in restoring flexion stability of the MCP joint. Tendon transfers that replace the deep head of the flexor pollicis brevis and oblique head of the adductor pollicis pass directly over the volar aspect of the MCP joint and are in a better position to stabilize and increase flexion power at this joint. However, they use weaker motors and have a very oblique, poor angle of approach for restoration of palmar adduction.

When powerful pinch is needed, the most effective surgical procedure is tendon transfer to replace the adductor pollicis transverse head, as described by Smith.[41,43] An incision is made over the insertion of the extensor carpi radialis brevis onto the base of the third metacarpal. The tendon is detached, mobilized, and prolonged with a tendon graft of palmaris longus or plantaris. An incision is made along the ulnar side of the thumb MCP joint. The tendon graft then is passed through the second intermetacarpal space, dorsal to the transverse muscle belly of the adductor pollicis, and inserted into the adductor pollicis tendinous insertion. The transfer is sewn into position with the wrist in neutral position and the radial side of the thumb in the plane of the palm. The transfer is immobilized with the wrist in full dorsiflexion and the thumb in abduction. Through insertions of the adductor pollicis, force will be applied to initiate MCP joint flexion and IP joint extension. Stabilizing the IP joint to keep it from assuming a hyperflexed attitude on power pinch will often increase pinch force by at least 907 g (2 pounds).[11] If the transfer itself does not effectively accomplish this, either a separate transfer to augment the flexor pollicis brevis or fusion of the thumb IP joint may be done. Volar transfer as described by Zancolli[52] into the radial intrinsics of the index and middle fingers is indicated if these two fingers are involved with clawing deformity or if their additional contribution to power pinch is desired.

In cases where muscular motors for tendon transfer to restore power pinch are not available, a Zancolli[52] volar plate capsuloplasty of the MCP joint is performed to stabilize the MCP joint in mild flexion. At the same time the first annular pulley at the MCP joint is released to allow bowstringing and increased flexion moment arm. Arthrodesis of the IP joint in 15 degrees of flexion is performed to prevent a Froment's hyperflexion deformity[24] and to transfer the flexion force of the flexor pollicis longus to the MCP joint.

Weakness of grasp

Weakness of grasp is consistently a major complaint among patients with ulnar nerve palsy. With high ulnar nerve palsy, grip strength is decreased by 60% to 80%.[41] Because the strength of the ulnar innervated intrinsics is equal to almost half that of the extrinsic finger flexors,[41] low ulnar nerve palsy also causes significant weakness. Flexion force of the important ring and small fingers is more severely affected than that of the index and middle digits, whose median innervated lumbricals are still functioning. Procedures to augment grip strength do so by either redistributing motors within the hand or bringing new motor strength to the hand.

Asynchronous finger flexion

Patients with low ulnar nerve palsy can only flex the MCP joints of their ring and small fingers after flexion of the more distal joints is almost completed. On the patient's attempt to grasp a large object, the object is pushed out of the palm by the already flexed IP joints. There is also great difficulty in handling small objects. Pulp-to-pulp or pulp-to-side pinch is very awkward, since the distal joint cannot be held extended at the same time that the MCP joint is flexed. (See Figs. 32-9 and 32-10.) Even in patients with nonexistent or minimal clawing deformity the inability to flex the MCP joints independent of IP joint flexion will usually require surgical correction. This disability has been labeled *asynchronous finger flexion*[42] or *rolling finger flexion*.[52]

SURGICAL TREATMENT OF DEFORMITY, WEAKNESS OF GRIP, AND ASYNCHRONOUS FINGER FLEXION

Treatment considerations for deformity, weakness of grip, and asynchronous finger flexion are intricately related and, in planning, need to be considered together. Treatment planning is made according to the clinical-surgical classification proposed by Zancolli.[52] Intrinsic palsy with claw hand deformity is classified on the basis of the *Bouvier*[2] maneuver, or *extrinsic test* (Fig. 32-13). If the extensor digitorum communis tendon can adequately extend the IP joints while MCP joint hyperextension is prevented, this test is considered positive and the claw hand deformity classified as simple. If, despite preventing MCP joint hyperextension, the extrinsic extensor tendons cannot adequately extend the IP joints, the test is negative and the claw hand deformity classified as complicated. *Treatment of claw hand deformity depends on either starting with a simple claw hand deformity or converting a complicated claw hand deformity to one that is considered simple.*

All complications of claw hand deformity must be corrected by therapy or surgery. *Each patient must be individually evaluated and treatment planned according to*

SECTION 9 TENDON TRANSFER PROBLEMS

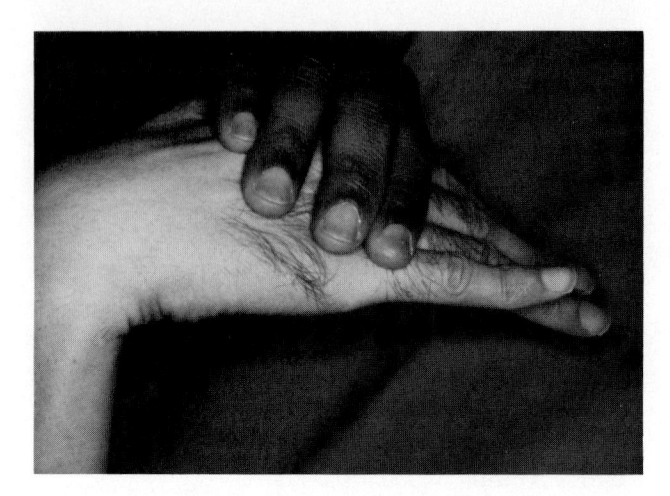

FIG. 32-13. Bouvier[2] maneuver (extrinsic test). In this positive test, prevention of MCP joint hyperextension enables patient in Fig. 32-10 to fully extend IP joints.

the particular variables pertaining to the case, such as the following:
1. Subjective and objective appraisal of the patient's functional disabilities and needs
2. Relative degree of joint laxity
3. Relative degree of clawing deformity
4. Presence or absence of high ulnar or combined motor palsy
5. Availability of donor motors for tendon transfers

Planning appropriate treatment will depend on an understanding of these considerations, a knowledge of the treatment options available, and a sound knowledge of the indications and contraindications for each of the potential procedures.

Motors for tendon transfer not available

In diffuse motor palsy or combined motor paralysis, motors may not be available for restoration of powerful finger flexion or synchronous finger flexion. In these situations the patient and surgeon may have to settle for prevention of clawing deformity alone. Procedures to accomplish this include the following:
A. Splints
  1. Static—lumbrical bar[21]: passively prevents MCP joint hyperextension of ring and little fingers for low ulnar nerve palsy; somewhat awkward to wear
  2. Dynamic
    a. Wynn Parry[21,50]: more comfortable and practical than lumbrical bar; prevents MCP joint hyperextension; by spring action, initiates MCP joint flexion; made for either ring and little fingers or index through little fingers
    b. Dynamic MCP flexion slings[21]: rubber bands attaching volar wrist cuff to slings over proximal phalanges; dynamically flexes MCP joints; impractical since interferes with grasping of objects
B. Surgical procedures
  1. Static
    a. Zancolli[52] volar plate capsuloplasty with bone fixation: simple concept but technically difficult; ideal for diffuse palsy or combined motor palsy without available motors
    b. Fascio-dermadesis[10]: originally used as an adjunct for the initial Zancolli[52] capsuloplasty without bone fixation; no longer needed with new method of volar plate fixation to bone
    c. Howard[15]-Mikhail[33] bone block: bone block graft inserted into metacarpal head to physically prevent hyperextension of the proximal phalanx; use discontinued because of complications with union of the bone graft and interference with joint function
    d. Tenodesis
      (1) Zancolli[52]: tendon graft from metacarpal origin, passing volar to the transverse intermetacarpal ligament, and inserted into the proximal and distal conjoint extensor tendons
      (2) Riordon[38]: portion of extensor carpi radialis longus or extensor carpi ulnaris used as a graft, reflected distally still attached to its insertion, routed through the intermetacarpal spaces, volar to the transverse intermetacarpal ligament, and inserted into the radial lateral bands
  2. Dynamic—tenodesis (Parkes[36]): tendon graft from volar aspect of wrist flexor retinaculum through the lumbrical canals and inserted into radial lateral bands

Howard[15] and later Mikhail[33] described creating a bone block to prevent hyperextension at the MCP joint. This procedure has not worked well. There are several tenodesis procedures that, with active MCP joint extension, act to extend the IP joints by their tenodesis effect. They offer no power to MCP joint flexion. Common to all the tenodesis procedures is a route volar to the transverse intermetacarpal ligament. Fowler's tenodesis[22] has a similar route but, by virtue of its origin proximal to the wrist, can function actively to flex the MCP joint when the wrist is palmar flexed.

Zancolli's initial volar plate capsuloplasty without bony fixation[51] secured the volar plate with the MCP joint in 20 degrees of flexion. More than 6% of these cases relapsed into recurrent hyperextension at the

Table 32-4. Procedures to prevent clawing deformity, provide synchronous MCP and IP motion, and augment power of MCP joint flexion

Procedure	Donor	Route	Insertion
Mild strength contribution			
Bunnell[13] and Fowler[22]	Extensor indicis proprius, extensor digiti minimi	Through intermetacarpal spaces, volar to transverse intermetacarpal ligament	Radial lateral bands
Fritschi[23] (palmaris longus)	Palmaris longus with tendon graft	Through lumbrical canals	Lateral bands
Moderate strength contribution			
Zancolli[52] lasso	Flexor digitorum superficialis	Lasso around A₁ pulley	Lasso around A₁ pulley into itself proximally
Modified Stiles-Bunnell[14]	Flexor digitorum superficialis	Through lumbrical canals	Radial lateral bands (ring and little fingers)
Greatest strength contribution			
Brand[4-6]	Extensor carpi radialis brevis or longus with tendon graft	Dorsal, through intermetacarpal spaces, volar to transverse intermetacarpal ligaments	Lateral bands
		Volar, through carpal canal, through lumbrical canals	Lateral bands
Burkhalter and Strait[16]	Extensor carpi radialis brevis or longus with tendon graft	Dorsal, through intermetacarpal spaces, volar to transverse intermetacarpal ligaments	Lateral bands
Brooks and Jones[8]	Flexor carpi radialis with tendon graft	Volar, through carpal canal	A₁ pulley
Riordan[38]	Flexor carpi radialis with tendon graft	Dorsal, through intermetacarpal spaces, volar to transverse intermetacarpal ligaments	Lateral bands

MCP joint.[52] The procedure was modified to include the additional incision of 2 cm of dermis or excision of fascia and dermis.[10] The procedure, as now done by Zancolli[52] with bony fixation of the volar plate, is very simple by design, technically difficult, but yields predictable, excellent results. The Zancolli volar plate capsuloplasty with bony fixation is the procedure of choice when motors for tendon transfer are not available. The flexor tendon sheath is opened over the MCP joint, and a longitudinal incision is made in the volar plate. The volar plate is detached proximally from its metacarpal neck origin, advanced proximally, and fixed directly into bone with the MCP joint flexed 5 degrees. Postoperatively the patient is placed in a cast for 5 to 6 weeks with the MCP joint protectively flexed 30 degrees and the IP joints free to flex and extend. With this procedure clawing deformity, even when severe, is corrected. This procedure does not restore power or synchrony to finger flexion.

Motors for tendon transfer available

When motors are available for tendon transfer, reconstruction to prevent clawing, provide power for finger flexion, and provide MCP joint flexion independent of IP flexion can and should be done. If there is a high ulnar nerve palsy or combined ulnar and median nerve palsy, weakness will be substantial. Additional motors to provide power for finger flexion will be needed. When only low ulnar nerve palsy is present, weakness will be less disabling, and using local motors from each finger is simpler, more predictable, and usually quite adequate. If the aforementioned deformity complications of ulnar nerve palsy are successfully treated prior to tendon transfer, there is no need to insert the transfer into the extensor apparatus. Prevention of MCP joint hyperextension and provision for increased force of MCP flexion alone will suffice. There is less risk of inducing scarring and dysfunction of the extensor apparatus and little to no risk of creating muscular imbalance and hyperextension at the PIP joint. Insertion of the tendon transfer into the lateral bands is needed only when attempts to correct or convert a complicated claw hand deformity to a simple claw hand deformity have been unsuccessful and there remains an extension lag at the PIP joint on Bouvier[2] maneuver. Insertion into the lateral bands is contraindicated when the patient has hypermobile lax fingers. All the procedures listed in Table 32-4 will successfully correct clawing, restore the ability to flex the MCP joint independent of IP joint flexion, and restore a varying amount of power to MCP joint flexion.

Reconstruction of mild grasp strength

Patients with low ulnar nerve palsy and low demands for grasp strength can be successfully treated by many of the procedures for mild strength listed in Table 32-4. In most situations tendon transfers with greater strength contribution can be used and are preferable. The extensor indicis proprius and the extensor digiti minimi tendon transfers[13,22] are best used when there is little or no need for increased grip strength and more powerful motors are not available. Since in many hands the extensor digiti minimi is the only significant extensor of the little finger MCP joint, transfer of this tendon should be avoided if possible. In addition, its length is usually inadequate for transfer into a more distal insertion. The extensor indicis proprius is more expendable and has greater length for transfer to the ring and little fingers. It is particularly useful when there has been scarring along the volar side of the wrist and hand or when the flexor digitorum superficialis is unsuitable for transfer because of a previous laceration or scar.

Reconstruction of moderate grasp strength

When tendon transfer to provide better strength for MCP joint flexion is possible, either the Zancolli[52] lasso procedure or the modified Stiles-Bunnell procedure[14] can be used. The Zancolli lasso procedure is somewhat simpler to perform, is more predictable, and provides greater strength for MCP joint flexion because of its increased moment arm. In most cases this is the treatment of choice for low ulnar nerve palsy. The modified Stiles-Bunnell tendon transfer is contraindicated when the PIP joints are hyperextensible and lax or when weakness of grip is a major complaint. PIP joint hyperextension deformity after the modified Stiles-Bunnell procedure can be avoided by transfer of the flexor digitorum superficialis of the middle finger to the ring and little fingers in low ulnar nerve palsy and by leaving an adequate proximal stump of the flexor digitorum superficialis at the PIP joint to adhere and prevent hyperextension. Burkhalter and Strait's modification[16] of the Stiles-Bunnell procedure avoids some of these disadvantages by using a bony insertion. Both the Zancolli lasso procedure and the modified Stiles-Bunnell procedure are of no use in high ulnar nerve or ulnar and median nerve palsy where weakness is substantial. Neither procedure can be used in cases of extensive scarring or injury to the flexor digitorum superficialis in the wrist or hand, in Volkmann's contracture with compromise to the flexor digitorum superficialis motors, or when a wrist flexion contracture weakens the effectiveness of these potential donor muscles.

The Zancolli[52] lasso procedure is carried out by making an incision between the A_1 and A_2 pulleys, dividing the flexor digitorum superficialis just distal to its decussation into two slips, bringing the flexor digitorum superficialis out of the sheath between the A_1 and A_2 pulleys, and sewing it back onto itself proximal to the A_1 pulley. The tension is set at full passive distraction excursion while the MCP joint is held in neutral position. Slightly less tension is used in the lax hand and slightly greater tension in the hand with stiffness at the PIP joint. Ideally the flexor digitorum superficialis is used in transfer to the same digit to retain greater flexion power and independence of function. Postoperatively the patient is immobilized in a short-arm plaster cast with the wrist in neutral position and the MCP joints flexed 20 degrees. The IP joints are left free to move, minimizing the risk of stiffness at these joints.

The modified Stiles-Bunnell procedure[14] in low ulnar nerve palsy is preferably done using the flexor digitorum superficialis of the middle finger in transfer to the ring and little fingers. Incision is made along the distal palmar crease from the middle finger to the little finger with proximal extension to the midpalm. The flexor tendon sheath is opened proximal to the A_1 pulley, and the flexor digitorum superficialis is identified. The tendon is retracted proximally and divided just distal to its decussation. In the midpalm the tendon is withdrawn from the sheath of the middle finger, split into two slips, and directed out through the respective lumbrical canals of the ring and little fingers. A separate incision is made dorsoradially over the proximal aspect of each finger, and the transfer is inserted into the radial lateral bands of the ring and little fingers. Particular care is taken in suturing the transfer to the extensor apparatus to avoid injury to the periosteum, which would later limit excursion of the oblique lateral band fibers. The transfer is sewn in with no tension while the wrist and MCP joints are held fully flexed. Tension should not be so excessive that full passive extension of the fingers cannot be achieved. In stiffer fingers greater tension is used. Postoperatively the patient is protected with the wrist in neutral position and the MCP joints fully flexed. Although the insertion is into the lateral bands, relaxation is sufficient to allow for active PIP joint motion during the immobilization period.

Reconstruction of maximal grasp strength or in cases of high ulnar or combined palsy

When there is high ulnar nerve palsy, combined median and ulnar nerve palsy, or when maximal restoration of grasp strength is needed, a more powerful motor such as a wrist extensor or flexor is needed. The Brand[4-6] transfer uses the extensor carpi radialis brevis or extensor carpi radialis longus prolonged with a "four-tailed" plantaris graft that is passed from the dorsal aspect of the hand, through the intermetacarpal spaces, volar to the transverse intermetacarpal ligaments, and inserted into

CHAPTER 32   LOW ULNAR NERVE PALSY: EVALUATION AND TREATMENT CONSIDERATIONS

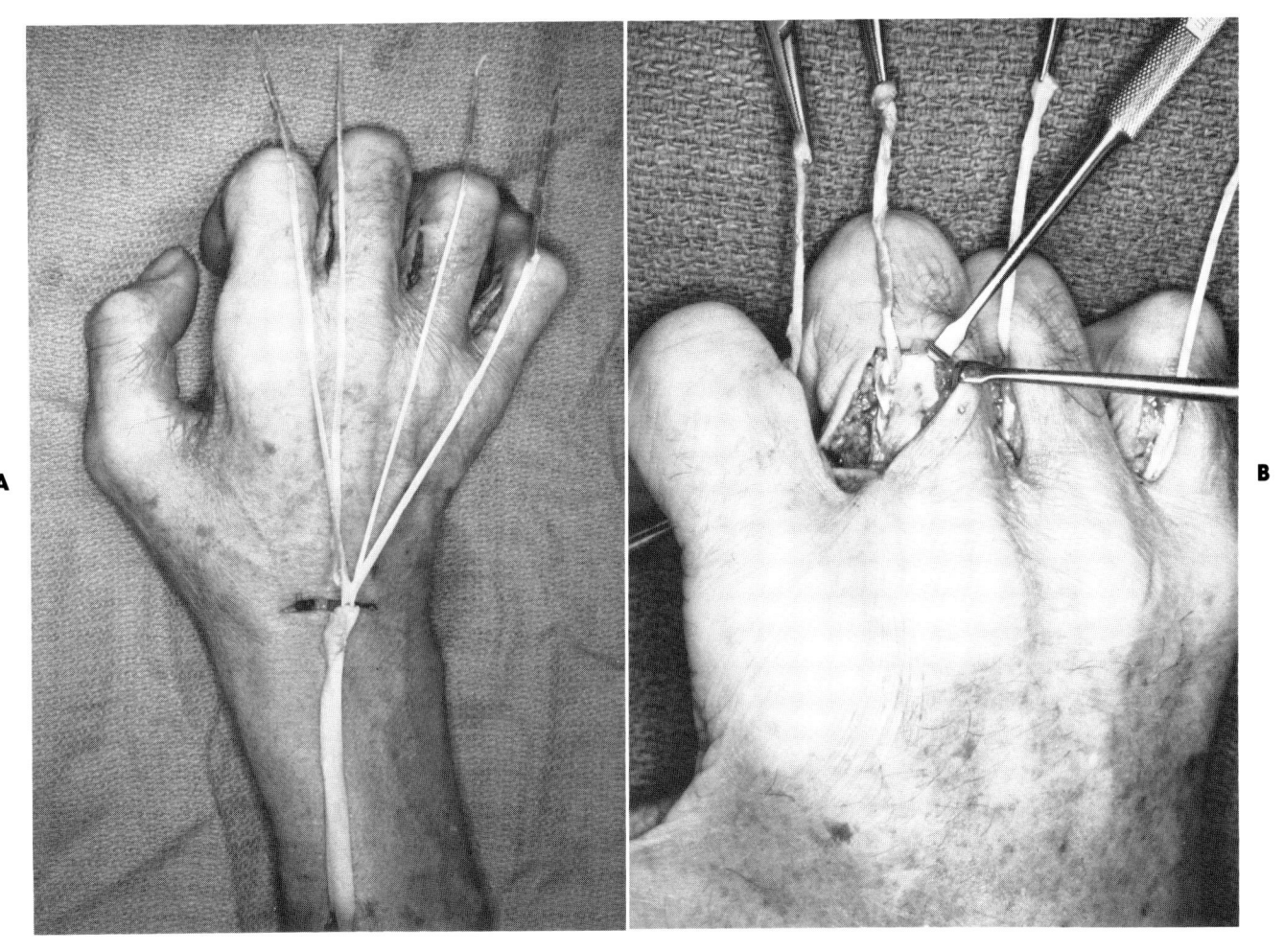

FIG. 32-14. Brand[4-6] intrinsic tendon transfer (dorsal route). **A,** Extensor carpi radialis brevis is prolonged with "four-tailed" plantaris tendon graft. **B,** Tendon grafts are sewn into index ulnar lateral band and radial lateral bands of middle, ring, and little fingers. (Courtesy James B. Steichen, M.D.)

the ulnar lateral band of the index finger and radial lateral bands of the middle, ring, and little fingers (Fig. 32-14). The dorsal route is particularly useful when there has been a Volkmann flexion contracture or scarring through the volar wrist area. Patients with long-standing ulnar nerve palsy often will markedly flex their wrist while extending their fingers.[42] Because this transfer removes a wrist dorsiflexor and also has an additive tenodesis effect with volar flexion of the wrist, this pattern of wrist flexion may be accentuated. In addition, this dorsal route transfer is prone to adhesions at its course through the intermetacarpal spaces. Because of this, it is more advantageous to bring the transfer volar through the carpal canal. Since the transfer is volar to the axis of the MCP joint, it may be safely inserted into the radial lateral band of the index finger for greater stabilization of the index on pinch without fear of it slipping dorsal to the joint axis. The volar route is particularly useful in patients who have developed a volar flexion wrist pattern on digital extension. Theoretically, because it increases the volume within the carpal canal, compression of the median nerve in this area is possible. It cannot be used when there is marked scarring within the volar wrist area. Burkhalter and Strait[16] have advised bony insertion of the four-tailed grafts into the proximal third of the proximal phalanx, which provides a greater moment arm for MCP joint flexion and has no risk of producing PIP joint hyperextension. If the power of wrist dorsiflexion is impaired, a volar wrist motor such as the flexor carpi radialis is used to avoid weakening the wrist by use of a dorsiflexion motor.[8,38]

CONCLUSIONS

Ulnar nerve injury is a result of a variety of causes. Despite modern techniques of decompression and neurorrhaphy, full return of intrinsic motor function is still unusual. Even though gross finger extension and flexion are preserved, the unique balance between the extrinsic extensors and flexors is disrupted and fine coordination of the IP joints lost. In many patients functional disability will be profound.

The diversity of reconstructive procedures reflects the extent and great variability of involvement seen. The reconstructive surgeon must have a solid understanding of the pathomechanics involved and a knowledge of the treatment options available and their relative indications and contraindications. A thoughtful evaluation of each patient and appropriate treatment will successfully restore balance and strength to the hand.

REFERENCES

1. Blacker, G.J., Lister, G.D., and Kleinert, H.E.: The abducted little finger in low ulnar nerve palsy, J. Hand Surg. **1**:190, 1976.
2. Bouvier, M.: Note sur une paralysie partielle des muscles de la main, Bull. Acad. Nat. Med. **18**:125, 1851.
3. Boyes, J.H.: Bunnell's surgery of the hand, ed. 5, Philadelphia, 1970, J.B. Lippincott Co.
4. Brand, P.W.: Paralytic clawhand with special reference to paralysis in leprosy and treatment by the sublimis transfer of Stiles and Bunnell, J. Bone Joint Surg. **40B**:618, 1958.
5. Brand, P.W.: Tendon grafting illustrated by a new operation for intrinsic paralysis of the fingers, J. Bone Joint Surg. **43B**:444, 1961.
6. Brand, P.W.: Deformity in leprosy. In Cochrane, R.G., and Devey, T.F., editors: Leprosy in theory and practice, ed. 2, Bristol, England, 1964, John Wright & Sons, Ltd.
7. Brand, P.W.: Tendon transfers for median and ulnar nerve paralysis, Orthop. Clin. North Am. **1**:447, 1970.
8. Brooks, A.L., and Jones, D.S.: A new intrinsic tendon transfer for the paralytic hand, J. Bone Joint Surg. **57A**:730, 1975.
9. Brooks, H.S.: Variations in the nerve supply of the lumbrical muscles in the hand and foot, with some observations on the innervation of the perforating flexors, J. Anat. Physiol. **21**:575, 1887.
10. Brown, P.W.: Zancolli capsulorrhaphy for ulnar claw hand, J. Bone Joint Surg. **52A**:868, 1970.
11. Brown, P.W.: Reconstruction for pinch in ulnar intrinsic palsy, Orthop. Clin. North Am. **5**:233, 1974.
12. Bruner, J.M.: Tendon transfer to restore abduction of the index finger using the extensor pollicis brevis, Plast. Reconstr. Surg. **3**:197, 1948.
13. Bunnell, S.: Repair of tendons in the fingers and description of two new instruments, Surg. Gynecol. Obstet. **26**:103, 1918.
14. Bunnell, S.: Surgery of the intrinsic muscles of the hand other than those producing opposition of the thumb, J. Bone Joint Surg. **24**:1, 1942.
15. Bunnell, S.: Surgery of the hand, Philadelphia, 1944, J.B. Lippincott Co.
16. Burkhalter, W.E., and Strait, J.L.: Metacarpophalangeal flexor replacement for intrinsic-muscle paralysis, J. Bone Joint Surg. **55A**:1667, 1973.
17. Cannieu, J.M.A.: Note sur une anastomose entre la branche profunde du cubital et le median, Bull. Soc. Anat. Physiol. **18**:339, 1897.
18. Capener, N.: Lively splints, Physiotherapy **53**:371, 1967.
19. Duchenne, G.B.: Reserches electro-physiologiques et pathologiques sur les muscles de la main, et sur les extenseurs communs des doigts, extenseurs propes de l'index et du petit doigt, Arch. Gen. Med. **25**:361, 1851.
20. Duchenne, G.B.: Physiology of motion, Philadelphia, 1949, J.B. Lippincott Co. (Translated by E.B. Kaplan.)
21. Fess, E.W., Gettle, K.S., and Strickland, J.W.: Hand splinting, principles and methods, ed. 1, St. Louis, 1981, The C.V. Mosby Co.
22. Fowler, S.B.: Extensor apparatus of the digits, J. Bone Joint Surg. **31B**:477, 1949.
23. Fritschi, E.P.: Reconstructive surgery in leprosy, Baltimore, 1971, William & Wilkins Co.
24. Froment, J.: La paralysie de l'adducteur du pouce et le signe de le prehension, Rev. Neurol. **28**:1236, 1914.
25. Goldner, J.L.: Deformities of the hand incidental to pathological changes of the extensor and intrinsic muscle mechanisms, J. Bone Joint Surg. **35A**:115, 1953.
26. Goldner, J.L.: Tendon transfers in rheumatoid arthritis, Orthop. Clin. North Am. **5**:425, 1974.
27. Gruber, W.: Über die Verbindung des Nervus medianus mit dem Nervus ulnaris am Unterarme des Menschen und der Säugethiere, Arch. Anat. Physiol. Med. Leipzig **37**:501, 1870.
28. Jeanne, M.: La déformation du pouce dans la paralysie cubitale, Bull. Mem. Soc. Chir. **41**:703, 1915.
29. Littler, J.W.: Tendon transfers and arthrodeses in combined median and ulnar nerve paralyses, J. Bone Joint Surg. **31A**:225, 1949.
30. Mannerfelt, L.: Studies on the hand in ulnar nerve paralysis, Acta Orthop. Scand (Suppl.) **87**:4, 1966.
31. Martin, R.: Tal om Nervers allmänna Egenska per i Människans Kropp, Stockholm, 1763, L. Salvius.
32. Masse, L.: Contribution a l'étude de l'achon des interosseus, J. Med. (Bordeaux) **46**:198, 1916.
33. Mikhail, I.: Bone block operation for claw hand, Surg. Gynecol. Obstet. **118**:1077, 1964.
34. Monrad-Krohn, G.H.: Clinical examination of the nervous system, ed. 9, London, 1948, H.K. Lewis & Co., Ltd.
35. Omer, G.: Tendon transfers in combined nerve lesions, Orthop. Clin. North Am. **5**:377, 1974.
36. Parkes, A.R.: Paralytic claw fingers—a graft tenodesis operation, Hand **5**:192, 1973.
37. Riche, P.: Le nerf cubital et les muscles de l'éminence thénar, Bull. Mem. Soc. Anat. **5**:251, 1897.
38. Riordan, D.C.: Surgery of the paralytic hand. In American Academy of Orthopaedic Surgeons: Instructional Course Lectures, vol. 16, St. Louis, 1959, The C.V. Mosby Co.
39. Rowntree, T.: Anomalous innervation of the hand muscles, J. Bone Joint Surg. **31B**:505, 1949.
40. Seddon, H.T.: Surgical disorders of the peripheral nerves, ed. 1, Baltimore, 1972, Williams & Wilkins Co.
41. Smith, R.J., and Hastings, H.: Principles of tendon transfer to the hand. In American Academy of Orthopaedic Surgeons: Instructional Course Lectures, vol. 29, St. Louis, 1980, The C.V. Mosby Co.

42. Smith, R.J.: Surgical treatment of the clawhand. In American Academy of Orthopaedic Surgeons: Symposium on Tendon Surgery in the Hand, St. Louis, 1975, The C.V. Mosby Co.
43. Smith, R.J.: ECRB adductor-plasty, Presented to the American Society for Surgery of the Hand, Las Vegas, Feb. 24, 1981.
44. Stopford, J.S.B.: The variation in distribution of the cutaneous nerves of the hand and digits, J. Anat. **53**:14, 1918.
45. Sunderland, S.: Nerves and nerve injuries, ed. 2, Edinburgh, 1978, Churchill Livingstone.
46. Thompson, T.C.: A modified operation for opponens paralysis, J. Bone Joint Surg. **24**:632, 1942.
47. Tubiana, R.: Anatomic and physiologic basis for the surgical treatment of paralysis of the hand, J. Bone Joint Surg. **51A**:643, 1969.
48. Von Lanz, T., and Wachsmuth, W.: Praktische anatomie, arm, vol. 1, Berlin, 1959, Springer-Verlag.
49. Wartenberg, R.: A sign of ulnar palsy, J.A.M.A. **112**:1688, 1939.
50. Wynn Parry, C.B., et al.: New types of lively splints for peripheral nerve lesions affecting the hand, Hand **2**:31, 1970.
51. Zancolli, E.A.: Claw-hand caused by paralysis of the intrinsic muscles, J. Bone Joint Surg. **39A**:1076, 1957.
52. Zancolli, E.A.: Structural and dynamic bases of hand surgery, ed. 2, Philadelphia, 1979, J.B. Lippincott Co.
53. Zweig, J., Rosenthal, S., and Burns, H.: Transfer of the extensor digiti quinti to restore pinch in ulnar palsy of the hand, J. Bone Joint Surg. **54A**:51, 1972.

Chapter 33 Hand reconstruction and tendon transfer problems

H. Kirk Watson

THE HAND AS A MECHANICAL UNIT

The rebuilding of the hand is accomplished considering it as a mechanical unit. The purely mechanical aspect of the hand may be divided into three basic components: pinch, space grasp, and placement. Pinch is obvious; it entails the ability of two sections of the hand to meet under control and power for the manipulation of objects.

Space grasp is not curently given the importance that it deserves. Space grasp is the ability to encompass the largest object possible for that hand. It is usually the injured hand or the less-developed hand (in cases of congenital abnormalities) that requires the greatest possible space grasp ability. It is this assisting hand which will hold objects so that specific manipulations and functions (e.g., winding a clock) may be carried out by the more normal hand. It is the assisting hand that requires space grasp to hold the clock while the winding and setting are one by the more dexterous, normal hand. A factory worker often must hold an object in one hand while working on it with the other. There should be an increased emphasis on the development of space grasp capabilities in the more injured or deficient hand. Pollicization, for instance, should be carried out on the assisting hand as well as on the major hand.

The third mechanical component is placement. Any reconstruction of mechanics of the hand must include consideration of the patient's ability to place the reconstructed hand in various functional positions in relation to the body and its surroundings.

"LABORER" PHILOSOPHY

The philosophy of the "laborer" relates to all hand surgery, not just tendon transfers. With the development of widely applied compensation laws, the increase in wages, and the increase in leisure time, the laborer concept, i.e., returning the patient to work in a week or two regardless of the reconstruction principles of hand surgery, has become obsolete. Most "laborers" have several weeks a year for vacation time, play golf, or are active with their particular hobbies on weekends and holidays and have activities outside of the laborer capacity that require the very best in hand function capability. This label can no longer be used as an excuse for expeditious but less than optimal reconstruction of the hand.

TENDON TRANSFER SURGERY

The motions of the hand belong to basically one of two categories: prefunctional or functional activities. This distinction separates the kinds of hand and finger activity that require very little power and are essentially prepositioning activities from the power function. An example that brings to light several prefunctional activities is a person about to take a half gallon of milk from the refrigerator. Finger extension and thumb opposition are required along with thumb abduction and thumb extension. This prepares the hand to encompass the full half gallon. The wrist would assume the position to align the open hand with the half gallon wherever it might be on the shelf. These are all prefunctional activities; they require little or no power but simply set the digits and joints in such a way that they are ready to carry out the functional part of the maneuver. Tendon transfers for these activities therefore can be accomplished with muscles from the lower portion of the absolute power scale. Once the full half gallon is encountered and grasped, the wrist is likely to come back to the dorsiflexion power position, and the finger flexors and thumb adductor must have sufficient power to carry out the function. These activities require tendon transfers from the upper portion of the absolute power scale and are labeled functional tendon transfers.

The adductor pollicis is the most important muscle in the hand. It is the muscle of pinch. There are other muscles that come into play, but the most powerful pinch is accomplished almost entirely by the adductor pollicis. This muscle has little or no tendinous component. It requires no change in direction of pull. The total muscle volume is significant, and the excursion is relatively low in relation to the muscle bulk, producing an ideal power situation. The loss of the adductor pollicis is a far more serious loss than that of the median innervated thenars. The prepositional function of the median innervated thenars is visible and obvious and therefore has commanded significant attention for a long time with many successful operations to reproduce thumb opposition (a prefunction). Currently there is no ideal tendon transfer to replace the lost adductor pollicis. This loss is not usually evident but is a major deficit to hand function. These thoughts have influenced surgery in several ways. During pollicization all small muscles are inserted on the ulnar side of the new thumb to act in the capacity of adductor pinch. There is little excuse for using one of the small muscles on the radial side of the hand for opposition when that muscle could be used to supply adductor pinch. The opposition can be easily restored with an extrinsic tendon, keeping in mind that opposition is indeed a prefunction.

The tendon transfer I use most commonly for opposition following pollicization is that of the extensor digiti minimi. The advantage here is in the use of an extrinsic tendon for opposition that has no pulley and a direct pull. The direct pull around the forearm without pulley mechanism seems to be a better arrangement, particularly when one is preparing an infant's hand for 60 or 70 years of function.

A major concept in transferring the extensor digiti minimi is the necessity of reestablishing or ensuring the existence of extensor digitorum communis function to the little finger. Often the little finger is supplied only with an intertendinous communicator and not a direct tendon out of the fourth dorsal compartment. This intertendinous communicator is insufficient for full active extension of the little finger. Usually there are several slips that make up the extensor digitorum communis tendon of the ring finger. One of these tendinous slips can be taken to the little finger to reestablish extensor digitorum communis function when transferring the extensor digiti minimi.

The brachioradialis is the second highest muscle on the absolute power scale, second only to the flexor carpi ulnaris. This motor makes a good tendon transfer as long as one understands the anatomy of this particular muscle. It is best to think of the brachioradialis as originating on the distal aspect of the radius and inserting on the humerus because indeed the entire tendon of the brachioradialis crosses no joint and therefore has no effective motion. The motion all takes place from the musculotendinous junction to its insertion on the humerus. If one considers this muscle in this "backward" fashion and realizes that the tendon has no motion in its normal state, then it becomes obvious that to use this muscle in a tendon transfer requires significant dissection. The tendon is freed from the distal side of the radius. It must be freed from the tight "envelope" all along its course, and the distal half of the muscle belly must be freed from its fascial envelope. The neurovascular structures enter the muscle on its inferior and medial surface and are usually not a concern until a third to half the way up the muscle belly. Once this muscle-tendon unit is mobilized in this fashion, it makes a good transfer donor particularly for functional transfers. It will do an adequate job of restoring power to the adductor pollicis when extended with a free-tendon graft passing between the middle and ring finger metacarpals to the front of the hand, then along the adductor and inserting at the adductor insertion. I usually use a small Silastic sheet between the metacarpals, since the free-tendon graft must make two 90-degree angles, one entering and one exiting the intermetacarpal space. After this transfer it is not easy to reeducate the hand for light thumb pinch activity; however, it does work well when heavy grasping adductor function is a requirement.

The flexor digitorum superficialis (or sublimis) is frequently taken for tendon transfers of various types. The removal of the superficialis from the finger must be done with care and consideration for the vascular anatomy of the remaining profundus tendon. The superficialis tendon should be taken at the proximal finger crease, not at the middle finger crease and, I believe, not any higher than its position midlateral on the profundus where the profundus passes through the superficialis. Taking the superficialis tendon no further distally will ensure protection of the vincular system that passes through and is part of the superficialis system before reaching the profundus.

When the profundus has been lacerated in a finger and the superficialis is intact, a late reconstructive technique advocated is a distal joint tenodesis. I feel that this is an applicable procedure on occasion but only in the ring finger. The index and middle fingers deserve profundus function. The little finger superficialis will provide a full range of motion of the little finger; however, it is inadequate as the lone power flexor of the finger. One of two things must be done: the superficialis must be attached to the profundus in the palm to restore the profundus power to the little finger in conjunction with the distal joint tenodesis; or, probably the better approach, the profundus function of the distal joint in the little finger must be reestablished. The little finger superficialis alone will produce adequate flexion, and photographs can be obtained of what appears to be nearly perfect finger function; however, the muscle bulk of the little finger superficialis is totally inadequate to run this finger by itself.

QUADRAREGIA SYNDROME

A typical patient with quadraregia syndrome might appear in the office following profundus surgery or finger amputation, complaining of pain with stressful use of the hand. The pain is usually of the volar aspect of the wrist or forearm. The complaints often are of long standing with the patient out of work and an irate insurance company and a history of regular medical examinations. The problem is a distal tethering of one profundus tendon, which creates a painful shearing effect at the intertendinous junctions of all four profundi. The pain is extreme and can be recreated in a normal hand by simply holding one finger, usually the ring or middle finger, in full extension while actively attempting to make a strong fist or by holding all fingers except the index in full extension and forcibly pinching it to the thumb. The condition is easily treated by releasing the offending profundus proximal to its lumbrical origin attachment. Awareness of this problem will save the day in an otherwise prolonged and difficult situation.

SECTION TEN PAIN PROBLEMS

Chapter 34 Reflex sympathetic dystrophy*

Harold E. Kleinert

Graeme J. Southwick

Reflex sympathetic dystrophy (RSD) is a syndrome complex involving the upper or lower extremity and characterized by the following: (1) pain, (2) swelling caused by edema, (3) stiffness, (4) osteoporosis, and (5) skin changes with altered sensitivity to pain and temperature. There are altered vasomotor, sudomotor, and nail and hair growth patterns.

Pain is the central feature of this syndrome and was well defined by the British Medical Research Council in 1920 as (1) spontaneous, (2) hot, burning, intense, diffuse, persistent, but subject to exacerbation, (3) being excited by stimuli that do not necessarily produce a physical effect on the limb, and (4) leading to profound changes in the mental state of the patient.

The stimulus to the development of RSD is most commonly trauma, be it iatrogenic from surgery or otherwise. Nerve damage may or may not be apparent. The stimulus may be unrelated to the involved limb. RSD may follow ischemic heart disease, a cerebrovascular accident, or neoplasia.

The incidence of RSD is reported to be about 5% of all peripheral nerve injuries. It affects males and females equally,[4] although some series report a predominance of females.[2] Whites are the main group affected, with a low incidence of involvement in the black population.[2,4] All age groups are affected, and there have been several recent reports of RSD in children.

CLASSIFICATION

For over 2 centuries there have been many reports documenting this syndrome complex. In so doing many aspects of RSD have been highlighted in a "hodgepodge" of terminology. The simplest classification is that reported by Lankford and Thompson[5] in 1977.

In 1867 Mitchell[8] coined the term *causalgia* from Greek, meaning burning pain, to describe the pain following a severe nerve injury. Mimocausalgia (from the Greek word *mimo*, to mimic) refers to those cases of RSD where there is no apparent nerve injury. Thus the following classification was developed:

A. Causalgia (apparent nerve damage)
   1. Major: a mixed nerve injury, commonly the median nerve
   2. Minor: purely sensory nerve injury, commonly the superficial branch of the radial nerve, the palmar branch of the ulnar nerve, or digital nerves
B. Mimocausalgia (no apparent nerve injury)
   1. Major traumatic dystrophy: may follow a major fracture with soft tissue damage or Colles' fracture producing acute carpal tunnel syndrome, presumably because of median nerve pressure injury
   2. Minor traumatic dystrophy: most common form, which follows minor trauma such as a fracture or crushed fingertip injury
C. Shoulder-hand syndrome (described by Steinbrocker, Spitzer, and Friedman[10] in 1947): involves the hand and shoulder, almost always avoiding the elbow; usually seen in the over-50 age group; no cause found in about 20% of cases, but more commonly associated with nontraumatic causes, especially ischemic heart disease, cerebrovascular accidents, and neoplasia

CLINICAL STAGES

RSD is a progressive disorder that is initially reversible, but when extensive structural changes intervene, an irreversible state is reached. Three stages can be described.

Stage 1: pain

Pain usually develops in the first 3 weeks after injury, but a high index of suspicion will allow an earlier diagnosis. There is severe burning pain that is out of proportion to the apparent injury. Hyperesthesia and trigger areas may be present. Soft tissue edema produces swelling

---
*From the Department of Surgery, University of Louisville School of Medicine, Louisville, Ky.

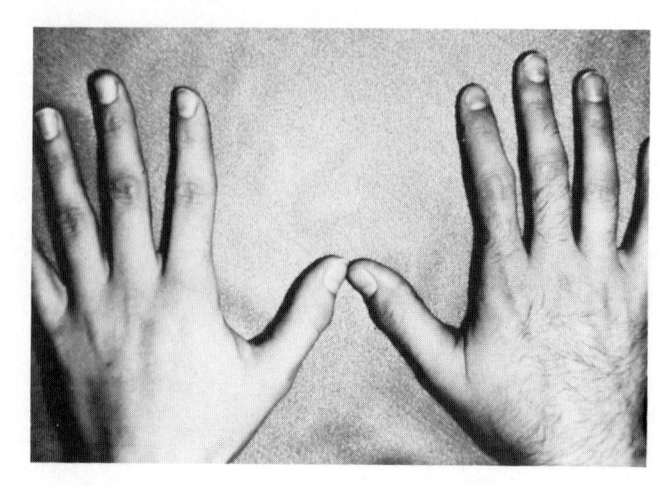

FIG. 34-1. Increased hair growth in patient with RSD.

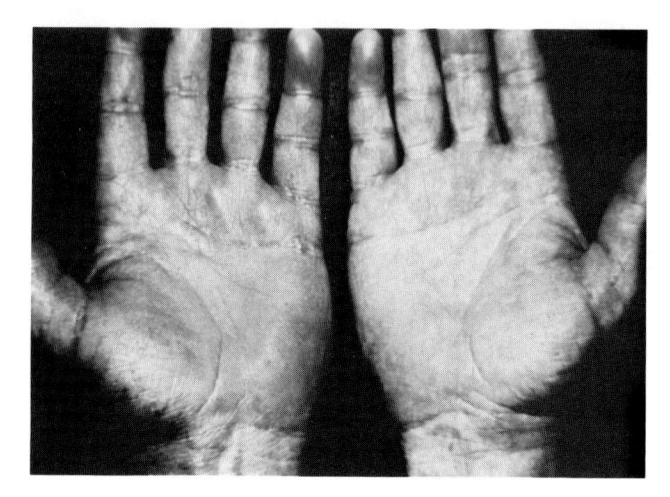

FIG. 34-2. Sluggish circulation in right hand, 1 minute after release of fist.

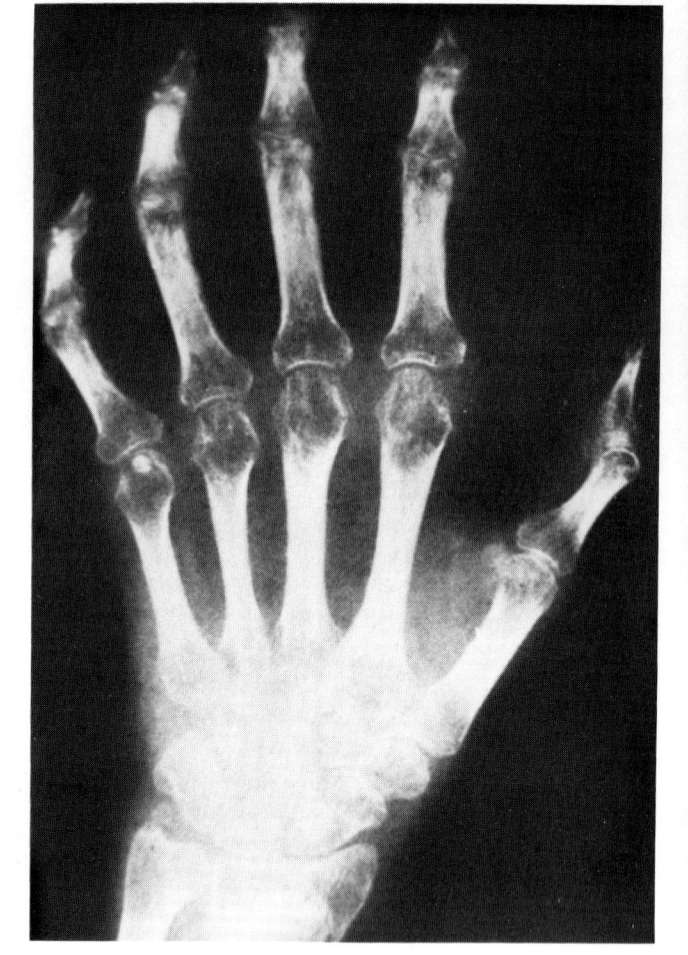

FIG. 34-3. Marked polar demineralization of long bones in RSD.

and stiffness of the hand. Because of these features, there is reluctance of the patient to move or use the limb. There is hyperthermia, hyperhidrosis, and an increase in nail and hair growth over the involved region (Fig. 34-1). Skin color will vary with vasomotor activity, being pale with arteriolar constriction, cyanotic with venous constriction, and bluish gray with both arterial and venous constriction. In the latter case capillary return is sluggish (Fig. 34-2). After about 1 month osteoporosis will develop, initially with spotty demineralization of carpal bones and polar demineralization of long bones (Fig. 34-3).

Stage 2: dystrophy

At about 3 months the skin becomes cool, pale, and tight with loss of skin creases. A brawny edema and fat atrophy develop, producing spindly "pencil-tapered" fingers. There is a decrease in hair over the limb, and the nails become brittle. Joint stiffness and immobility persist. Acute palmar fasciitis may develop. This occurs more commonly in females and is represented by tender palmar nodules, which are often associated with red streaks in the skin over the nodules. Steroid injections into the nodules may be efficacious in treatment, but surgical excision is contraindicated, since it exacerbates the condition.

Stage 3: atrophy

After about 6 to 9 months the condition reaches a relatively irreversible stage because of extensive structural damage. The limb is pale, cool, and dry with atrophic skin. The hand is stiff, and pain tends to be more diffuse. Osteoporosis is generalized in the bones of the limb with thinning of the cortex.

DIAGNOSIS

An early diagnosis is vital if treatment is to be effective. A high index of suspicion is important. The personality of the RSD-prone patient is almost stereotypic. They are usually dependent with hysterical affect. They are often insecure and fearful and may have secondary gains from their pain situation. It is important to remember that these patients are not malingerers.

Subjective clinical observations should prompt the physician to diagnose RSD, especially when pain is out of proportion to an injury. The objective clinical signs, as described, should make the diagnosis more definite. Attention to the finer details is important, such as increased hair and nail growth. Osteoporosis may be revealed on x-ray examination.

In the difficult diagnostic situation nerve blocks may help establish a diagnosis. These include: (1) local anesthetic infiltration to pain zones or areas of hyperesthesia, (2) stellate ganglion blocks, and (3) placebo block using Ringer's solution to help exclude the malingerer from the true RSD patient. Rarely, special investigative techniques will be required. These include thermography, plethysmography, bone scan, and blood flow studies. Electromyography, nerve conduction studies, and serum calcium and alkaline phosphatase assays are usually not helpful.

PATHOGENESIS IN RELATION TO TREATMENT

There have been many theories proposed for the mechanism of development of RSD based on nutritional, metabolic, bone, and vessel blood flow changes. Although the pathogenesis is still far from clear, the work of Livingston,[6a] Melzack and Wall,[6] and Doupe, Cullen, and Chance[1] has now gained wide acknowledgment, and much experimental evidence fits their models.

The normal somatic sensory nerve pathway passes from the peripheral receptor to the spinal cord internuncial pool of neurons and from there in a cephalic direction to the cerebral cortex via the thalamus. The peripheral nerve contains large myelinated fast-conducting type A fibers and small unmyelinated slow-conducting type C fibers. Trauma produces nerve injury, which results in cross-stimulation from sympathetic postganglionic efferents (which are type C nerve fibers) to somatic sensory type C nerve fibers in the peripheral nerve. Injury is associated with an increased sympathetic outflow, which in turn stimulates the type C fibers of the peripheral nerve via the cross-stimulation. In keeping with the gate control theory of pain[6] the type C fiber activity keeps the pain gate open. There is a heightened activity in the internuncial pool, which increases sensory input to the higher centers, resulting in the perception of poorly localized burning pain. Higher center response to pain increases sympathetic outflow, which also is increased by somatic sensory type C fiber stimulation of the spinal cord's internuncial pool of neurons. Thus this abnormal sympathetic reflex cycle is established, and the RSD syndrome results.

The cerebral cortex can modulate this reflex, and thus a susceptible personality, as previously described, will help propagate this syndrome.

Effective treatment therefore could be established by (1) inhibiting higher center facilitation of the system, (2) increasing type A somatic sensory nerve input to close the pain gate and overcome the type C fiber activity, (3) decreasing sympathetic outflow, (4) interrupting cross-stimulation between the sympathetic efferent and somatic afferent neurons, and (5) interrupting pain pathways to the higher center.

TREATMENT

With an understanding of the pathogenesis of RSD the efficacy of treatment regimens becomes obvious.

First, frequent intelligent use of graduated physical therapy programs will prevent stiffness and increase type A fiber input to the spinal cord. This will close the pain gate and dominate the activity of the type C abnormal reflex system. Transcutaneous nerve stimulation can aid the physical therapy program. This therapy also heightens type A fiber stimulation and thus pain gate closure.[11]

If physical therapy is too active, severe pain will result and negate these effects. Elevation of the limb, night splintage, and warm whirlpool baths may aid treatment. One should be cautious with whirlpool baths, since extreme temperatures will provoke an increased sympathetic outflow and exacerbate the condition.

Second, psychiatric guidance with the help of drugs that affect the central nervous system such as diazepam (Valium), chlordiazepoxide (Librium), trifluoperazine (Stelazine), or chlorpromazine (Thorazine) will inhibit higher center facilitation of RSD. Analgesics will act in a similar manner, but care should be taken to avoid addiction.

Third, nerve blocks will help break the reflex if the treatment just mentioned is unsuccessful. The peripheral sensory nerve may be blocked by local anesthetic injections into the painful or hyperesthetic regions. Relief as a result of this is rarely long lasting.

Stellate ganglion blocks often give good relief in the more resistant cases (later stage 1 and early stage 2). The anterior approach for stellate block is preferred in which the patient is supine with the neck extended, and a 1½-inch 25-gauge needle on a 10-ml control syringe is inserted at a point approximately 2.5 cm above the supra-

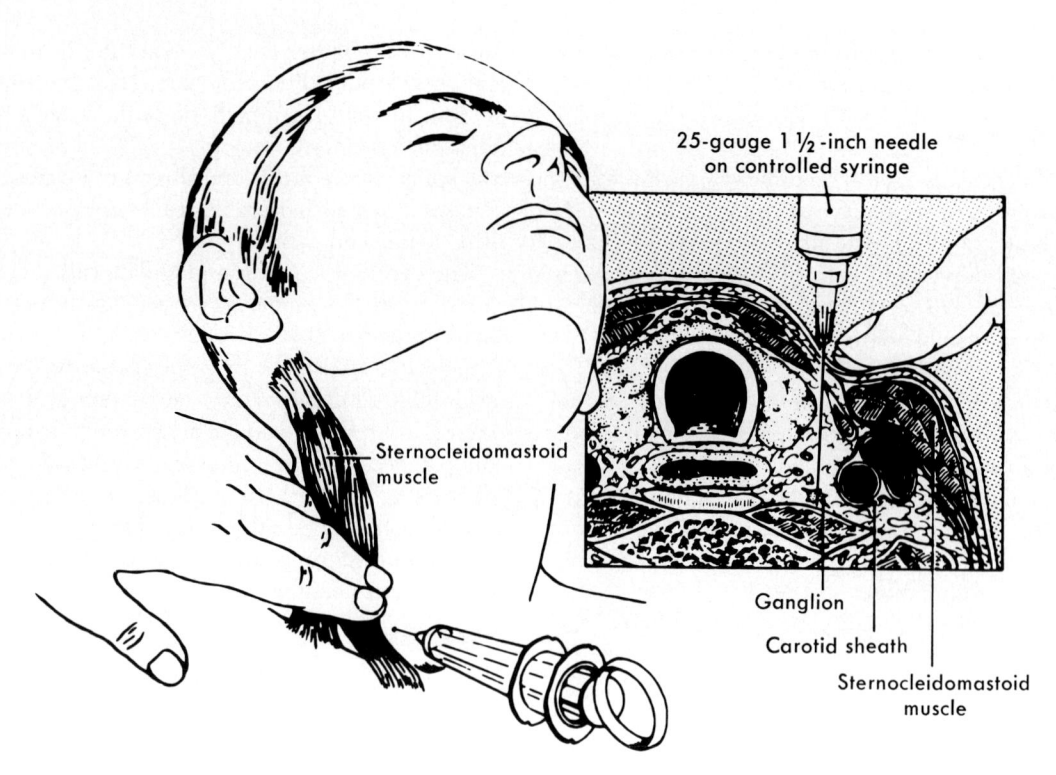

FIG. 34-4. Technique of stellate block, anterior approach. Sternocleidomastoid muscle and carotid sheath are retracted with fingertips. (From Kleinert, H.E., et al.: Orthop. Clin. North Am. **4:**917, 1973.)

sternal notch, between the trachea and the sternocleidomastoid muscle and carotid sheath, which are retracted laterally (Fig. 34-4). The needle is advanced to the transverse process of the sixth cervical vertebra, which is quite easily palpable; then it is withdrawn slightly and the injection made. The patient is immediately placed with the head and neck elevated to facilitate the gravitational flow of anesthetic material to the stellate ganglion. Normal precautions against intravascular injections are exercised. All blocks are performed in the hospital outpatient facility as a precaution against the infrequent complication of pneumothorax, which could require immediate resuscitative treatment not available in the nonhospital environment. Mepivacaine hydrochloride (Carbocaine) 1%, bupivacaine (Marcaine) 0.5%, and lidocaine (Xylocaine) hydrochloride 1% are the local anesthetics of choice, and the volume of injection ranges from 10 to 20 ml with each block. The presence of Horner's sign and vasodilatation of the hand are the criteria for an effective block. Stellate blocks are most commonly given on consecutive days in a series of three to five or less as indicated by relief of symptoms. In the more refractory cases hospitalization for the series of blocks is recommended to minimize external emotional stress and to permit intensive physical therapy during pain-free periods following an effective block.[4]

Tourniquet-controlled guanethidine limb perfusion has been used successfully.[3] An intravenous catheter is inserted into the forearm and a tourniquet applied to the arm. After limb elevation to promote venous drainage the tourniquet is inflated to above systolic blood pressure and 10 to 20 mg guanethidine given with 500 IU heparin in 25 ml of saline into the intravenous catheter. After 10 minutes intermittent deflation of the tourniquet allows slow release of unbound guanethidine into the general circulation. Slight hypotension may develop, and this treatment should not be used in patients with cardiac or renal impairment. Guanethidine displaces norepinephrine to be strongly bound by the postganglionic sympathetic nerves. In response to stimuli it is released as a false transmitter substance from these nerves. Thus guanethidine effectively blocks sympathetic outflow effects in the periphery and can break the abnormal reflex pattern with good relief from pain.

The beta blocker propranolol has been reported to help relieve pain when given orally; however, its mechanism of action in RSD is unknown.[9] Propranolol does have local anesthetic effects.

Corticosteroids and vasodilators have been employed with variable success. On cessation of steroid therapy a rebound of RSD may ensue.

Sympathectomy has given excellent results in patients

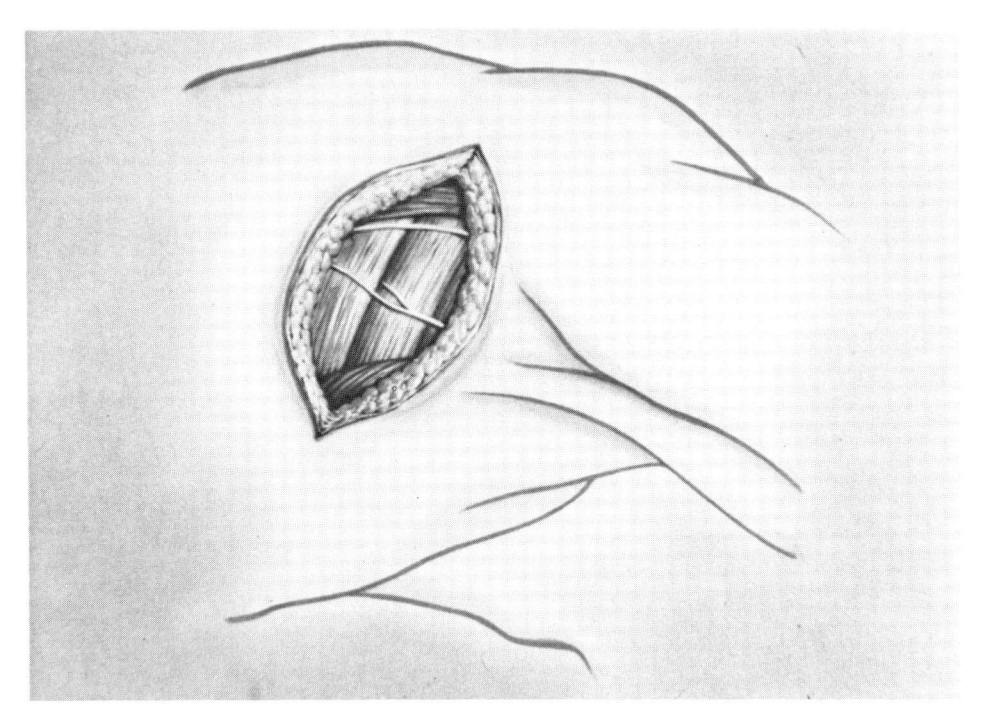

FIG. 34-5. After incision is made, intercostal brachial nerve is found running subcutaneously. Long thoracic nerve parallels anterior border of latissimus dorsi. (From Kleinert, H.E., et al.: Arch. Surg. **90**:612, 1965. Copyright 1965, American Medical Association.)

who respond well to sympathetic block but who failed to experience permanent relief. The transaxillary approach seems to offer the best exposure. The patient is placed on the side with a "doughnut" beneath the shoulder and the affected extremity abducted 100 to 120 degrees from the side and extended 30 degrees. Care must be taken not to exceed 120 degrees of abduction, since otherwise injury to the brachial plexus may result. The skin incision is made over the second intercostal space, extending from the anterior border of the latissimus dorsi to the pectoralis major muscle (Fig. 34-5). The axillary fat pad is swept cephalad, and the long thoracic nerve is identified at the anterior border of the lattissimus dorsi and carefully preserved. As the second and third intercostal spaces come into view, the intercostal brachial nerve is identified, arising mainly from the second space with some filaments occasionally coming from the third. This nerve can be seen passing subcutaneously to provide sensation to the medial aspect of the arm. The pleural cavity is entered through the second intercostal space. It is necessary to divide that portion of the intercostal brachial nerve arising from the third intercostal space, but those from the second are carefully preserved. The ribs are spread by a laminectomy retractor. The lung is packed caudally and the sympathetic chain identified on the heads of the ribs. The pleura is incised over the sympathetic chain from the first through the fourth thoracic ribs (Fig. 34-6). The second, third, and fourth ganglia with the lower third of the stellate ganglion are resected, as described by Palumbo[7] (Fig. 34-7). If there are any postganglionic filaments going to the arm from the remainder of the stellate ganglion, they also are divided. The pleura is left open over the bed of the sympathetic chain and the chest closed. If pleural adhesions were lysed on entering the chest, a tube is brought out through the sixth intercostal space and connected to a water-sealed drain. Rib closure is accomplished by paracostal or intracostal sutures placed to avoid the intercostal nerve. Accurate approximation of subcutaneous tissue and skin is necessary to obtain an airtight pleural cavity.[4]

Surgery of the affected part rarely is successful and may exacerbate the condition. However, occasionally release of nerve entrapment, revision amputation, or neuroma and fracture treatment may help (e.g., reduction of a Colles' fracture may relieve acute carpal tunnel pressure on the median nerve).

Rarely, when all else fails and pain is persistent and severe, pain-relieving neurosurgical procedures may be necessary.

SECTION 10 PAIN PROBLEMS

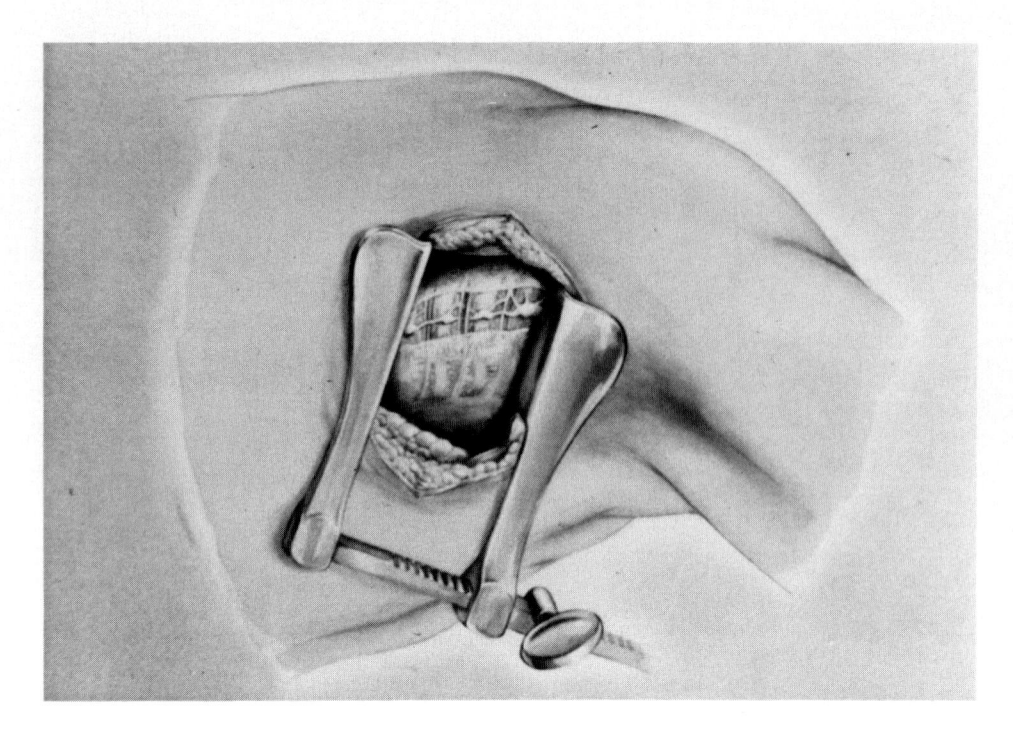

FIG. 34-6. Pleural cavity is entered through second intercostal space. Pleura over sympathetic chain is incised from first through fourth thoracic ribs. (From Kleinert, H.E., et al.: Arch. Surg. **90:**612, 1965. Copyright 1965, American Medical Association.)

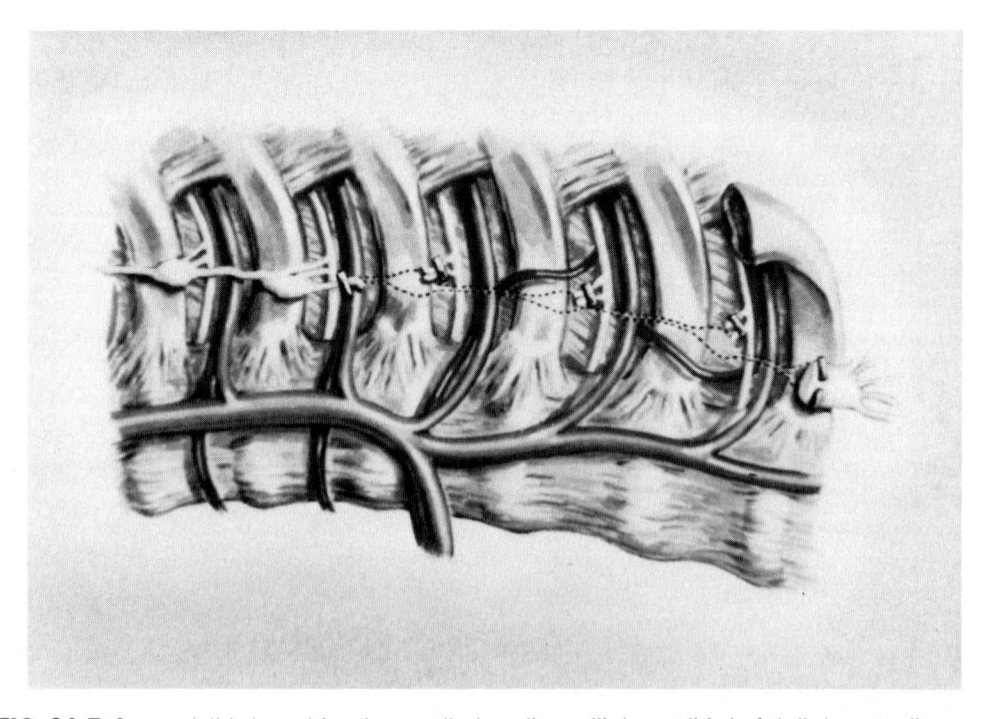

FIG. 34-7. Second, third, and fourth ganglia together with lower third of stellate ganglion are resected. (From Kleinert, H.E., et al.: Arch. Surg. **90:**612, 1965. Copyright 1965, American Medical Association.)

SUMMARY

Reflex sympathetic dystrophy is a syndrome complex with pain as its central feature. If left unchecked, it will result in a useless upper limb with irreversible structural damage and a patient who is mentally disturbed by the effects of chronic pain. Effective treatment is available, especially if an early diagnosis is made. A high index of suspicion is important, and one should pay particular attention to the patient who describes pain out of proportion to the injury. The pathogenesis of RSD, although not fully established, allows a better understanding of this condition and its treatment.

REFERENCES

1. Doupe, J., Cullen, C., and Chance, G.: Post-traumatic pain and the causalgic syndrome, J. Neurol. Neurosurg. Psychiatry 7:33, 1944.
2. Drucker, W., Hubay, C., Holden W., and Bukovnic, J.: Pathogenesis of post-traumatic sympathetic dystrophy, Am. J. Surg. 97:454, 1959.
3. Hannington-Kiff, J.: Intravenous regional sympathetic block with guanethidine, Lancet 1:1019, 1974.
4. Kleinert, H.E., Cole, N.M., Wayne, L., Harvey, R., Kutz, J.E., and Atasoy, E.: Post-traumatic sympathetic dystrophy, Orthop. Clin. North Am. 4:917, 1973.
5. Lankford, L., and Thompson, J.: Reflex sympathetic dystrophy, upper and lower extremity: diagnosis and management. In American Academy of Orthopaedic Surgeons: Instructional Course Lectures, vol. 26, St. Louis, 1977, The C.V. Mosby Co.
6. Melzack, R., and Wall. P.: Pain mechanisms: a new theory, Science 150:971, 1965.
6a. Livingston, W.K.: Pain mechanisms: a physiological interpretation of causalgia and its related states, New York, 1943, Macmillan, Inc.
7. Palumbo, L.: Upper dorsal sympathectomy without Horner's syndrome, Arch. Surg. 71:743, 1955.
8. Richards, R.: Causalgia, a centennial review, Arch. Neurol. 16:339, 1967.
9. Simson, G.: Propranolol for causalgia and Sudek's atrophy, J.A.M.A. 227:327, 1974.
10. Steinbrocker, O., Spitzer, N., and Friedman, H.H.: The shoulder-hand syndrome in reflex dystrophy of the upper extremity, Ann. Intern. Med. 29:22, 1947.
11. Stilz, R.J., Conn, H., and Sanders, D.B.: Reflex sympathetic dystrophy in a 6 year old: successful treatment by transcutaneous nerve stimulation, Anaesth. Analg. 56:438, 1977.

Chapter 35 Tenolysis: pain control and rehabilitation

James M. Hunter

Frank Seinsheimer III

Evelyn J. Mackin

The adherence of injured tendons to surrounding tissue is a frequent result of injury and operative repair. The resultant limitation of active motion is a significant cause of disability in these injured hands. For many patients the lysis of these adhesions, if successful, will dramatically end a period of hand disability. The gain in active range of motion of the fingers leads to a predictable increase in both the strength and the control of hand function.

There are two principal difficulties in obtaining a successful tenolysis result. First, during surgery it may be difficult to determine how extensive a tenolysis is necessary, and an incomplete lysis may result. Second, during the early postoperative period, pain may prevent the patient from achieving the full active potential until after the adhesions reform. In this situation the full active potential is never realized.

For the past 8 years we have performed tenolyses using neuroleptanalgesics (NLA) and anesthesia with active patient participation.[2,3] This technique allows us to be completely confident that a complete tenolysis has been performed, because we see when the patient finally attains the full active potential. In addition, the patient sees himself or herself moving through the full range of motion at the time of surgery, and this provides important psychologic help during postoperative therapy.

More recently we have introduced a new alternative in postoperative management: prn sensory analgesia. Bupivacaine 0.5% is administered by the patient via a soft Silastic catheter every 4 hours as needed to anesthetize the operative site. This allows active motion without pain. We feel that *control of pain* is the *key* to retaining the improved function gained in the operating room. This chapter reviews the technical details of the method of NLA-local anesthesia, the operative program for tenolysis, and the postoperative prn sensory analgesia program. This technique has been used successfully in over 30 cases.

METHOD
Preoperative preparation

Prior to tenolysis the hand should be prepared for maximal function: (1) fractures are healed; (2) wound healing is complete, and the skin is soft; and (3) passive joint motion is optimal. The indications for tenolysis are: (1) there is a significant difference between the passive range of motion and the active range of motion of the finger(s); (2) tendon gliding has not improved despite proper physical and occupational therapy; (3) the passive range of motion and the active range of motion are equal, but grip strength remains low and plateaued; and (4) during the performance of a joint contracture release (done under NLA-local anesthesia) passive range of motion increases, but active range of motion does not improve to equal the new passive range of motion. The patient should understand that if the tendon and tendon bed are severely scarred, a tenolysis will not be performed. Instead the tendon will be excised rather than lysed, and a stage-1 sheath-building implant will be inserted. Stage-2 tendon grafting will follow in 3 to 4 months.

NLA-local anesthesia[1a,3-6]

One half to 1 hour prior to surgery standard preoperative medication (morphine or meperidine and a barbiturate or tranquilizer) is administered at two thirds or less of the usual dosage. On arrival in the operating room, the patient undergoes an initial evaluation of pulse rate, blood pressure, and respiratory rate, and an intravenous infusion is started. Induction is begun with the intravenous infusion of 1 ml of Innovar. Innovar is a mixture of fentanyl and droperidol combined in a ratio of 1:50. Fentanyl is a potent synthetic narcotic reported to be 100 times more potent than morphine and has a short half-life. Droperidol is a potent and long-acting tranquilizer. Administration of a second and third ml of Innovar occurs at 4- to 5-minute intervals. The respiratory rate is closely monitored and usually decreases to 12 to 14 respirations per minute when adequate sedation and analgesia are attained. Although the recommended induction dose for Innover is 1 ml per 10 kg of body weight, we have found that a dose of 1 ml per 20 kg of body weight (between 3 and 5 ml) is usually sufficient.

Frequent monitoring of vital signs is carried out by the anesthesiologist. Severe respiratory depression and/or relative hypotension are rare and, when they occur, are usually the result of too rapid injections of Innovar. Maintenance of the analgesia with repeated doses of fentanyl is necessary to overcome tourniquet pain and the discomfort caused by prolonged immobility on the operating table. Small doses of fentanyl at suitable intervals to keep the respiratory rate depressed to 12 to 14 respirations per minute provide satisfactory analgesia.

Diazepam (Valium) may be used as the tranquilizer component of the NLA, provided that sufficient fentanyl is given for analgesia. This is particularly useful for outpatients in whom the prolonged effect of droperidol is troublesome. Diazepam should not be used instead of fentanyl during the maintenance phase of NLA.

After suitable skin preparation, sterile draping, and tourniquet application the skin incision is infiltrated with 1% lidocaine without epinephrine. We occasionally do intermetacarpal nerve blocks, but we avoid infiltrating any more proximal mixed sensory and motor nerves. This avoids paralysis on the intrinsic muscles of the hand and allows completely normal active function during surgery. Most patients have received between 3 and 5 ml of Innovar by this time. If the patient has been adequately sedated by the Innovar, there will be no withdrawal of the arm or other response during the injection of lidocaine. If there is a reaction to the injection, the patient is undermedicated, and surgery should be delayed until more Innovar is given.

Surgical technique

The arm is exsanguinated with an Esmarch bandage, and the tourniquet is inflated. One percent lidocaine is infiltrated into the line of the skin incision. If possible, the bulk of surgical investigation is carried out within the first 20 minutes, so that the patient can cooperate and move the fingers as needed. Tourniquet ischemia results in motor paralysis, which appears between 20 and 25 minutes following inflation of the tourniquet.

If longer dissection is required, the dissection can proceed without the active participation of the patient until a point is reached when active motion is desired. Then the tourniquet is released, and bleeding is controlled. After several minutes, when the patient has recovered motor function, active motion is evaluated. If considerable additional work is required, the tourniquet can be inflated and released multiple times. At all times direct communication between the surgeon and the patient is possible. It is important that the surgeon extend the dissection proximally and distally until the patient can produce active function that equals the passive range of motion. (We refer to this extra effort as "walking the last mile.") This eliminates the problem of incomplete tenolysis. Procedures as long as 3 to 4 hours have been eventually productive.

Incision

For flexor tenolyses the volar zigzag incision, as popularized by Julian Brunner,[1] is employed. The apex of the angles should fall over the neurovascular bundles and not to the midlateral border of the fingers. This exposure permits a thorough review of the tendon anatomy and allows the lysis of adherent structures under direct visualization. It also favors the vascular nutrition of injured or previously operated fingers. For extensor tenolyses and proximal interphalangeal (PIP) joint capsulectomies a dorsal curvilinear incision is used. These two incisions can be used at the same time in a patient who requires both extensor and flexor tenolyses.

Tourniquet

The Esmarch or Martin rubber bandage should be applied carefully from the finger up to the level of the tourniquet. In long procedures requiring multiple inflations and deflations of the tourniquet, soft tissue edema may be a problem. In this situation a small 2.5-cm wide piece of rubber may be cut from the rubber bandage and the finger or fingers wrapped separately prior to the application of the larger rubber bandage. Applying this technique in the operating room may permit early wound closure and uncomplicated healing.

Pulley system[6]

During flexor tenolysis every attempt should be made to preserve as much of the pulley system as possible. If possible, all five annular pulleys should be preserved. This includes the two fixed annular pulleys over the proximal and middle phalanges (A_2 and A_4) and the three adjusting annular pulleys attached to the volar plates of the metacarpophalangeal (MCP), PIP, and distal interphalangeal (DIP) joints (A_1, A_3, and A_5) (Fig. 35-1). When possible, the flexor tendon should be explored through the cruciate, or folding, pulley segments. Only critical adhesions are lysed, and frequent patient movement is helpful.

If the pulley system has been damaged by injury or previous surgery, the stress on the remaining pulleys is greater than normal during active patient function. In this situation weak, damaged pulleys may rupture in the postoperative period. Thus absence of pulleys or the presence of weak, attenuated pulleys is an indication for pulley reconstruction. This may be accomplished using

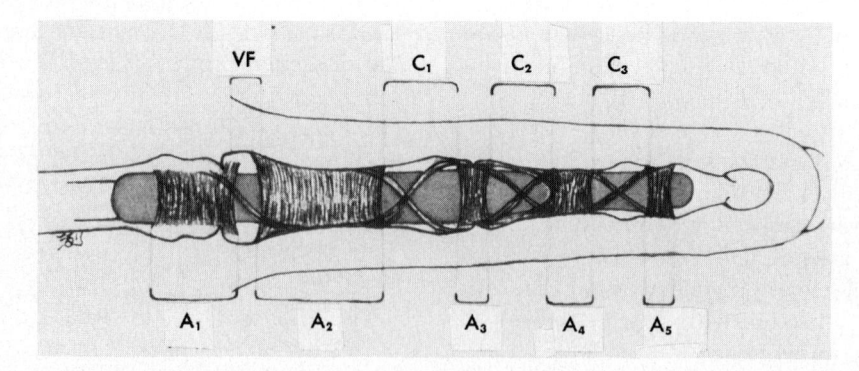

FIG. 35-1. Diagrammatic representation of pulley system.[2] When possible, flexor tendon should be explored through cruciate, or folding, pulley segments.

free-tendon grafts passed through drill holes or around the bone beneath the extensor tendon system. We believe that firm fixation to bone or around bone is necessary if the reconstructed pulley is to withstand the elevated stresses present in an injured pulley system. If the reconstruction of more than one pulley is necessary, then staged tendon reconstruction should be seriously considered rather than tenolysis.

Tendon quality

Large segments of tendon freed from adhesions may survive, provided that postoperative gliding is achieved and maintained. Cell systems will form early, stimulated by gliding, and will produce fluid nutrition while soft adhesions carrying blood vessels develop at segmental levels.

It is important to critically assess the quality of the tendon at the time of surgery. If 30% of tendon segments have been lost or the continuity of the tendon is only through a segment of scar, then this is a questionable case for tenolysis. The surgeon must exercise judgment, based on past experience, to decide when to change the reconstructive program from tenolysis to staged reconstruction using an active or passive Hunter tendon implant. The patient must be prepared for this possibility.

PRN sensory analgesia

Prior to closure of the wound a soft Silastic Jackson-Pratt catheter is laid proximal to the site of surgery over the sensory nerve branches. This is usually done in the palm through a separate stab incision. This is placed either in the midpalm to reach the sensory branches of the median nerve or in the ulnar side of the palm to reach the sensory branches of the ulnar nerve (Fig. 35-2). Occasionally, when tenolysis is carried out proximal to the wrist, the catheter is laid in the distal aspect of the forearm (Fig. 35-3). The terminal end of the catheter is sutured to the skin to hold it in place. Generally, 2 or 3 ml of 0.5% bupivacaine is instilled into the wound prior to closure. The syringe (20 ml) filled with the bupivacaine is taped to the forearm dressing, and the patient is shown how to self-administer 2 ml of bupivacaine every 4 hours to begin active motion in the immediate postoperative period. The skin is closed with multiple, closely spaced, interrupted sutures, which are left in place for 2 to 3 weeks.

Therapy

Postoperative therapy begins within a few hours after surgery in the patient's hospital room. The patient is shown how to inject the bupivacaine, and active assistive exercise is encouraged by the surgeon and the nursing staff. By controlling the pain with bupivacaine, early active exercise is possible even in children and patients with low tolerance for pain. The bupivacaine should be instilled into the wound slowly, since rapid instillation will produce pain. While the catheter is in place, the patient receives prophylactic systemic antibiotics.

On the morning after surgery the patient is discharged from the hospital and goes directly to a hand rehabilitation center. There the patient begins treatment under close supervision of the hand therapist. The large, bulky dressing applied at surgery is removed, and the patient's extremity is placed on a sterile field (with the therapist wearing sterile gloves). All therapy must take place in a sterile environment to protect the incision and catheter entrance site from contamination. The petroleum jelly gauze covering the incision line is left on as a protective covering for several days until it separates from the wound site. Whirlpool is not permitted for at least 2 weeks, until the wound has completely healed. The patient is seen daily by the therapist during the first postoperative week.

CHAPTER 35 TENOLYSIS: PAIN CONTROL AND REHABILITATION

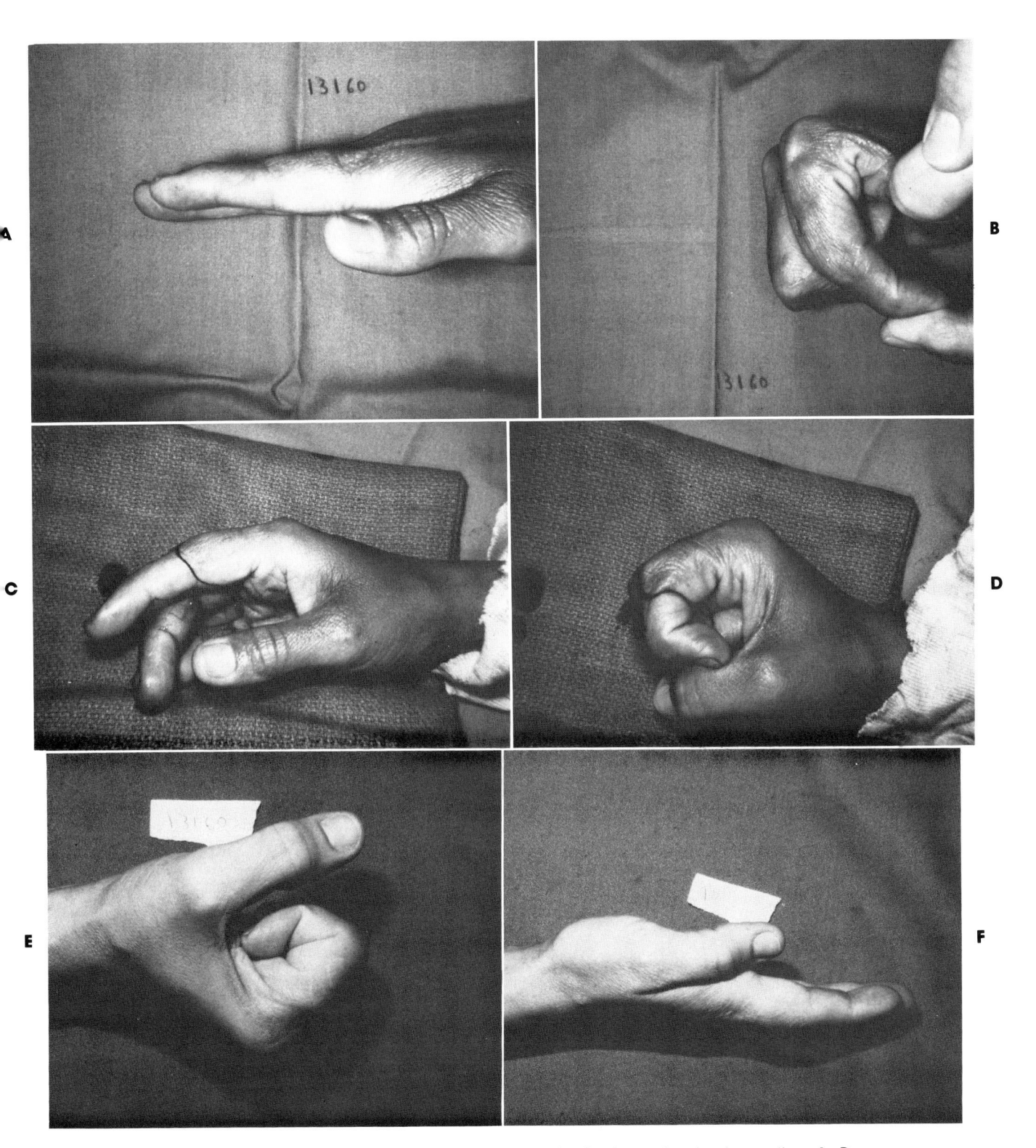

FIG. 35-2. Extension contracture 2 years after repair of extensor tendon laceration. **A,** Preoperative extension. **B,** Preoperative passive flexion. **C,** Intraoperative extension under NLA-local anesthesia. **D,** Following tenolysis and PIP joint capsulectomy, intraoperative flexion under NLA-local anesthesia. **E,** Five days following operation, Silastic catheter traverses center of palm extension. **F,** Flexion.

Continued.

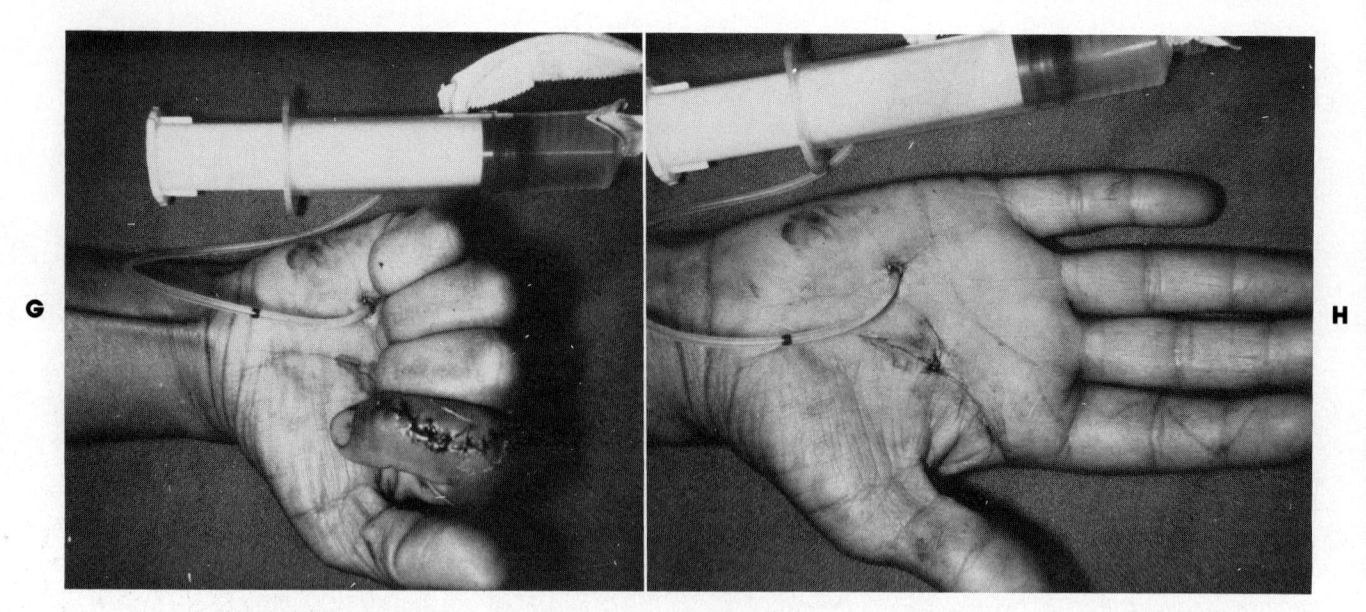

FIG. 35-2, cont'd. G and **H,** Four months after operation her active flexion actually exceeds that obtained at time of surgery.

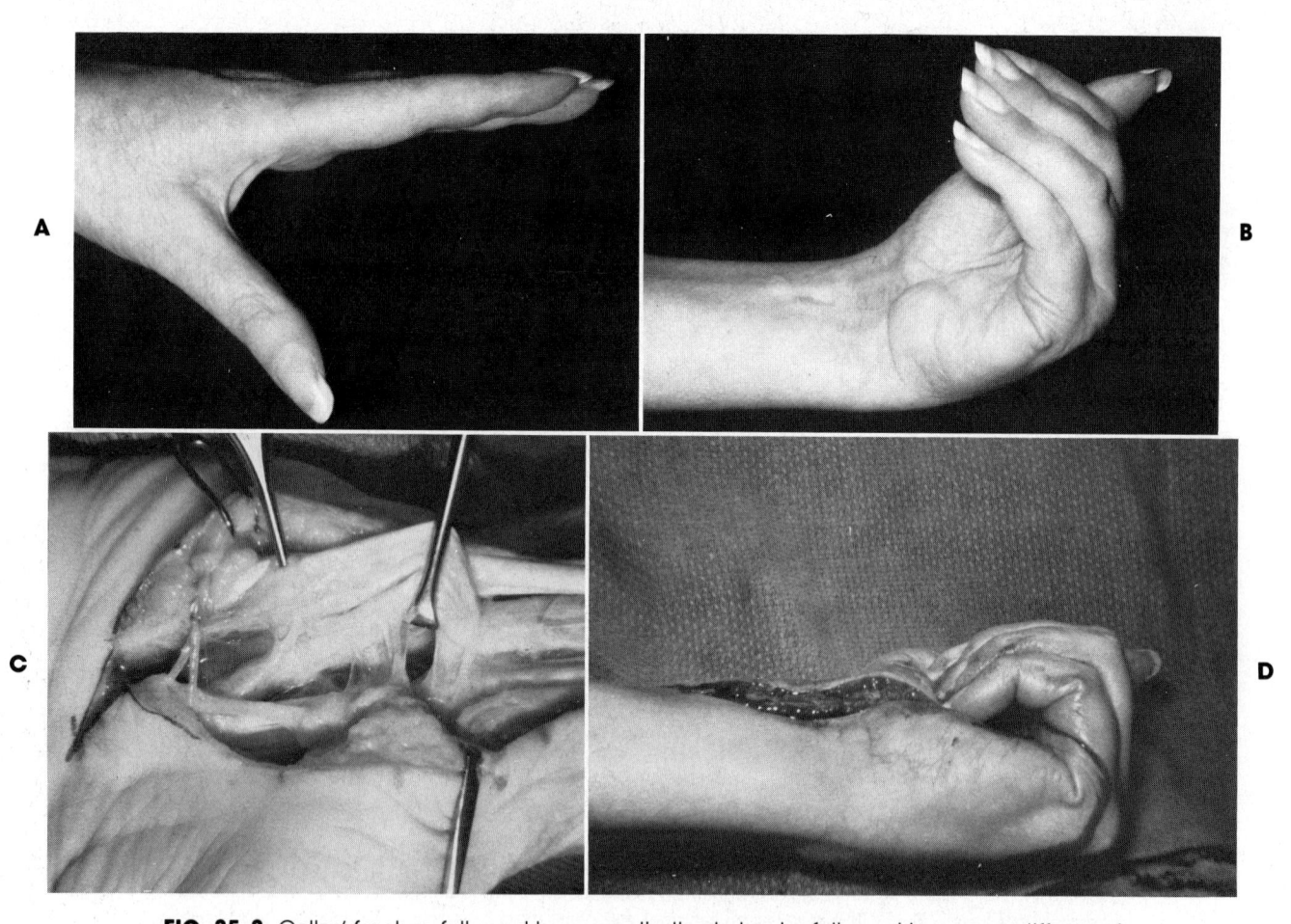

FIG. 35-3. Colles' fracture followed by sympathetic dystrophy followed by severe stiffness of hand. **A,** Preoperative active extension. **B,** Preoperative active flexion (passive flexion was near normal following hand therapy). **C,** Tendon adhesions seen at tenolysis. **D,** Intraoperative active flexion under NLA-local anesthesia. It was necessary to extend tenolysis proximally up into forearm before this amount of active flexion was achieved.

CHAPTER 35 TENOLYSIS: PAIN CONTROL AND REHABILITATION

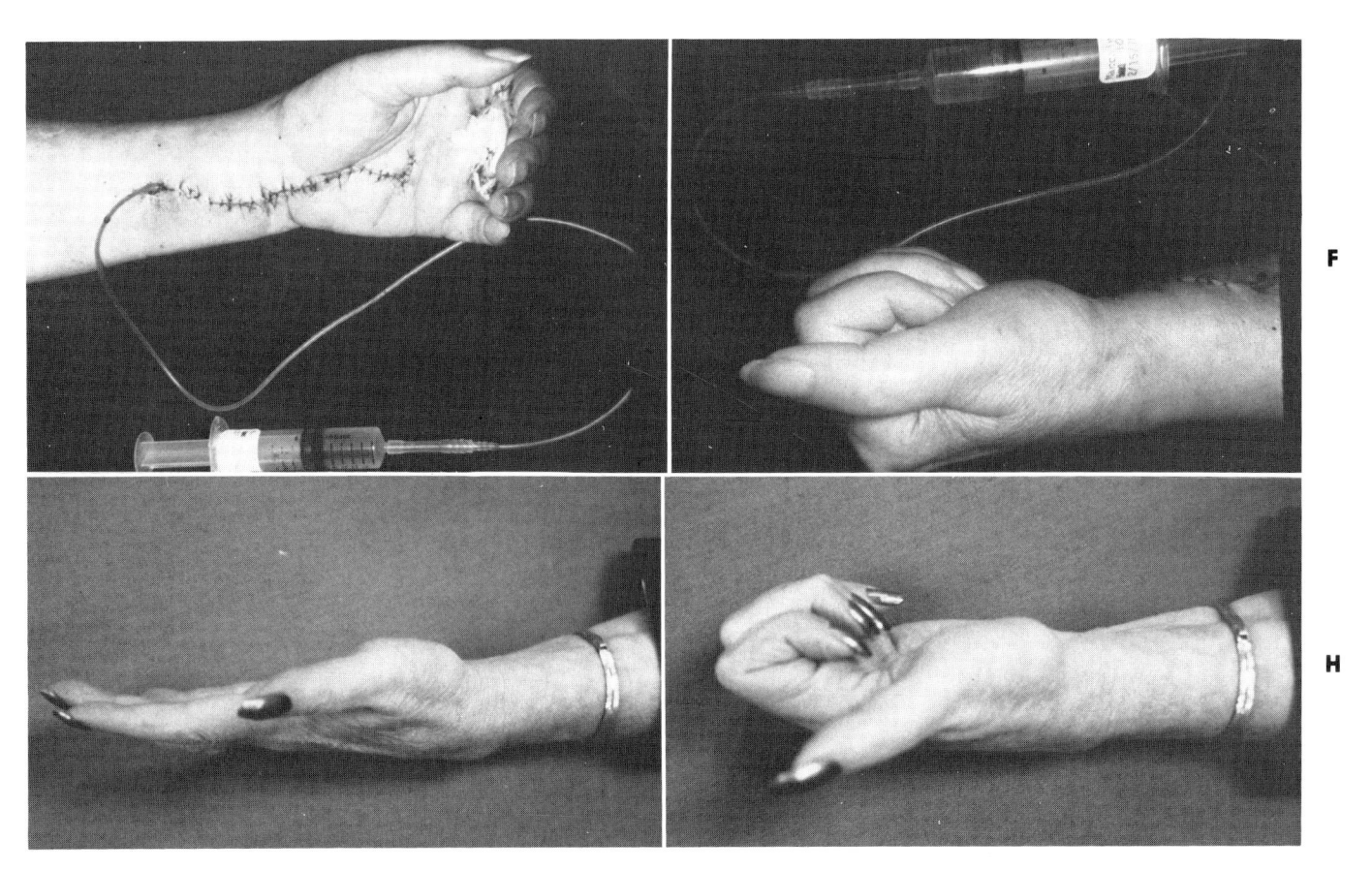

FIG. 35-3, cont'd. E, Five days after surgery Silastic catheter lays along carpal canal. **F,** Five days after surgery active flexion under bupivacaine analgesia. **G** and **H,** One-year follow-up findings.

It is extremely important that the exercise program be written out as well as explained verbally, since it will be carried out by the patient at home. The patient must fully understand that, if good results are to be obtained from the tenolysis procedure, active flexion exercises emphasizing full grip must be carried out immediately and on a regular basis at home during the first postoperative week.

The exact exercises vary according to the surgical procedure but may include the following:

1. Gentle, passive flexion of the involved DIP, PIP, and MCP joints
2. Active flexion of the involved DIP, PIP, and MCP joints
3. Gentle passive extension of any PIP joint contracture, with the wrist and MCP joint in flexion to protect the tendon
4. Active extension of the involved DIP, PIP, and MCP joints
5. Isolated flexor digitorum sublimis function
6. Passive fist making: pressing the involved hand into a fist with the uninvolved hand (or by the therapist) and then releasing the hand and trying to retain the fist with his or her own muscle power
7. Active flexion of the DIP joint by rolling the fingertips in to make a tight fist; the flexor digitorum profundus exercise

Following each daily therapy session an antibiotic ointment is applied along the incision and at the catheter entrance site. The patient is sent home with the limb in a light dressing with a protective posterior plaster splint. Only a light, sterile gauze wrap is placed around the involved fingers and palm so that full active range of motion is possible within the confines of the dressing. While at home the patient performs active and passive fist making 10 times each hour. The other exercises are each performed 10 times, four times a day, following the injection of the bupivacaine.

The catheter is removed on approximately the fifth postoperative day. The sutures are left in for 2 to 3 weeks. There have been no wound infections in over 30 cases treated with the prn sensory analgesia technique. In two patients the catheter was removed on the second or third postoperative day because of erythema. The erythema may have been a result of tissue reaction to the frequent instillation of bupivacaine. No infection developed.

Graded grip strengthening activities are begun 3 to 6 weeks following surgery. Heavy resistance exercise begins at 8 weeks following surgery. Return to heavy work is permitted after the eighth postoperative week.

Approximately two thirds of our patients reach their active potential by the end of the first week. Most of the other patients have even exceeded the active potential demonstrated at surgery. This may be because of improved joint mobility and increased muscle power, which are results of the intensive therapy after surgery. It may also be attributable to the fact that a sedated patient in the operating room will not exert the maximal force. There is a small group of patients in the salvage class who require extensor tenolysis, PIP capsulectomy, and flexor tenolysis. These patients often have suffered crush injuries to the finger(s) and comminuted fracture of the phalanges.

The extensive dissection required to gain active motion at surgery and the postoperative swelling that follows make it difficult to maintain the full active range of motion obtained at surgery. Nonetheless the final range of motion obtained is still significantly better than the preoperative status.

CONCLUSION

The approach to tenolysis presented in this chapter emphasizes (1) intraoperative control of pain, which allows an evaluation of the patient's active motion during surgery, and (2) postoperative control of pain, which allows the early active motion that we feel is the key to obtaining good results from tenolysis. If flexor tenolyses, extensor tenolyses, and releases of joint contractures are done with the patient under local anesthesia, the problem of incomplete release can be eliminated completely. This method of anesthesia also may be useful in tendon transfers, in repairs of boutonniere deformity, and in the diagnostic evaluation of complex hand problems. The use of prn sensory analgesia program provides *control of pain*, which we believe is the *key* to obtaining early postoperative motion following tenolysis and the release of joint contractures. If early full active motion is obtained, it will be maintained in most cases. We have emphasized the role of hand therapy in this chapter, since hand therapy plays an integral role in the achievement of good results in this type of surgery. This type of surgery should not be performed without a commitment to frequent, regular therapy sessions. Not only does the use of local Innovar anesthesia improve results by allowing a better understanding of the dynamics of hand function, but it also makes the performance of the surgery more demanding, challenging, and rewarding.

REFERENCES

1. Bruner, J.M.: The zig-zag volar-digital incision for flexor tendon surgery, Plast. Reconstr. Surg. **40:**571, 1967.
1a. Erickson, J.C., III, Hunter, J.M., and Schneider, L.H.: Neuroleptanalgesia and local anesthesia for a dynamic approach to surgery of the hand, Exhibit shown at the International Anesthesia Research Society, Phoenix, 1976; American College of Surgeons, Chicago, 1976; American Academy of Orthopaedic Surgeons, Las Vegas, 1977; Rehabilitation of the Hand Course, Philadelphia, 1976, 1977, and 1978.
2. Hunter, J.M., Cook, J., Ochiai, N., Merklin, R.J., Konikoff, J., and Mackin, G.A.: The pulley system, Presented at meeting of the American Society for Surgery of the Hand, Atlanta, Feb. 1980.
3. Hunter, J.M., Schneider, L.H., Dumont, J., and Erickson, J.C., III: A dynamic approach to problems of hand function, Clin. Orthop. **104:**112, 1974.
4. Martin, S.J., Murphy, J.D., Colliton, R.J., and Zeffiru, R.G.: Clinical studies with Innovar, Anesthesiology **28:**458, 1967.
5. Morgan, M., Lumley, J., and Gillies, I.D.S.: Neuroleptanalgesia for major surgery, Br. J. Anaesth. **46:**288, 1974.
6. Siker, E.S., Wolfson, B., Stewart, W.D., and Ciccarelli, H.E.: The effects of fentanyl and droperidol, alone and in combination, on pain thresholds in human volunteers, Anesthesiology **29:**834, 1968.

SUGGESTED READINGS

Hunter, J.M.: In American Academy of Orthopaedic Surgeons: Symposium on Tendon Surgery in the Hand, St. Louis, 1975, The C.V. Mosby Co.

Hunter, J.M., and Jaeger, S.H.: Tendon implants: primary and secondary usage, Orthop. Clin. North Am. **8:**473, 1977.

Hunter, J.M., and Salisbury, R.E.: Flexor tendon reconstruction in severely damaged hands: a two-stage procedure using a silicone-Dacron reinforced gliding prosthesis prior to tendon grafting, J. Bone Joint Surg. **53A:**829, 1971.

Chapter 36 The painful neuroma

George E. Omer, Jr.

Painful neuromas are enigmatic lesions without specific histologic characteristics to differentiate them from nonpainful neuromas. Painful amputation neuromas are characterized by a focal increase in volume, primarily resulting from fibrous tissue. There is a disorganized mass of fibroblasts, Schwann cells, and disoriented axons. Cajal[3] emphasized the predominance of small axons that are within and outside the original perineurial limits. Axon counts and size frequency histograms from varied levels have been obtained in humans, but it remains unknown whether nonpainful neuromas show any distinctive features when compared with painful neuromas.[20]

The electrophysiology of painful neuromas has been explained by several theories. Noordenbos[19] advanced the fiber dissociation theory, which states that the selective loss of large-diameter afferents releases extra output from small-diameter sensory axons that conduct impulses related to pain. Noordenbos's concept was based on clinical observations in postherpetic neuralgia. Melzack and Wall[15] gave support to the fiber dissociation concept with their gate control theory of pain. The hypothesis that an external physical injury can produce a breakdown of normal biophysical nerve insulation with resulting abnormal "artificial synapse" has clinical support.[7,11] Pain afferents would be ephaptically cross-excited by normal ascending or descending (somatic and autonomic) impulses. Ephaptic excitation at an artificial synapse has been shown electrophysiologically in laboratory animals,[8] but Wall, Waxman, and Basbaum[27] failed to confirm long-lasting cross-excitation following experimental nerve injury. No comparable studies are available in humans. In addition to the fiber dissociation and artificial synapse theories, a third concept implicates the spontaneous generation of impulses in abnormal axons.[25,26] The abnormal generators are immature sprouts from small-diameter afferent axons. Structural defects, such as inadequate myelin, stimulate the abnormal impulses.[4] Many patients suffer from chronic pain from neuromas, and yet we know very little about the mechanisms involved in the sensory experience.

Excessive scarring, infection, poor tissue nutrition, or thin skin is found in some cases of painful neuroma,[2] but there is little evidence that any of these complications of injury contributes to the formation of a neuroma. Pain is a complex sensory experience related to the mechanisms of injury, the location of the pathologic lesion, the length of time that pain has been present, and the patient's personality. A neuroma can become the trigger point for prolonged spontaneous pain with resultant narcotic addiction and emotional deterioration of a susceptible individual.

DIFFERENTIAL LOCALIZATION

Injuries have associated edema and fibrosis, and the resulting ischemic changes or traumatic arthrosis may confuse the clinical diagnosis of a painful neuroma.

There is little doubt that severe acute ischemia or chronic compression ischemia can produce pain. The patient's history must include the presence or absence of vascular pathosis. Pulse volume recorder readings, skin temperature levels, thermography, cold tolerance tests, and the relationship of all these tests to pain must be determined.[18] I follow the method of Porter and associates[22]: the patient sits quietly for 30 minutes in a warm room with the temperature about 24° C. The digital pulp temperature is determined with an electronic telethermometer. The patient's hands are then immersed in an ice water mixture for 20 seconds, and after they are dried, the digital pulp temperature is measured until the temperature returns to the pre–ice water level or 45 minutes have passed. The usual recovery time is 10 minutes, with a range of 5 to 20 minutes. The digital pulp temperature test can be supplemented with arteriography to differentiate arterial spasm from organic obstructive disease. If digital flow is abnormal, medication to decrease local sympathetic reflex activity is indicated.

A variety of drugs have been used, including the alpha-receptor blocking drug tolazoline hydrochloride, the beta-adrenergic receptor blocking drug propranolol hydrochloride, and the neuronal norepinephrine depletor reserpine. Porter and associates[22] obtained acceptable patient response with repeated brachial artery injections of 0.25 mg reserpine at approximately 2- to 3-week intervals. Griseofulvin also has been used because it has a direct vasodilator action exclusive of sympathetic innervation.

Chemical sympathetic nerve block procedures provide information concerning alterations in total blood flow to the extremity. I perform a central chemical sympathetic block with either lidocaine hydrochloride 1% or mepivacaine hydrochloride 1% solutions. Subsequent blocks may use an anesthetic agent with a longer duration of action, such as prilocaine hydrochloride 1% or bupivacaine 1% solutions. When the burning pain resolves completely, a surgical sympathectomy should be performed. The effectiveness of sympathectomy is not related to interrupting a sensory pathway from the extremity but is related to eliminating the sympathetic efferent discharge to the peripheral arteries and sweat glands. Sympathectomy will relieve only burning pain, and associated arthritic pain or painful neuromas will not be affected.

Painful inflammatory stiffness may respond to pharmacologic agents. Corticosteroids are useful for the patient with inflammatory arthrosis. I have used a tourniquet and an intravenous regional block with 30 ml lidocaine hydrochloride 1% and 40 mg methylprednisolone sodium succinate.[31] During the 20 to 30 minutes of analgesia one can manipulate stiff joints and stretch contracted web spaces. An alternate technique used at the Hospital for Special Surgery in New York is a 10-day program where 25 mg of prednisone is given orally each day for 5 days, and then the dosage is decreased 5 mg each day for 5 days. A similar 10-day program is 250 mg of hydrocortisone sodium succinate intravenously each day for 5 days with the dosage decreased to 100 mg each day for 5 days. As the pain subsides, salicylates should be given to abort ongoing inflammatory metabolic pathways.

Other medications are reported effective in patients with inflammatory fibrosis. Carbamazepine is an anticonvulsant that has been used in the treatment of diabetic neuropathy.[32] Carbamazepine, 800 mg daily, has been combined with phenytoin sodium, 300 mg daily, for the treatment of severe inflammatory pain such as scleroderma with necrotic fingertips.[1] Alternate programs are phenytoin sodium (600 mg daily) with amitriptyline hydrochloride (75 mg at bedtime) or fluphenazine hydrochloride (3 mg daily) with amitriptyline hydrochloride (75 mg at bedtime).[1] These drugs must be diligently monitored and the patients carefully evaluated for adverse reactions. They are ineffective in the patient with a painful neuroma.

Pain secondary to a neuroma is usually well localized and can be elicited by percussion or massage.

TREATMENT TO RELIEVE PAIN

There are only two principles in the treatment of an established painful neuroma: (1) relieve the pain, and (2) institute active use of the involved extremity. Possible treatment programs are the following:
A. To relieve pain
  1. Peripheral (local) procedures
    a. Transcutaneous electric stimulation
    b. Continuous nerve block
    c. Surgical translocation of neuroma
  2. Central procedures
    a. Acupuncture and hypnosis
    b. Surgical ablation
B. To restore functional activity
  1. Passive physical modalities
    a. Static splints
    b. Contrast temperature baths
    c. Alternating pressure splints (Jobst)
    d. Percussion or massage
  2. Contact participation
    a. Dynamic splints
    b. Activities of daily living
    c. Tools for games and work
    d. Normal work activities

Transcutaneous electric stimulation

Transcutaneous electric stimulation is used as a peripheral method for the production of local analgesia. The technique attempts to selectively stimulate large myelinated sensory axons and control pain by activating the inhibitory mechanisms. The direct current stimulator delivers a modified square-wave pulse with controllable frequency, pulse width, and voltage. The intensity should be varied by the patient because stimuli that are too intense overcome the inhibitory mechanism and produce additional pain. Loeser, Black, and Christman[12] reported on 198 patients; 68% obtained partial or short-term relief, and 12.5% used the stimulator for long-term pain control. Long[13] has studied 400 patients with pain of diverse origins; 33% of these patients found the stimulating device to be of sufficient value to use it as the only method of pain therapy, whereas an additional 44% found stimulation a valuable adjunct in an overall treatment program that included behavior modification, drug withdrawal, and a physical activity program.

The best results are obtained when the treatment is given within 3 months of the onset of pain. In our patients with established pain for 3 months or longer the percutaneous electric stimulator has produced subjective improvement if it is operated continuously; however, it has not been effective enough to produce objective improvement such as increased grip or pinch strength or endurance pull without supplemental analgesia. At Massachusetts General Hospital in Boston operative placement of the electrodes directly on involved peripheral nerves and prolonged stimulation have resulted in lasting relief from pain in 30% of 44 patients who were monitored for at least 6 months. An additional 31% had initial pain relief, but pain returned as scar tissue formed around the electrodes.[30] Another study at Duke University[17] reported lasting relief from pain in 36% of 20 patients monitored for 30 months after surgical implantation of the electrodes directly on involved peripheral nerves.

Acupuncture and hypnosis

Acupuncture seems to be effective in the susceptible individual. However, there is no scientific evidence, anatomic or physiologic, that acupuncture points, or meridians, exist.[5] In the latter part of the eighteenth century the German physician Franz Anton Mesmer developed modern techniques for hypnosis. Experiments in hypnosis have shown that subjects can distort perception as well as motor movements, and through hypnosis one can produce partial to total anesthesia. Successful acupuncture and hypnosis both require the cerebral cortex to activate complex conditioned reflexes that raise pain thresholds, remove anxiety and tension, and relieve depression.[16]

Local anesthetic injections

Local anesthetic injections, with long-acting medications, may diminish the intensity of the pain. When the patient is first examined, the extremity should be palpated and tapped very gently from distal to proximal aspects to demonstrate any trigger points of extreme irritation. If a trigger point is found, the area is prepared for surgery and marked with a sterile pen. After local cutaneous anesthesia a 16-gauge needle is inserted into the area of irritation. Fluid is aspirated to avoid blood-vessel penetration, and a flexible 18-gauge polyethylene intravenous catheter is inserted through the 16-gauge needle. If inserted in this manner, the intravenous catheter should not penetrate a nerve or blood vessels. The large-bore 16-gauge needle is then removed, leaving the catheter in place. One-half milliliter of 0.5% lidocaine hydrochloride is then injected into the intravenous catheter for anesthetic effect. If the trigger-point pain is relieved, the venous catheter is capped and taped in place. The anesthetic block usually is insufficient for complete motor or sensory paralysis, and the pain-free patient is asked to exercise the extremity, to walk, and to perform the assigned physical therapy program. If the anesthetic block is not effective, then one additional milliliter of lidocaine is injected; if this also is not effective, the intravenous catheter is withdrawn. If the anesthetic block is effective, additional periodic injection of lidocaine solution is based on the time of pain-free activity. The patient decides the frequency of injection, dependent on pain relief. The usual regimen has been 0.5 ml of 2% lidocaine hydrochloride solution with 1:100,000 of epinephrine or mepivacaine hydrochloride every 4 hours. The volume for each injection has ranged from 0.5 to 1 ml, and the time range between injections has been 1 to 10 hours. The average time range between injections was 2.2 hours during the acute stage, lengthening to 3.4 hours as the effect of the periodic peripheral infusion decreased pain and muscle strength improved. The periodic infusion is injected through the catheter without need for further skin puncture and has been continued for 2 weeks in a few cases.[21] If there is more than one area of irritation, separate catheters should be used for each trigger point. In contrast to a central chemical stellate block, the periodic peripheral infusion is a ward procedure that can be performed simultaneously with other modes of treatment. The peripheral infusion will relieve painful symptoms for a variable period but will not produce permanent relief from pain. It is much less effective where the pain has been untreated and unrelieved for 3 or more months after injury. It is ineffective in the patient who has a lesion involving the brachial plexus.

Percutaneous injection of triamcinolone acetonide about the neuroma after a cutaneous anesthetic block with 2% lidocaine hydrochloride has been reported to relieve the pain symptoms in 50% of patients after one injection and in 80% of patients after multiple injections.[23] It was surmised that softening of the fibrous tissue about the neuroma was the basis for the relief from pain.

Percussion

Percussion or massage of painful neuromas has been a clinical procedure for military amputees since World War I. Controlled clinical studies[9] have indicated that the technique is very useful in selected cases. Rubber mallets, mechanical vibrators, and ultrasonic treatments can be used to provide the repetitious percussion. Local anesthesia may be necessary over the area of trigger pain at the beginning of the treatment program; then later the percussion or massage can be done without local anesthesia.

Prevention of neuroma formation

A variety of physical and chemical methods have been used to prevent the formation of a painful neuroma. Ligation of the proximal stump with silk, wire, fascia, or other suture materials has not been successful. The proximal nerve stump has been implanted under fascia or into muscle, bone, veins, and even its own proximal nerve trunk.[24] The proximal stump has been capped with sheaths of glass, gold foil, tantalum, silver, Millipore, methyl methacrylate, and silicone. Initial clinical success was reported with all ensheathing materials, but all except silicone have been abandoned.[28,29] Electrocoagulation, freezing, steroids, or injection with phenol, alcohol, nitrogen mustard, tannic acid, gentian violet, and many other chemicals has not prevented painful neuromas. Snyder has estimated that more than 150 physical and chemical methods have been used, but none has had consistent success.[24]

Surgical treatment

The best objective guide in selecting patients whose painful neuromas can be relieved by local surgery is a diagnostic nerve block. The local anesthetic can be injected about the neuroma or more proximally about the nerve trunk. The pain must be completely relieved. One should do a short series of nerve blocks, using a placebo of normal saline for one block to evaluate the patient's emotional reaction.

The best surgical approach for a painful neuroma is transfer of the entire neuroma and the proximal nerve stump to a new tissue bed where compression is unlikely and traction is minimal. The neuroma should be placed in an area of good circulation with a thick subcutaneous layer that is free to scar. Success has been reported in 82% of patients treated with this technique.[10] A repeat excisional neurectomy is indicated one time in those cases with continued pain.[24]

The nerve trunk has been divided at one or more sites proximal to the terminal neuroma and resutured with an epineural technique. The indication for proximal neurotomy is axon degeneration at several levels and a resultant inability to form the terminal neuroma. This is effective only if there is considerable length of nerve distal to the neurotomy.[14]

A painful neuroma-in-continuity can occur following contusion or compression of a peripheral nerve. The traumatic episode may be isolated, as in radial nerve compression from "Saturday night palsy." More often the trauma is repetitious, as in bowler's thumb or the cubital and carpal tunnel syndromes. Surgery for a neuroma-in-continuity can be either intraneural neurolysis or excision of the neuroma. Meticulous intraneural neurolysis is helpful if the cause is repeated compression with retention of distal function, as inmedial nerve pain from carpal tunnel syndrome.[6] When there is significant paralysis distal to the lesion, it is best to excise the neuroma-in-continuity and suture the nerve trunk under minimal tension. The resection must be complete.

If there is no relief after local surgery, an anterolateral chordotomy may be indicated in the patient threatened with permanent dysfunction and narcotic addiction. However, White and Sweet[30] have recorded that postchordotomy analgesia cannot be expected to last longer than 6 months, with somewhat better results in those cases involving the lower extremity than in those involving the upper. Rhizotomy, posterior column tractotomy, postcentral gyrectomy of the sensory cortex, and frontal leukotomy all have been ineffective for sustained relief from pain. Initial success has been reported after cingulumotomy,[14] but evaluation of sustained relief from pain after this procedure is incomplete. Most of the surgical procedures for the central nervous system interrupt the spinothalamic tract, which projects pain to the ventroposterolateral nucleus of the thalamus and to the parietal cortex. The return of pain after surgery is related to the increased activity of polysynaptic systems (paleospinothalamic system or spinoreticulothalamic system) that are highly developed and widespread in the brain stem and thalamus. These polysynaptic systems are infinitely complex and diffuse and eventually frustrate any ablation procedure.

FUNCTIONAL ACTIVITY OF THE EXTREMITY

The second principle in the treatment program in use of the involved extremity. Available physical modalities are divided into passive and active types. The passive activities will improve circulation, decrease edema, and prepare the patient for active voluntary participation in the active exercise program. Passive modalities include percussion, static splints (Orthoplast), faradic muscle stimulation, ice packs, hot paraffin packs, combined contrast baths, and massage. For the apprehensive patient the passive modalities may need to be preceded by very delicate passive techniques. The skin can be lightly stroked with a feather, followed by very gentle massage, with progression to hot paraffin baths before percussion and similar passive modalities will be tolerated.

The more important phase is active functional contact, which can be assisted with dynamic splints, supportive exercise slings, and special handles for tools. Function can be developed with diversionary games, assigned work, and activities of daily living. It is most important that physicians, physical therapists, occupational therapists, and other attendants be compassionate and yet obtained maximal effort from the patient. The best functional activity for a patient is to return to usual work. Ultimately the patient "cures" his or her own painful neuroma.

REFERENCES

1. Benson, W.F.: Medications in the control of intractable pain syndromes, American Society for Surgery of the Hand Newsletter 1977-50, Sept. 16, 1977.

2. Bunnell, S.: Surgery of the hand, ed. 3, Philadelphia 1956, J.B. Lippincott Co.
3. Cajal, S.R.: Degeneration and regeneration of the nervous system, London, 1928, Oxford University Press.
4. Calvin, W.H., Loeser, J.D., and Howe, J.F.: A neurophysiological theory for the pain mechanism of tic douloureux, Pain 3:147, 1977.
5. Cantrell, J.R.: Acupuncture: a form of psychologic healing, Southwest Med. 63:14, 1975.
6. Curtis, R.M., and Eversmann, W.W., Jr.: Internal neurolysis as an adjunct to the treatment of the carpal-tunnel syndrome, J. Bone Joint Surg. 55A:733, 1973.
7. Doupe, J., Cullen, C.H., and Chance, G.Q.: Post-traumatic pain and causalgic syndrome, J. Neurol. Neurosurg. Psychiatry 7:33, 1944.
8. Granit, R., and Skoglund C.R.: Facilitation, inhibition and depression at the artificial synapse formed by the cut end of a mammalian nerve, J. Physiol. 103:435, 1945.
9. Grant, G.H.: Methods of treatment of neuromata of the hand, J. Bone Joint Surg. 33A:841, 1951.
10. Herndon, J.H., Eaton, R.G., and Littler, J.W.: Management of painful neuromas in the hand, J. Bone Joint Surg. 58A:369, 1976.
11. Kleiman, A.: Causalgia: evidence of the existence of crossed sensory sympathetic fibers, Am. J. Surg. 87:839, 1954.
12. Loeser, J.D., Black, R.G., and Christman, A.: Relief of pain by transcutaneous stimulation, J. Neurosurg. 42:308, 1975.
13. Long, D.M.: Electrical stimulation for the control of pain, Arch. Surg. 112:884, 1977.
14. Mathews, G.J., and Osterholm, J.L.: Painful traumatic neuromas, Surg. Clin. North Am. 52:1313, 1972.
15. Melzack, R., and Wall, P.D.: Pain mechanisms: a new theory, Science 150:971, 1965.
16. Murphy, T.M., and Bonica, J.J.: Acupuncture analgesia and anesthesia, Arch. Surg. 112:896, 1977.
17. Nashold, B.S., Jr., Goldner, J.L., and Bright, D.S.: Direct electrical stimulation of the peripheral nerves for relief of intractable pain, J. Bone Joint Surg. 57A:729, 1975.
18. Nashold, B.S., Jr., Goldner, J.L., and Bright, D.S.: Electrical stimulation of peripheral nerves with micro-electrical implants for pain relief. In Omer, G.E., Jr., and Spinner, M., editors: Management of peripheral nerve problems, Philadelphia, 1980, W.B. Saunders Co.
19. Noordenbos, W.: Pain, Amsterdam, 1959, Elsevier.
20. Ochoa, J.: Nerve fiber pathology in acute and chronic compression. Omer, G.E., Jr., and Spinner, M., editors: Management of peripheral nerve problems, Philadelphia, 1980, W.B. Saunders Co.
21. Omer, G.E., Jr., and Thomas, S.R.: The management of chronic pain syndromes in the upper extremity, Clin. Orthop. 104:37, 1974.
22. Porter, J.M., et al.: The diagnosis and treatment of Raynaud's phenomenon, Surgery 77:11, 1975.
23. Smith, J.R., and Gomez, N.H.: Local injection therapy of neuromata of the hand with triamcinolone acetonide, a preliminary study of 22 patients, J. Bone Joint Surg. 52A:71, 1970.
24. Tupper, J.W., and Booth, D.M.: Treatment of painful neuromas of sensory nerves in the hand: a comparison of traditional and newer methods, J. Hand Surg. 1:144, 1976.
25. Wall, P.D., and Gutnick, M.: Ongoing activity in peripheral nerves: the physiology and pharmacology of impulses originating from a neuroma, Exp. Neurol. 43:580, 1974.
26. Wall, P.D., and Gutnick, M.: Properties of afferent nerve impulses originating from a neuroma, Nature 248:740, 1974.
27. Wall, P.D., Waxman, S., and Basbaum, A.I.: Ongoing activity in peripheral nerve: injury discharge, Exp. Neurol. 45:576, 1974.
28. Weeks, P.M., and Wray, R.C.: Management of acute hand injuries: a biological approach, St. Louis, 1973, The C.V. Mosby Co.
29. Weissman, G.: Pain mediators and pain receptors. In Bonica, J.J., editor: Considerations in management of acute pain, New York, 1977, Hospital Practice Publishing Co.
30. White, J.C., and Sweet, W.H.: Pain and the neurosurgeon: a 40 year experience, Springfield, Ill., 1969, Charles C Thomas, Publisher.
31. Wiley, A.M., Poplawski, Z.B., and Murray, J.: Post-traumatic dystrophy of the hand, Orthop. Rev. 6:59, 1977.
32. Wilton, T.D.: Tegretol in the treatment of diabetic neuropathy, South African Med. J. 48:869, 1974.

Chapter 37   The surgical management of painful neuromas in the hand

Thomas L. Greene

James B. Steichen

Painful neuromas in the hand and forearm may be encountered frequently in a hand surgery practice and are difficult to treat successfully. Trauma, frequently work related, or nerve injury during surgical procedures about the hand usually accounts for the formation of these neuromas. The neuroma typically involves a named sensory nerve of the hand or wrist. The palmar cutaneous branch of the median nerve and the superficial sensory branch of the radial nerve are particularly prone to the formation of painful neuromas. The presence of a symptomatic neuroma can be a considerable disability. A variable loss of function results and may lead to a pattern of complete avoidance of use of part of or all the upper extremity.

An injury to a nerve that disrupts the Schwann cell–endoneurial barrier will inevitably form a neuroma.[5] After the breakdown of this barrier the fine regenerating axons will branch and grow in a disorganized fashion among the fibroblasts, Schwann cells, organized blood clot, and the epineurial tissue of the severed nerve end. The result is a neuroma of variable size, which is primarily dependant on the extent of axon growth.[5] The distinguishing features of a neuroma that becomes painful versus one that does not, under similar circumstances, are unfortunately unknown.

PREVENTION OF THE PAINFUL NEUROMA

The correct initial management of a nerve injury offers the best opportunity for preventing the consequences of a painful neuroma. Adherence to the basic surgical principles of gentle distal retraction of a nerve, sharp proximal transection, and allowing nerve retraction into an unscarred tissue bed away from the primary wound is of great importance in dealing with digital amputations and irreparable nerve injuries. Allowing the inevitable neuroma that forms to reside in a pressure-free, well-vascularized bed away from continuous trauma will reduce the incidence of symptomatic neuromas.[1]

When conditions allow, neurrorrhaphy offers the best chance of minimizing neuroma formation by directing the regenerating axons to reinnervate the distal nerve trunk and to be confined by the perineurium. This properly directed regeneration will limit the usual disorganized axonal growth that occurs at the free severed nerve end.

A good deal of effort has been expended over the years in an attempt to either limit axonal growth from the severed nerve end or to contain the growth that inevitably occurs. Over 150 chemical and physical means have been described, none of which is reliably or consistently effective.[5]

TREATMENT OF THE PAINFUL NEUROMA

Several approaches to the management of the established painful neuroma in the hand have evolved. Nonoperative methods include repeated massage or desensitization programs, transcutaneous nerve stimulation, sympathetic blockade, and injection of various materials about the neuroma, including local anesthetics, alcohol, and steroids. Injection of a neuroma with steroid preparations has some theoretic basis in view of their effects on limiting collagen formation. Smith and Gomez[4] have reported the results of steroid injections in 34 painful neuromas in the hand. Symptoms of tenderness, spontaneous pain, paresthesia, and hyperesthesia were evaluated before and after the injection. Thirteen of 24 neuromas with tenderness were completely relieved, and five were partially relieved. Paresthesia was unrelieved in 10 of 23 neuromas (43%). Even less encouraging results were obtained for hyperesthesia and spontaneous pain, with virtually 100% failure. It would seem therefore that injection of painful neuromas with steroids is not effective enough to justify its use.

Some painful neuromas will respond to conservative treatment, but many will eventually require surgery. The operative management of the painful neuroma can be divided into methods that resect the neuroma, those which leave it intact, and those which attempt to eliminate reformation of the neuroma by neurorrhaphy.

Excision of the neuroma and allowing the divided nerve end to retract into a healthy protected tissue bed have been applied to the care of neuromas as well as to irreparable primary nerve injuries. This treatment is most often associated with those neuromas resulting from amputation of the digits. A retrospective review of 316 neuromas in the hand treated by one or more neurectomies has been reported by Tupper and Booth.[7] Results were categorized as excellent (no or minimal tenderness), satisfactory (mild to moderate tenderness without functional limitations), or unsatisfactory (severe tenderness and functional limitations). Crush injuries achieved a combined average of 78% excellent and satisfactory results if a second neurectomy was performed. Semisharp injuries (e.g., from power saws) and sharp injuries gave combined averages of 94% and 42% excellent and satisfactory results, respectively, if a second neurectomy was performed. For all injury types this gives 71% excellent and satisfactory results. The reasons for the rather poor results following sharp injuries to a nerve are not readily apparent.

Neurectomy and covering the nerve end with silicone rubber (either a silicone tube [Ducker-Hayes] or cap [Frackelton]) have enjoyed some popularity. Tupper and Booth[7] found, however, a combined average of 53% excellent and satisfactory results if a second neurectomy and capping were done, making this technique less satisfactory then neurectomy alone. Frackelton, Teasley, and Taurus[2] found that the best results of capping were with those neuromas which were transposed as well. Twenty digital nerve neuromas treated by neurectomy and silicone capping, combined with retraction of the nerve into protected soft tissues or transposition, have been reported by Swanson, Boeve, and Lumsden.[6] Pain relief was obtained in 85% of the neuromas, and tenderness was relieved in 65%. Although these results are better than those of Tupper and Booth for the same procedures, comparable results are obtainable with neurectomy or transposition alone.

Neurorrhaphy may be employed, with a nerve graft if needed, particularly in a digital nerve injury. There may be some functional return of sensation, but more important is a limitation of axon regeneration to endoneurial tubes, thereby limiting painful-neuroma formation.

One of the best approaches to the management of the painful neuroma is transposition of the intact neuroma. In this technique the intact neuroma with sufficient nerve length is mobilized and transferred to another location in the soft tissues, usually toward the dorsum of the hand. The neuroma may be secured in its new location by a suture placed through the fibrous tissue covering about the nerve end. The neuroma comes to lie in a protected area, thereby eliminating the irritating effects of pressure, traction, and friction. Herndon, Eaton, and Littler[3] have reported their results using this technique for painful neuromas of the hand. Eight-two percent of the amputees' and 63% of the nonamputees' neuromas achieved a level of no or minimal pain and no limitation of activity following transposition. The result is an average 72% combined success rate for the two groups. Transposition of the intact neuroma into bone is another alternative, particularly in areas such as about the dorsal aspect of the wrist where satisfactory soft tissue protection is not afforded.

CASE HISTORIES

The following case histories demonstrate several methods of surgical management of painful neuromas in the hand.

SECTION 10　PAIN PROBLEMS

Case 1

A 23-year-old, right-handed man sustained a comminuted fracture of the distal aspect of the radius. Treatment consisted of closed reduction and internal fixation by means of a Rush pin placed through the radial styloid. Following this he had numbness over the dorsum of the hand in the distribution of the superficial branch of the radial nerve. The wound at the site of pin placement was painful and extremely sensitive to touch (Fig. 37-1, A). Use of the hand was severely limited. The fracture went on to heal uneventfully. Eventual surgical exploration of the area of tenderness revealed a large neuroma-in-continuity of a majority of the superficial branch of the radial nerve (Fig. 37-1, B). An internal neurolysis of the nerve was performed using the operating microscope. After resection of the neuroma and isolation of the intact portion of the nerve a neurorrhaphy was accomplished (Fig. 37-1, C). Six months after the procedure the area of original injury, although improved, was still hypersensitive and painful, and he could not return to work. Further treatment is being contemplated.

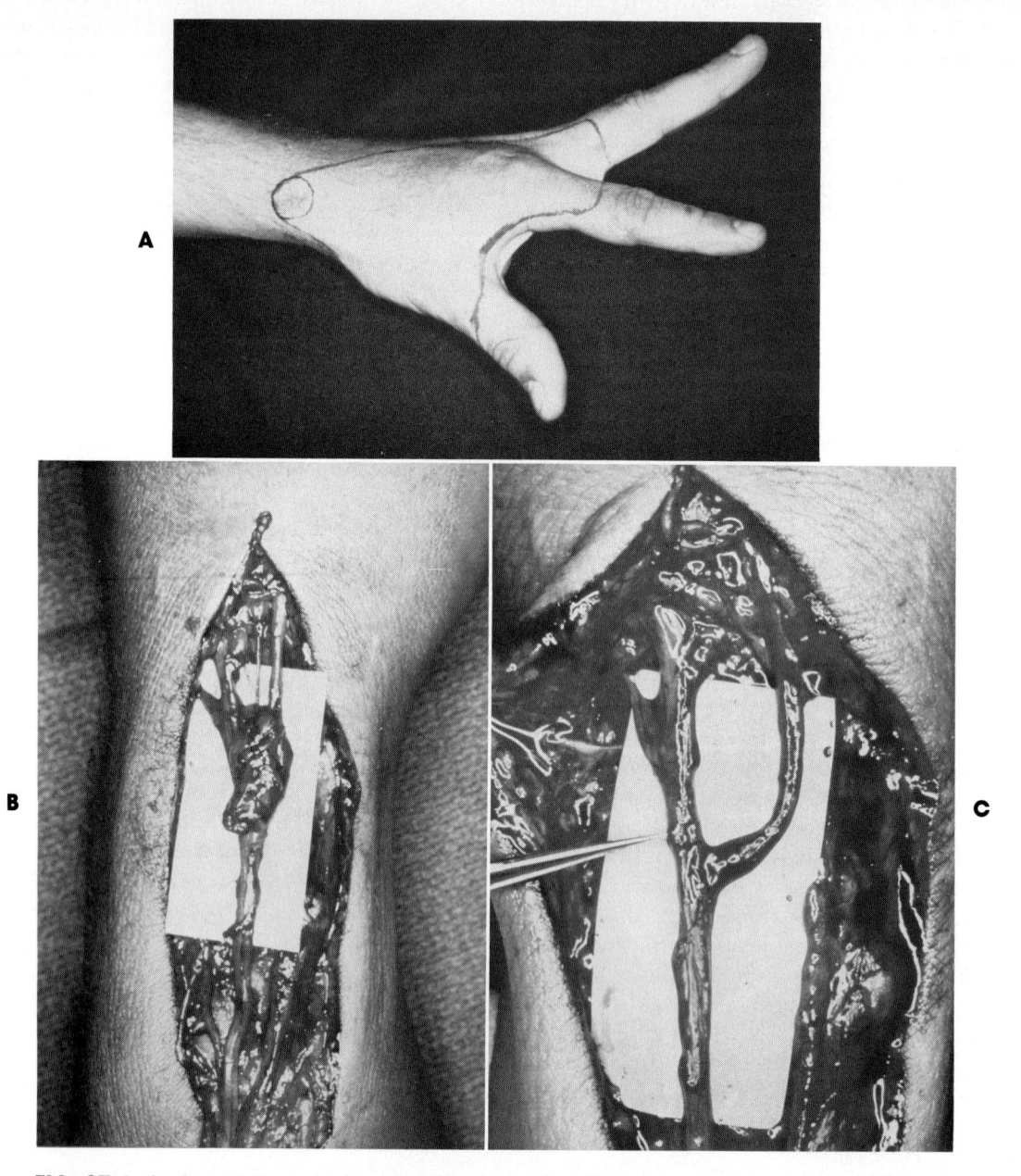

FIG. 37-1. A, Case 1. Injury to superficial branch of radial nerve at wrist occurred following Rush pin fixation of radius. Area of sensory loss over dorsum of hand is outlined and site of percutaneous pin placement circled. **B,** Large neuroma-in-continuity following partial severance of superficial sensory branch of radial nerve. **C,** After internal neurolysis of neuroma was performed using operating microscope, neuroma was resected, and neurorrhaphy was performed at site pointed out by microsurgical forceps.

Case 2

A 48-year-old, right-handed man sustained a crush injury to the left index finger in an industrial accident. Following unsuccessful reconstructive surgery he had a ray resection of the index finger. One month after the amputation the surgical incision was hypersensitive and produced "electric shocks" on percussion. Five months later a resection of the digital neuromas to the index finger was performed. Pain and hypersensitivity in the palm continued. One year after the neurectomy, transposition of two large digital neuromas toward the dorsum of the hand to lie between the muscle bellies of the intrinsic muscles was performed (Fig. 37-2). He had complete relief from the pain and returned to work 30 months after the original injury.

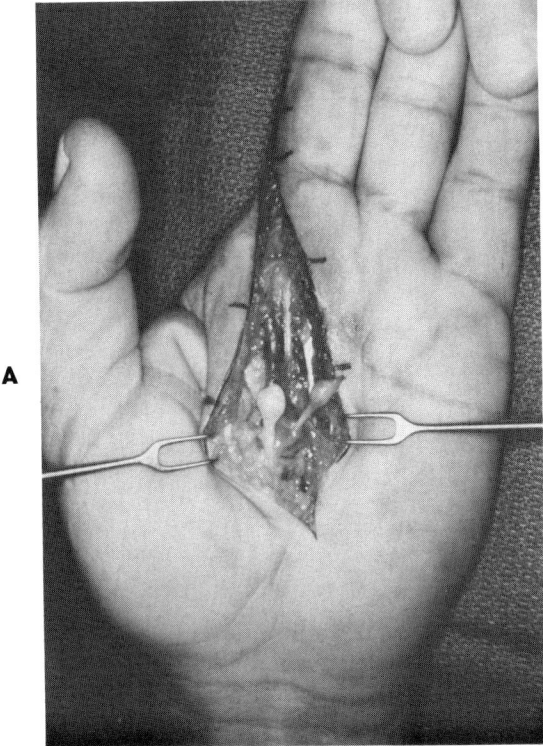

FIG. 37-2. A and **B,** Case 2. Neuromas of digital nerves to index finger present in palm following ray resection of index finger and subsequent neurectomies for painful neuromas. **C,** Neuromas were transposed toward dorsum of hand to lie between muscle bellies of intrinsic muscles.

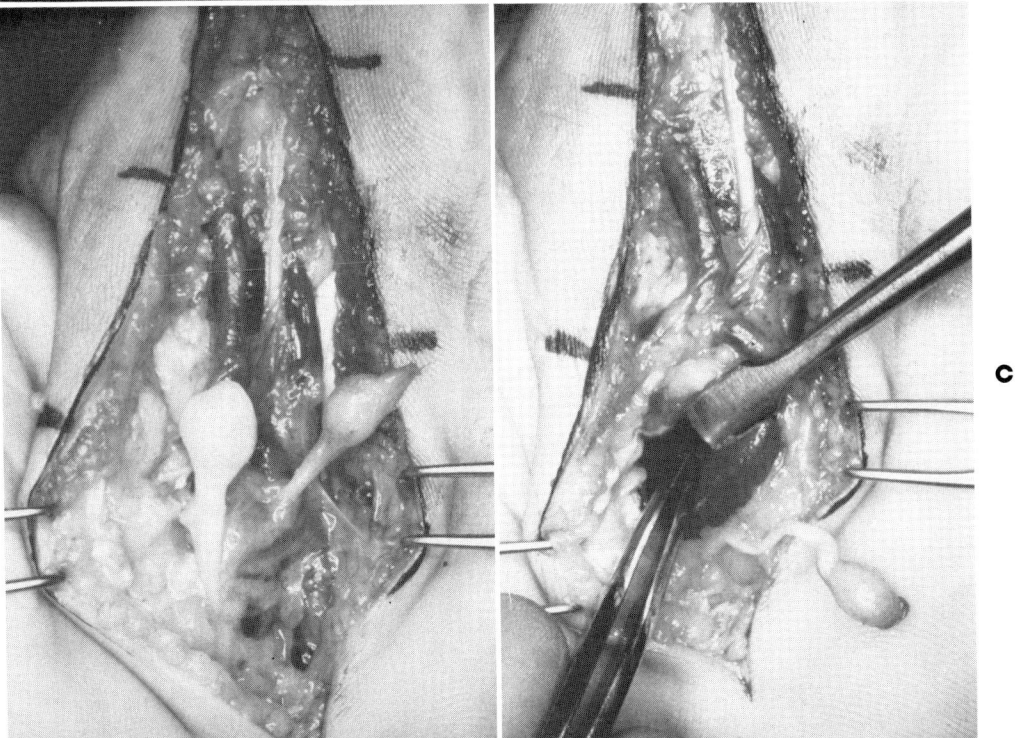

SECTION 10 PAIN PROBLEMS

Case 3

A 20-year-old, right-handed man sustained an amputation of the left small finger proximal to the proximal interphalangeal joint on a power saw while at work. The initial treatment involved digital neurectomies and closure. Two months later he developed tender digital neuromas in the finger, which were treated by amputation revision and digital neurectomies. Over the next year he continued to develop progressively sensitive neuromas in the amputation stump (Fig. 37-3, A). These neuromas were transposed toward the dorsum of the hand along the radial margin of the hypothenar muscles in the palm (Fig. 37-3, B). In follow-up analysis 5 months later he continued to exhibit complete relief from the painful neuroma symptoms and had returned to work.

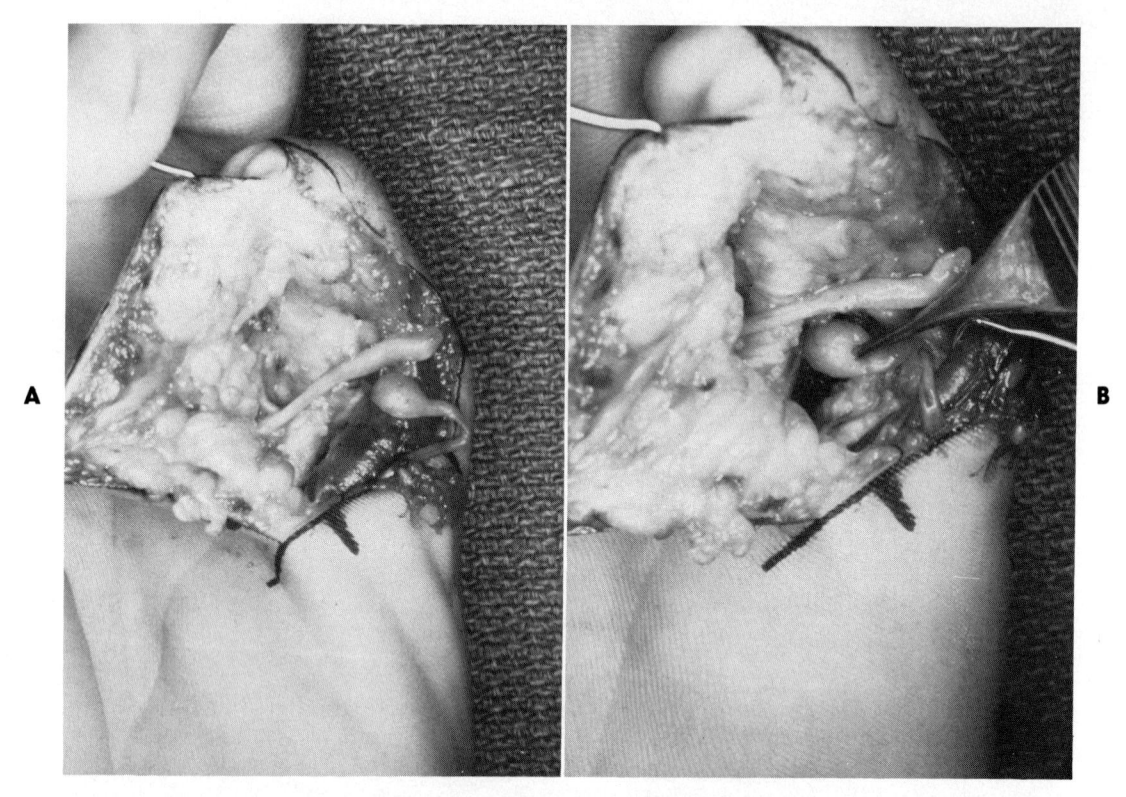

FIG. 37-3. A, Case 3. Two neuromas have been dissected out of amputation stump of small finger prior to transposition. **B,** Transposition of two digital neuromas of small finger toward dorsum of hand between flexor sheath and hypothenar muscles in distal aspect of palm.

Case 4

A 23-year-old, right-handed woman had a dorsal carpal ganglion excised from the right wrist through a transverse incision. Two weeks later she began to have abnormal tenderness along the radial extent of the incision. A very sensitive mass developed in this same area. Four months later a recurrent ganglionectomy and a neurectomy of a terminal division of the superficial branch of the radial nerve in the area were performed. She continued to be quite symptomatic from the new neuroma that formed. One injection of this neuroma with a steroid resulted in no change in symptoms. Nine months after the initial neurectomy a large neuroma of a branch of the superficial radial nerve was transposed intact into the distal aspect of the radius (Fig. 37-4). Subsequently she has had total relief from the neuroma pain.

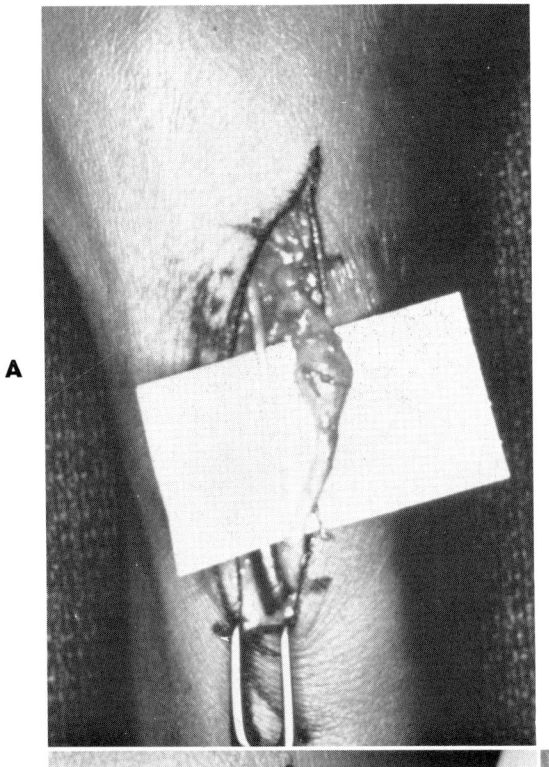

FIG. 37-4. A, Case 4. Most dorsal division of superficial branch of radial nerve developed large neuroma following dorsal ganglionectomy. **B,** Mobilization of neuroma and nerve branch and preparation of site in distal aspect of radius to accept neuroma. **C,** Neuroma has been buried in distal aspect of radius and secured by suture placed through bone.

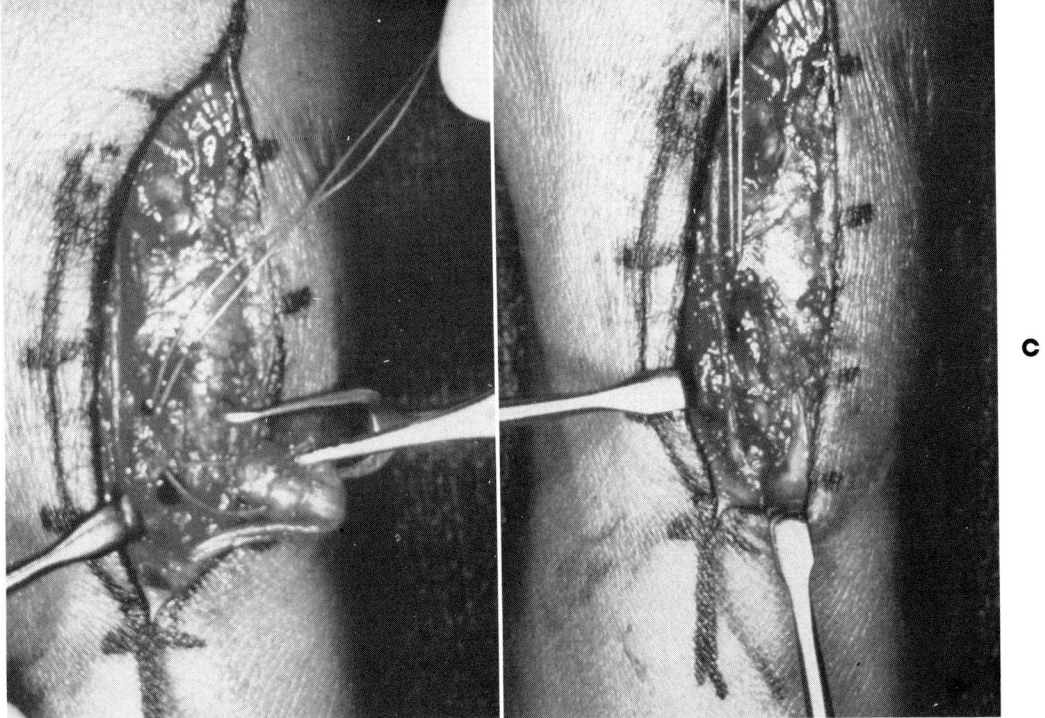

SECTION 10 PAIN PROBLEMS

Case 5

A 49-year-old, right-handed woman sustained a crushing amputation of the left index fingertip in a punch press. Initial management required distal interphalangeal joint disarticulation and digital neurectomies. The amputation stump remained very sensitive, especially on the ulnar side, which prohibited use of the finger. Three months later a revision of the amputation and digital neurectomies were performed. Delayed healing of the wound was encountered. Seven months passed, during which time the index finger was used little primarily because of ulnar tip pain and sensitivity. Another revision of the amputation with excision of bulbous neuromas after distal retraction and proximal severance of the digital nerves was performed (Fig. 37-5). The third neurectomy completely relieved the pain in the digit, and she was able to return to her previous occupation.

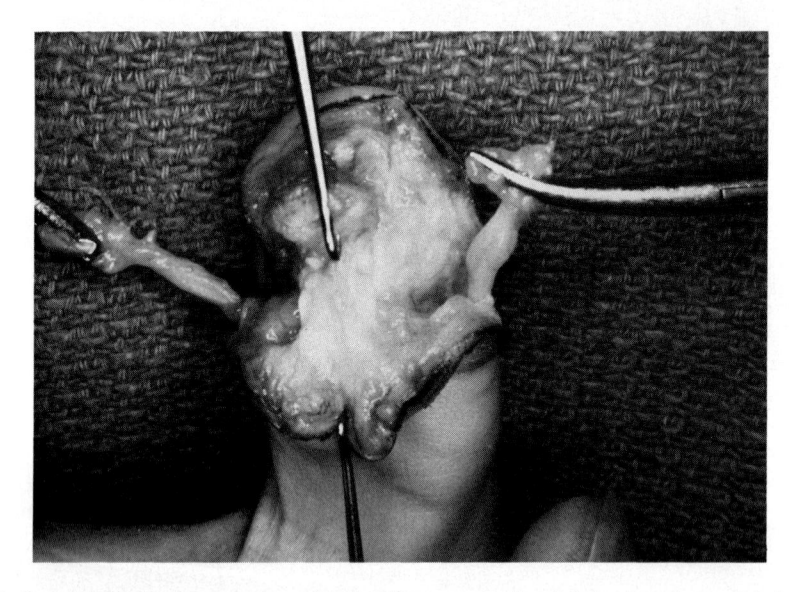

FIG. 37-5. Case 5. Digital neuromas of index finger prior to distal retraction and sharp proximal division. Nerves are not divided until level of osseous amputation and skin coverage are established.

SUMMARY

The formation of a neuroma is the inevitable consequence of a nerve injury that disrupts the Schwann cell–endoneurial barrier. Why some neuromas become symptomatic and require treatment and others do not is unknown. Proper initial management of a nerve injury can minimize the number of symptomatic neuromas that develop. Early recognition and treatment of a neuroma can possibly prevent the establishment of a chronic pain syndrome and return the patient to a functional role in society. Surgical management by neurectomy (multiple if needed) or transposition into protected soft tissue or bone offers the best prospects for useful recovery.

Admittedly there will continue to be some neuromas refractory to present treatment modalities. The future may hold an answer for these only by a better understanding of nerve regeneration and its control.

REFERENCES

1. Boyes, J.H., editor: Bunnell's surgery of the hand, ed. 4, Philadelphia, 1964, J.B. Lippincott Co.
2. Frackelton, W.H., Teasley, J.L., and Taurus, A.: Neuromas in the hand treated by nerve transposition and silicone capping, J. Bone Joint Surg. **53A**:813, 1971.
3. Herndon, J.H., Eaton, R.G., and Littler, J.W.: Management of painful neuromas in the hand, J. Bone Joint Surg. **58A**:369, 1976.
4. Smith, J.R., and Gomez, N.H.: Local injection therapy of neuromata of the hand with triamcinolone acetonide, J. Bone Joint Surg. **52A**:71, 1970.
5. Sunderland, S.: Nerves and nerve injuries, ed. 2, New York, 1978, Churchill Livingstone.
6. Swanson, A.B., Boeve, N.R., and Lumsden, R.M.: The prevention and treatment of amputation neuromata by silicone capping, J. Hand Surg. **2**:70, 1977.
7. Tupper, J.W., and Booth, D.M.: Treatment of painful neuromas of sensory nerves in the hand: a comparison of traditional and newer methods, J. Hand Surg. **1**:144, 1976.

SECTION ELEVEN WRIST PROBLEMS

Chapter 38 Limited wrist arthrodesis

H. Kirk Watson

Arthrodesis of units in the wrist, as opposed to complete arthrodesis, has been well described.[1-5,8] This approach to wrist problems leaves the wrist with some motion while obliterating the damaged or painful joints.[15a]

Congenital fusions of most adjacent carpal bones (all but scaphoid to trapezium) have been described.[9,10] These are asymptomatic, and they last throughout the person's life without contributing to degenerative changes. Obtaining a limited wrist fusion is difficult, and the technique is one of those procedures in hand surgery requiring exacting attention to detail.

This chapter covers (1) the anatomy, briefly as it relates to limited wrist arthrodesis, (2) the indications, and more important, definite contraindications to limited wrist arthrodesis, (3) the surgical technique, including graft donor, pin placement, and the important pitfalls, (4) the postoperative management, and (5) the handling of complications.

ANATOMY

The anatomy of the wrist is too complex to be fully discussed here; however, some current functional concepts of wrist motion are worth considering. Because of the construction of the carpals and their ligaments, certain motion theories have come to be accepted. Certain bones are expected to work with others in specific patterns. The scaphoid is generally expected to move with the lunate, and the joint between them primarily allows a bending moment in the coronal plane. In radial deviation they both move dorsally, palmar flex, and tend to flatten their common curve. In ulnar deviation they both move volarly, dorsiflex, and slightly increase the outer arch that fits the radius. However, fusing the lunate to the radius and then evaluating the wrist with cineradiography demonstrate a significant motion in flexion-extension of the wrist, i.e., rotation at the scapholunate joint. Put another way, there are guidelines of motion that apply in the normal state, but underlying these is an adaptability in the face of fusion of two or more wrist bones, which does not surface until there has been a limited fusion plus 9 months to a year of postsurgical mobility. This increased motion probably represents a maximizing of available adaptive capsule stretch rather than any increase of normal ligament length. Certain patterns of fusion are demonstrating very effective planes of adaptability and increased motion.

One patient, 11 years after scapholunate-to-radius arthrodesis, demonstrates a motion plane through the triscaphe joint (scaphotrapeziotrapezoid) then across the capitate-scaphoid joint, the capitate-lunate joint, and the triquetral-lunate joint with 70 degrees of motion and no signs of degenerative joint disease. Certainly in the normal wrist there is much less motion through this pathway.

Motion between scaphoid and capitate after triscaphe fusion permits exceptionally good wrist function. This fusion pattern results in 80% of normal flexion-extension in the wrist and 66% of normal radioulnar deviation in the wrist. These are the figures for the overall series and are better still in the noncrushed, nontrophic younger patient with, e.g., rotary subluxation of the scaphoid. Wrists with capitate-lunate fusion gradually increase the motion of the lunate on the radius well beyond what is seen in a normal wrist. This happens slowly but steadily following fusion of the capitate-lunate joint. The hamate-triquetral or triquetral-lunate fusion for ulnar wrist instability injuries is new and promises very little total motion loss. The hamate is often added to the capitate without major change in expected wrist motion. The thumb carpometacarpal (CMC) joint probably should not be fused along with a triscaphe arthrodesis or when one is already present. This does not interfere particularly with wrist function but does interfere with thumb mobility.

Another general concept which must be borne in mind is that sufficient bone union must be achieved to carry the expected loads or pain will result. The classic example of this problem is a fused distal phalanx that is painful under load. X-ray examination will reveal that only one corner or a portion of the contact surface between the middle and distal phalanx is solidly fused. In this situation there is insufficient bone to carry the loading on the distal phalanx, and, although solid, the arthrodesis is painful. This problem applies when attempting a scaphoid-lunate fusion. I feel there is limited indication for this particular limited wrist arthrodesis. It is very difficult to obtain adequate bone to carry the loads, which tend to change the convexity of these two bones during loaded radial and ulnar deviation.

The story is by no means complete on which limited wrist arthrodeses will produce greater motion than anticipated, nor is it clear whether degenerative arthritis will be found in specific joints during long-term follow-up analysis on any particular limited wrist arthrodesis.[11-14] It seems at this time that at least 5 to 10 years will pass before other joints demonstrate degeneration. This is encouraging in that a fully stressed joint which is being badly insulted should exhibit any problems in a reasonably short time. The converse is also true, i.e., a joint that has a constant added load because of a nearby fusion by all rights should develop changes sooner than a contralateral normal joint.

Limited wrist combinations

The *thumb CMC* joint is well covered in general literature and is not discussed here.

Triscaphe arthrodesis

Triscaphe arthrodesis, i.e., fusion of the scaphoid, trapezium, and trapezoid joints, represents the most common form of limited wrist arthrodeses.[16] This is an easily achieved fusion that leaves very little residual disability and, to date, has demonstrated no tendency to destroy the surrounding joints. There are three indications for triscaphe arthrodeses: degenerative arthritis of the triscaphoid joint with a good thumb CMC joint, radial hand dislocations, and rotary subluxation of the scaphoid. Degenerative joint disease of this three-bone unit is common. The disease is limited to these three bones, and the rest of the wrist is uninvolved. This may represent a long-standing disruption of the ligaments supporting the distal pole of the scaphoid, allowing it to tilt forward out from under the trapezium and trapezoid. Long-standing rotary subluxation of the scaphoid can be present with painful degenerative arthritis of only the triscaphe joint. This is an atypical pattern.

Radial hand dislocation occurs in a common repeating pattern. The plane of displacement passes between the index and middle metacarpals, between the capitate and the trapezoid, and across and between the trapezoid, trapezium, and scaphoid joints. Thus the thumb and index rays dislocate dorsally with the trapezium and trapezoid. This usually appears to be a result of a severe crush in the radioulnar plane. These dislocations are often missed and are then impossible to relocate satisfactorily without fusing the triscaphe joint.

The third indication for triscaphe arthrodesis is rotary subluxation of the scaphoid. This procedure is new. The mechanical advantage of rotating the scaphoid on inline wrist loading is extreme, and ligamentous reconstructions of any type are notoriously unsuccessful for maintaining complete reduction of the rotated scaphoid. Complete reduction and triscaphe arthrodeses have demonstrated very encouraging initial results. One can expect better than 80% of the normal range of flexion-extension and better than 66% of the normal range of radial and ulnar deviation following a triscaphe arthrodesis. Slight volar or dorsal lunate instability does not seem to contraindicate this procedure.

Capitate-lunate arthrodesis

Capitate-lunate arthrodesis is indicated in localized degenerative disease of the capitate-lunate joint and as an adjunct to handling nonunion of the coronal plane fracture of the lunate. Capitate-lunate arthrodesis is not generally indicated in Kienböck's disease. The lunate must be uncollapsed and fused to the capitate in its normal relationship for adequate wrist function. The flexion-extension range of motion increases surprisingly when one considers the amount of motion that takes place between the capitate and lunate. This arthrodesis has been useful several times where the scaphoid has either an old nonunion or rotary displacement with severe long-standing degenerative arthritis and erosion between the radius and the scaphoid and secondary destruction of the capitate-lunate joint. This presents a major problem in that one has disease in the radiocarpal joint as well as of the intercarpal joint. This problem is successfully solved by doing a limited wrist arthrodesis of the capitate-lunate joint combined with a Silastic scaphoid implant. The wrist functions on the radiolunate joint and is positioned and supported by the implant. To be successful, one must have good cartilage on the proximal radiolunate joint. Fortunately this is usually present under these conditions.

Scaphocapitate-lunate arthrodesis

Scaphocapitate-lunate arthrodesis is more of a salvage procedure and is indicated when there is change or destruction in the intercarpal plane with good radiocarpal joints. Rotary subluxation of the scaphoid with severe volar and dorsal lunate instability with displacement should be handled by scaphocapitate-lunate rather than triscaphe arthrodesis, since the latter will not restabilize the lunate. Some lunate displacement is not uncommon with a displaced scaphoid, and triscaphe arthrodesis is sufficient.

Capitate-hamate-lunate-triquetral arthrodesis

Limited wrist arthrodesis of the capitate-hamate-lunate-triquetrum joint is usually used with panintercarpal degenerative arthritis with a free scaphoid, with adequate joint surfaces, and a good radiocarpal joint surface. This is seen after infection and occasionally with generalized degenerative joint disease in the carpals. The motion here is not dissimilar from that in a capitate-lunate arthrodesis.

Hamate-triquetral or lunate-triquetral arthrodesis

Arthrodesis of the hamate-triquetrum or lunate-triquetrum for ulnar wrist instability has been carried out successfully in several cases. One or the other will successfully repair this instability pattern.

The problem here is a diagnostic one. Radiographic demonstration of ulnar wrist instability is notoriously difficult. The problem is often dynamic rather than static; i.e., the bones tend to be normally related to one another, and the ligamentous instability only occurs with significant loading. Static deformities can be readily seen on standard films. Occasionally a line on the proximal surface of the scaphoid and lunate will not continue on the proximal surface of the triquetrum but will intersect or pass through the triquetrum, increasing suspicions of a lunate-triquetral instability pattern.[7] When there is convincing clinical evidence that one of these two joints is symptomatically unstable, then the final decision is made at surgery.

Carpometacarpal arthrodesis

Unlike the thumb, the index and middle finger metacarpals may be added to limited wrist arthrodeses if destruction has occurred in these joints. The ring and little finger metacarpals are usually better handled by an arthroplasty technique rather than fusion. These are almost always done after traumatic situations.

Scaphoradial and lunate-radial arthrodesis

These arthrodeses are typically done after traumatic situations where there is a defect in the radius, producing instability and degenerative joint disease of the wrist on the radial side. Fractures through the distal articular surface of the radius can occur in almost any plane. The two major problems occur when the volar articular surface is destroyed or fractured away and when the distal radial articular surface is centrally depressed. Pain-free stability is achieved by fusing the scaphoid or lunate to the radius. A Silastic prosthesis, of course, has no place in this type of injury. One should look carefully at a severe scaphoradial degenerative arthritis, since often there will be significant cartilage loss and degenerative change between the capitate-lunate joint, as well. In this situation a scaphoradial arthrodesis should not be attempted, and this situation is best handled as described under capitate-lunate arthrodesis. For isolated degenerative disease of the scaphoradial joint a Silastic implant is preferred, since the inline loading will be handled by the capitate-lunate and lunate-radius joints, and function is usually painless and adequate for all but the heavy, 8-hour-a-day laborer, who should expect periodic synovitis dependent on duration and severity of loading.

Scapholunate-radial arthrodesis

This arthrodesis is simply an extension of the scaphoradial or lunate-radial one. More extensive radiocarpal destruction and/or degenerative disease and loss of stability are the indications for fusing both of the key proximal row bones to the radius. A reasonable plane of motion can be expected to develop along the distal edge of the scapholunate bones.

Kienböck's disease

Kienböck's disease must be divided into two groups: the uncollapsed and the collapsed lunate. When the lunate has not collapsed, a capitate-lunate arthrodesis may enhance revascularization of the lunate, but a better approach is to protect the lunate from compressive forces of the capitate by fusing the triscaphe or capitate-scaphoid joints.

When the lunate has collapsed, there is usually some degree of rotary subluxation of the scaphoid and proximal migration of the capitate. If the articular cartilage of the proximal lunate is good, then capitate-lunate-scaphoid arthrodesis may be indicated. More commonly I use a Silastic lunate to triscaphe arthrodesis.

Contraindications

Scapholunate arthrodesis is difficult to achieve, and the fusion between scaphoid and lunate must have sufficient bone volume, or pain can be expected. Seldom will one be faced with degenerative joint disease isolated to the scapholunate joint.

The ulna should never be included in any limited wrist arthrodesis.

Carpal boss is not an indication for limited wrist arthrodesis.[15] This condition is a highly localized, congenital abnormality that produces degenerative arthritis in a very localized fashion, often in the very young and involving the index and middle finger metacarpals and capitate and trapezoid. This localized area is easily resected, leaving excellent stability and normal joints.

Nonunion of the scaphoid is not in itself an indication for limited wrist arthrodesis. This is best handled by obtaining satisfactory reduction and fusion of the scaphoid itself. Once secondary changes have occurred between the ununited scaphoid fragments and the surrounding bones, then various forms of limited wrist arthrodesis can be considered, as described. Both fragments can be fused to the capitate, but only if all the changes are on the intercarpal side with a good scaphoradial joint.

SURGICAL PRINCIPLES

1. Analysis and planning is everything.
2. Fuse only the minimal joints necessary.
3. Cancellous bone-graft packing arthrodesis must be used.
4. The external dimensions of the fused unit must equal the external dimensions of the same bones in their normal state.
5. Use sufficient bone graft.
6. Pin only the arthrodesed unit.

SURGICAL TECHNIQUE

The wrist is prepared for the operation in the usual manner. A transverse incision is made on the dorsum of the wrist over the area of fusion. After the skin incision only forceful spreading with scissors is used. Nerves, veins, and tendons are retracted, and another transverse incision is made into the wrist joint. The capsule of the joint to be fused is reflected. The articular cartilage remnants and subchondral bone is removed with a dental rongeur. This leaves broad cancellous bone on each opposing surface. These surfaces will not be pressed together. The bones will be set in such a way that their remaining cartilage surfaces will be in their normal relationship to the adjacent bones, usually leaving a wide gap up to about 8 or 9 mm between these cancellous surfaces.

Bone grafting is accomplished from the distal aspect of the radius.[17] By retracting the skin proximally, or by making a second, more proximal transverse incision, the distal side of the radius is approached between the extensor carpi radialis longus and the extensor pollicis brevis. The periosteum is incised and elevated between these first and second dorsal compartments. This exposes a flat area of cortical bone that can be used as a cortical graft. The cancellous portion of the distal part of the radius is removed by curettage to obtain sufficient bone for the arthrodesis. This is not a styloidectomy.

The bones to be fused are held in their normal positions with respect to the surrounding bones, while 0.045-inch diameter Kirschner wires are prepositioned in retrograde fashion. Each pin is sharp on both ends and inserted backward or preset in one bone (i.e., the trapezium) so that the point is just at the fusion surface. The operator can readily see exactly where the pin will cross and strike the opposite fusion surface (i.e., the scaphoid). This ensures that the pin will be exactly where needed after the grafts have been packed in and one cannot visually monitor the pin's position as it is being driven across. The minimum is usually three pins, but as many as eight have been useful. Occasionally it is necessary to pin other than across the fusion itself. In rotary subluxation of the scaphoid the proximal pole of the scaphoid is depressed until the proximal dorsal surface is aligned and level with the dorsal surface of the lunate. The distal pole is pulled dorsally if necessary, and two pins are then driven through the scaphoid into the capitate to maintain reduction. Do not overreduce.

Special care is taken never to pass any pins from an intercarpal arthrodesis into the radius or ulnar, since this would greatly decrease motion in the radiocarpal joint, which serves as a safety valve during healing. Any inadvertent loads are absorbed as free motion at the radiocarpal joint and do not stress the arthrodesis.

The spaces between bones are filled with cancellous bone graft. It is mandatory that the bones being arthrodesed have a normal relation with the rest of the wrist. They must not be pressed together. The external dimensions of the completed fusion unit must be the same as the external dimensions of those bones in the normal wrist.

A cortical graft often is used to dorsally bridge the fusion site and is carefully fitted or notched into position. The pins are then driven across the former joint surfaces. With intercarpal arthrodesis, wrist motion is checked to be certain no pin is crossing the radiocarpal joint. The pins are then clipped off so that their ends are just below the skin surface. The wound is closed, and a bulky dressing with a long-arm plaster splint is applied.

POSTOPERATIVE MANAGEMENT

The bulky dressing is maintained for a week. At the end of the week the sutures are removed, and a long-arm plaster cast is applied. The circular cast includes the thumb and a volar extension to support the index and middle fingers, preferably in the intrinsic-plus position. The elbow is at a 90-degree angle. This long-arm plaster cast is maintained for 4 weeks. The results in limited wrist arthrodesis correlate very nicely with the degree of immobilization achieved in the first 4 postoperative weeks. It is at this stage that small vascular connections are making their way through the trabecular graft between the bones. The slightest motion between these trabecular fragments ruptures the small capillaries, and the process must begin again. Once the initial vascular connections have been established, osteocytes will form, and new bone will be laid down between the graft trabeculae and between the graft and arthrodesing carpals. At 4 weeks there is reasonable continuity between the bones, and the arthrodesis need only be protected from any significant motion or stress. It is at this stage that the fingers can be freed from the cast, and the cast can be cut below the elbow to a gauntlet-type including the thumb and extending from the distal palmar confluence to the proximal third of the forearm. Supination-pronation may be allowed as long as none of the pins have crossed into the ulna. At the end of 6 weeks x-ray determination of healing is made, and either the gauntlet cast or a volar plaster splint is used for an additional week, depending on the reliability of the patient, the appearance of the x-ray films, and other factors. Full mobilization without external support is then allowed. Motion will be limited initially, and in fact motion will steadily increase for 9 months to a year following the surgery. There is an adaptive change of the joints surrounding a limited wrist arthrodesis, which demonstrates a slow, progressive increase. If significant swelling or shoulder-hand-arm dystrophy is present, a stress program is begun. Stress is accomplished by scrubbing a 1-yard section of the floor for three 10-minute sessions a day and carrying a weighted briefcase or satchel in the affected hand at all times when mobile. The dystrophy syndrome responds nicely to stress loading. No motion exercises are necessary as long as activity is steadily increased. Rarely, serial plasters can be used to derive early motion.

COMPLICATIONS

Complications of limited wrist arthrodeses, with the exception of a few technical problems, can be eliminated in the planning stage of the operation. One must be alert not to fuse joints that will put stress on other joints that already demonstrate degenerative arthritis. If the planning is correct, the technical complications are minimal.

Nonunion is recognized at 6 to 8 weeks and should probably be handled aggressively. If there is clear-cut evidence of nonunion, the patient should be alerted to the fact, and plans should be made to regraft immediately. In my experience no amount of hopeful casting will convert a nonunion to a union. The contralateral radius can be used if a significant amount of bone is needed; otherwise the same radius can be opened again for more cancellous bone, as necessary.

A nonunion between two bones often has significant fibrous stability. This stability can be used in handling the nonunion by creating a large groove between the two bones while maintaining the intrinsic fibrous stability of the nonunion and grafting. It must be borne in mind that sufficient bone must exist to carry the expected loads. Occasionally one might choose to add an additional carpal(s) to the limited wrist nonunion, such as adding the hamate and triquetrum to a nonunion of the capitate-lunate to significantly increase the surface arthrodesis and ensure fusion with a minimal change in expected motion.

Infection should be handled as in any other situation, usually with closed irrigation and continued immobilization.

Occasionally a pin cannot be retrieved with the use of lidocaine (Xylocaine) and a small skin nick in the office. Under these circumstances I do not hesitate to take the patient to the operating room on a short-stay admission and remove the pins. This complication can be avoided by leaving the pins long enough to lie immediately beneath the skin without significant tenting. If the pins tent the skin, they usually will erode the skin while in plaster casts and often have to be pulled early.

I have not yet had to add other joints to the limited wrist arthrodeses because of subsequent degeneration, although this certainly must be borne in mind as a definite long-term possibility.

SUMMARY

Limited wrist arthrodesis is the surgical fusion of selected bones of the wrist. In each case the extent of the fusion is determined by the extent of the disease process. Limited wrist arthrodesis is an alternative to complete wrist fusion when there is a localized area of degenerative change or instability in the carpus. It relieves pain yet still allows a good range of motion.

REFERENCES

1. Campbell, C.J., and Keokarn, T.: Total and subtotal arthrodesis of the wrist, J. Bone Joint Surg. **46A**:1520, 1964.
2. Cockshott, W.P.: Pisiform hamate fusion, J. Bone Joint Surg. **51A**:778, 1969.
3. Fenollosa, J., and Valverde, C.: Resultats des arthrodeses intracarpiennes dans le traitement des necroses du semilunaire, Rev. Chir. Orthop. **56**:745, 1970.
4. Gordon, L.H.: Partial wrist arthrodesis for old ununited fractures of the carpal navicular, Am. J. Surg. **102**:460, 1969.
5. Graner, O., Lopes, E.I., Carvalho, B.C., and Atlas, S.: Arthrodesis of the carpal bones in the treatment of Kienböck's disease, painful ununited fractures of the navicular and lunate bones with avascular necrosis, and old fracture-dislocation of carpal bones, J. Bone Joint Surg. **48A**:767, 1966.
6. Deleted in galleys.
7. Linsheid, R.L.: Personal communication, 1976.
8. Mazet. R., and Hohl, M.: Fractures of the carpal navicular, J. Bone Joint Surg. **45A**:82, 1963.
9. Peterson, H.A., and Lipscomb, P.R.: Intercarpal arthrodesis, Arch. Surg. **95**:127, 1967.
10. Ricklin, P.: L'Arthrodese radiocarpienne partielle, Ann. Chir. **30**:909, 1976.
11. Rosemeyer, B.: Differenzierte Arthrodesen im Karpalbereich, Z. Orthop. **111**:483, 1973.
12. Schwartz, S.: Localized fusion at the wrist joint, J. Bone Joint Surg. **49A**:1591, 1967.
13. Sutro, C.J.: Treatment of nonunion of the carpal navicular bone, Surgery **20**:536, 1946.
14. Szaboky, G.T., Muller, J., Melnick, J., and Tamburro, R.:

Anomalous fusion between the lunate and triquetrum, J. Bone Joint Surg. **51A**:1001, 1969.
15. Watson, H.K., and Cuono, C.B.: The carpal boss: surgical treatment and etiological considerations, J. Plast. Reconstr. Surg. **63**:88, 1979.
15a. Watson, H.K., Goodman, M.L., and Johnson, T.R.: Limited wrist arthrodeses. II. J. Hand Surg. **6**:223, 1981.
16. Watson, H.K., and Hempton, R.F.: Limited wrist arthrodeses. I. The triscaphoid joint, J. Hand Surg. **5**:320, 1980.
17. Watson, H.K., and McGrath, M.H.: Late results with local bone graft donor sites in hand surgery, J. Hand Surg. **6**:234.

Chapter 39 Scapholunate dissociation

Julio Taleisnik

Subtle varieties of carpal instability are probably more common than was previously recognized. In my experience the functional dissociation between scaphoid and lunate secondary to rotatory subluxation of the scaphoid is the most frequent form of carpal instability. Since the early references to scaphoid participation in carpal instability by MacConaill[14] and by Gilford, Bolton, and Lambrinudi[8] and reports by Cave,[4] Russell,[17] and Vaughan-Jackson[23] considerable progress has been made toward understanding the pathogenesis of this form of collapse deformity, as well as toward the treatment of the chronic subluxations. The search continues, however, for a reliable solution to the scapholunate dissociation that has been allowed to progress untreated into the chronic stage. Therefore the most persistent problem is still the lack of recognition of this entity in its early stages, since rotatory subluxation of the scaphoid diagnosed in the acute phase still offers the most consistent opportunity for successful correction.

REVIEW OF THE ANATOMY

MacConaill[14] and Gilford and associates[8] first stressed the role the scaphoid plays as a connecting rod between the proximal and distal carpal rows, protecting the wrist against the imbalance that is inherently built into the intercalated segment of a three-link system.[11] The loss of scaphoid support through fracture or ligamentous injury allows the carpus to collapse under compression loads and to assume a stance variously described as a *crumpling*,[8] *zigzag*,[11] or *concertina* deformity[7] (Fig. 39-1). The scaphoid is stabilized at its proximal pole by the deep radioscapholunate and both volar and dorsal scapholunate interosseous ligaments[15,19,21] (Figs. 39-2 and 39-3). The distal pole is controlled by the radial collateral

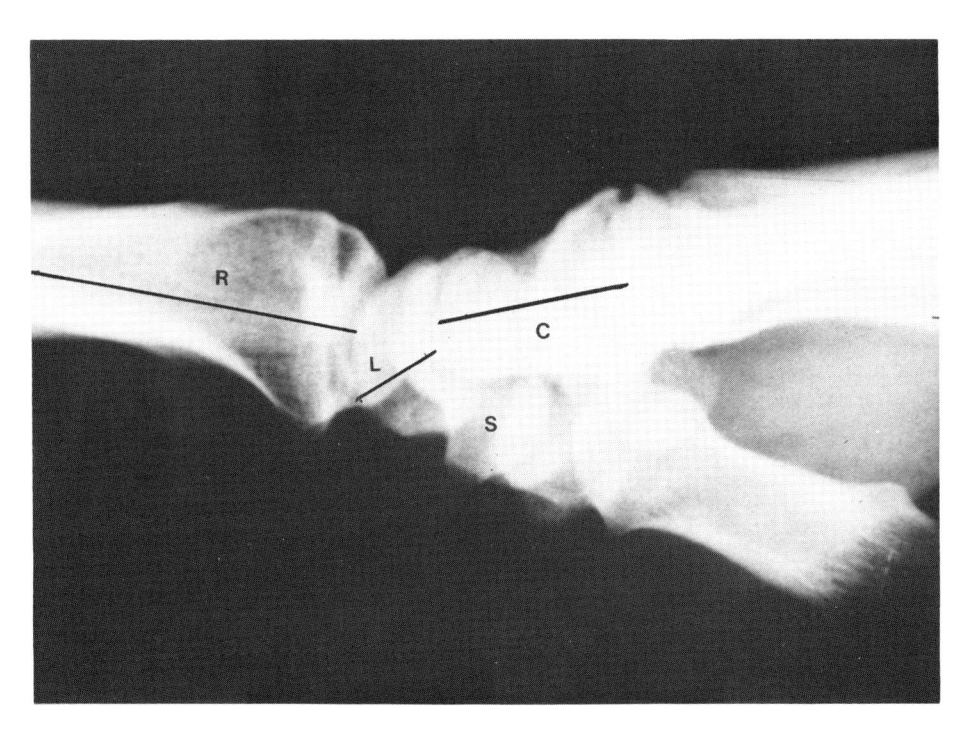

FIG. 39-1. Crumpling, zigzag, or concertina deformity. *R*, Radius; *L*, lunate; *S*, scaphoid; *C*, capitate.

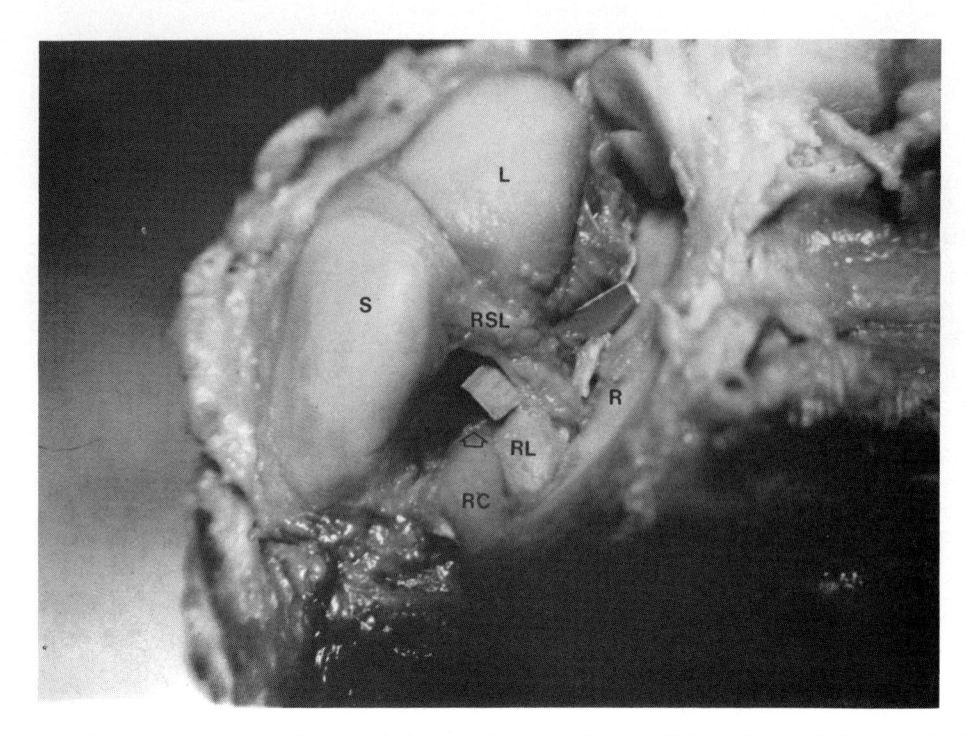

FIG. 39-2. Deep volar radiocarpal ligaments seen from within wrist joint. *S,* Scaphoid; *L,* lunate; *R,* articular surface of radius; *RL,* radiolunate ligament; *RSL,* deep radioscapholunate ligament; *RC,* radiocapitate ligament, here detached from scaphoid *(arrow).*

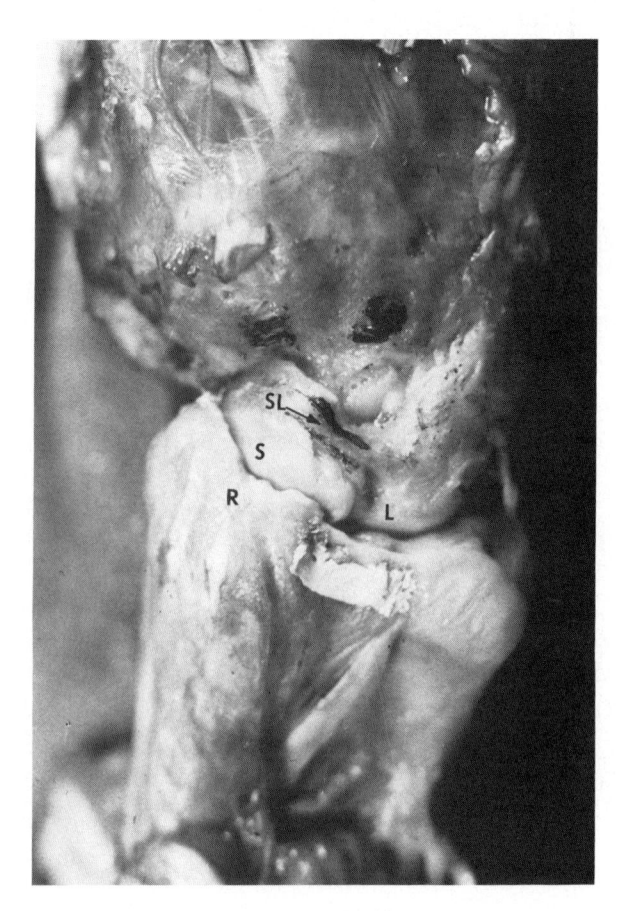

FIG. 39-3. Intrinsic dorsal scapholunate ligament *(SL).* *S,* Scaphoid; *L,* lunate; *R,* radius. (From Taleisnik, J.: J. Hand Surg. **1:**110, 1976.)

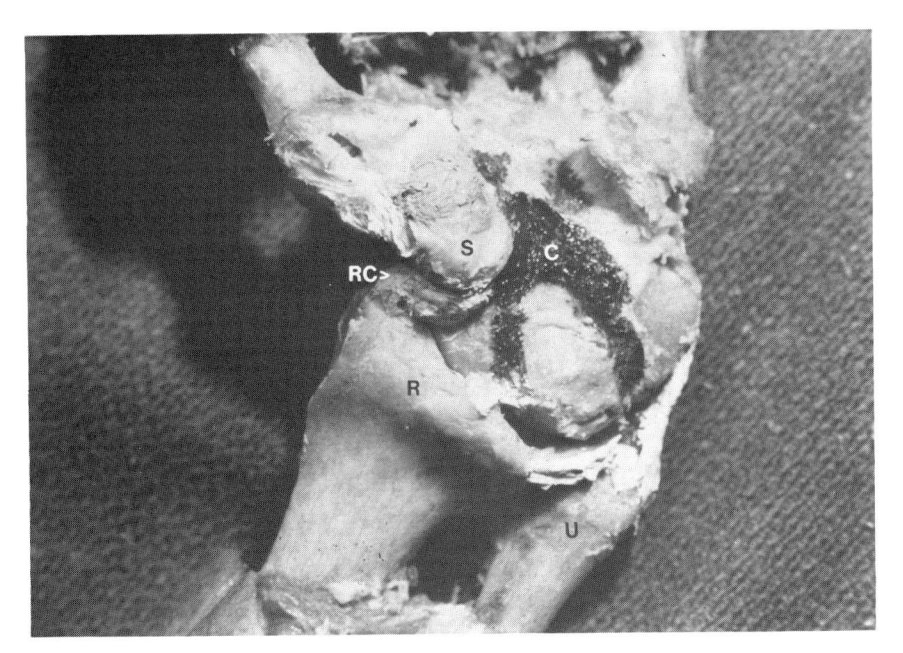

FIG. 39-4. Volar aspect of wrist specimen. Radiocapitate, or *sling*, ligament *(RC)*. *S*, Scaphoid; *C*, capitate; *R*, radius; *U*, ulna. (From Taleisnik, J.: J. Hand Surg. **1:**110, 1976.)

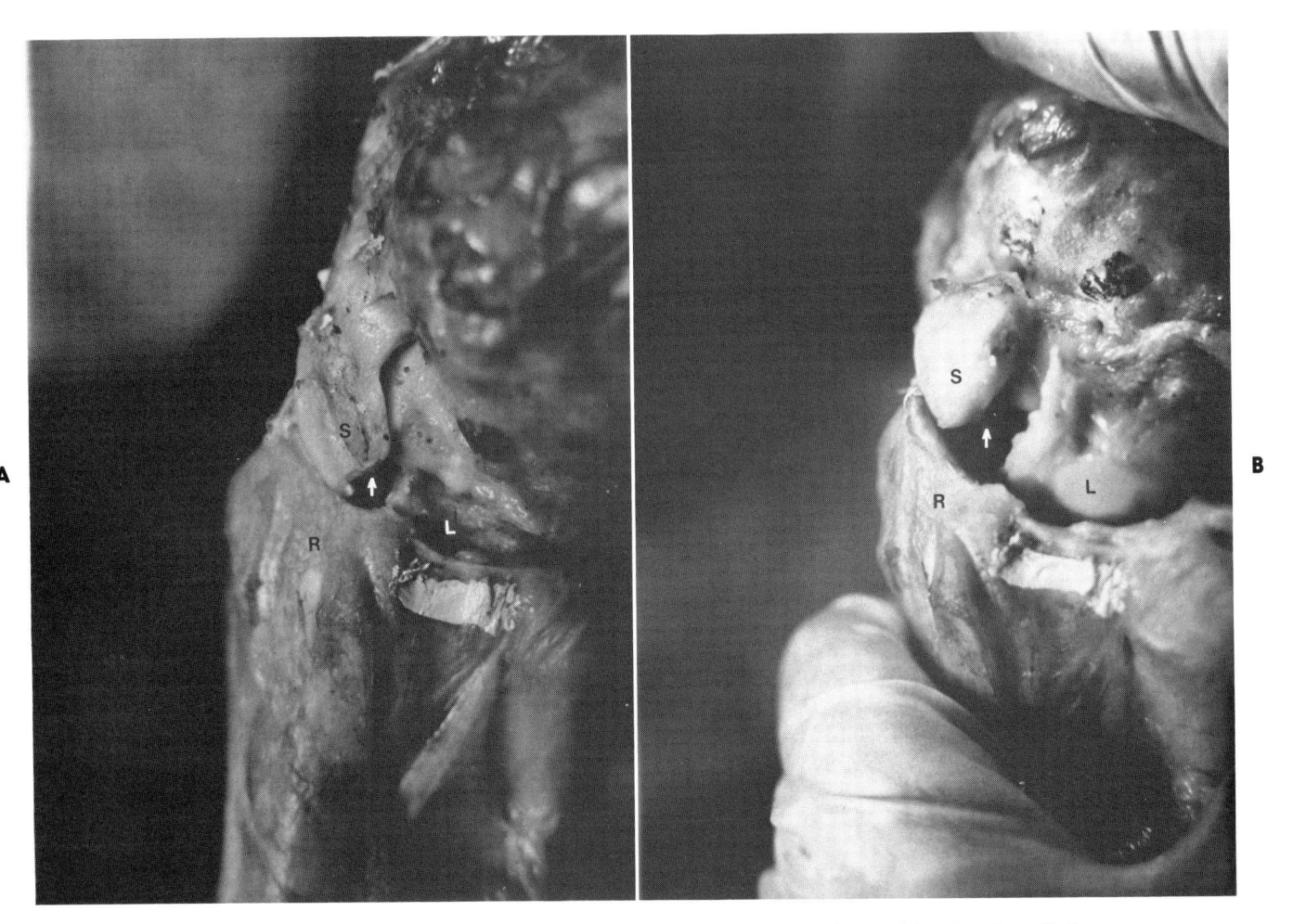

FIG. 39-5. A, Division of all scapholunate ligaments allows gap *(arrow)* to develop. **B,** For scaphoid *(S)* to subluxate dorsally *(arrow)*, volar stabilizers of proximal pole (deep radio-scapholunate and radiocapitate ligaments) also must be severed. *L*, Lunate; *R*, radius.

and lateral arm of the V or deltoid ligament. Considerable scaphoid motion is allowed by these ligaments, from scaphoid dorsiflexion during full wrist ulnar deviation and dorsiflexion to scaphoid volar flexion at the extreme of wrist radial deviation or volar flexion. The scaphoid rotates on a volar, central, waist-level ligamentous sling originating from the volar margin of the radius and inserting on the capitate, with a weak scaphoid attachment on the way (radiocapitate ligament) (Fig. 39-4). For the proximal pole to subluxate dorsally and dissociate from the lunate, there must be a disruption of all volar proximal pole support, as well as a detachment from the weak scaphoid connection to the sling ligament (Fig. 39-5). These volar ligaments are best recognized if visualized from within the joint.[12] (See Fig. 39-2.) Both the radiocapitate and the radioscapholunate ligaments are strong fascicles, although the latter's insertion on the scaphoid is weaker than that on the lunate.[21]

MECHANISM OF INJURY

Patients who recall the mechanism of their injury report a force applied to the palm of their hand, particularly at the hypothenar area, with the wrist in dorsiflexion and ulnar deviation (Fig. 39-6). Not infrequently a cylindric object (e.g., racket handle or motorcycle handlebar) was held in the hand at the time of injury.[2,3] Isolated subluxation of the scaphoid may be considered the initial stage of an injury that, if allowed to progress, would result in a perilunate carpal dislocation, just as a fracture of the scaphoid, if subjected to continuation of the injury force, would lead to a transscaphoid perilunate fracture-dislocation. Therefore scapholunate dissociation could be a *primary injury*, when the load applied to the wrist stopped short of producing a perilunate dislocation, or else a *secondary* finding, residual of a reduced major carpal injury.[2,22] For these instability patterns to develop, excessive midcarpal laxity may need to be present, secondary to either a systemic hypermobility involving multiple joints[18] or a local carpal anatomic weakness. Fisk's assumption[7] that deficient volar capitate-lunate support may facilitate intercarpal dislocation correlates well with the frequent anatomic absence of a capitate-lunate ligament and the dorsal-stress instability present in the uninjured wrists of patients who have sustained scapholunate dissociations.[19] With the wrist in dorsiflexion and ulnar deviation the scaphoid is directly in the path of a force applied to the hypothenar region. The scapholunate articulation is the weak link, receiving the full impact of this force. The proximal pole of the scaphoid, as the less supported of the two components of this joint, becomes destabilized when the weaker attachments of the radiocapitate and deep radioscapholunate ligaments tear. This allows the scaphoid to be driven dorsally by the injury force, whereas the lunate remains

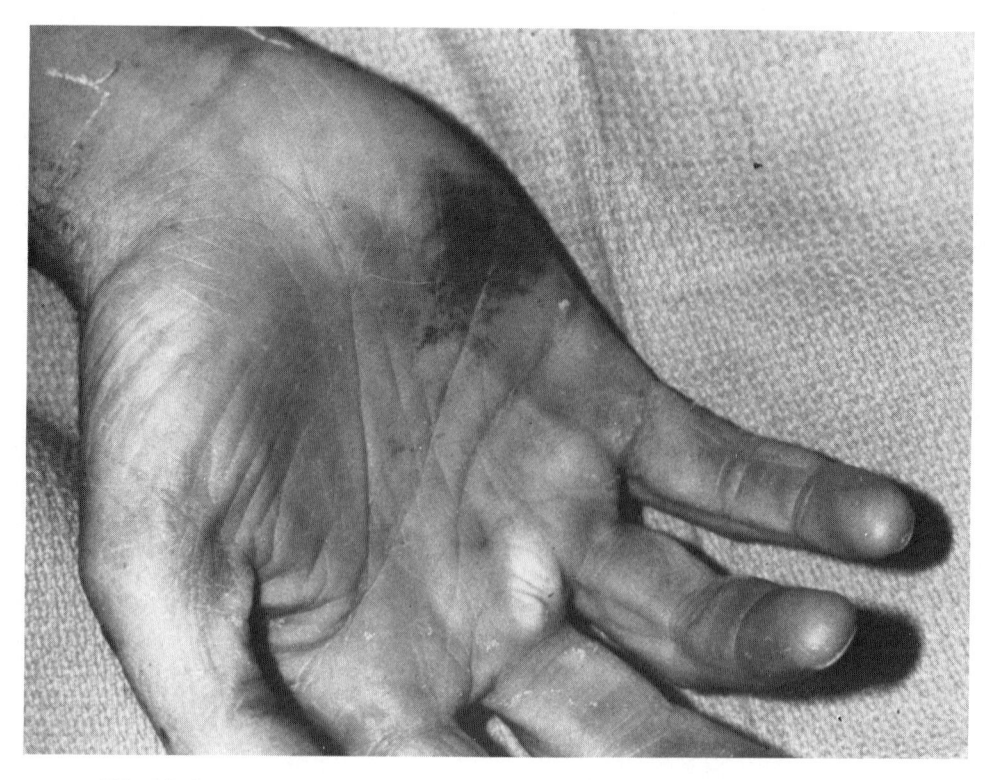

FIG. 39-6. Hypothenar abrasion in patient with scapholunate dissociation.

CHAPTER 39 SCAPHOLUNATE DISSOCIATION

under the protective dome of the radius. In the anatomy specimen, division of the interosseous scapholunate ligaments alone fails to produce a subluxated scaphoid, until the volar proximal pole support from the radiocarpal ligaments is divided as well. The subluxated scaphoid now lies away from the lunate, its longitudinal axis perpendicular to that of the radius.

DIAGNOSIS

Early recognition of scapholunate dissociation is most important for the successful treatment of this injury. Although the diagnosis may be suspected by the patient's description of the accident, it is confirmed only after radiographic and, at times, cineradiographic studies are obtained. The patient with a scapholunate dissociation is frequently a young adult with excessive carpal laxity on the uninjured wrist. The primary form of rotatory subluxation of the scaphoid is frequently traced to a deceivingly minor injury, at times so minor that is difficult to remember. Secondary rotatory subluxations are usually residual of major carpal injuries (reduced perilunate and lunate dislocations) that leave behind the telltale radiologic signs of scapholunate dissociations. Because of the major nature of the initial injury in the secondary subluxations, medical care is sought earlier, and the diagnosis of dissociation is less frequently delayed. Patients with primary subluxations, on the other hand, do not seek medical help until much later, partly because of the apparent insignificance of the injury itself and partly because symptoms may not become disabling until several weeks later. Progressive grip weakness is the most consistent complaint. There is pain on motion, but not infrequently these patients are surprisingly free from discomfort. At times a painful, loud snap can be reproduced, usually during volar flexion and secondary to the subluxation of the proximal pole of the scaphoid as it rides dorsal to the dorsal margin of the radius. Severe limitation of motion is rarely encountered early. Because of the disturbed mechanics of radiocarpal motion, these patients' wrists are very susceptible to the rapid onset of

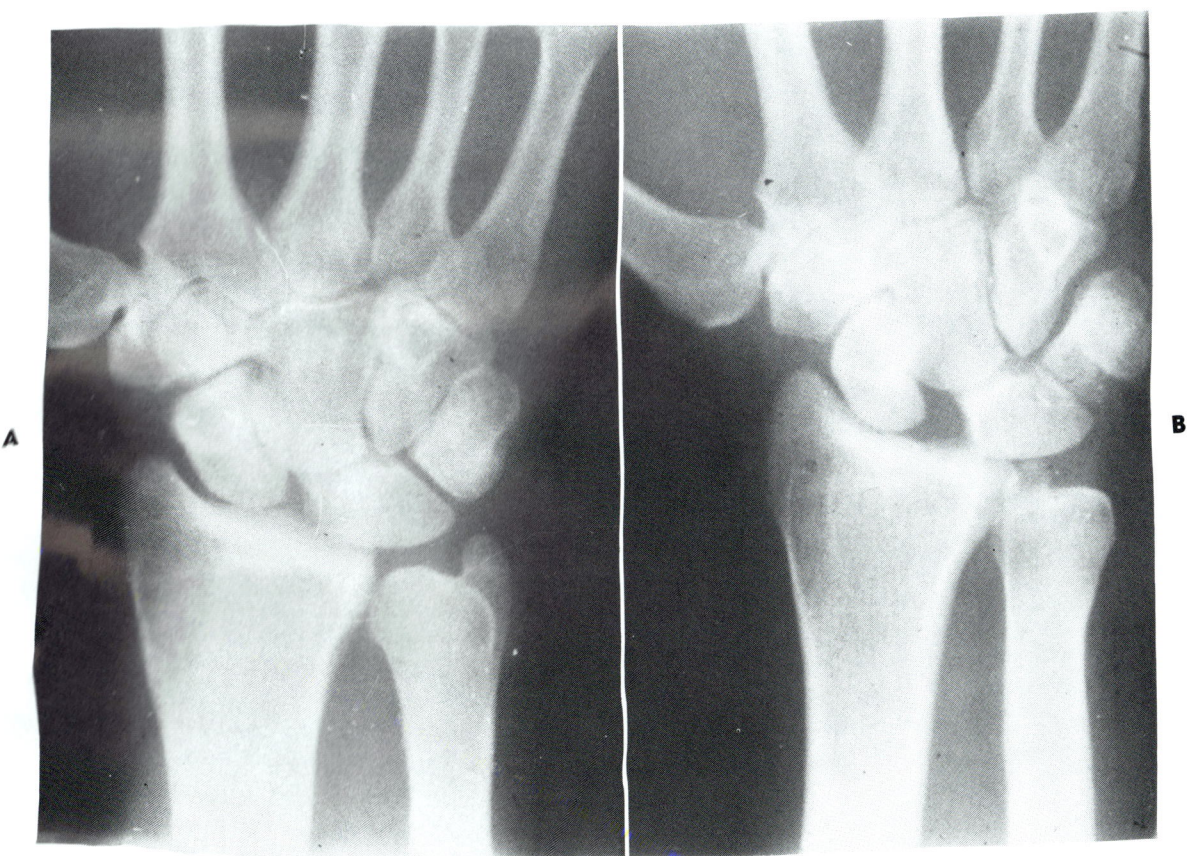

FIG. 39-7. A, Anteroposterior roentgenogram with hand pronated suggests scaphoid subluxation. **B,** Anteroposterior roentgenogram with hand supinated shows wider scapholunate gap in same patient. (From Taleisnik, J.: Wrist: Anatomy, function, and injury. In American Academy of Orthopaedic Surgeons: Instructional Course Lectures, vol. 27, St. Louis, 1978, The Mosby Co.)

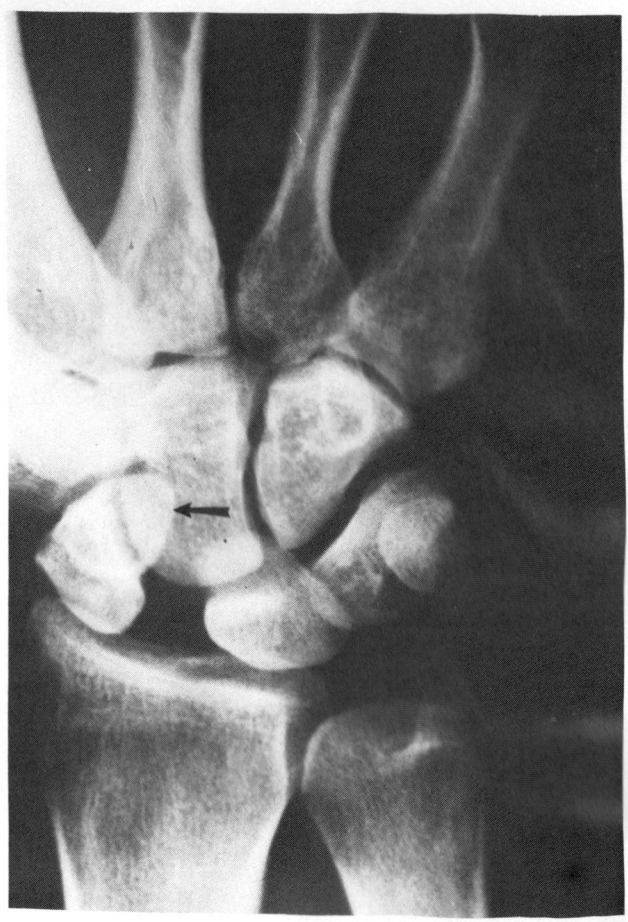

FIG. 39-8. Cortical ring image created by visualization from end of distal pole of scaphoid (arrow). (From Taleisnik, J.: Wrist: anatomy, function, and injury. In American Academy of Orthopaedic Surgeons: Instructional Course Lectures, vol. 27. St. Louis, 1978, The C.V. Mosby Co.)

degenerative changes, particularly between the radial styloid and the subluxated scaphoid. As arthrosis develops, limitation of motion and pain become more constant and disabling.

The diagnosis is established by appropriate radiologic studies.* Frontal x-ray views show a gap between the scaphoid and lunate, wider than that in the opposite uninjured wrist; this is usually more noticeable if the roentgenogram is obtained with the hand and wrist in supination[22] (Fig. 39-7). The distal pole of the abnormally perpendicular scaphoid is visualized from the end, creating a typical cortical ring image[5] (Fig. 39-8). For this same reason the anteroposterior views show foreshortening of the scaphoid outline. Additional views with the wrist in ulnar deviation and in radial deviation and with a longitudinal compression load created by having the patient make a tight fist[6] can assist in identifying the widened scapholunate gap. The importance of obtaining a proper frontal projection was stressed by Hudson, Caragol, and Faye[10]; a projection was considered ideal when the distal ends of the ulna and radius did not overlap. Increased overlapping suggested unwanted obliquity, at times enough to obscure the presence of a scapholunate dissociation. The lateral projection shows best the perpendicular position of the scaphoid (Fig. 39-9). The normal values of the angles between the axes of all the components of the radiocarpal link have been thoroughly discussed by Linscheid, Dobyns, and associates.[6,13] Normally the long axis of the scaphoid and a line drawn tangential to the volar flare of the distal aspect of the radius are closely parallel to each other. In the abnormally volar-flexed scaphoid these lines converge at an acute angle. For the same reason the volar cortical outlines of the scaphoid and the styloid, which normally create a wide C o sign open anteriorly, change into a s the scaphoid is subluxated.

---

*References 2, 5, 6, 9, 10, and 22.

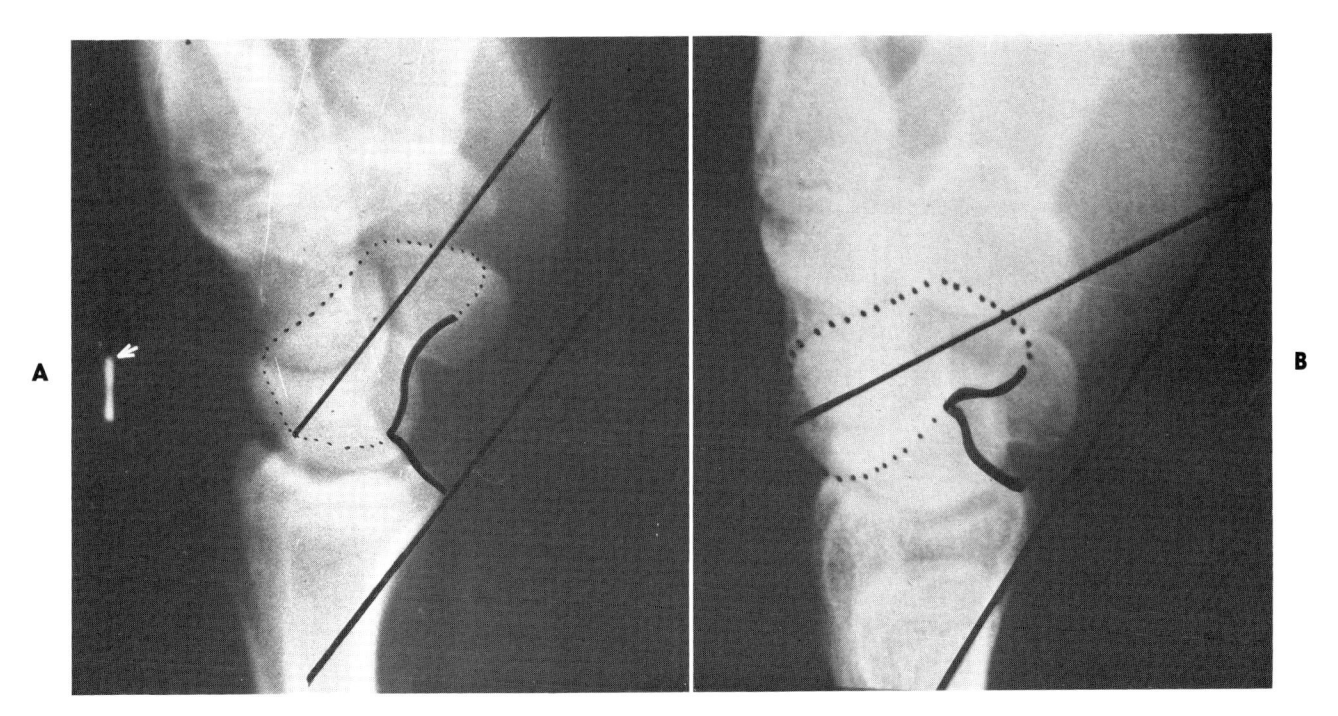

FIG. 39-9. A, Lateral view of normal but sprained wrist. Metal marker *(arrow)* is placed at point of maximal tenderness. Longitudinal axis of scaphoid and line tangential to volar flare of radius are nearly parallel. Volar outlines of scaphoid and radial styloid create bracket shape. **B,** Subluxated scaphoid. Scaphoid axis and line tangential to radial flare are convergent. Volar scaphoradial styloid outline is in shape of V. (From Taleisnik, J.: Wrist: anatomy, function, and injury. In American Academy of Orthopaedic Surgeons: Instructional Course Lectures, vol. 27, St. Louis, 1978, The C.V. Mosby Co.)

Cineradiographs may help to demonstrate the mechanical disturbance created by the scapholunate dissociation.[1] During ulnar and radial deviation there is a loss of the synchronous motions of scaphoid and lunate. The abnormal widening of the scapholunate space, as well as the dorsal subluxation of the scaphoid, usually can be documented. In the lateral projection during dorsiflexion and volar flexion, cineradiographs show the relative immobility of the lunate, which remains dorsiflexed (dorsal intercalated segment instability deformity[13]) throughout most of the movements.

TREATMENT

The best treatment for scapholunate dissociation is the early treatment, performed within the initial 3 weeks after injury. Although secondary dissociation may require surgical repair of torn ligaments, the primary rotatory subluxation of the scaphoid may be successfully handled by blind pinning and prolonged immobilization. Manipulation of the scaphoid in attempts to maintain position by immobilization in a plaster cast alone are usually insufficient because of the "paradox" of closed reduction[15]: when the wrist is volar flexed to relax the torn volar ligaments and facilitate their healing, the proximal pole of the scaphoid is placed in an undesirable, unstable position of presubluxation; conversely, if the scaphoid is reduced with the wrist in dorsiflexion, healing of the torn volar ligaments is either prevented or delayed. A satisfactory solution to this paradox may consist of reducing the scaphoid with the wrist in dorsiflexion and, under cineradiographic control, securing this reduction by appropriate Kirschner wire fixation of the scaphoid to the rest of the carpus. With scaphoid and lunate under control, the radiocarpal joint is volar flexed to afford relaxation to the torn volar ligaments. The wrist is then placed in a long-arm thumb spica cast for a period of 6 weeks, followed by 4 weeks in a similar short-arm cast. At the end of this period all the Kirschner wires are removed, and mobilization is started.

The treatment of the chronic scapholunate dissociation is difficult and not consistently successful. Stabilization of the scaphoid is possible by ligament reconstruction techniques, but it is difficult to maintain because of the considerable amount of force exerted by the scaphoid as it tends to return to its subluxated position (which it may do in spite of plaster and internal fixation). Different techniques of ligament reconstruction have been described.[6,9,16,20] All share a common goal: to create a scapholunate ligament and restore a more normal scapholunate relationship. In some cases[20] an attempt is made to further reproduce the normal anatomy by reconstructing a volar radioscaphoid "suspensory" ligament, as well, to tether the proximal pole of the scaphoid and keep it from subluxating dorsally. All these procedures are technically difficult, unreliable as to the objective correction that is obtained and the degree of patient satisfaction, and frequently disappointing because of late complications after prolonged follow-up monitoring.

A simpler surgical approach has been proposed[24] that is designed to control proximal pole rotation by a limited arthrodesis of the *distal* pole to the trapezium and trapezoid. Although the long-range effect of this localized fusion on the remaining carpal joints has not yet been determined, this technique has been more satisfactory in providing a stable, pain-free wrist, at the expense of some loss of motion.

REFERENCES

1. Arkless, R.: Cineradiography in normal and abnormal wrists, Am. J. Roentgenol. **96:**837, 1966.
2. Armstrong, G.W.D.: Rotational subluxation of the scaphoid, Can. J. Surg. **11:**306, 1968.
3. Bindi, R.: La luxacion del escafoides carpiano, Bol. Trabajos Soc. Argentina Ortop. Traum. **29:**194, 1964.
4. Cave, E.F.: Retrolunar dislocationo of the capitate with fracture or subluxation of the navicular bone, J. Bone Joint Surg. **23:**830, 1941.
5. Crittenden, J.J., Jones, D.M., and Santerelli, A.G.: Bilateral rotational dislocation of the carpal navicular: case report, Radiology **94:**629, 1970.
6. Dobyns, J.H., Linscheid, R.L., Chao, E.Y.S., Weber, E.R., and Swanson, G.E.: Traumatic instability of the wrist. In American Academy of Orthopaedic Surgeons: Instructional Course Lectures, vol. 24, St. Louis, 1975 The C.V. Mosby Co.
7. Fisk, G.R.: Carpal instability and the fractured scaphoid, Ann. R. Coll. Surg. Engl. **46:**63, 1970.
8. Gilford, W.W., Bolton, R.H., and Lambrinudi, C.: The mechanism of the wrist joint; with special reference to fractures of the scaphoid, Guy's Hosp. Rep. **92:**52, 1943.
9. Howard, F.M., Fahey, T., and Wojcik, E.: Rotatory subluxation of the navicular, Clin. Orthop. **104:**134, 1974.
10. Hudson, T.M., Caragol, W.J., and Faye, J.J.: Isolated rotatory subluxation of the carpal navicular, Am. J. Roentgenol. **126:**601, 1976.
11. Landsmeer, J.M.: Studies in the anatomy of articulation. I. The equilibrium of the "intercalated" bone, Acta. Morphol. Neerl. Scand. **3:**287, 1961.
12. Lewis, O.J., Hamshere, R.J., and Bucknill, T.M.: The anatomy of the wrist joint, J. Anat. **106:**539, 1970.
13. Linscheid, R.L., Dobyns, J.H., Beabout, J.W., and Bryan, R.S.: Traumatic instability of the wrist, J. Bone Joint Surg. **54A:**1612, 1972.
14. MacConaill, M.A.: Mechanical anatomy of the carpus and its bearing on some surgical problems, J. Anat. **75:**166, 1941.
15. Mayfield, J.K., Johnson, R.P., and Kilcoyne, R.F.: The ligaments of the human wrist and their functional significance, Anat. Rec. **186:**417, 1976.
16. Palmer, A.K., Dobyns, J.H., and Linscheid, R.L.: Management of post-traumatic instability of the wrist secondary to ligament rupture, J. Hand Surg. **3:**507, 1978.
17. Russell, T.B.: Inter-carpal dislocations and fracture-dislocations: a review of 59 cases, J. Bone Joint Surg. **31B:**524, 1949.
18. Sutro, C.J.: Hypermobility of bones due to "overlengthened" capsular and ligamentous tissues, Surgery **21:**67, 1947.
19. Taleisnik, J.: The ligaments of the wrist, J. Hand Surg. **1:**110, 1976.
20. Taleisnik, J.: Wrist: anatomy, function, and injury. In American Academy of Orthopaedic Surgeons: Instructional Course Lectures, vol. 27, St. Louis, 1978, The C.V. Mosby Co.
21. Testut, L., and Latarjet, A.: Tratado de anatomia humana, ed. 9, vol. 1, Barcelona, 1951, Salvat Editores, S.A.
22. Thompson, T.C., Campbell, R.D., Jr., and Arnold, W.D.: Primary and secondary dislocation of the scaphoid bone, J. Bone Joint Surg. **46B:**73, 1964.
23. Vaughan-Jackson, O.J.: A case of recurrent subluxation of the carpal scaphoid, J. Bone Joint Surg. **31B:**532, 1949.
24. Watson, H.K., Johnson, T.R., Hempton, R.F., and Jones, D.S.: Limited wrist arthrodesis, Presented at thirty-fourth meeting of the American Society for Surgery of the Hand, San Francisco, Feb. 20, 1979.

Chapter 40 Static and dynamic forces on the multiple-linked carpus as an explanation for wrist deformity

Ronald L. Linscheid

The wrist is subject to a variety of injuries and developmental abnormalities. The increased severity of the deformities that result is largely related to internally generated forces from the musculotendinous structures that cross the wrist. The complex anatomy of the wrist joint may be analyzed as a multiple-linked cantilever system that, under compressive load, seeks the position of least potential energy.[1,4-6,8] It is the purpose of this chapter to review a variety of clinical wrist deformities from the point of view of biomechanics and to suggest some possible treatment modalities.

The wrist is most often injured when exposed to impulse loads of 100 to 400 kg of force (960 to 3840 N).[8] The carpus is forced past the constraints to maximal angular excursion, resulting in ligamentous or osseous failure as the energy-absorption capacities of the viscoelastic structures are exceeded. The modulus of elasticity increases from muscle through ligaments to bone with failure strength of bone and osseoligamentous junctures approaching one another. Dorsiflexion injury is most common because of the specific protective adaptations associated with upright posture. The failure position is determined by attitudinal orientation of the hand and wrist at impact, and this position in turn determines the resolution of forces imposed across the carpus. Imposed stresses become maximal on the osseoligamentous elements responsible for constraint at each position of the wrist, which determines a reasonable specificity of injury for each loading position. Both ligamentous and osseous failures occur primarily in tension. Compressive stresses and shear strain applied across the articular cartilage, however, may exceed the tolerable limits and fail first, or combined failure modes may result in osseous, osseoligamentous, and cartilage injury.

The muscular tensile forces across the wrist are exerted continuously as a result of resting tension but are increased markedly by forceful contraction.[3] A tetanic contraction of all the transcarpal musculature in the adult male might exceed 350 kg, with normal activities generally below this. Such forces acting across weakened or distorted anatomy induce abnormal positioning and/or kinematics.

SCAPHOID NONUNION

Scaphoid nonunion poses a continuing clinical problem that can be treated by adequate early immoblization as a preventive measure and by osteosynthesis when it is seen late. The scaphoid appears to fail in tension at the volar aspect of the waist cortex, most often from a dorsiflexed radially deviated stress.[8] The scaphoid, which acts as a link by obliquely crossing the intercarpal joint, is responsible for maintaining the integrity of carpal stability. The intercarpal joint assumes a collapsed position of varying degrees, depending on topographic and ligamentous stability of the middle flexion-extension column as well as on the stability of the fracture.[7] The common tendency of the lunate to assume the dorsiflexed instabil-

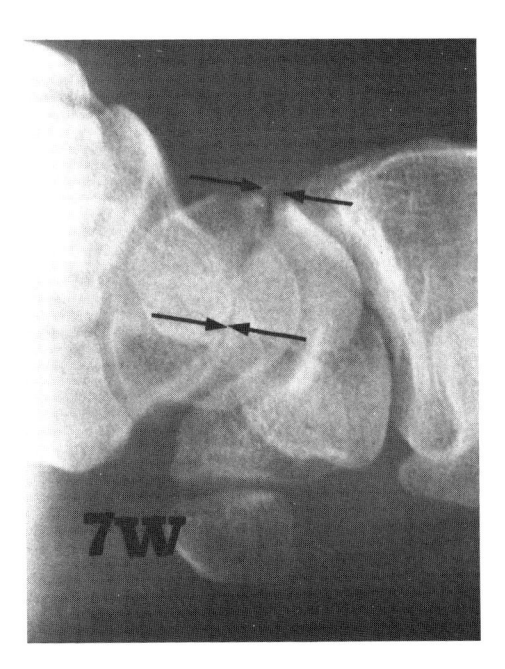

FIG. 40-1. A 35-year-old trucker with known scaphoid nonunion on right of five years' duration and recent fracture of left scaphoid secondary to fall. Oblique view of scaphoid shows palmar surface of fracture site compressed, with dorsal surfaces distracted. Failure to obtain correction of angulation of scaphoid fragments leads to scaphoid nonunion or malunion.

349

ity pattern in unstable scaphoid fractures induces angular changes at the fracture surfaces (Fig. 40-1). It appears that this most often distracts the dorsal cortices while compressing the volar ones. This may lead to malunion of the scaphoid in a "hunchback" position or progressive absorption of the volar cortex with the intermittent compressive angulation motions. This angular distraction of the dorsal cortex may be seen on oblique or tomographic views of the scaphoid or strongly suspected by a capitate-lunate angle exceeding 10 to 15 degrees.

Preventive treatment is immobilization in which the emphasis is placed on molding of the plaster to correct intercarpal alignment. Late treatment may succeed best where the scaphoid is aligned with the least distraction of the fracture site. The success of the volar Matti-Russe approach may be explained on this basis.

SCAPHOLUNATE DISSOCIATION

Scapholunate dissociation has progressed from a clinical curiosity to a treatable deformity in which the most persistent problem is a lack of early recognition. It should be considered a partial perilunate dislocation in which the scapholunate interosseous membrane tears.[2,5] The scaphoid may be rendered more unstable by attenuation of its ligamentous tether to the volar cortex of the radius (radioscapholunate ligament). The degree or length of interruption of the interval between radioscaphoid and radiolunate ligaments (space of Poirier) is also a determinant of stability. The disruption of the scapholunate linkage permits the scaphoid to radially dissociate from the lunate and adapt a palmar flexed position, while the lunate dorsiflexes within its intercalated position, a classic example of intercalated segment collapse under compressive stress (dorsiflexed intercalated segment instability, or DISI).[4] If it is recognized early and suitably stabilized, at least partial healing of this ligamentous complex may allow suitable return of function. Stabilization by molded plaster casts, transcutaneous pinning, or open reduction is more apt to be successful by overcorrection of carpal alignment.[2] Late reconstruction poses problems essentially related to substitution for the scapholunate interosseous ligamentous complex.

VOLAR INSTABILITY PATTERN

The pathomechanics of the collapse deformity in which the proximal row palmar flexes as an intercalated segment have only recently been elucidated. A partial perilunate dislocation in which the volar ligamentous complex between lunate and triquetrum is attenuated appears to be the specific defect (Fig. 40-2). This area is

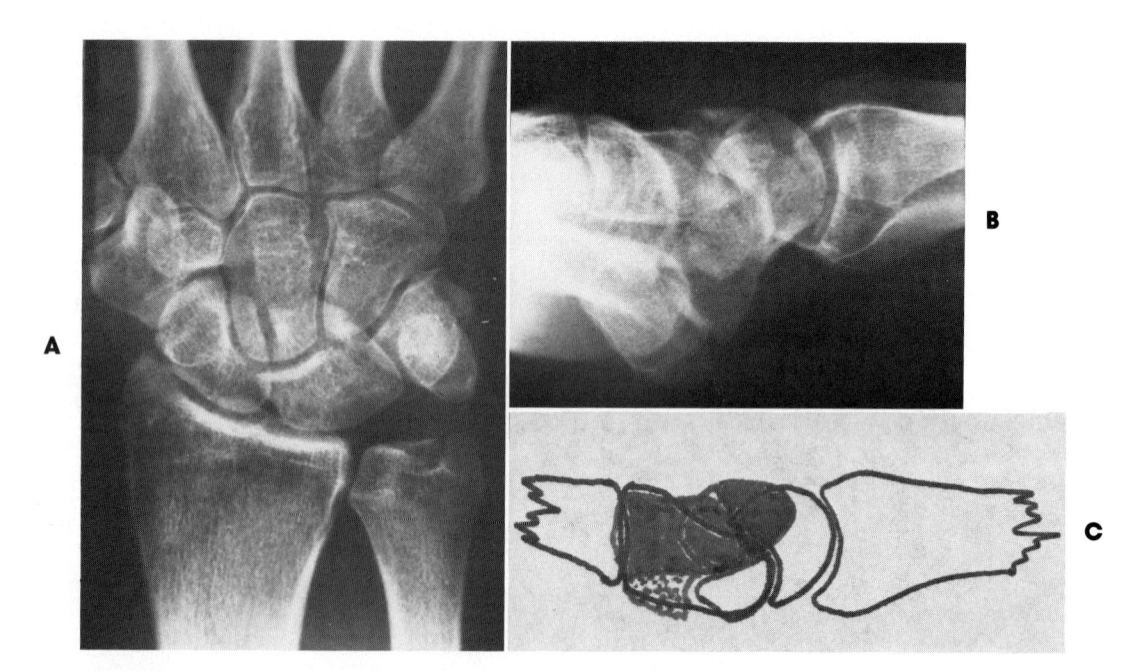

FIG. 40-2. Anteroposterior view of right wrist suggests foreshortening of scaphoid, triangular pattern of lunate, and break in smooth line between lunate and triquetrum. On lateral view following excision of fractured hook of hamate, note volar instability pattern of capitate-lunate angle. Triquetrum is angled only slightly in comparison to lunate. This suggests a lunate-triquetral dissociation from attenuation of lunate-triquetral interosseous membrane and ligament. Patient continued to have discomfort and weakness secondary to volar intercalated segment instability pattern.

contiguous with the ulnar termination of the space of Poirier and proximally is bounded by the strongest palmar ligament of the wrist, which spans obliquely from the radial styloid volar surface through the lunate volar pole to the triquetrum. It is also contiguous with the lunate-triquetral interosseous membrane. Disruption may occur with ligamentous attenuation or fracture of the radiovolar lip of the triquetrum. Tear of the interosseous membrane may be associated. The topographically determined contact areas of the carpus in this situation appear to dictate the volar flexed intercalated segment instability (VISI). One recent example appears to indicate that the triquetrum in normal alignment, with the scapholunate palmar flexed, provides an ulnar equivalent of the dissociation pattern. When it is recognized, stabilization by methods similar to those aforementioned should suffice. Late reconstruction by dorsal tendinous tethers has been disappointing. Volar reconstruction awaits a satisfactory surgical approach.

ULNAR TRANSLATORY RADIOCARPAL SUBLUXATION

Ulnar translatory radiocarpal subluxation is obviously related in etiology and pathology to the two previous problems. Attenuation of the radiolunate-triquetral ligament and perhaps the radiocarpal allows the carpus to translate ulnarly. The resolution of forces acting at the radiocarpal articulation would appear to dictate a substantial vector force favoring ulnar translation down the inclined slope of the radius. Treatment modalities similar to those mentioned previously would appear rational.

DORSAL SUBLUXATION OF THE CARPUS

Dorsal subluxation of the carpus is usually associated with a dorsal rim and/or radial styloid fracture or an intraarticular fracture of the radius with proximal displacement of the dorsal fragment. The lunate follows the dorsal fragment, distorting the length relations of the palmar capsular ligaments. Changes in the kinematics of carpal motion as a consequence of this distortion and the mechanical blocking of the lunate are symptom producing. A particular aspect of this would appear to be a marked snap in the wrist occurring during the excursion from radial to ulnar deviation and to a lesser extent in the excursion of dorsopalmar flexion. The normal conjunct rotation of the proximal row occurring smoothly through the motion is rendered abrupt and disquieting by the altered mechanics. Early recognition is often missed because of unsuitable roentgenograms in the emergency room and unfamiliarity with and disdain for the consequences associated with apparent minimal displacements. Anatomic restoration should be the goal of treatment.

SUBLUXATION OF THE RADIOULNAR JOINT

Subluxation of the radioulnar joint has not been considered as a multiple-linked collapse pattern deformity. The relation of the carpus to the distal radioulnar joint is accorded scant recognition. The ulnar rotation column of the carpus, however, is intimately associated with the distal aspect of the ulnar through the contiguity of the radioulnar ligaments, the enclosed discus articularis (triangular fibrocartilage), ulnar collateral ligaments, and the ulnotriquetral ligamentous complex. Dorsal subluxation of the ulna is usually associated with an interfibrillar stretching of the dorsal radioulnar capsule with torsional stress applied with the forearm in pronation and the wrist in dorsiflexion. Recently I have seen a palmar tear of the radioulnar capsule as well. A secondary consequence of this instability is a relative supination of the carpus on the radioulnar complex, resulting in an ulnocarpal dissociation. Clinical examination is usually more diagnostic than is radiologic examination. Early treatment with reduction in full supination is usually effective. Late reconstruction techniques are numerous but successes few. A modification of an undescribed Bunnell technique is offered for consideration in which correction of the ulnocarpal dissociation is considered paramount to successful reconstruction.

Deformities of the wrist seem approachable from a biomechanical standpoint in which the internal forces acting across a multiple-linked cantilevered structure provide a means of analysis and rational therapeutics.

REFERENCES

1. Dobyns, J.H., et al.: Traumatic instability of the wrist. In American Academy of Orthopaedic Surgeons: Instructional Course Lectures, vol. 24, St. Louis, 1975, The C.V. Mosby Co.
2. Green, D.P., and O'Brien, E.T.: Open reduction of carpal dislocations: indications and operative techniques, J. Hand Surg. **3:**250, 1978.
3. Ketchum, L.D., Brand, P.W., Thompson, D., and Pocock, G.S.: The determination of moments for extension of the wrist generated by muscles of the forearm, J. Hand Surg. **3:**205, 1978.
4. Linscheid, R.L., et al.: Traumatic instability of the wrist: diagnosis, classification and pathomechanics, J. Bone Joint Surg. **54A:**1612, 1972.
5. Mayfield, J.K., Johnson, R.P., and Kilcoyne, R.F.: The ligaments of the human wrist and their functional significance, Anat. Rec. **186:**417, 1976.
6. Sarrafian, S.K., Melamed, J.L., and Goshgarian, G.M.: Study of wrist motion in flexion and extension, Clin. Orthop. **126:**153, 1977.
7. Sebald, J.R., Dobyns, J.H., and Linscheid, R.L.: The natural history of collapse deformities of the wrist, Clin. Orthop. **104:**140, 1974.
8. Weber, E.R., and Chao, E.Y.S.: An experimental approach to the mechanism of scaphoid waist fractures, J. Hand Surg. **3:**142, 1978.

Chapter 41 Arthrodesis of the wrist (position and technique)

Mack L. Clayton

Arthrodesis of the wrist is an established procedure. Even though arthroplastic procedures are gaining popularity, there is still a definite place for the time-proven procedure of arthrodesis.[1-3,5,8]

The general recommendation has been fusion with the wrist in some degree of dorsiflexion (Haddad and Riordan[5] 10 degrees and Boyes[2] 20 to 30 degrees). Bilateral cases have had one wrist dorsiflexed and one palmar flexed for sanitary toilet functions.

I recommend fusion in the neutral position for unilateral or bilateral cases (Fig. 41-1). Neutral is defined as 0 degrees on the lateral plane with about 10 degrees of ulnar deviation. If one makes a clenched fist and rapidly opens the hand, this is the position attained.

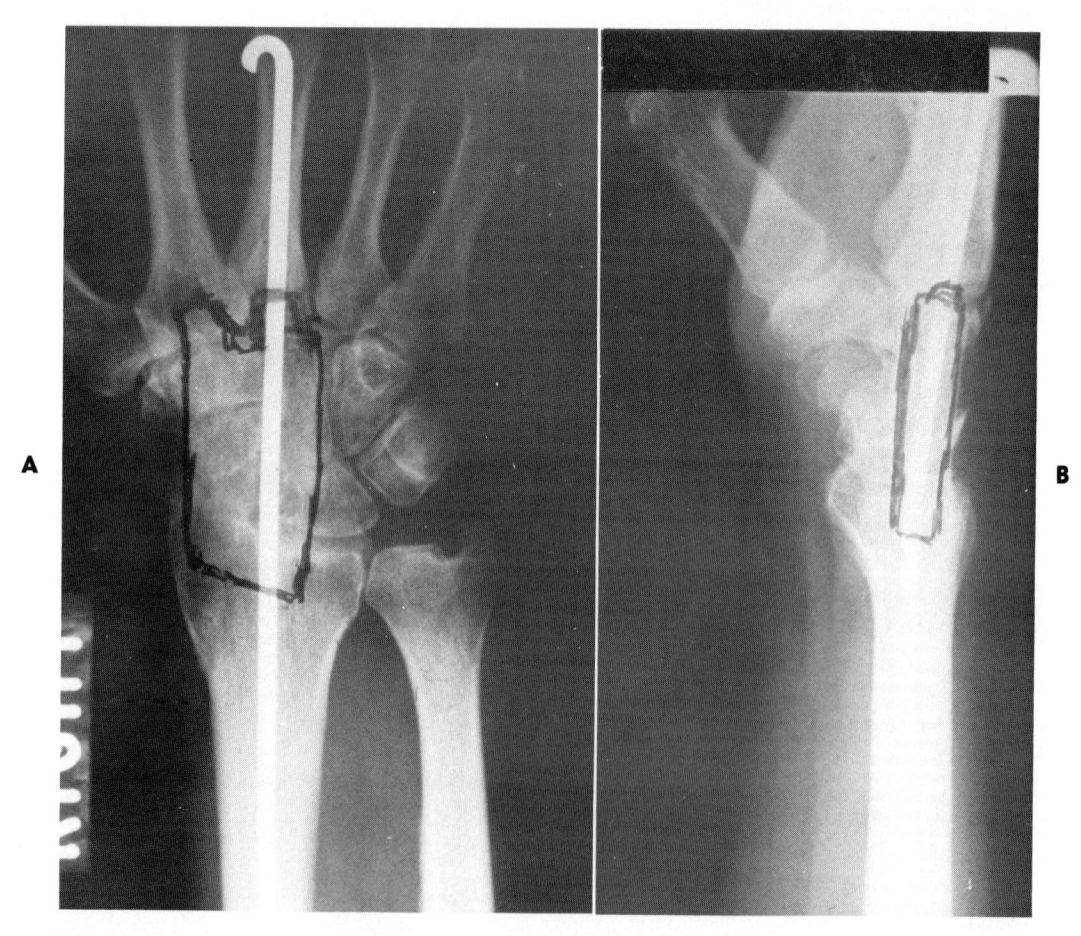

FIG. 41-1. A 61-year-old rancher with disabling osteoarthritis of wrist and good distal radioulnar function had dorsal iliac bone graft inlayed from base of second and third metacarpals into radius; intramedullary Rush pin through third metacarpal and through bone graft gave good stability in "automatic" neutral position. Radioulnar joint was not disturbed. His pain was relieved, and he was able to do heavy work with his hand.

With the wrist placed at neutral the arc of motion of pronation and supination substitutes for palmar and dorsiflexion without shoulder or elbow substitution (Fig. 41-2). This is very helpful in working at a desk or tabletop. In this position the axis of pronation and supination is down the central forearm and along the third metacarpal, and tip pinch of the thumb and index finger is about 7.5 cm below the axis in pronation. Supination will give an arc of elevation of 15 cm without awkward movement of the shoulder or elbow. The normal arc of palmar flexion to dorsiflexion in pronation only is about 20 cm; with added supination the arc only increases to 22.5 cm.

With dorsiflexion of 20 to 30 degrees fingertip pinch is essentially along the axis of rotation of the forearm and gives a minimal arc of about 5 cm with pronation and supination alone. This makes desk, table, or bench work much more awkward. One function of the wrist is to effectively position the fingers in space, and using a global concept only about one third of function is lost by fusion at neutral compared with two thirds lost with fusion at 30 degrees dorsiflexion.

Neutral position provides a good gripping position for use of tools and does not cause any distal digital imbalance; a carpenter can still use a hammer. Cosmetically it is also pleasing. It allows one to reach in pockets easily and is suited for sanitary toilet functions.

TECHNIQUE

I treated a patient with an unstable wrist from a "loose" type of rheumatoid arthritis and obtained a nonunion from a lateral Smith-Petersen[8] fusion in the 1950s. About 1962 a method of fusion utilizing an intramedullary pin with a local or iliac bone graft was devised, and this method has been continued successfully with minor variations.[3,4,6,7] Pronation and supination are essential for good function. If the radioulnar joint is deranged, the distal aspect of the ulna is excised; conversely, if the radioulnar joint is good, it is avoided during the fusion.

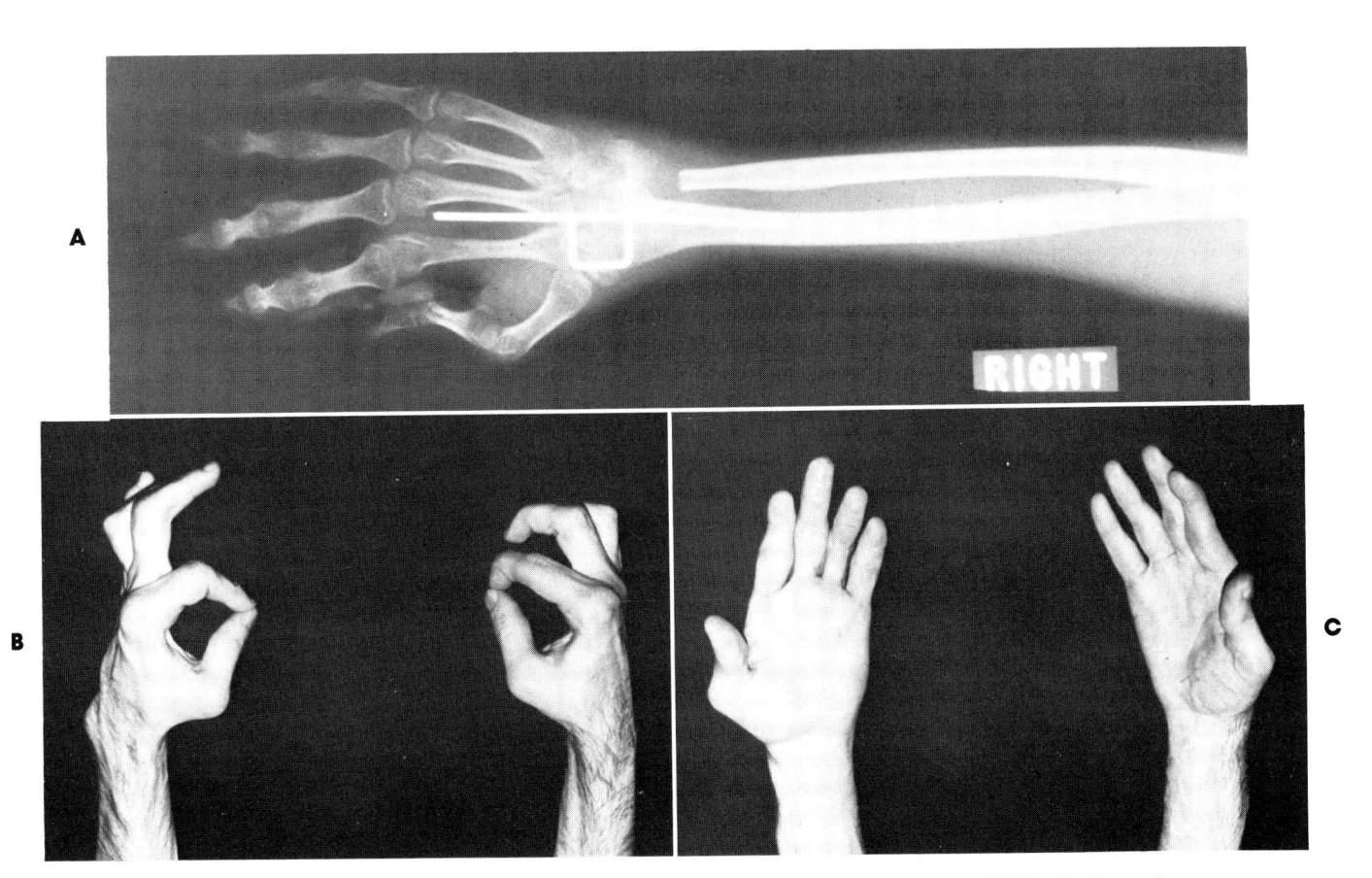

FIG. 41-2. **A,** A 23-year-old senior medical student with juvenile rheumatoid arthritis and metacarpals too small for intramedullary fixation: pin fixation obtained by retrograde pinning with $3/32$-inch pin and staple gave compression and rotary stabilization. Distal aspect of ulna was excised. Short-arm splint only was used. **B** and **C,** He has bilateral wrist fusions in neutral position. Note cosmetic appearance, functional positions, and arc of rotation. He has finished his internship, and has had no difficulty in use of his hand.

PRINCIPLES

The principles of arthrodesis are the following:
1. Neutral position
2. Internal fixation
3. Bony contact (bone graft)
4. Compression
5. Obtain or maintain rotation of forearm

A dorsal approach is used with essentially a long, straight incision extending distally between the second and third metacarpals, which gives excellent exposure and can be extended if necessary. As few dorsal veins as possible are ligated. Dissection is carried directly to the dorsal retinaculum, and all fat is carefully reflected with the skin, since wide exposure is necessary. The incision is essentially between sensory nerves, and these should be protected. Skin must be handled very carefully.

The dorsal carpal ligament is reflected like the page of a book in about 5-cm width; if the distal radioulnar joint is deranged, the dorsal carpal ligament is incised directly over the ulna and reflected radially, and the distal 2 cm of the ulna is resected subperiosteally. If the distal radioulnar joint is good, the dorsal carpal ligament may be reflected from its radial attachment; care is taken not to disturb the radioulnar joint. A longitudinal incision in the capsule of the wrist is extended to expose the bases of the second and third metacarpals and distal aspect of the radius; a good bony bed must be prepared to connect these areas. Some bone may have to be removed to gain decent contact and position. With rheumatoid arthritis local bone graft from the ulnar head and/or a sliding radial graft will suffice, with an iliac graft if necessary. Fixation is obtained with a ⅛-inch Rush pin introduced at the distal end of the third metacarpal from the radial side and into the radius for about 15 to 20 cm. Any bone graft is shaped and placed so that the pin holds it in position. Manual compression is then applied, and a staple can be driven into the second metacarpal and radius to maintain contact-compression and prevent rotation (or buried Kirschner wires also can be used). This allows use of a short-arm cast or a removable splint after surgery.

In traumatic cases an iliac graft is used, and a slot is sawed dorsally in the carpus from the base of the second and third metacarpals to the radius, to a depth of 1.0 to 1.2 cm and width of 2.5 cm. (See Fig. 41-1.) An opening is undercut into the radius and the bones of the second and third metacarpals. A unicortical inner table iliac graft is removed and shaped to fit the prepared bed and tightly wedged proximally and distally; the Rush pin is driven across, either through or dorsal to the bone graft, holding it in position. If it is rigid enough, no transfixion is necessary. (Special length staples can be made from small pins and used for compression.)

The wrist is positioned automatically at neutral with this technique; if a few degrees of alteration are desired, the intramedullary pin can be bent manually after insertion. The dorsal capsule of the wrist is closed and the dorsal carpal ligament passed beneath the long thumb and finger extensors. If the ulnar head has been excised, the dorsal carpal ligament is repaired snugly to stabilize the distal end.

The tourniquet is usually released, hemostasis obtained, and a drain inserted; closure with skin staples is excellent. With conforming bulky, light compression dressing with nonadherent gauze over the incision the hand is immobilized to the fingertips for a few days. Drains are removed at 48 hours. Finger motion is allowed in 3 to 10 days according to the status of the wound; often proximal interphalangeal joint motion is allowed at 2 or 3 days because this gives minimal long extensor tendon motion at the incision. Sutures remain at least 2 weeks. A short-arm cast or a simple volar splint is then used as protection if the internal fixation is rigid. If a large graft and no cross-fixation are used, a long-arm cast will be necessary for about 6 weeks. Union is obtained between 2 and 3 months.

I have used intramedullary fixation with bone graft for 16 years in over 30 cases, with union obtained in all. (One patient, in whom difficulty in inserting the pin was encountered, was treated with dorsal bone graft without rigid intramedullary fixation and developed a nonunion.)

Fusion should extend to the base of the second and third metacarpals. In one patient with rheumatoid arthritis, fusion was obtained and the pin removed; instability developed with destructive changes in all carpometacarpal joints.

A painless, mobile, stable, balanced wrist arthroplasty is to be desired over a wrist fusion, but it cannot always be obtained or maintained. There is still a place for arthrodesis of the wrist in selected cases.

REFERENCES

1. Abbot, L.C., Saunders, J.B.deC.M., and Bost, F.C.: Arthrodesis of the wrist with use of grafts of cancellous bone (from ilium), J. Bone Joint Surg. 24:883, 1942.
2. Boyes, J.H.: Bunnell's surgery of the hand, ed. 5, Philadelphia, 1970, J.B. Lippincott Co.
3. Clayton, M.L.: Surgery of the wrist in rheumatoid arthritis, J. Bone Joint Surg. 47A:741, 1965.
4. Clayton, M.L.: Wrist arthrodesis and tendon reconstruction in rheumatoid arthritis, Chicago, 1966, American Film Academy of Orthopaedic Surgeons Film Library. (Film.)
5. Haddad, R.J., Jr., and Riordan, D.C.: Arthrodesis of the wrist, J. Bone Joint Surg. 49A:950, 1967.
6. Mannerfelt, L., and Malmsten, M.: Arthrodesis of the wrist in rheumatoid arthritis: a technique without external fixation, Scand. J. Plast. Reconstr. Surg. 5:124, 1971.
7. Millender, L.H., and Nalebuff, E.A.: Arthrodesis of the rheumatoid wrist, J. Bone Joint Surg. 55A:1026, 1973.
8. Smith-Petersen, M.N.: A new approach to the wrist joint, J. Bone Joint Surg. 22:122, 1940.

Chapter 42 Management of the radial clubhand

William B. Kleinman

One of the most difficult management problems in reconstructive congenital hand surgery is failure of formation of the radius. Recommendations for the treatment of this longitudinal intercalary deficiency of forearm growth have been described in the literature since 1733, yet to this day it remains a controversial therapeutic challenge.

The deformity is an unsightly one, associated with generalized forearm shortening and severe radial deviation of the wrist (Fig. 42-1). Usual findings include gross instability of the wrist with progressive ulnocarpal displacement, deviation of the radial side of the wrist of an average of 75 degrees, volar carpal displacement secondary to the unopposed pull of the flexor carpi radialis muscle, and either failure of formation or hypoplasia of the thumb (Fig. 42-2).

TREATMENT OBJECTIVES

The general treatment plan in management of the radial clubhand is quite straightforward: improve the position of the hand-forearm unit, increase the apparent length of the limb, and enhance general function of the limb as a unit.[17]

The advantages of any reconstruction plan to improve apparent forearm length, reduce a severely dislocated and unstable wrist for better alignment of the hand-forearm unit, perform a pollicization of an index ray, or release an elbow or wrist contracture must be carefully weighed against the preoperative function of a so-called ulnar-oriented hand. The radial clubhand is oriented with the more functional ulnar-border digits positioned toward objects to be manipulated (Fig. 42-3). Both the structure and function of digits in this congenital deformity improve toward the ulnar border of the hand. O' Rahilly[16] has noted that in the majority of these patients the radial portion of the carpus (scaphoid and trapezium) is absent. In contrast, the roentgenographic appearance of the fingers may be normal, suggesting normal joint surfaces (including those of the index and long fingers). Limited motion appears to be related to extraarticular causes, involving perhaps the extensor or flexor mechanism of the fingers.[21]

The surgical approach to the radial clubhand should direct itself toward whether a straightened wrist with good stability can afford the child any functional or cosmetic advantages over the ulnar-oriented hand. The problem for the hand surgeon is how best to improve the appearance of this unsightly limb without interfering with overall function. Since instability of the wrist is a

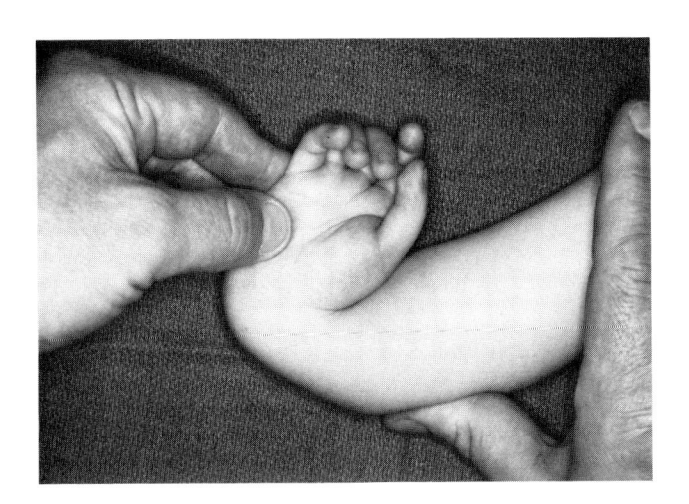

FIG. 42-1. Radial clubhand: severe radial deviation of wrist and forearm shortening.

SECTION 11 WRIST PROBLEMS

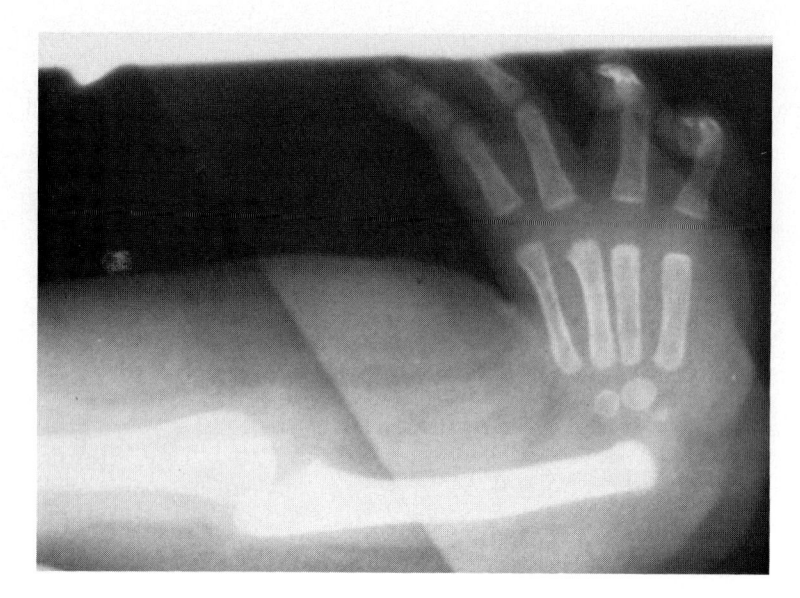

FIG. 42-2. Radiograph demonstrating complete failure of formation of thumb ray and profound radial deviation of hand on forearm (elbow in full extension).

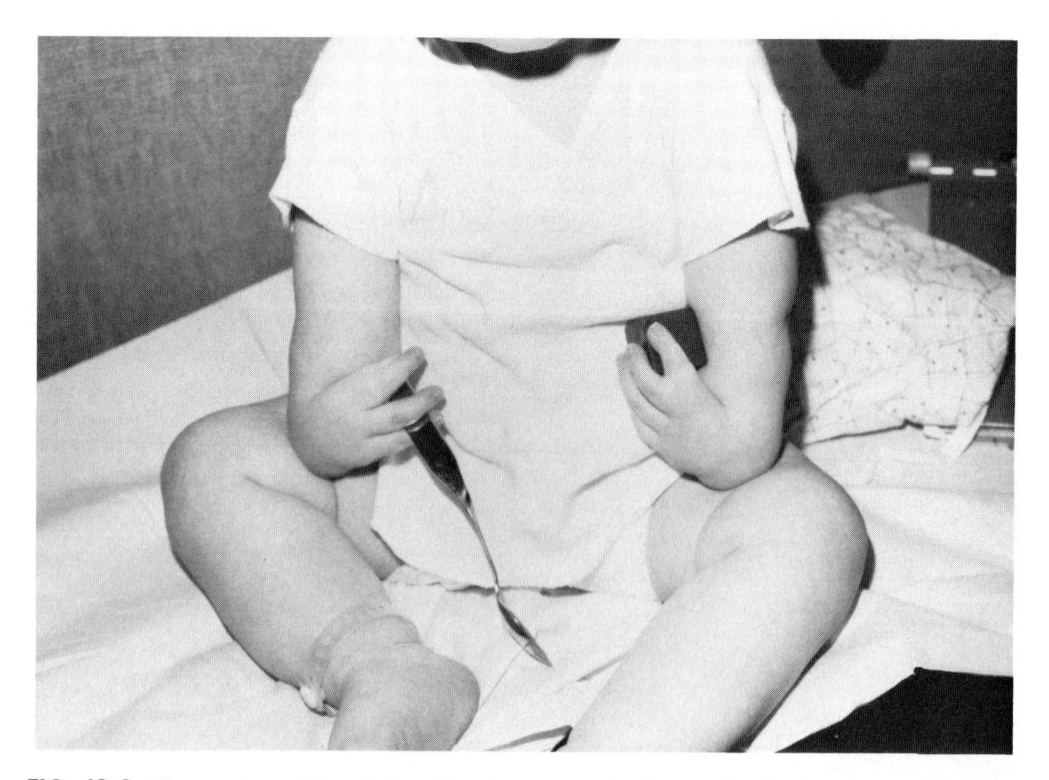

FIG. 42-3. *Ulnar-oriented hand:* functional compromise least affects ulnar-border digits; a child often preferentially uses this side of the hand.

PROCEDURES TO CORRECT HAND-FOREARM MALALIGNMENT AND WRIST INSTABILITY

1. Soft tissue release
   (with or without ulnar osteotomy)

2. Substitution for radius
   (strut bone grafting or epiphyseal transplant)

3. Centralization of ulna

4. Wrist arthrodesis

Sayre,[20] 1893
Bardenheuer, 1894
Antonelli, 1904
Ryerson, 1924
Albee, 1928
Starr,[22] 1945
Riordan, 1955,[18] 1963
Carroll,[4] 1966
Lidge,[15] 1969
Delorme,[6] 1969
Bora, Nicholson, and Cheema,[1] 1970
Lamb,[13,14] 1972, 1977
Goldberg and Meyn,[9] 1976

regular feature of the untreated deformity, much has been contributed to the literature over the past 90 years regarding surgical procedures that align and stabilize the position of the hand-forearm unit. These procedures can be placed in four general categories. (See accompanying box.)

SURGICAL PROCEDURES
Soft tissue releases with or without osteotomy of the ulna

In cases of severe radial deviation and volar carpal disloation, wide Z-plasty of the skin overlying the radial aspect of the wrist, followed by capsulotomy, tenotomy, or step-cut lengthening of contracted tissue, may be necessary as a preliminary procedure before further definitive reconstruction can begin.[2,5] In his Founder's Lecture to the American Society for Surgery of the Hand in 1975, Lamb[14] reviewed the works of Hoffa, Sayre,[20] Romano, and Bardenheuer, all published at the turn of the twentieth century; each advocated osteotomy of the ulna in association with soft tissue release. Long-term follow-up studies showed that soft tissue release and ulnar osteotomy alone were ineffective in maintaining a stable ulnocarpal relationship, even with postoperative splint management.[14]

Replacement of the aplastic radius

In 1945 Starr[22] popularized earlier works by Albee and by Ryerson in an effort to substitute local or distant autogenous bone graft for the absent radius. Problems associated with lysis of the autogenous tibial graft used by Albee led Ryerson to split off a large longitudinal length of ulna, transposing it to the radial side of the forearm as a strut. Similarly Starr, and Riordan[18] again in 1955, advocated that the entire proximal fibula with intact epiphyseal plate be used as a radial strut, with expectation of proximal fibular growth after transplantation. Long-term follow-up analysis by Carroll[4] in 1966 of 18 patients with limbs undergoing transplantation, as advocated by Riordan, showed that the "transplanted fibula does not keep pace with growth of the ulna," and that the fibular physis closes rapidly, allowing recurrence of the deformity and wrist instability and the subsequent need for surgical revision. Kutz[12] has recently suggested that free vascularized pedicle transplantation of the proximal fibula might be effective in maintaining the growth potential of the open epiphyseal plate and stability of the hand-forearm unit.

Centralization

Almost 100 years ago Sayre[20] proposed what has only recently been accepted as the foundation for achieving the basic goals in management of this deformity. In his original article Sayre recommended centralizing the severely radially displaced hand and carpus onto the distal end of the ulna in a small notch made at the proximal carpal level. The fundamentals proposed by Sayre were biomechanically described by Lidge[15] in 1969, and his method is now generally recommended. Sayre's basic philosophy is still used, modified by centralizing the distal aspect of the ulna deeply into the carpus by resection of the entire lunate and capitate, with the longitudinal axis of the hand (the long finger metacarpal) oriented perpendicular to the distal epiphyseal plate of the centralized ulna. In some cases additional resection of a portion of the radial aspect of the triquetrum is necessary to ensure that the breadth and depth of the channel created for the distal portion of the ulna are equal.

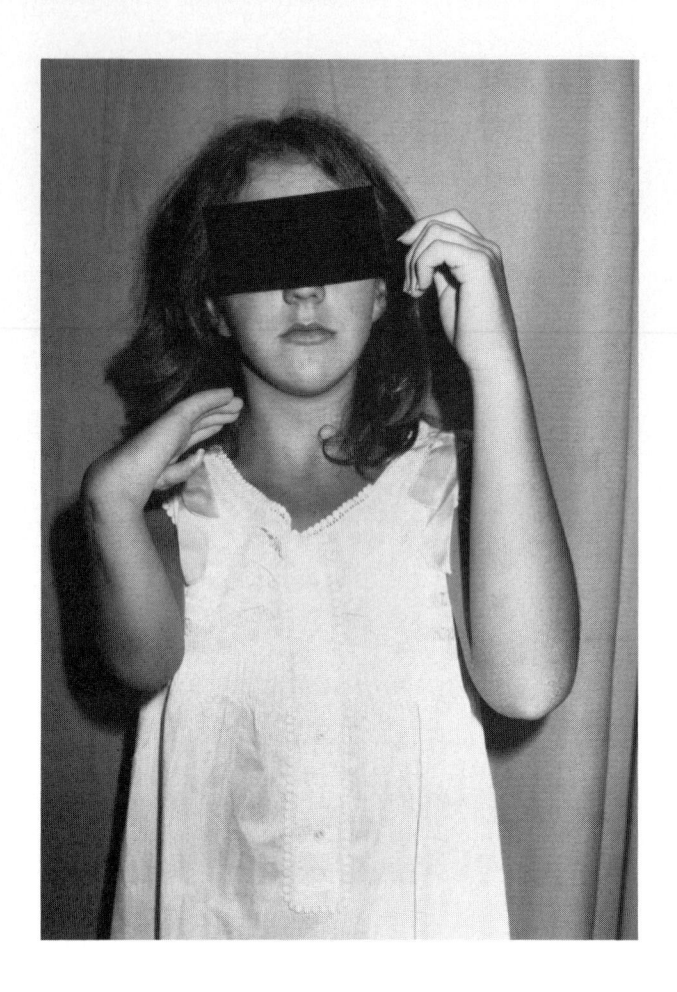

FIG. 42-4. Normally, length ratio between humerus and ulna is 1:1. In radial clubhand, because of profound forearm shortening, this ratio may be 3:2 or as high as 2:1.

Use of a nonvascularized proximal fibular graft to support the hand on the forearm has been generally abandoned. In his critical 1959 analysis Heikel[11] suggested:

[Although] a permanent correction of the position will be achieved if bony ankylosis between the ulna and the carpus on the metacarpals is produced . . . , no ankylosis between the ulna and the carpus or metacarpus can be achieved . . . without complete or partial destruction of the distal growth of the ulna, with resultant arrest or disturbed growth in length of the latter.

Both Heikel[11] and Lamb,[14] in their independent statistical reviews, showed that the retained length of the forearm in complete radial agenesis was approximately 60% of normal and that the ratio of the length of the humerus to that of the ulna (normally about 1:1) was 3:2, or as high as 2:1 (Fig. 42-4). With centralization in the manner suggested by Lidge,[15] growth of the ulna from the distal growth plate may be seen, but I agree with Flatt[7] that unpredictable growth from this area following centralization is a small price to pay for satisfactory stability of the hand.

Wrist arthrodesis

In the patient with congenital clubhand deformity, fusion of the wrist joint is the final definitive procedure to ensure wrist stability *after growth has ceased*. To avoid any further compromise to the growth potential of the distal aspect of the ulna, this procedure should not be performed prior to closure of the epiphyseal plate; thereafter it is an excellent procedure to both correct angular deformity at the wrist and to improve wrist stability (Fig. 42-5). Lamb[14] has pointed out, however, that arthrodesis in the *bilateral*, previously untreated adolescent patient with radial clubhands gives a poor result. The child is unable to allow "a satisfactory pattern of prehension to develop" as an adolescent with bilateral wrist arthrodesis, unlike the infant with bilateral centralizations.

SURGICAL RECONSTRUCTION: THE PHILOSOPHY

Improvement in limb appearance without loss of limb function is the goal of any reconstructive effort in radial

CHAPTER 42 MANAGEMENT OF THE RADIAL CLUBHAND

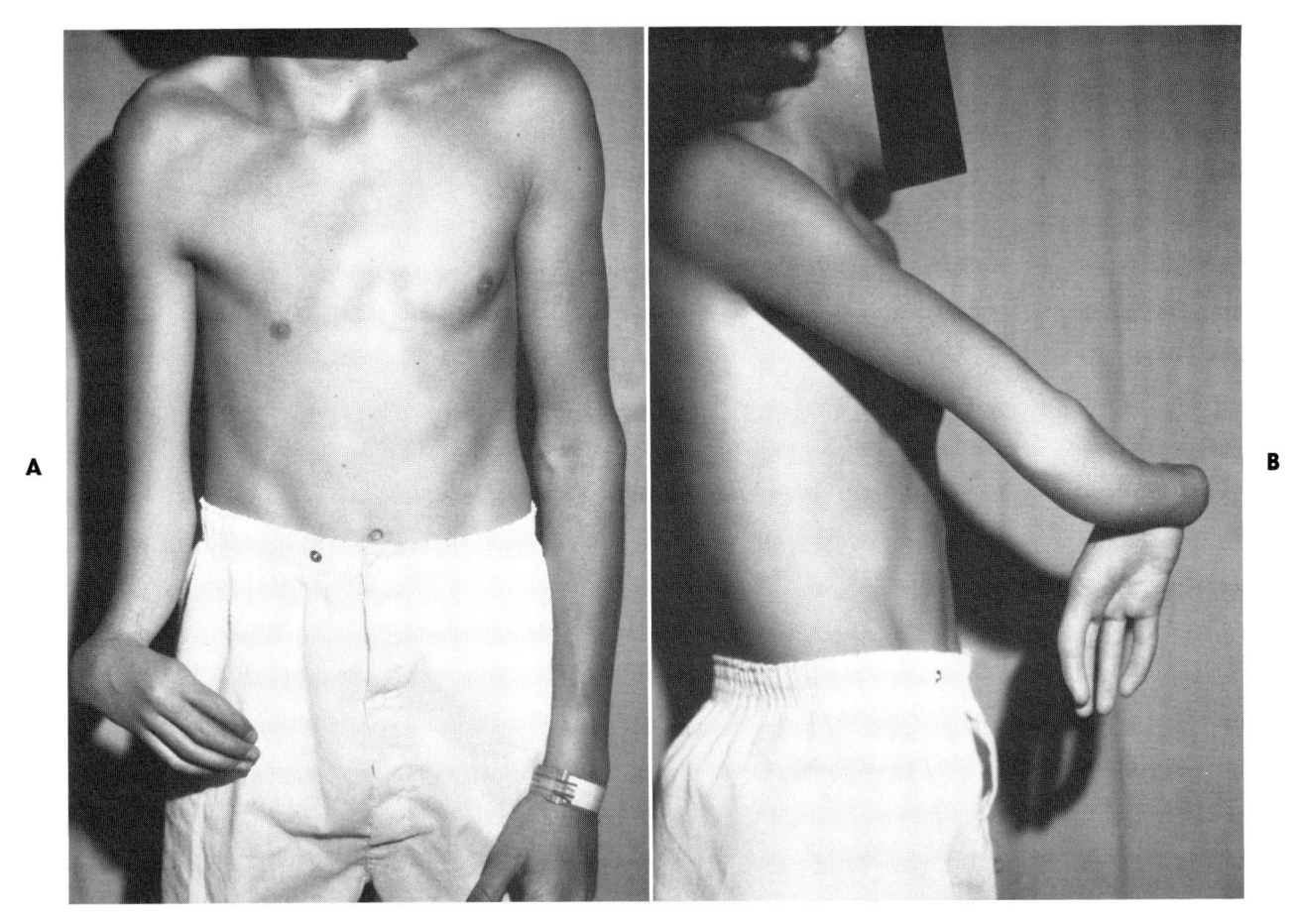

FIG. 42-5. A, Untreated adolescent clubhand is refractory to conservative splinting techniques. **B,** Alignment and stabilization by wrist arthrodesis should be considered in these cases.

clubhand. Straightening the wrist and eliminating the ulnar orientation of the hand do not seriously compromise function, nor does surgical correction of the deformity cause serious shortening of the forearm, even if the ulna must be centralized to the level of the metacarpal bases. My own experience is similar to that of Lamb.[13,14] Even in those cases in which preoperative elbow stiffness (active flexion less than 90 degrees) has been a problem, I have used posterior capsulotomy with or without anterior transposition of the triceps to restore functional elbow flexion subsequent to centralization, with satisfactory results. Lamb has reported similar successful reconstructive efforts even in bilateral cases. Frankel, Goldner, and Stelling,[8] however, suggest that, in patients with bilateral deformity and limited elbow motion, centralization and loss of wrist motion secondary to ankylosis between the carpus and ulna make this procedure a contraindication.

Whether stability of the hand provides the greatest potential for digital movement in the patient with radial clubhand is still controversial. Flatt[7] feels that not only will movement be maximized, but also "early stabilization should allow the maximum grasp in partially stiff hands." The concept of the ulnar-oriented hand suggests that the most functional medial-border digits are oriented *toward* the object to be grasped by the patient, frequently with the only prehensile ability available to them. Heikel[11] states that wrist position does not affect finger function, and Lamb's meticulous functional assessments[13,14] by experienced occupational therapists bear this out. Delorme[6] and Bora and associates[1] even report a measurable improvement in fine prehensile activities and grip strength after wrist stabilization. In my own cases I have found that preoperative digital function is not affected by early centralization.

CENTRALIZATION: IS THERE AN IDEAL TIME?

Assuming, then, that ulnar centralization in the radial clubhand affords functional and cosmetic improvement, when should the procedure be performed? The literature on radial clubhands is consistent; all authors recommend *splinting of the untreated clubhand from birth* or as soon as the infant is seen by a specialist; soft tissue contractures along the volar and radial side of the wrist should be avoided. Under ideal circumstances Riordan[18] operates on a patient as young as 6 weeks to 6 months old; Flatt[7] suggests that any time during the second year of life is satisfactory, but beyond 2 years of age is late; Salter[19] and Tachdjian[23] both suggest "early" centralization. Lidge,[15] who studied 25 patients and who designed the technique now used by most hand surgeons, felt the best time for centralization was 2 to 3 years of age. It appears from Lamb's work[13,14] that predictable cessation of distal ulnar growth is a problem only if the procedure is carried out at a late date (more than 7 years of age) when the ulnar epiphysis is near spontaneous closure in these children.

I feel that, ideally, serial corrective casting should begin at birth. After alignment is attained by soft tissue stretching, night bracing should continue until centralization can be performed. After the age of 1 year, when tissues are larger and less friable and the child less an anesthetic risk, a very successful centralization can be carried out with little total risk to the patient. It should be kept in mind that bracing alone usually becomes ineffective after 3 years of age, as the carpus progressively slides off the distal aspect of the ulna with forearm growth and increasing soft tissue tightness.

THE RECALCITRANT HAND

Because of extrinsic muscle imbalance, certain patients with radial agenesis may be predisposed to recurrence of the deformity even after centralization has been completed. To avoid this problem, Bora and associates[1] advocate a two-stage treatment program to stabilize the wrist: centralization at the age of 6 to 12 months, followed by tendon transfers 6 to 12 months later to balance muscle forces about the wrist. Their method uses either one or both of the flexor digitorum superficialis tendons to the ring and small finger (when available), transferred around the ulnar border of the wrist to the dorsal index and middle finger metacarpals for stability. Superficialis tendons are chosen to eliminate their contribution to progressive wrist subluxation and ulnar bowing in some cases. Transfer of these tendons not only weakens the deforming force but also creates a degree of wrist extensor power helpful in maintaining the hand-forearm relationship following centralization. In contradistinction, in only five of Lamb's 31 cases[14] was tendon transfer employed to eliminate a *strong* deforming force, and these transfers were performed at the time of centralization. In most cases of radial clubhand, the extensor carpi radialis brevis and longus musculotendinous units are absent, and frequently the flexor carpi radialis is deficient or vestigial. If the flexor carpi ulnaris or superficial extrinsic finger flexors are truly deforming forces, this should be recognized at the time of surgery and eliminated. Either the flexor carpi ulnaris or the flexor digitorum superficialis of the middle, ring, or little finger will function quite well as a dorsal carpal stabilizer, but I have found that tendon transfer should *only* be performed if a strongly deforming force is observed at the time of centralization.

RECONSTRUCTION OF THE THUMB IN RADIAL APLASIA

Once stabilization of the hand-forearm unit has been completed by centralization of the ulna, attention can be directed toward the child's prehensile ability. Each patient with radial agenesis will have some thumb involvement, ranging within the hypoplasia spectrum from the grossly unstable "floating thumb" *(pousse flotant)* to simple terminal tendon deficiency. In my own experience complete radial aplasia is usually associated with complete failure of formation of the thumb (Fig. 42-6). There is little doubt that in those cases in which the thumb is absent or in which a classic floating thumb

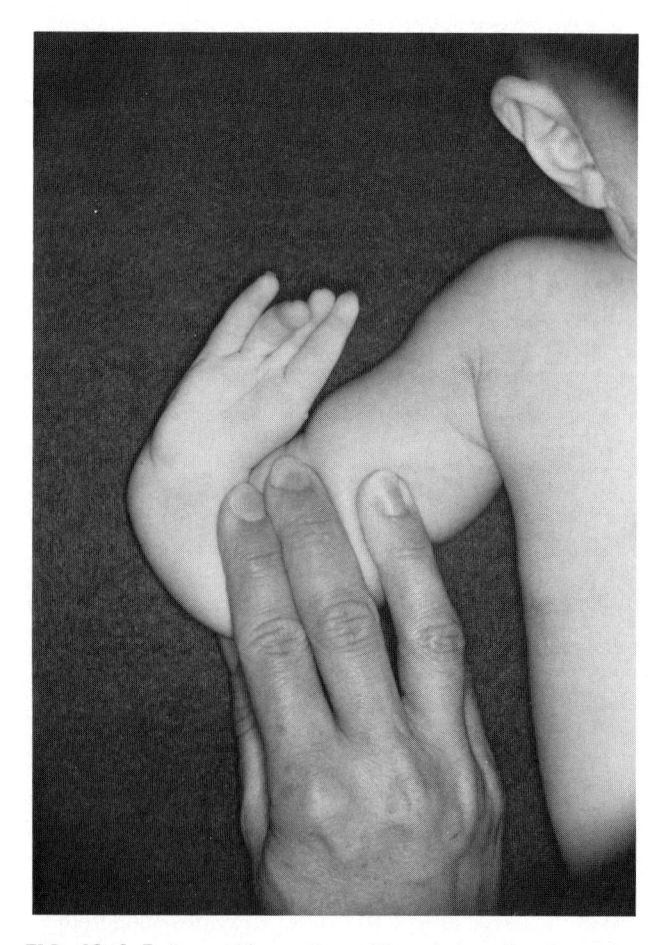

FIG. 42-6. Failure of formation of thumb is quite characteristic in cases of complete absence of radius.

is present, pollicization of the index finger will greatly improve not only prehensile function but also the function of the limb in general (Fig. 42-7). Salter[19] and others have suggested that in bilateral cases of radial agenesis pollicization should be limited to one hand. It is my own feeling that improvement in hand function is so noticeable after pollicization that unilateral and bilateral cases should be approached similarly. This has been Lamb's experience[14] also: "whenever the overall condition of the limb and hand justifies confidence that functional improvement will be possible," pollicization should be considered, whether unilateral or bilateral. Harrison[10] in 1970 suggested that, since there is an ulnar-oriented approach to function in these severely compromised limbs, pollicization might best be performed on the *ulnar* border of the hand. Flatt[7] also feels this to be an interesting suggestion. The child's function is usually so compromised that the most workable parts (i.e., the more medial side of the hand) might best be used for improved function. I have no personal experience with this approach.

Although index finger stiffness is a frequently observed problem in radial agenesis, pollicization of the index finger should improve the prehensile capability of the limb, especially after centralization, when the ulnar-oriented hand is stable and considerably less radially deviated, and the index finger, after pollicization, is in a better position for prehensile function. The technique I have used combines the skin incision described by Carroll,[5] the carpometacarpal stabilization and position described by Buck-Gramcko,[3] and the principles of intrinsic rearrangement outlined by Riordan.[18]

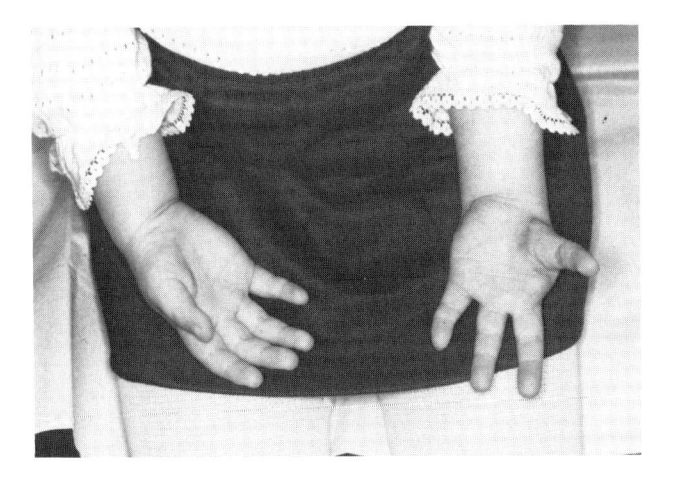

FIG. 42-7. Pollicization of index finger in cases of absence or hypoplasia of thumb provides improvement in function, even in bilateral cases.

WRIST STABILIZATION

Stabilization of the wrist in the radial clubhand by centralizing the carpus on the distal end of the ulna increases the apparent limb length, improves the cosmetic appearance of the limb, and usually results in no loss of preoperative hand function. It must be kept in mind that these patients have no available forearm pronation and supination,[21] and often the grossly radially deviated and unstable preoperative wrist joint is the only factor that enables the child to bring the hand to the face or mouth or hygiene and personal care. Some surgeons' reluctance to perform bilateral centralization in cases of bilateral radial agenesis is based on the severe functional compromise that wrist straightening and stabilization might have. I feel that, as long as shoulder and elbow stiffness are not factors, bilateral centralization will not impair function (Fig. 42-8). Even in cases of elbow flexion less than 90 degrees good results have been achieved recently in my patients when centralization is preceeded by posterior capsulotomy of the elbow either alone or in combination with a triceps tendon transfer to restore an active arc of elbow flexion.

DIFFICULT PROBLEMS WITH CENTRALIZATION: RECURRENCE

The most frequent problem after centralization is recurrence of the original deformity. These unsatisfactory results are most often related either to failure to achieve proper alignment at the time of surgery or to a gross extrinsic motor imbalance with a net vector toward reproduction of the deformity. Lidge[15] and Lamb[13,14] have both emphasized the critical importance of alignment of the longitudinal axis of the hand perpendicular to the distal ulnar growth plate (Fig. 42-9). Once this critical relationship is achieved, transepiphyseal intramedullary fixation as advocated by Delorme[6] and Goldberg and Meyn[9] has been satisfactory in my patients in maintaining alignment (with or without tendon transfers) until ankylosis is ensured (Fig. 42-10). The surgeon must decide at the time of centralization if there indeed is a persistent deforming force and, if so, whether hypothenar muscle transfer,[18] extensor carpi ulnaris transfer through a distal ulnar pulley,[9] flexor digitorum superficialis "wraparound,"[1] or simple use of the extensor carpi ulnaris as an unlar collateral ligament reinforcement[15] is indicated.

SUMMARY

The treatment plan for radial agenesis should ideally begin at birth, with serial casting until alignment is attained by soft tissue stretching along the radial and volar borders of the wrist. This should be followed by continuous night bracing until centralization can be performed, any time after 1 year of age, understanding that bracing

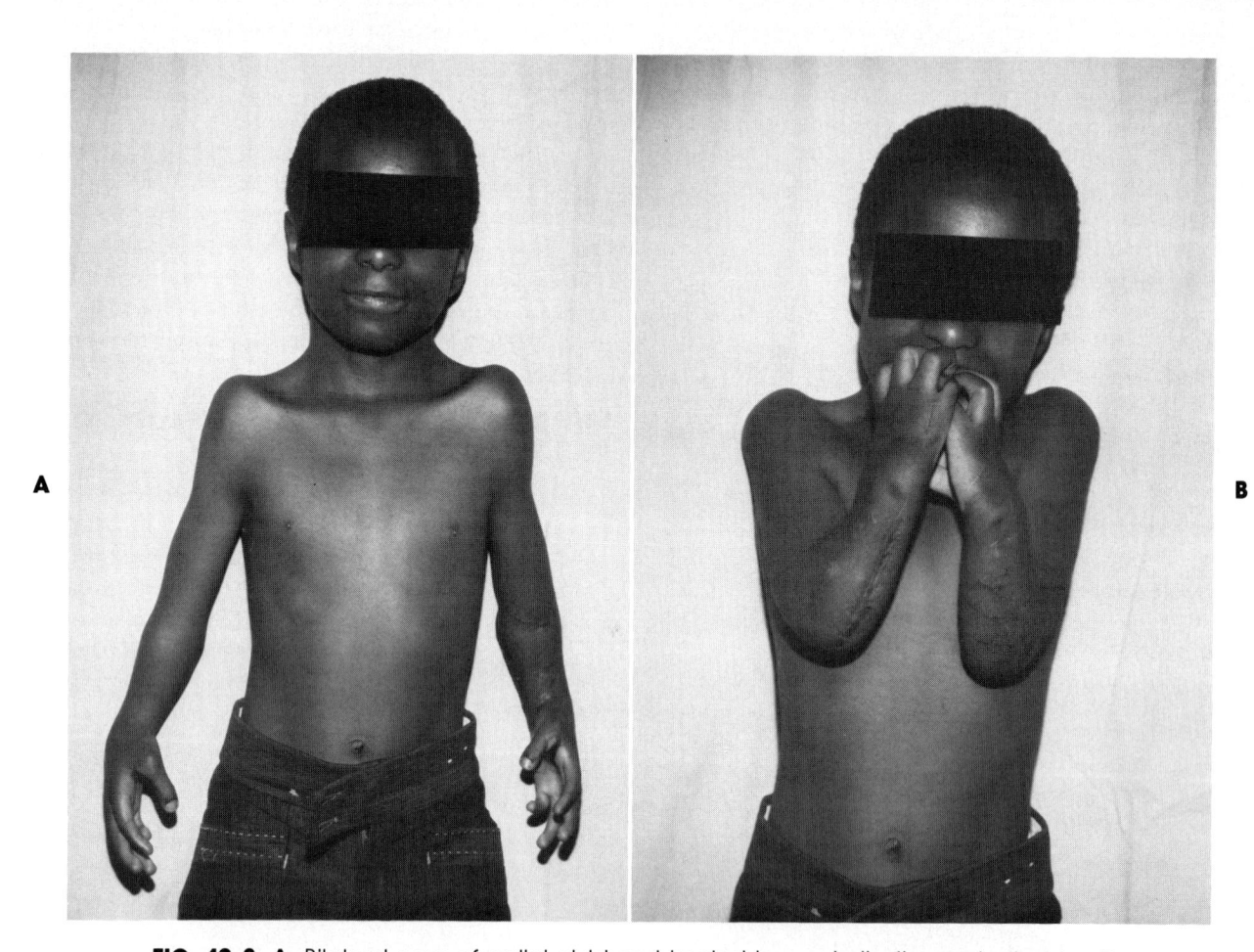

FIG. 42-8. A, Bilateral case of radial clubhand treated by centralization on both sides. **B,** Ability to bring hands to mouth or face for regular hygiene is unimpaired. (Note functional arc of elbow flexion.)

CHAPTER 42 MANAGEMENT OF THE RADIAL CLUBHAND

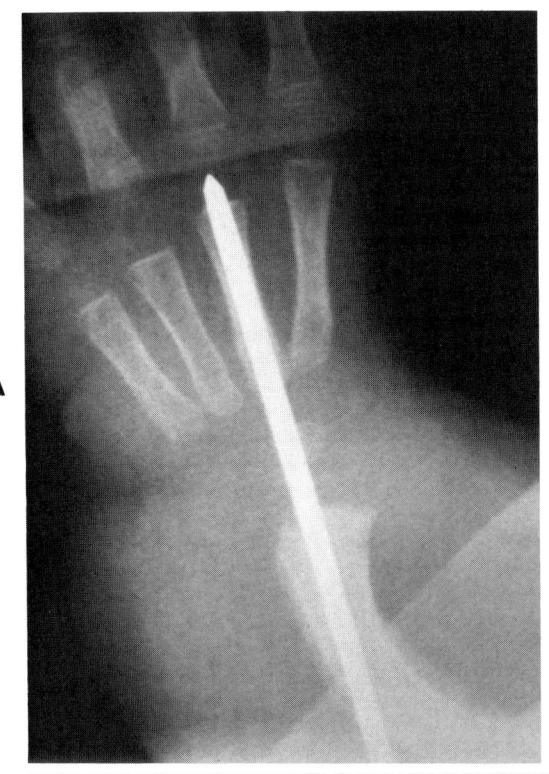

FIG. 42-9. A, Alignment of longitudinal axis of hand (third metacarpal) perpendicular to epiphyseal plate of distal aspect of ulna ensures good relation of hand-forearm unit, with least risk to forearm growth from their center. **B,** This technique has been described by Lidge,[15] Lamb,[13,14] and Delorme.[6]

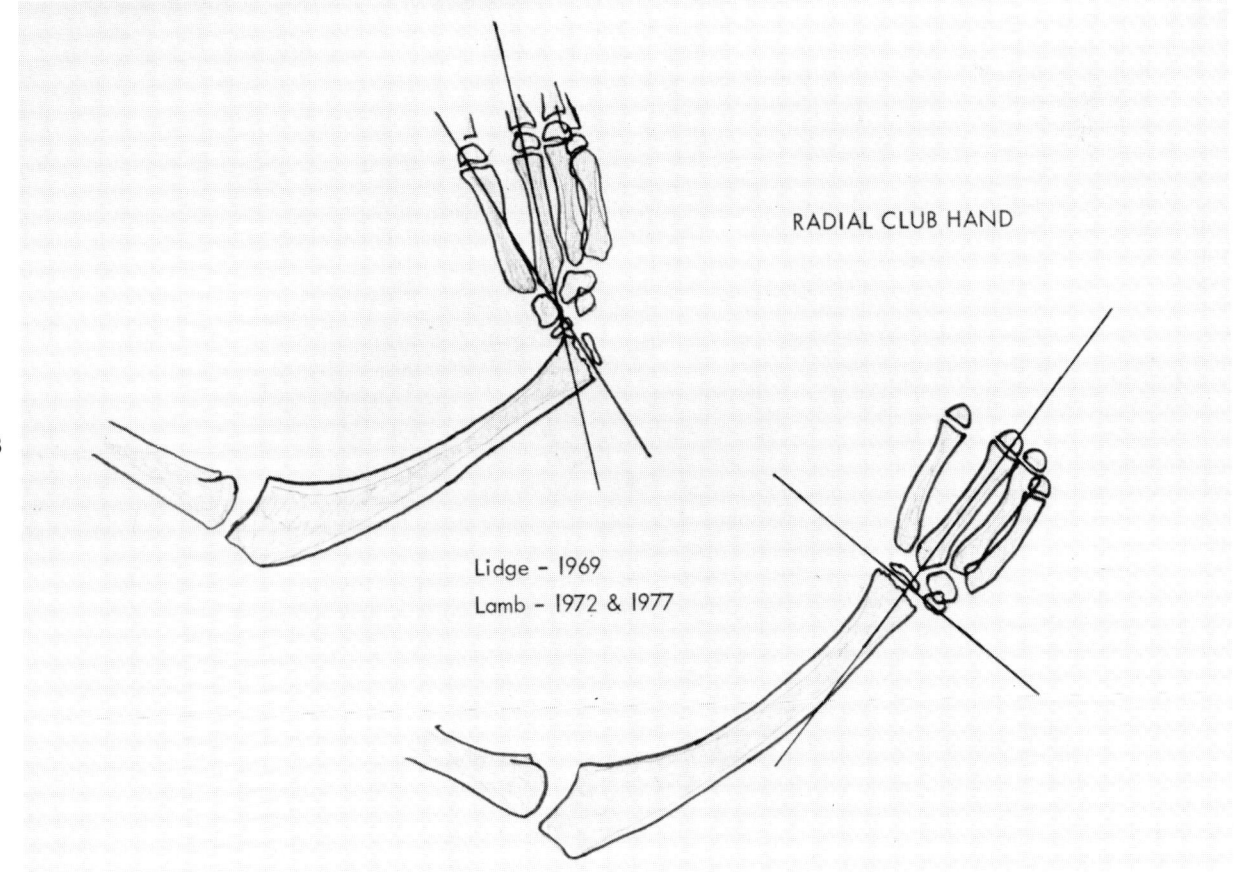

Lidge - 1969
Lamb - 1972 & 1977

RADIAL CLUB HAND

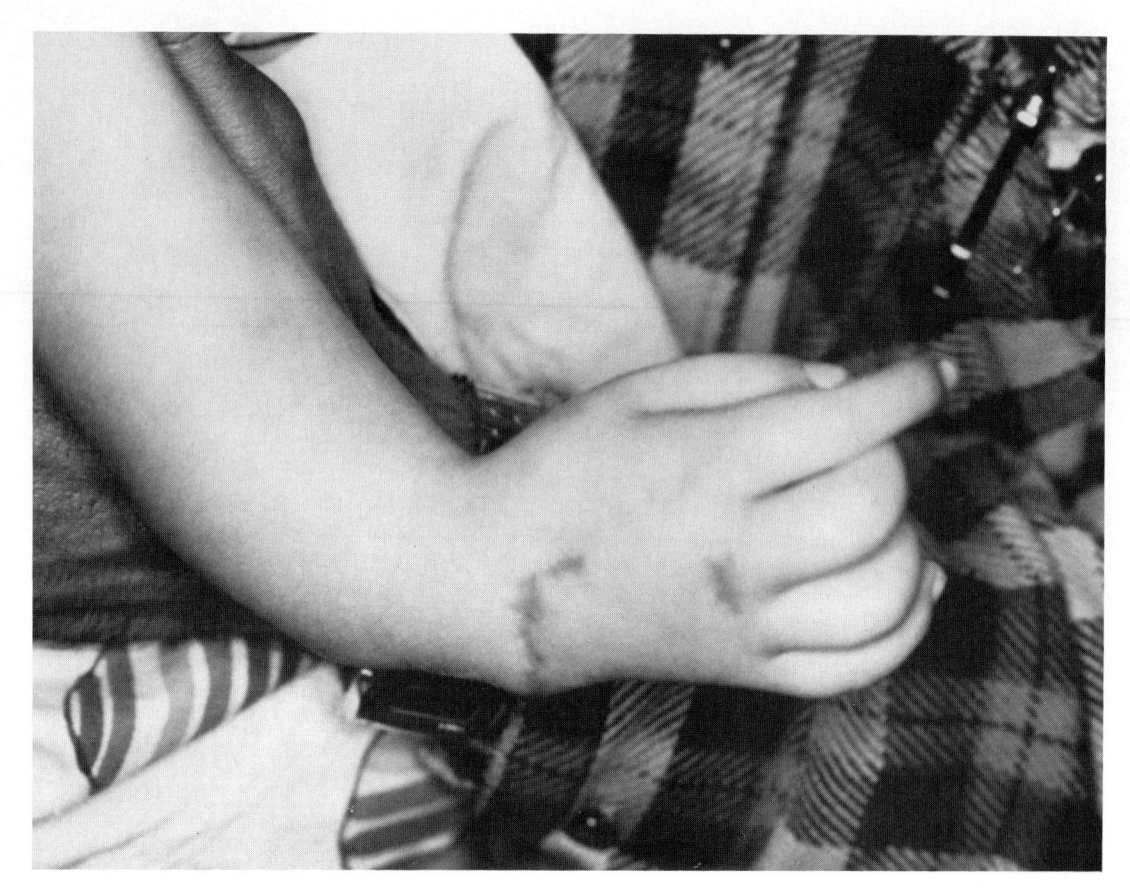

FIG. 42-10. Hand-forearm relation in radial clubhand, seen 1 year following centralization of ulna in same case shown in Fig. 42-1.

becomes ineffective alone after age 3. Centralization of the carpus on the ulna after age 7 or 8 is usually followed by rapid growth arrest of the ulna.

If elbow flexion is deficient in range or strength, this should be treated by soft tisue releases or tendon transfers before dealing with the wrist deformity. The after-centralization plan should be either continuous night bracing (after 3 months in plaster) or second-stage tendon transfers, as recommended by Bora and associates.[1] As the untreated age of patient advances, severe soft tissue tightening makes the patient refractory to conventional casting and splinting techniques. (See Fig. 42-5.) Boyes[2] and later Carroll[5] have recommended a single large radial Z-plasty of the skin and tenotomies as necessary for length. The median nerve, however, is frequently the most limiting structure in soft tissue releases because of its superficial attitude in these deficient limbs. Carroll's approach to this problem uses recession of the entire flexor origin from the proximal ulna and elbow, followed by preliminary casting and subsequent splinting in turnbuckle braces.

The most difficult challenge in radial agenesis is, then, the untreated adolescent. Complete soft tissue release from the radial aspect of the unla should be followed by wrist arthrodesis only after all longitudinal growth from the distal end of the ulna is complete. Primary wrist arthrodesis in adolescence represents an effective but frequently a salvage procedure for partial correction of hand-forearm malalignment.

If the hand surgeon adheres to the principles reviewed in this chapter, wrist stability with continued forearm growth can be satisfactorily attained in the young patient with radial agenesis, with improvement in the cosmetic appearance of the limb without functional compromise.

REFERENCES

1. Bora, F.W., Nicholson, J.T., and Cheema, H.M.: Radial meromelia: the deformity and its treatment, J. Bone Joint Surg. **52A:**966, 1970.
2. Boyes, J.H.: Bunnell's surgery of the hand, ed. 5, Philadelphia, 1970, J.B. Lippincott Co.

3. Buck-Gramcko, D.: Pollicization of the index finger: method and results in aplasia and hypoplasia of the thumb, J. Bone Joint Surg. **53A**:1605, 1971.
4. Carroll, R.E.: Use of the fibula for reconstruction in congenital absence of the radius, J. Bone Joint Surg. **48A**:1012, 1966.
5. Carroll, R.E.: Personal communication, 1978.
6. Delorme, T.L.: Treatment of congenital absence of the radius by transepiphyseal fixation, J. Bone Joint Surg. **51A**:117, 1969.
7. Flatt, A.E.: The care of congenital hand anomalies, St. Louis, 1977, The C.V. Mosby Co.
8. Frankel, M.E., Goldner, J.L., and Stelling, F.H.: Radial club hand: is centralization necessary? A rational surgical approach, J. Bone Joint Surg. **53A**:1026, 1971.
9. Goldberg, M.J., and Meyne, M.: The radial clubhand, Orthop. Clin. North Am. **7**:341, 1976.
10. Harrison, S.H.: Pollicization in cases of radial club hand, Br. J. Plast. Surg. **23**:192, 1970.
11. Heikel, H.V.A.: Aplasia and hypoplasia of the radius, Acta Orthop. Scand. (Suppl.) **39**:1, 1959.
12. Kutz, J.: Personal communication, 1977.
13. Lamb, D.W.: The treatment of radial club hand, Hand **4**:22, 1972.
14. Lamb, D.W.: Radial club hand, J. Bone Joint Surg. **53A**:1, 1977.
15. Lidge, R.T.: Congenital radial deficient club hand, J. Bone Joint Surg. **51A**:1041, 1969.
16. O'Rahilly, R.: Radial hemimelia and the functional anatomy of the carpus, J. Anat. **80**:179, 1946.
17. Pulvertaft, R.G.: Watson-Jones lecture, J. Bone Joint Surg. **49B**:587, 1967.
18. Riordan, D.C.: Congenital absence of the radius, J. Bone Joint Surg. **37A**:1129, 1955.
19. Salter, R.B.: Textbook of disorders and injuries of the musculoskeletal system, Baltimore, 1970, Williams & Wilkins Co.
20. Sayre, R.H.: A contribution to the study of club-hand, Trans. Am. Orthop. Assoc. **6**:208, 1893.
21. Skerik, S.K., and Flatt, A.E.: The anatomy of congenital radial dysplasia, Clin. Orthop. **66**:126, 1969.
22. Starr, D.E.: Congenital absence of the radius: a method of surgical correction, J. Bone Joint Surg. **27**:572, 1945.
23. Tachdjian, M.O.: Pediatric orthopaedics, Philadelphia, 1972, W.B. Saunders Co.

SECTION TWELVE NERVE PROBLEMS

Chapter 43 The neuroma-in-continuity

George E. Omer, Jr.

The timing of nerve exploration and suturing in an open injury is complicated by associated trauma. Nerves are only as functional as the residual sensory receptors and muscle-tendon motor units.[8] Nerve suturing should not be done when there is vascular insufficiency, because tissue homeostasis cannot be restored. Soft tissue coverage with a skin flap may be necessary. A disrupted skeleton prevents an active range of motion for muscle-tendon units. Infection will compromise circulation and contribute to muscle fibrosis and joint stiffness. A successful neurorrhaphy requires elimination of associated tissue problems. However, the longer the delay before nerve suturing, the poorer the prognosis for good clinical recovery.[9] In the delayed exploration the gross appearance, secondary to fibrotic response about the nerve lesion, may be misleading.

A closed injury with associated nerve dysfunction is usually observed, since approximately 85% of these nerve lesions have spontaneous clinical recovery within 4 months.[9,10] However, the proximal (high) nerve injury presents a difficult problem. It may be considerable distance from the site of the nerve lesion to the first motor point to be reinnervated. From the time of injury there is progressive distortion and degeneration of the distal motor and sensory end-organs, with associated slowing of the regenerative process for axon regrowth. If the nerve is disrupted, the distal stump will shrink and prejudice successful reentry of regenerating axons. Expectant management could be prolonged to the time when suture of a previously unrecognized severed nerve would be without hope for good clinical recovery. Therefore it is appropriate at 3 months to explore the clinically complete nerve lesion above the elbow or knee. However, the gross appearance of the nerve is not indicative of the actual number of functioning axons.

Seddon[12] introduced a simple classification of traumatic injuries to peripheral nerves. The minimal injury is termed *neurapraxia* and may be secondary to localized ischemic demyelination. The moderate injury is termed *axonotmesis* and is characterized by interruption of the axons and their myelin sheath; but the endoneurial tubes remain intact and guide the regenerating axons to their proper peripheral connections. The severe injury is termed *neurotmesis* and describes a nerve that either has been severed completely or is so seriously disorganized that spontaneous regeneration is impossible. The abortive natural repair following a traumatic nerve lesion leads to the development of a neuroma—a lesion composed of misdirected axonal sprouts, Schwann cells, and proliferating connective tissue from the epineurial, perineurial, or endoneurial layers of the nerve.

Clinical studies[6] indicate that the majority of traumatic injuries do not transect the involved nerve but leave it in continuity. The evaluation of a neuroma-in-continuity is one of the more difficult problems in peripheral nerve surgery because the surgeon must decide whether the lesion is a neurapraxia, and thus reversible, or a neurotmesis, and thus demanding surgical intervention.

INSPECTION AND PALPATION

The appearance and consistency of a neuroma-in-continuity can be misleading. A bulbous neuroma may be the result of epineurial scar with a relatively organized intrafascicular pattern of regenerating axons. In contrast, a smooth lesion, perhaps secondary to an injection injury, may have severe intrafascicular disorganization and minimal potential for regeneration.[1] If the neuroma is fusiform, swelling to less than twice the normal diameter indicates either axonotmesis or neurotmesis, but swelling to more than twice the normal diameter usually indicates neurotmesis. Lateral neuromas suggest partial transection. The very firm neuroma suggests massive internal scar and neurotmesis. In general, the internal architecture of the neuroma-in-continuity is more disorganized than it appears on inspection and palpation.[13]

NEUROLYSIS

External neurolysis is unreliable. I[9] studied 59 nerves where an external release procedure was performed and found that only 36% had any clinical function outside the time range for spontaneous recovery for neurapraxia (1 to 4 months) or axonotmesis (3 to 8 months). External neurolysis is simple freeing of the nerve from the scarred epineurium and surrounding tissue without transposition of the nerve to a healthy vascular bed.

Injection of normal saline solution or a contrast medium into a damaged nerve near a neuroma-in-continuity has been used to demonstrate scar tissue.[11] This seems to be a rather gross procedure, since the fibrosis preventing axon regeneration is intrafascicular rather than perineurial. Kline and Nulsen[7] state that saline injection may eliminate recordable electric activity.

With the common fusiform neuroma Zachery and Roaf[15] advised experimental section cutting through the epineurial scar until intact axons are encountered. This has been a hazardous procedure in my experience, even with adequate magnification, because the continuity of the axons cannot be determined through a transverse incision.

Internal neurolysis is a useful procedure when an isolated area of intraneural scarring is found, as in compression syndromes, crush injuries, or injection accidents. A longitudinal incision is made in the normal nerve on the proximal side of the neuroma-in-continuity. The epineurium is carefully freed with small dissecting scissors. As the area of the neuroma is approached, the epineurium thickens and becomes lost in the entrapping scar and must be resected. The intraneural isolation of fascicular groups is initiated proximally and carefully traced into the neuroma. Microsurgical techniques must be used to free the fascicular groups from the strangulating scar tissue and to confirm the continuity or disruption of individual groups of fascicles (axons). It is difficult to determine exactly when intact fascicular bundles have been freed and to avoid unnecessary dissection with sacrifice of intact axons. If a portion of the perineurium is intact and free from gross scar and fascicular group continuity is maintained through the neuroma area, an internal neurolysis should be successful. There is no available anatomic method to evaluate the functional status of the nerve following internal neurolysis of a neuroma-in-continuity. Kline and Hackett[6] reported a series of 213 nerve lesions in which 80% were in continuity, yet clinical recovery did not occur in any patient where a neurolysis was performed but the nerve-action potential response was negative on stimulation.

ELECTRIC STIMULATION

Stimulation of a regenerating nerve proximal to a neuroma-in-continuity may produce distal muscular function even though the patient cannot voluntarily contract the same muscles. However, a positive electric test will antedate voluntary contraction by only a few weeks at most,[2] because some axons must reach the motor endplate before the muscle will respond to electric stimulation. Stimulation may travel retrograde and activate muscles with innervation proximal to the neuroma-in-continuity and give a misleading appearance of function. A positive response could not be obtained in a proximal (high) axonotmetic lesion, even though it is regenerating, until the axons reach the motor endplate. Therefore the test is of little value in a high median or ulnar nerve lesion if exploration and stimulation are undertaken at 3 months after injury.

Since axons may regenerate through a neuroma-in-continuity and into the distal stump without measurable muscular activity, the electric property of the nerve itself has been used as a diagnostic tool. Kline[4,5,7] has recorded the nerve-action potential across the neuroma-in-continuity. Necessary equipment includes bipolar stimulating and recording electrodes. The electrode tips are stainless steel or platinum alloy, no. 18 in caliber, and bent in an arc, like a shepherd's crook, to fit the nerve. The tips are soldered to shielded bipolar wire and passed through a Plexiglas rod. A stimulator and stimulus isolation unit is used, and recording is done by a differential amplifier and oscilloscope. Kline uses a Polaroid camera to record the trace (Figs. 43-1 to 43-4).

The nerve is exposed proximal to the neuroma-in-continuity, and both the stimulating and recording electrodes are placed proximally. If the stimulating and recording system is functional, a nerve-action potential can be recorded from the proximal stump. The recording electrode is then moved distal to the neuroma-in-continuity to determine if a nerve-action potential can be evoked through the injury. It is a good technique to elevate the nerve away from surrounding soft tissues by means of the electrodes. If a potential is recorded just distal to the neuroma-in-continuity, then the recording electrodes are moved further distally to determine how far the regenerating axons have extended.

Nerve action–potential responses recorded 6 or more months after injury that require very high amplification (10 μV per division) and conduct less than 20 m per second indicate poor regeneration and may require resection and suture despite the presence of a nerve-action potential.[3]

When there is a lateral neuroma-in-continuity or a partial clinical loss, the nerve can be split into fascicular (axonal) bundles for isolated recordings. Williams and Terzis[14] have described intraoperative single fascicular recordings. On the basis of conduction velocity, amplitude of response, and the shape of the action potential, an objective decision can be reached.

The tourniquet should be deflated at least 15 minutes before the recording is attempted. In addition, a paralyzing anesthetic should not be used.

The nerve-action potential is the best available technique for evaluation of the neuroma-in-continuity. There are some current problems: (1) difficulty in obtaining appropriate stimulating and recording electrodes, and

CHAPTER 43 THE NEUROMA-IN-CONTINUITY

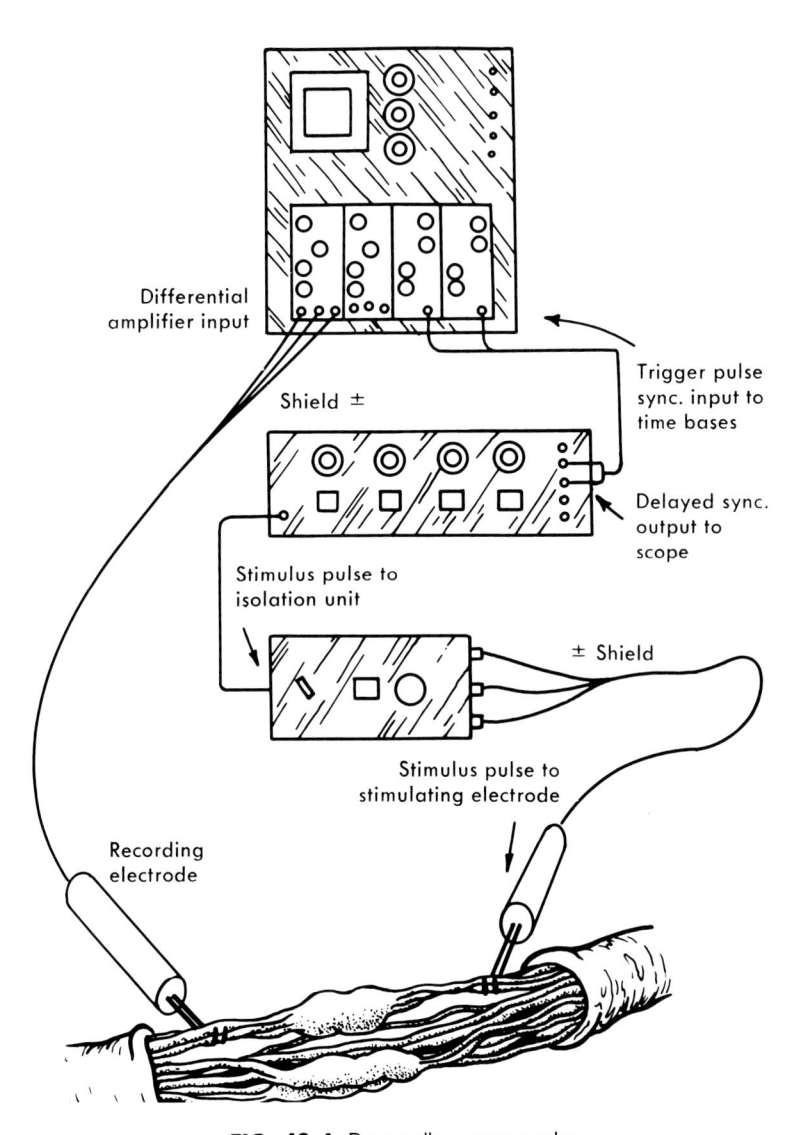

FIG. 43-1. Recording apparatus.

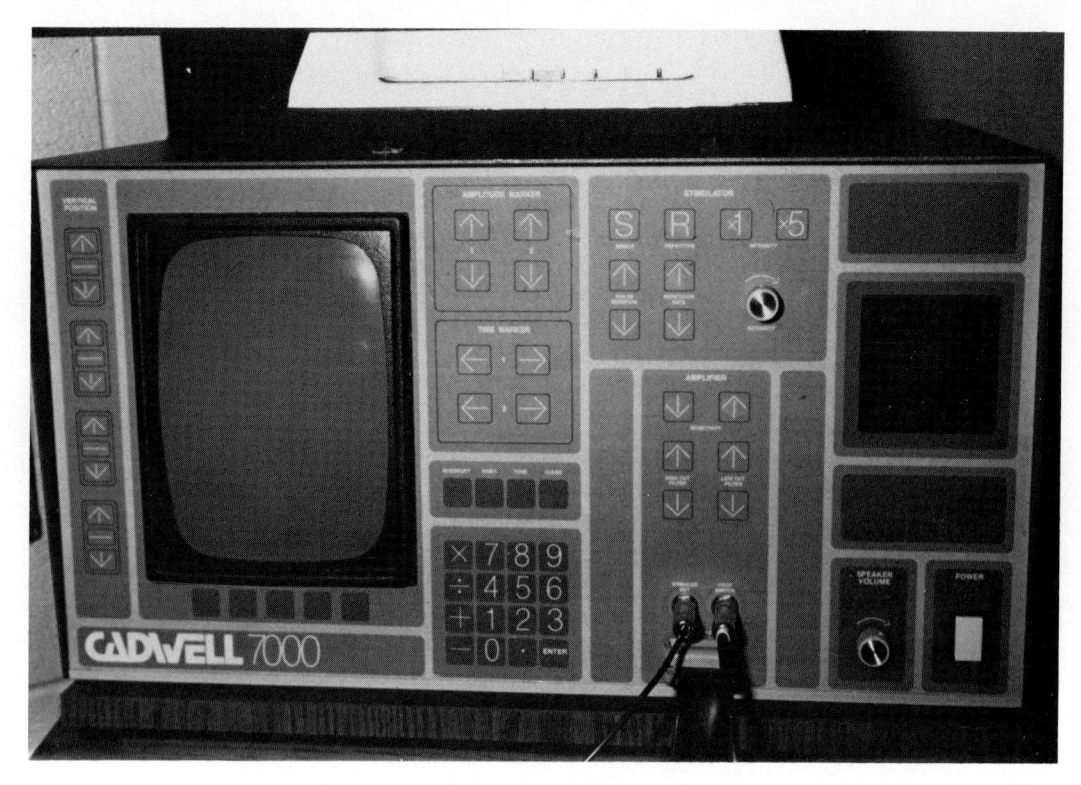

FIG. 43-2. Console for equipment, including computer for storing information.

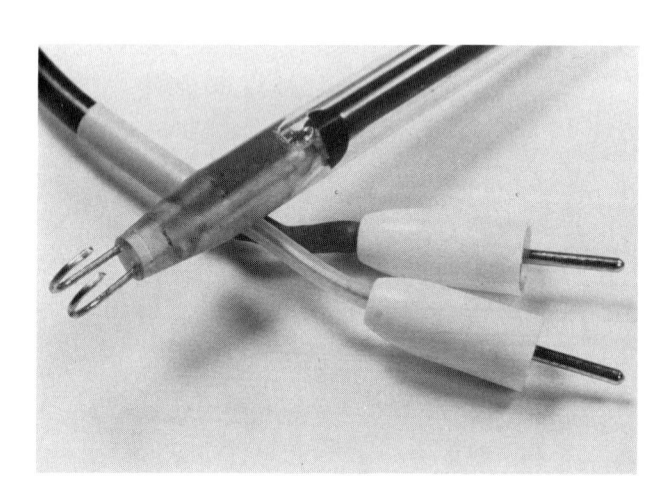

FIG. 43-3. Individually constructed stimulating and recording electrodes.

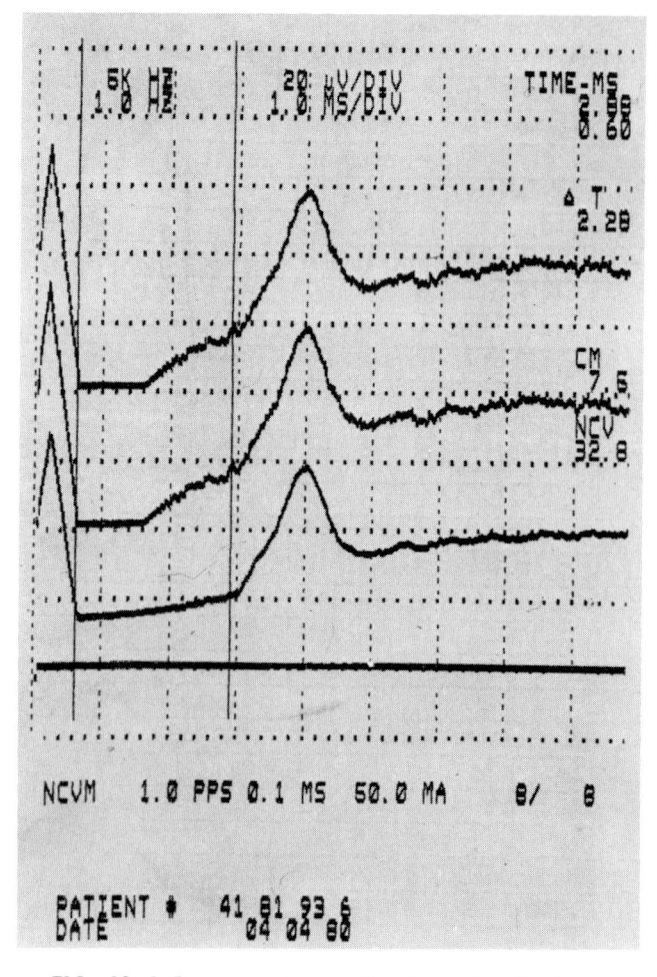

FIG. 43-4. Permanent recording for patient's chart.

(2) expensive equipment. In addition, the best measurements are made by comparison with computer-banked potential patterns, and (3) the intraoperative technique can be time consuming.

REFERENCES

1. Clark, K., Williams, P., Willis, W., and McGavran, W.: Injection injury of the sciatic nerve, Clin. Neurosurg. **17**:111, 1970.
2. Grundfest, H., Oester, Y. and Beebe, G.W.: Electrical evidence of regeneration. In Woodhall, B., and Beebe, G.W., editors: Peripheral nerve regeneration, Washington, D.C., 1957, Veterans Administration Medical Monograph, U.S. Government Printing Office.
3. Kline, D.G.: Evaluation of the neuroma in continuity. In Omer, G.E., and Spinner, M., editors: Management of peripheral nerve problems, Philadelphia, 1980, W.B. Saunders Co.
4. Kline, D.G., and DeJong, B.R.: Evoked potentials to evaluate peripheral nerve injuries, Surg. Gynecol. Obstet. **127**:1239, 1968.
5. Kline, D.G., and Hackett, E.R.: Value of electrophysiologic tests for peripheral nerve neuromas, J. Surg. Oncol. **2**:299, 1970.
6. Kline, D.G., and Hackett, E.R.: Reappraisal of timing for exploration of civilian peripheral nerve injuries, Surgery **78**:54, 1975.
7. Kline, D.G., and Nulsen, F.E.: The neuroma in continuity: its pre-operative and operative management, Surg. Clin. North Am. **52**:1189, 1972.
8. Omer, G.E., Jr.: Evaluation and reconstruction of the forearm and hand after acute traumatic peripheral nerve injuries, J. Bone Joint Surg. **50A**:1454, 1968.
9. Omer, G.E., Jr.: Injuries to nerves of the upper extremity, J. Bone Joint Surg. **56A**:1615, 1974.
10. Omer, G.E., and Spinner, M.: Peripheral nerve testing and suture techniques. In American Academy of Orthopaedic Surgeons: Instructional Course Lectures, vol. 24, St. Louis, 1975, The C.V. Mosby Co.
11. Razemon, J.P., Petyt, B., and Bonte, G.: Neurography in lesions of the peripheral nerves. In Michon, J., and Moberg, E., editors: Traumatic nerve lesions of the upper limb, London, 1975, Churchill Livingstone.
12. Seddon, H.J.: Three types of nerve injury, Brain **66**:237, 1943.
13. Seddon, H.J.: Surgical disorders of the peripheral nerves, ed. 2, Baltimore, 1975, Williams & Wilkins Co.
14. Williams, H.B., and Terzis, J.: Single fascicular recordings: an intraoperative diagnostic tool for the management of peripheral nerve lesions, Plast. Reconstr. Surg. **57**:562, 1976.
15. Zachery, R.B., and Roaf, R.: Lesions in continuity. In Seddon, H.J., editor: Peripheral nerve injuries, London, 1954, HMSO Medical Research Council Special Report, Series 282, p. 57.

Chapter 44 The ulnar nerve at the elbow

George E. Omer, Jr.

ANATOMY

The ulnar nerve extends from the medial cord of the brachial plexus and lies medial to the brachial artery in the upper half of the arm. In the midportion of the arm the ulnar nerve pierces the medial intermuscular septum and descends subfascially on the medial side of the triceps muscle. At the elbow the nerve is accompanied by the superior ulnar collateral artery as it passes along the posterior aspect of the condylar groove between the medial epicondyle of the humerus and the olecranon and enters the cubital tunnel.[7] In this area a condensation of connective tissue has been reported to extend from the nerve to the subcutaneous fascia and skin.[12]

The floor of the cubital tunnel is the medial collateral ligament (ulnar lateral ligament) of the elbow joint, and the sides are formed by the two heads of the flexor carpi ulnaris muscle. The roof is formed by an aponeurotic band (arcuate ligament) that extends from the medial epicondyle to the medial aspect of the olecranon.[1,22,23] The capacity of the cubital tunnel is greatest when the elbow is in extension, because the aponeurotic band is slack. Measurements in cadaveric material demonstrate that the distance between the humeral and ulnar attachments of the aponeurotic band lengthens 5 mm for each 45 degrees of flexion.[28] At 90 degrees of elbow flexion the proximal edge of the aponeurotic band is rigidly taut. In addition, the floor of the tunnel is elevated during flexion by the bulging medial collateral ligament.[14]

After the ulnar nerve passes through the cubital tunnel, it remains in the interval between the humeral and ulnar heads of the flexor carpi ulnaris muscle. The nerve gives motor branches to the flexor carpi ulnaris and the ulnar portion of the flexor digitorum profundus. There are several small articular branches and two sensory branches—the palmar cutaneous and dorsal cutaneous. Fibrous bands have been described that compress the ulnar nerve distal to the cubital tunnel.[12]

ETIOLOGY

Acute ulnar compression neuropathy can follow a single episode of blunt trauma such as a fracture or dislocation of the elbow. Tardy ulnar nerve palsy present in the adult as a consequence of injury about the elbow joint in childhood has been well documented.[9,11] However, tardy ulnar palsy in the child is an infrequent occurrence.[11] Congenital cubitus valgus deformity will result in chronic compression and dysfunction.[3] Childress[4] studied 2000 ulnar nerves in 1000 normal subjects and found an incidence of 16% of subluxation of the ulnar nerve from the humeral epicondylar groove during elbow flexion. Childress defined two types of subluxation of the ulnar nerve: (A) the nerve moves onto the tip of the epicondyle when the elbow is flexed to or beyond 90 degrees; and (B) the nerve passes completely across and anterior to the epicondyle when the elbow is completely flexed. Approximately 75% of nerves with recurring subluxation are type A.

Excursion of the ulnar nerve across the epicondyle makes it more accessible to trauma from direct pressure.[16] Compression of the nerve can occur from compression fascial bands or from lesions within the cubital tunnel, such as arthritic spurs, rheumatoid synovitis, muscle anomaly (anconeus epitrochlearis),[25] and ganglions and other soft-tissue tumors.

Reported cases have followed elective surgery or confinement to bed for a variety of reasons.[30] Certain positions, such as marked elbow flexion, put the ulnar nerve within the cubital tunnel at risk during operations. A prolonged period of extreme elbow flexion should be avoided in all chair-bound and bedridden patients. Whether the neuropathy is a result of mechanical deformation or ischemia or a combination of both is uncertain.

DIAGNOSIS

The first symptoms of ulnar neuropathy are paresthesias in the little and ring fingers, which often are related to repetitive exercises involving the elbow. Patients complain of numbness, tingling, or "falling asleep." Severe pain in the hand is not as common as in carpal tunnel syndrome, and night pain is unusual.[8] However, the patient often reports associated tenderness of the elbow with radiation of the pain into the shoulder and neck (Valleix's phenomena). The exact distribution of sensory loss should be determined, because involvement of the dorsal cutaneous branch of the ulnar nerve establishes the lesion proximal to the wrist.

Patients complain of weakness and loss of dexterity for handling objects. A more recognizable clinical feature is atrophy of the intrinsic muscles with clawing of the ring and little fingers. When weakness of the extrinsic flexor carpi ulnaris and the flexor digitorum profundus to the little finger is demonstrated, the ulnar neuropathy can be localized at the elbow. Sunderland's studies[27] of the intraneural topography of the ulnar nerve show that the sensory axons and the intrinsic motor axons lie in a more vulnerable superficial position within the ulnar nerve at the elbow, whereas the motor axons to the flexor carpi ulnaris and flexor digitorum profundus muscles are deep within the nerve and relatively protected from pressure.

Prolonged elbow flexion may cause an increase in numbness or tingling in the hand.[14] Tinel's sign may be positive secondary to percussion at the elbow. Electromyographic studies may show denervation potentials in the ulnar innervated muscles. A nerve conduction velocity study should show a slowing in the rate of conduction at the elbow in comparison with the normal contralateral elbow. Other causes of ulnar neuropathy, such as metabolic neuropathies, must be excluded. It is important to remember that a peripheral nerve can be trapped simultaneously at two levels.[21] Electromyographic studies are less effective than nerve conduction velocities in the determination of a double lesion.

Roentgenographic studies should be done to determine the degree of cubitus valgus or bony lesions compromising the cubital tunnel. Wadsworth[29] described a cubital tunnel view: a slightly oblique anteroposterior view with the elbow in full flexion and the arm externally rotated about 20 degrees.

McGowan[18] developed a clinical classification of ulnar neuropathy: Grade I has no detectable motor weakness in the hand, Grade II has weakness of the interossei and two ulnar lumbricals, and Grade III demonstrates paralysis of one or more of the ulnar intrinsic muscles. Wadsworth[29] classifies the cubital tunnel syndrome on an etiologic basis: (I) acute and subacute external compression, and (II) chronic internal compression caused by space-occupying lesions or lateral shift of the ulna (injury of the capitular epiphyses in childhood).

TREATMENT
Conservative treatment

Conservative treatment of ulnar neuropathy at the elbow includes padding the elbow, maintaining the elbow in extension, applying local heat and ultrasound, and locally administering steroids.[6] In hospitalized patients with instructions for strict bed rest, lamb's wool elbow pads are useful, and the overhead "monkey bar" should be used to move about the bed.[14] The arms should be extended during the recovery period as well as during an operation. One should avoid repetitive flexion and extension of the elbow, such as when a carpenter uses a hammer. Experience indicates that once an ulnar nerve becomes symptomatic, either spontaneously or secondary to identified trauma, the symptoms persist. The accepted treatment of an established ulnar neuropathy at the elbow has been surgical.

Surgical treatment

Nerve decompression. In every case the ulnar nerve must be released from tight fibrous bands. Proximal to the medial epicondyle, the medial intermuscular septum forms a taut ridge (Fig. 44-1). A section of this fascial septum must be excised to prevent kinking of the nerve.[16] The ulnar nerve should be freed for at least 8 cm proximal to the medial epicondyle to determine if the nerve is compressed in the arcade of Struthers.[25,26] Failure to release the nerve proximally may lead to an ulnar neuropathy at the level where the nerve passes from the anterior to the posterior plane of the arm.

During elbow flexion the ulnar nerve elongates approximately 4.7 mm.[1] Fixation of the nerve at the level of the medial epicondylar groove can result in traction neuritis.[1,12,31] Condensations of connective tissue and aponeurotic bands should be released. Bone fragments should be removed. The groove should be carefully inspected, because friction neuritis can develop with repeated movement of the ulnar nerve against osteophytes or bony spurs of the distal aspect of the humerus.

The aponeurotic roof of the cubital tunnel should be incised and the area inspected. An hourglass compres-

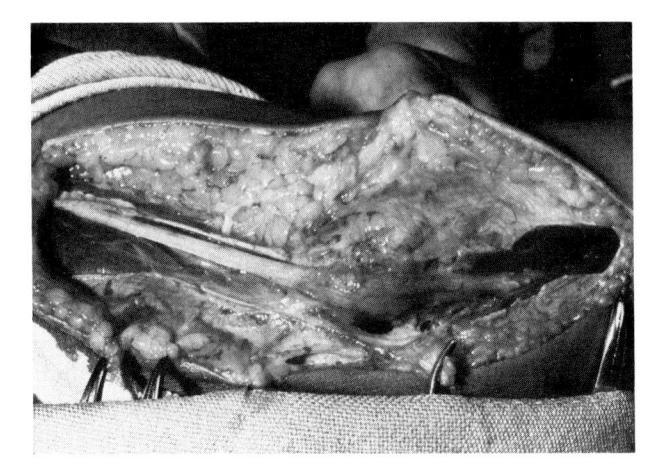

FIG. 44-1. Ulnar neuropathy secondary to subacute trauma: medial intermuscular septum is taut fibrotic ridge just anterior to ulnar nerve, proximal to medial epicondyle. Nerve is fixed in subcutaneous fibrous tissue in condylar groove.

sion of the ulnar nerve at the proximal edge of the aponeurotic roof suggests an intraneural neurolysis. Both saline neurolysis and epineurotomy have been advocated.[8,29] My experience has been that epineurotomy is useful in restoring a circulatory blush across a compressed segment, but there is no direct relation between intraneural neurolysis and improved sensory or motor function of the ulnar nerve. A more reliable indicator is the duration of clinical symptoms, and a McGowan[18] Grade-III lesion does not recover function following intraneural neurolysis.

The aponeurotic roof of the cubital tunnel may be excised or sewn deep to the nerve.[23] One should avoid injury to the superior ulnar collateral artery, which accompanies the ulnar artery in the condylar groove. I prefer to leave the ulnar nerve attached to the soft tissue in the depth of the groove and within the cubital tunnel, provided this vincula-like tissue is elastic and not fibrotic.

After the nerve is decompressed, the elbow should be extended and flexed to observe the position of the nerve. The nerve may be compressed against the side or posterior aspect of the medial epicondyle.

Epicondylectomy. If the ulnar nerve does not dislocate from the condylar groove but does compress against the medial epicondyle on functional flexion, an epicondylectomy is indicated.[8,13] The nerve is decompressed without releasing it from its bed, as previously described. A short incision, as described by Neblett and Ehni,[20] is not indicated. The medial epicondyle is exposed by incision of the origin of the flexor muscle mass and sharp detachment of the fibers from the epicondyle (Fig. 44-2). The dissection should not continue when the medial collateral ligament is exposed. The epicondyle is removed with an oscillating saw or a thin osteotome, while the nerve is protected with a broad-blade retractor. The medial collateral ligament and its bony attachments must remain intact. Bony spurs are removed with

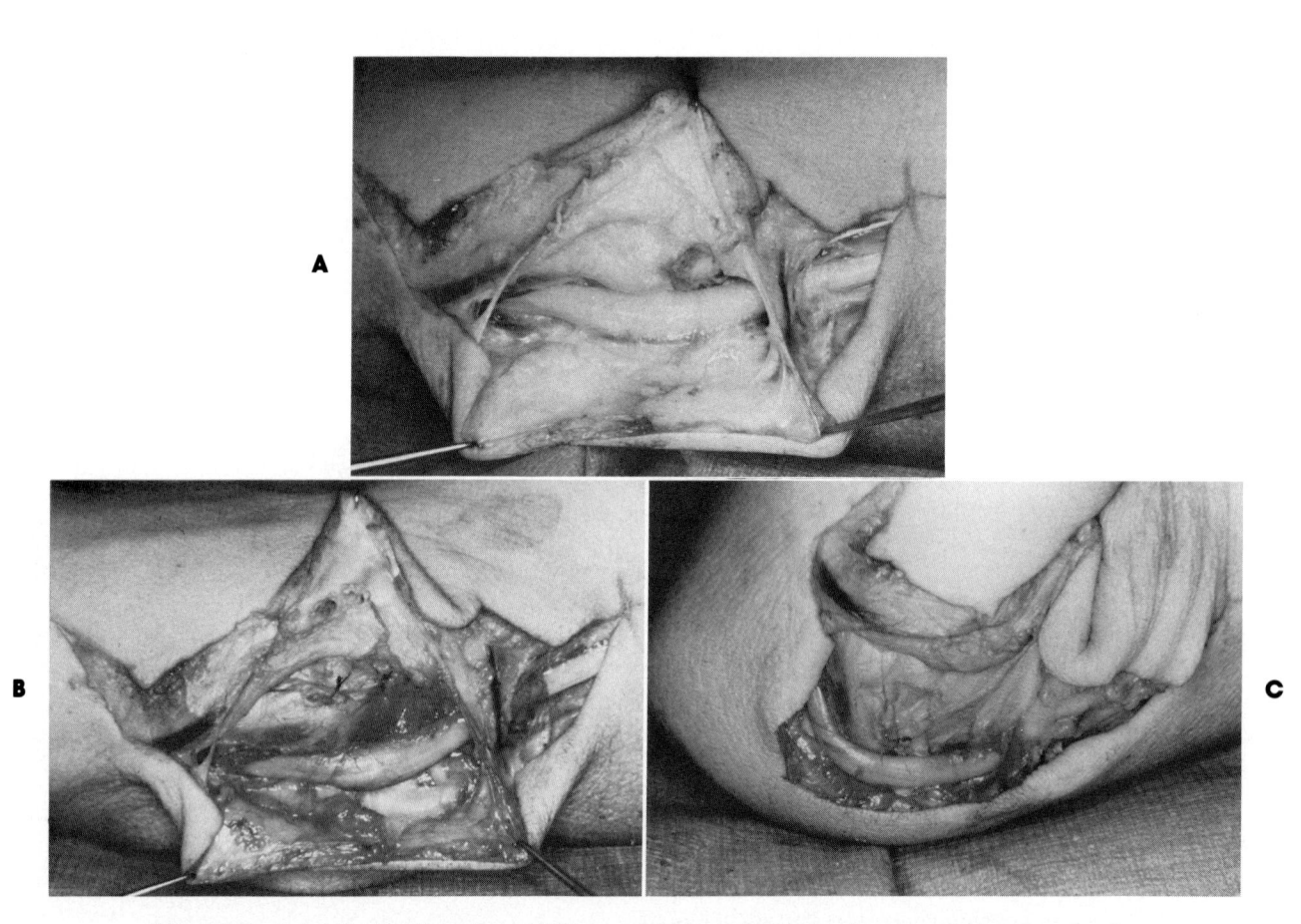

FIG. 44-2. A, Adult with diabetes and 18-month history of sensory changes and motor atrophy. Nerve has been decompressed from medial intermuscular septum and cubital tunnel. On flexion, there is compression against medial epicondyle. **B,** Epicondylectomy has been performed, and elbow is in full extension. **C,** Epicondylectomy has been performed, and elbow is in full flexion. There is minimal compression against medial epicondyle, and nerve is not subluxating from condylar groove.

a rongeur. The flexor muscle flap is reattached to the redundant periosteal flaps, leaving a smooth bed for the ulnar nerve. The nerve should not be compressed by the medial epicondyle during flexion. I deflate the tourniquet and ensure hemostasis before subcutaneous and skin closure. A bulky soft dressing is used for 24 to 48 hours and is replaced with a posterior plaster splint with the elbow in 90 degrees of flexion for 2 to 3 weeks. Active range of motion exercises are initiated with emphasis on regaining full extension of the elbow.

Anterior transposition. Curtis is reported[2,6] to have described in 1898 a technique for subcutaneous anterior transposition of the ulnar nerve, and the procedure was standardized by Platt[24] in 1928. Anterior transposition of the ulnar nerve is indicated for a Childress[4] type-B subluxation, where the nerve passes completely across and anterior to the epicondyle when the elbow is completely flexed. In addition, anterior transposition should be considered in cases with severe hypertrophic osteoarthritis[28] (Fig. 44-3).

Fasciodermal sling. Eaton, Crowe, and Parkes[6] decompress the ulnar nerve from the point where it penetrates the medial intermuscular septum to the distal portion of the cubital tunnel. The nerve is dissected from the condylar groove, mobilizing the accompanying veins, until the nerve is displaced anterior to the medial epicondyle. An epineurotomy is performed if there is constriction of the nerve. A flap of antebrachial fascia 1 cm wide and 1 cm long, based on the medial epicondyle, is then raised and reflected medially. The fascial flap passes posterior to the transposed ulnar nerve and is sutured to the subcutaneous tissue anterior to the medial epicondyle, preventing the ulnar nerve from returning to its original position. Once the fascial flap is completed, the skin is closed, and the limb is splinted with the elbow in 90 degrees of flexion for 2 weeks.

Subcutaneous slings have resulted in constriction or kinking of the ulnar nerve,[2,17] and the procedure is not indicated until there is symptomatic subluxation.

Submuscular transposition. Learmonth[15] decompresses the ulnar nerve from the point where it penetrates the medial intermuscular septum to the distal por-

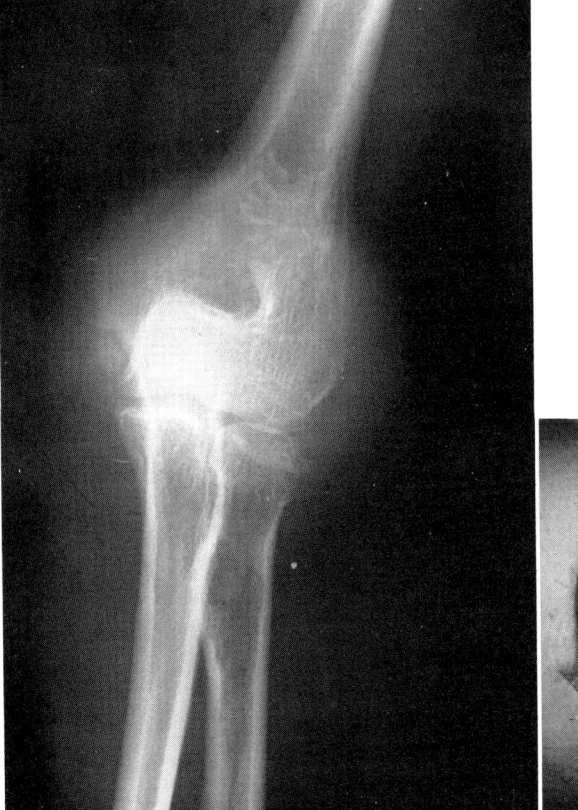

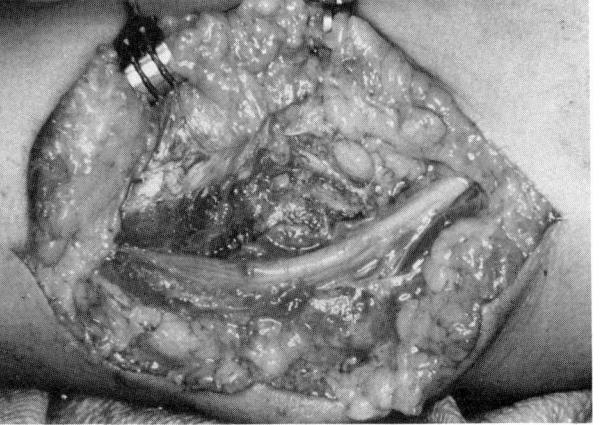

FIG. 44-3. A, Violin player who had acute dislocation of right elbow. Traumatic osteoarthritic spurs filled condylar groove. **B,** Nerve has been decompressed from medial intermuscular septum and cubital tunnel. Raw surface of humerus is shown following partial medial epicondylectomy.

tion of the cubital tunnel. The flexor-pronator muscle mass is detached from the medial epicondyle and turned distally to expose the median nerve. The ulnar nerve is transposed to lie alongside the median nerve on the brachialis muscle. The flexor-pronator muscle origin is reattached to the medial epicondyle. Broudy, Leffert, and Smith[2] immobilize the elbow in 90 degrees of flexion with the forearm fully pronated. The initial bulky dressing is replaced by a long-arm plaster dressing for 3 weeks. Del Pizzo, Jobe, and Norwood[5] note that that this procedure permits arthrotomy of the elbow and inspection of the medial collateral ligament. Levy and Apfelberg[16] modify the procedure by performing an osteotomy of the medial epicondyle, with the attached flexor muscles, and then reattaching the epicondyle with screw fixation.

Fibrous constriction of the ulnar nerve has been observed following submuscular transposition.[8]

RESULTS

Most reports of the results of surgical treatment have been optimistic.[16,18,28] Pain is usually relieved, and other sensory symptoms show consistent improvement. However, weakness tends to persist, and muscular atrophy is least likely to improve.[8,10,19] There is little prognostic difference between successful surgical procedures, but a guarded prognosis always should be given with secondary transposition.[2] The potential for full motor recovery after operation is greatly reduced in those patients in whom preoperative symptoms have been present for more than 1 year.

REFERENCES

1. Apfelberg, D.B., and Larson, S.J.: Dynamic anatomy of the ulnar nerve at the elbow, Plast. Reconstr. Surg. **51**:76, 1973.
2. Broudy, A.S., Leffert, R.D., and Smith, R.J.: Technical problems with ulnar nerve transposition at the elbow: findings and results of reoperation, J. Hand Surg. **3**:85, 1978.
3. Burman, M.S., and Sutro, C.J.: Recurrent luxation of the ulnar nerve by congenital posterior position of the medial epicondyle of the humerus, J. Bone Joint Surg. **21**:958, 1939.
4. Childress, H.M.: Recurrent ulnar-nerve dislocation at the elbow, Clin. Orthop. **108**:168, 1975.
5. Del Pizzo, W., Jobe, F.W., and Norwood, L.: Ulnar nerve entrapment syndrome in baseball players, Am. J. Sports Med. **5**:182, 1977.
6. Eaton, R.G., Crowe, J.F., and Parkes, J.C., III: Anterior transposition of the ulnar nerve using a non-compressing fasciodermal sling, J. Bone Joint Surg. **62A**:820, 1980.
7. Feindel, W., and Stratford, J.: Cubital tunnel compression in tardy ulnar palsy, Can. Med. Assoc. J. **78**:351, 1958.
8. Froimson, A.I., and Zahrawi, F.: Treatment of compression neuropathy of the ulnar nerve at the elbow by epicondylectomy and neurolysis, J. Hand Surg. **5**:391, 1980.
9. Gay, J.R., and Love, J.G.: Diagnosis and treatment of tardy paralysis of the ulnar nerve, J. Bone Joint Surg. **29A**:1087, 1947.
10. Harrison, M.J.G., and Nurick, S.: Results of anterior transposition of the ulnar nerve for ulnar neuritis, Br. Med. J. **1**:27, 1970.
11. Holmes, J.C., and Hall, J.E.: Tardy ulnar nerve palsy in children, Clin. Orthop. **135**:128, 1978.
12. Inglis, A.E., and Kinnett, G.: Ulnar neuropathy at the elbow. In Proceedings of American Society for Surgery of the Hand, J. Hand Surg. **3**:290, 1978.
13. King, T., and Morgan, F.: Treatment of traumatic ulnar neuritis, Aust. N.Z. J. Surg. **20**:33, 1950.
14. Lazaro, L., III: Ulnar nerve instability: ulnar nerve injury due to elbow flexion, South. Med. J. **70**:36, 1977.
15. Learmonth, J.R.: A technique for transplanting the ulnar nerve, Surg. Gynecol. Obstet. **75**:792, 1943.
16. Levy, D.M., and Apfelberg, D.B.: Results of anterior transposition for ulnar neuropathy at the elbow, Am. J. Surg. **123**:304, 1972.
17. Lluch, A.L.: Ulnar nerve entrapment after anterior transposition at elbow, N.Y. State J. Med. **75**:75, 1975.
18. McGowan, A.J.: The results of transposition of the ulnar nerve for traumatic ulnar neuritis, J. Bone Joint Surg. **32B**:293, 1950.
19. Macnicol, M.F.: The results of operation for ulnar neuritis, J. Bone Joint Surg. **61B**:159, 1979.
20. Neblett, C., and Ehni, G.: Medial epicondylectomy for ulnar palsy, J. Neurosurg. **32**:55, 1970.
21. Omer, G.E., Jr.: Pitfalls in the management of peripheral nerve injuries, Bull. N.Y. Acad. Med. **55**:829, 1979.
22. Osborne, G.V.: The surgical treatment of tardy ulnar neuritis. In Proceedings of the British Orthopaedic Association, J. Bone Joint Surg. **39B**:782, 1957.
23. Osborne, G.V.: Compression neuritis of the ulnar nerve at the elbow, Hand **2**:10, 1970.
24. Platt, H.: The operative treatment of traumatic neuritis at the elbow, Surg. Gynecol. Obstet. **47**:822, 1928.
25. Spinner, M.: Injuries to the major branches of peripheral nerves of the forearm, ed. 2, Philadelphia, 1978, W.B. Saunders Co.
26. Spinner, M.: Management of nerve compression lesions of the upper extremity. In Omer, G.E., Jr., and Spinner, M., editors: Management of peripheral nerve problems, Philadelphia, 1980, W.B. Saunders Co.
27. Sunderland, S.: The intraneural topography of the radial, median, and ulnar nerves, Brain **68**:243, 1945.
28. Vanderpool, D.W., Chambers, J., Lamb, D.W., and Whiston, T.B.: Peripheral compression lesions of the ulnar nerve, J. Bone Joint Surg. **50B**:792, 1968.
29. Wadsworth, T.G.: The external compression syndrome of the ulnar nerve at the cubital tunnel, Clin. Orthop. **124**:189, 1977.
30. Wadsworth, T.G., and Williams, J.R.: Cubital tunnel external compression syndrome, Br. Med. J. **1**:662, 1973.
31. Wilson, D.H., and Krout, R.: Surgery of ulnar neuropathy at the elbow: 16 cases treated by decompression without transposition, J. Neurosurg. **38**:780, 1973.

Chapter 45 Selection of type of peripheral nerve repair

James R. Urbaniak

The recent deluge of information on neurorrhaphy contributes to the confusion about which type of nerve repair should be selected. With the worldwide popularity of microsurgery in all surgical specialities, recent emphasis has been placed on using the operating microscope, perineurial or individual funicular repair, and interfascicular nerve grafting to achieve the best results. Does the application of these techniques in fact result in better nerve function after repair? Improved functional results are being obtained in peripheral nerve repair today because of refinements in instrumentation and suture material and needles, use of magnification and microsurgical techniques, and better understanding of nerve anatomy and physiology. It has not been proved that one particular type of nerve repair is the champion; the outcome of neurorrhaphy is more dependent on careful tissue handling, proper alignment, and accurate approximation of the nerve ends than on the particular selection of one type of repair.[11]

Despite these advancements and the inherent capacity of the severed peripheral nerve to regenerate, normal functional nerve recovery is not possible after repair, especially in the adult. The nerve surgeon should be cognizant that certain types of nerve repairs are more feasible than others in particular situations. The surgeon's familiarity with the different types of nerve repairs and the ability to apply them in suitable situations should produce more gratifying results in the management of nerve injuries.

PRACTICAL ANATOMY

The surgeon who participates in the repair of injured peripheral nerves must be knowledgeable about the complex anatomy of the peripheral nerve. The cell body of the peripheral nerve is located in the spinal cord (motor neuron) or the posterior root ganglion (sensory neuron). The neuron is an extremely long cell, with the nerve *axons* being extensions of the cytoplasm (axonplasm) of the cell.

The *Schwann sheath*, a series of alternated nucleated cells, envelopes a single axon or group of axons. *Nerve fibers* may be classified as *myelinated* and *unmyelinated* fibers. The myelin sheath is a distinct feature of large nerve fibers. Schwann cells enclose only one axon in these large fibers. In myelinated fibers the sheath consist of Schwann cells, myelin, and an outer connective tissue layer, the *endoneurium* (Fig. 45-1). The *nodes of Ranvier* are the segments of the axon devoid of myelin sheath. The nerve fiber (axon and sheath) is the smallest functional unit of the peripheral nerve.

From the practical standpoint of the surgeon, the *fasciculus* is the smallest surgical unit. The fasciculus is a group of nerve fibers (Fig. 45-2). The terms *funiculus*, *fasciculus*, and *fascicle* are synonymous. The *perineurium* is a fine but relatively strong connective tissue sheath that encases the fasciculus. Each fasciculus usually contains a mixture of motor, sensory, and sympathetic fibers, but one or two types of the fibers may be absent.

Sunderland[9] has emphasized that a great amount of cross-linking usually occurs in the groups of fascicles.

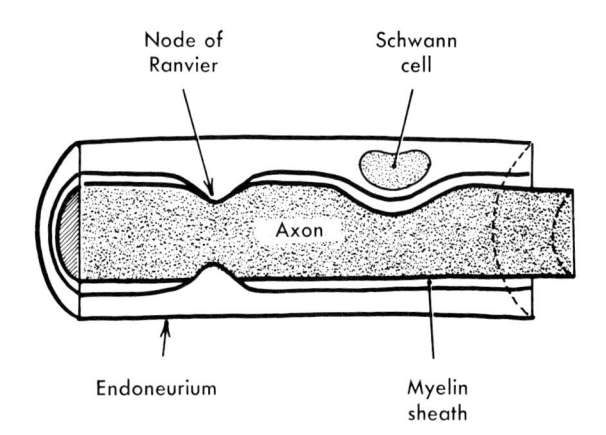

FIG. 45-1. Basic anatomy of myelinated nerve fiber. (From Urbaniak, J.R., and Warren, F.H.: Application of microsurgical techniques in the care of the injured peripheral nerve. In American Academy of Orthopaedic Surgeons: Symposium on Microsurgery, St. Louis, 1979, The C.V. Mosby Co.)

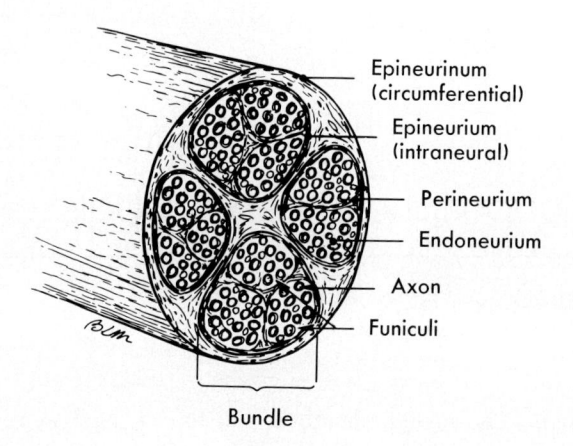

FIG. 45-2. Structures of peripheral nerve that are of practical importance to surgeon.

However, the amount of cross-linking appears to vary with particular peripheral nerves and at various levels in the extremity.[6] Groups of fasciculi are enclosed by a loose areolar sheath—the *epineurium* (intraneural epineurium). This epineurial tissue may make up 25% to 85% of the cross-sectional area of a peripheral nerve. The blood vessels and lymphatics are contained in this tissue. The strong, thick outer layer of a peripheral nerve is actually a condensed layer of epineurium (circumferential epineurium, or epineurial sheath).

Lucid understanding and correct usage of this terminology are necessary for an interchange of ideas, techniques, and results neurorrhaphy. In addition, an appreciation of the nerve structure and the ability to skillfully restore this anatomy of the severed nerve greatly aid in obtaining good results in surgical repair.

NERVE REGENERATION AFTER INJURY

The surgeon may take advantage of the activity of at least five areas of the nervous system to upgrade functional return following the repair of a peripheral nerve. Recovery of peripheral nerve function is influenced by the anatomic, physiologic, and biochemical properties in the following areas: (1) cell body, (2) axon, (3) suture line, (4) motor and sensory receptor sites, and (5) cortical representation.

Nerve regeneration is related to the capacity of the *cell* body to synthesize protein.[8] During successful regeneration a nerve can replace up to 100 times the organic material contained in the cell body.[3] The more proximal the injury, the more metabolic activity must occur in the cell body, since more of the axon has to be replaced. In proximal, crushing, or avulsing injuries more neuronal body injury or death can be expected. Also there is less likelihood of the regenerating axons reaching their appropriate motor and sensory target organs.

In the *axon* both the proximal and distal ends of the severed nerve swell within a few hours after injury. This swelling persists for about a week and then subsides. Proximal axonal budding begins about 4 days after severance in a sharply cut nerve in the distal portion of the extremity.[9] However, in a crushed or avulsed nerve in the proximal portion of the extremity, proximal axonal budding may be delayed until 14 to 21 days after injury.

In the axon sheath distal to the injury *wallerian degeneration* assisted by Schwann cell activity removes the debris from the tubules by 2 to 8 weeks.[9] After this period the empty sheaths begin to shrink, and by 2 years the cross-sectional area may be as little as 1% of the normal size if the nerve has not been repaired.[7,8]

Electronmicroscopic studies have demonstrated that a minimizing of scar tissue at the *suture line* and a maximal capturing of sprouting axons by the distal empty tubules will result in a more physiologically ideal repair process.[5] Although difficult to achieve at times, proper alignment of the corresponding proximal and distal fascicles by the surgeon is ideal.

A 4- to 20-day delay may occur before proximal axonal regeneration begins, and then the axonal growth proceeds at a rate of 1 to 3 mm per day, depending on the level of injury and the particular nerve injured.[9] A 30-day delay may occur at the suture line, and additional delays occur at the motor and sensory receptor organs.

Even if the axons manage to reach their proper end-organs, normal function may not occur. *Cortical representation*, or *reorientation*, appears to influence the functional result. Although in young persons axonal regeneration seems to occur more rapidly and effectively, the ability of the young for more potent cortical reorientation may account for the better functional results in this group.[9] Sensory reeducation may influence these central and peripheral receptor areas.

EQUIPMENT FOR NERVE REPAIR

Peripheral nerve surgeons universally agree that magnification is definitely beneficial in obtaining optimal results in neurorrhaphy. Surgical telescopic loupes of 3.5-power magnification are suitable for most epineurial repairs. An operating microscope capable of at least 10-power magnification is advisable for bundle, fascicular, or interfascicular nerve grafting.

Monofilament nylon or Prolene from 8-0 to 11-0 with 150 to 50 μ needles are needed. Basically, if greater than 8-0 suture is required, the nerve is being repaired under too much tension.

The basic instruments for the microtechnique include jeweler's forceps, tying forceps, spring-loaded needle holders and microscissors, and small sharp surgical blades (or razor).

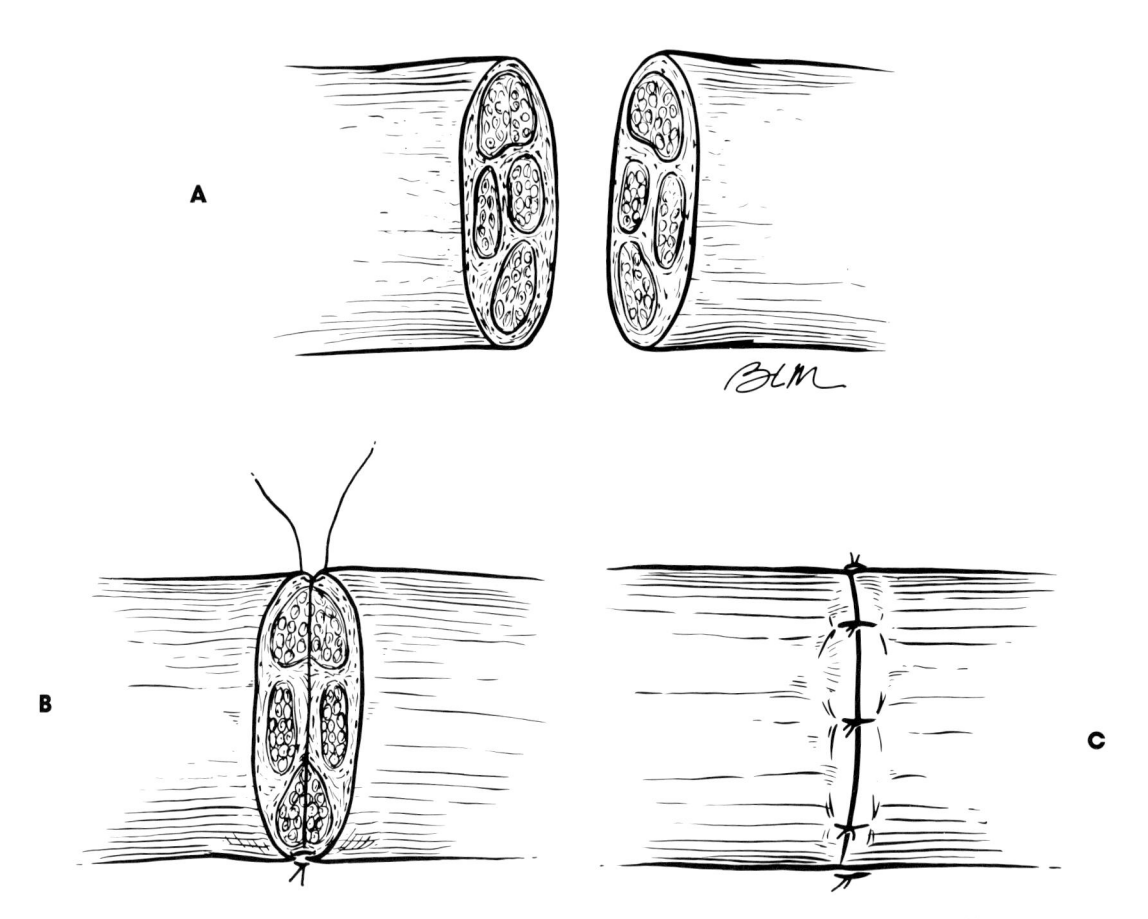

FIG. 45-3. Epineurial repair: under magnification, appropriate alignment of matching bundles is obtained. **A,** Nerve ends are sharply trimmed until healthy, pouting fascicles are visualized. **B,** Corresponding bundles are coapted with accurately placed epineurial stay sutures. **C,** Interrupted epineurial sutures complete repair.

SELECTION OF TYPE OF NEURORRHAPHY

The surgeon who participates in the reconstruction of peripheral nerves must be knowledgeable about several different types of nerve repair to achieve accurate geographic alignment of the bundles of fascicles of the severed nerve ends with a minimal scarring at the suture site. The terminology of the different types of nerve repair is confusing; the following classification is an attempt to simplify the types of repairs commonly used from an anatomic standpoint:
1. *Epineurial repair:* placement of sutures through the circumferential epineurium
2. *Group fascicular repair:* repair of matching groups (bundles) of fascicles
3. *Combined epineurial and group fascicular repair:* epineurial repair with a few sutures in matching bundles to achieve alignment
4. *Fascicular* (funicular or perineurial) *repair:* suturing of individual fascicles
5. *Interfascicular nerve grafting:* bridging of groups of fascicles with small nerve grafts

The goals of peripheral nerve repair are to restore the anatomy and reestablish neuron function. The particular type of repair selected is not as important as careful tissue handling, proper alignment, and accurate approximation of the nerve ends. Discussions of specific indications for each type of nerve repair follow.

Epineurial repair

Epineurial repair is the traditional type of neurorrhaphy, and most injured nerves are still considered suitable for repair by this method. The nerve ends are coapted by inserting the interrupted sutures through the circumferential epineurium (Fig. 45-3). There is no need to use suture material (nylon or polypropylene) stronger than 6-0, since no tension should be present at the suture line. Magnification (loupes of 2.5 to 3.5 times) is necessary for identifying healthy pouting fasciculi, proper bundle alignment, and accurate suture placement.

Most nerves can be repaired by this technique, and, to date, there is no convincing evidence that other types

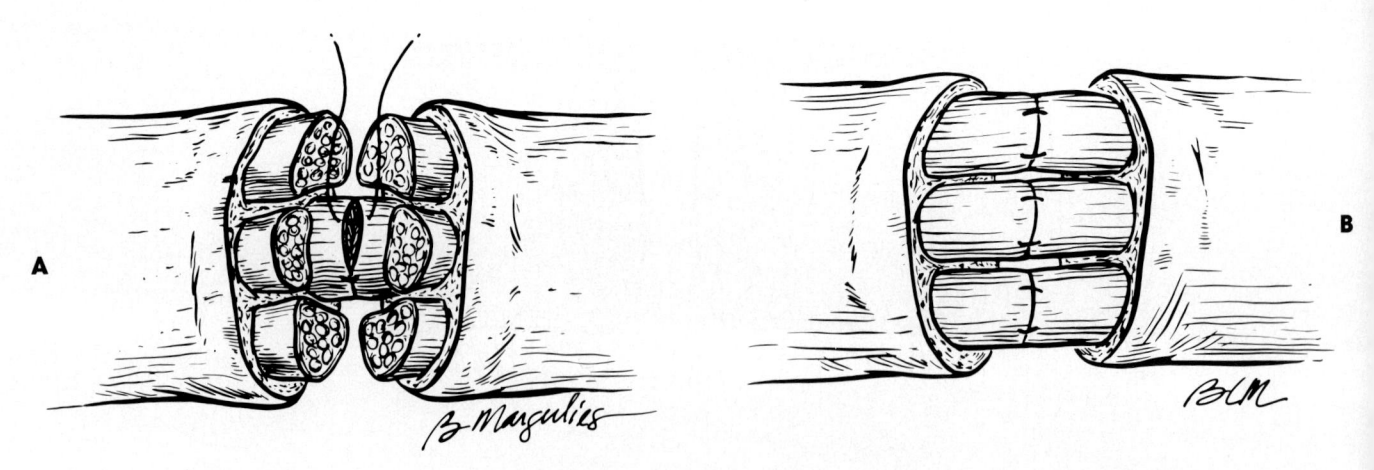

FIG. 45-4. Group fascicular repair: operating microscope is mandatory for this type of repair. **A,** Epineurial sheath is trimmed, and matching bundles are identified and paired. **B,** Usually two sutures are placed in intraneural epineurium of each bundle.

of nerve repairs are superior under usual conditions. Nerves that are basically pure motor or pure sensory nerves, e.g., radial nerve, median nerve at the wrist, and digital nerves, are ideal for epineurial repair. Nerves that have been sharply or evenly cut are usually best repaired by this method. Bone shortening is not passé, especially if two major nerves have been injured in the humeral region. In addition, significant gaps can be made up by judicial proximal mobilization of the nerve.[2] For example, the simple transposition of the nerve anterior to the humerus provides an additional 4 cm of proximal nerve. Epineurial repair should not be discarded, particularly when magnification and the microtechnique are used to obtain geographic bundle alignment. Perhaps there is less scarring stimulated by this method than by any other approach.

Group fascicular repair

For group fascicular repair the circumferential epineurium is excised at the severed ends, and matching groups of fascicles are identified and paired on the proximal and distal stumps (Fig. 45-4). Magnification of at least 6 power should be used for placement of 8-0 to 10-0 monofilament nylon or polypropylene suture through the *epineurium* around each bundle. Tourniquet ischemia is used for the initial dissection and proper orientation; then the tourniquet is released for the suturing so that fibrin clotting or adhesion will aid in the coaptation of the paired bundles. The suture line must be tension free.

This method of repair theoretically obtains ideal fascicular alignment, since the cross section of a nerve usually contains more collagen material (epineurium) than axons. It generally should be reserved for large nerves, uneven transections, avulsion injuries, and especially mixed (motor and sensory) nerves in which the surgeon can accurately identify and align the motor and sensory bundles.

Combined epineurial and group fascicular repair

The principle of combining epineurial and group fascicular repair is efficacious in the repair of mixed major nerves when a slight amount of tension is present. With the aid of magnification the severed nerve ends are sharply cut until pouting fascicles are apparent. Matching bundles are properly aligned and approximated with 9-0 or 10-0 nylon. To provide additional strength, 6-0 to 8-0 nylon (or polypropylene) sutures are placed in the circumferential epineurium.

This combined reattachment does ensure more accurate bundle alignment while providing immediate strength at the suture line. The technique is especially useful for the repair of severed mixed major nerves that have undergone some retraction, e.g., median or ulnar nerves about the elbow that are repaired several days after the injury. A disadvantage of this repair may be the creation of additional scar at the suture line, stimulated by the bundle sutures.

Fascicular repair

The fascicles are the smallest nerve units that can be isolated and connected by the surgeon. This repair is accomplished by placing 10-0 or 11-0 nylon sutures on a 50 μ needle through the *perineurium* using at least 10-power magnification (Fig. 45-5). The individual fascicles are exposed by excising the circumferential and intraneural epineurium. The fascicles should be stripped to a length about equal to the diameter of the nerve.[10] Visualization and handling of the fascicles are aided by using a

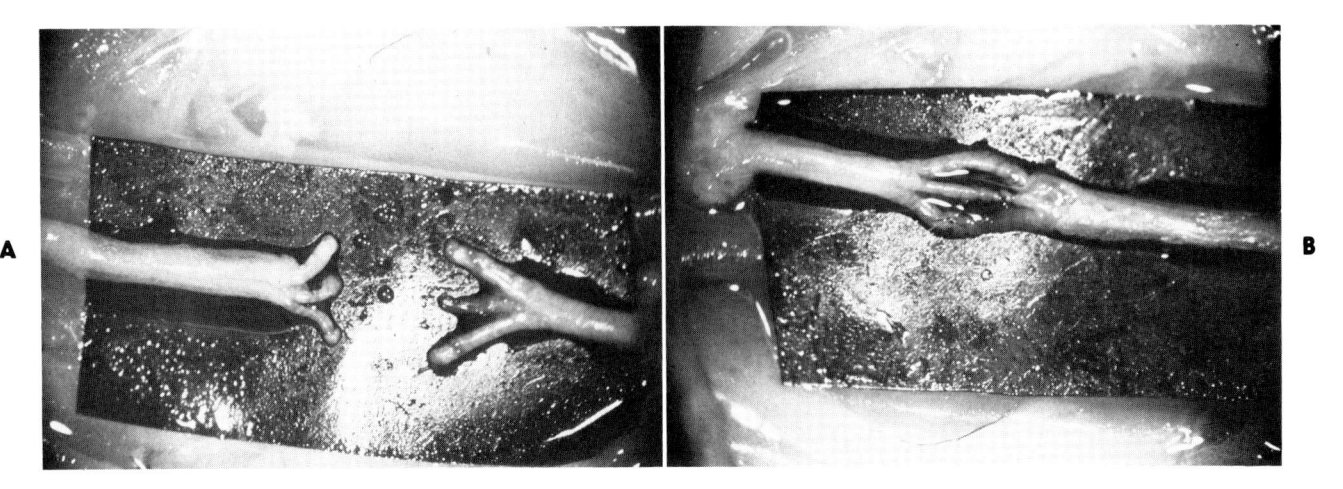

FIG. 45-5. Fascicular repair. **A,** Three fascicles are identified on each end of severed digital nerve. **B,** Fascicles are each connected using microsurgical techniques with two sutures of 10-0 nylon without tension at suture line. (From Urbaniak, J.R., and Warren, F.H.: Application of microsurgical techniques in the care of the injured peripheral nerve. In American Academy of Orthopaedic Surgeons: Symposium on Microsurgery, St. Louis, 1979, The C.V. Mosby Co.)

light blue or green rubber background (balloon) and frequent flushing with saline. The large fascicles are paired first, and then the remaining corresponding smaller fascicles are more easily matched.

No undue tension should exist at the suture line. Usually two sutures are necessary for each fascicular repair, since one suture will allow twisting and poor alignment. Fibrin clotting from the released tourniquet aids the approximation. This method is useful when repairing some injured fascicles of a neuroma-in-continuity, partially severed nerves (particularly digital nerves), and a "blowout" nerve injury such as a gunshot wound. This technique is tedious and time consuming, and, to date, there is no convincing evidence that it produces better results than a skillfully performed conventional epineurial repair in most severed nerves.[9]

Interfascicular nerve grafting

The primary indication for interpositional nerve grafting is to overcome undue tension at the suture line when a large gap is present. Nerve gaps of 3 to 7 cm in the arm and forearm can frequently be overcome by well-planned mobilization and slight joint flexion. An alternative to extensive nerve mobilization and transposition is interfascicular nerve grafting, as popularized by Millesi[7] and Mellesi, Meissel, and Berger.[8] This method does allow tension-free repair; however, the regenerating axons must cross two suture sites. Proponents of this technique point out that excessive mobilization of the nerve diminishes the nerve's blood supply, but it must be realized that the segments of the grafted nerve are totally avascular. Multiple interpositional grafts of small caliber are used to allow early revascularization of the grafts.

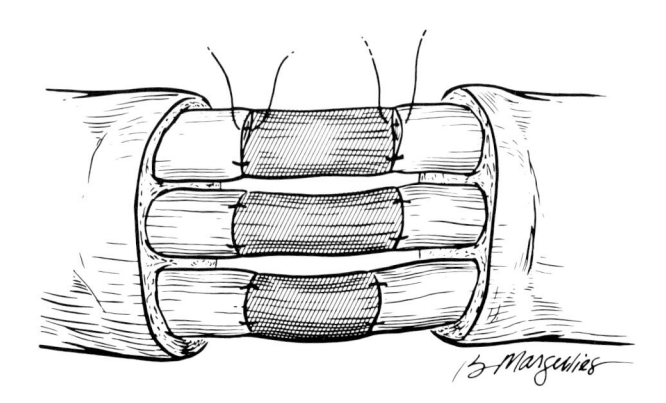

FIG. 45-6. Interfascicular nerve grafting: three strands of sural nerve *(dark segments)* are used as grafts to matching bundles. Epineurial sheath has been trimmed, and two sutures of 10-0 nylon are used at suture lines of each bundle.

The favored donor site is the sural nerve, since the diameter is ideal and the loss negligible, and usually sufficient length (up to 45 cm) may be obtained without difficulty. The median antebrachial cutaneous nerve at the elbow is a good donor for the digital nerves. It can be obtained from the ipsilateral arm with the patient under local anesthesia; it is the proper caliber, and the loss of this nerve has not been a problem for the patients.

With use of the microscope 1 cm of epineurium should be dissected free from the bundles, and matching bundles are identified on the proximal and distal stumps (Fig. 45-6). The bundles are bridged by the strands of grafts and usually require two sutures of 10-0 nylon for each connection. The suture line should be free from

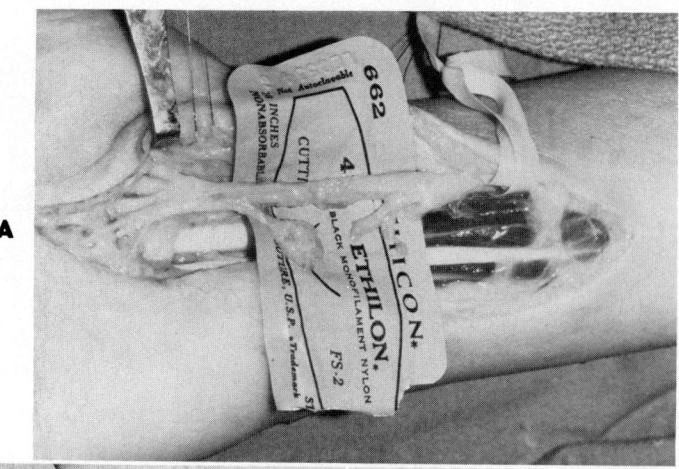

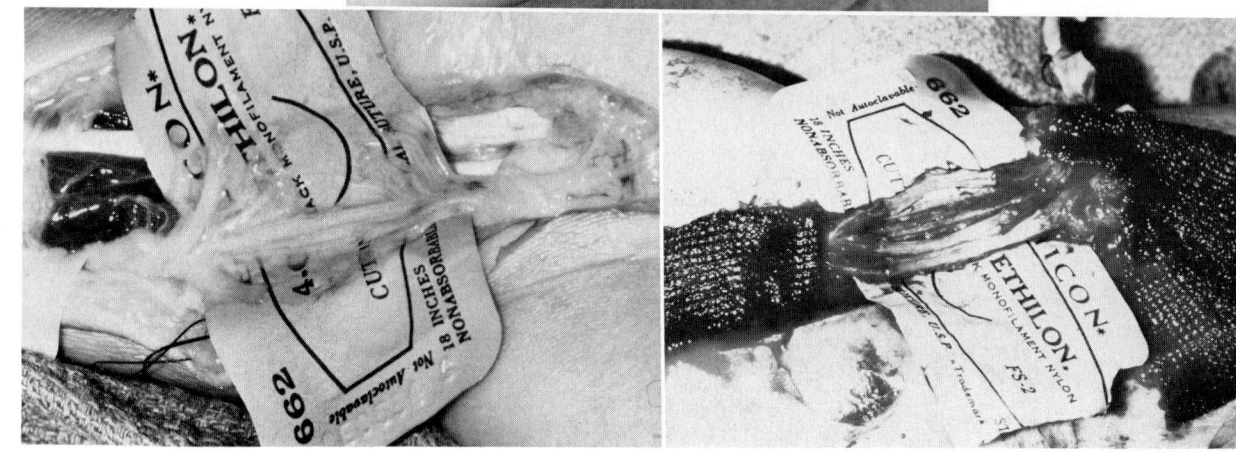

FIG. 45-7. A, Gunshot wound has caused partial severance of median nerve at wrist of 23-year-old woman. **B,** Three weeks after injury, with operating microscope, fascicles are easily separated into transected and intact fascicles. **C,** Injured fascicles are repaired by sural interfascicular nerve grafts. Intact fascicles are dark ones in center. (From Urbaniak, J.R., and Warren, F.H.: Application of microsurgical techniques in the care of the injured peripheral nerve. In American Academy of Orthopaedic Surgeons: Symposium on Microsurgery, St. Louis, 1979, The C.V. Mosby Co.)

tension, and usually three or four segments of such nerve graft are needed for bridging the median or ulnar nerves.

The results of nerve grafting are generally not as good as those of direct end-to-end repairs, but nerve grafting is usually reserved for the avulsed, crushed, or "blowout" injuries (Fig. 45-7). Properly executed nerve grafts do result in partial nerve recovery; protective sensibility and weak motor function can be achieved in nerve grafts as long as 10 to 15 cm.

Primary or secondary neurorrhaphy

The advantages of primary repair are as follows:
1. Only one surgical procedure is necessary.
2. Proper bundle alignment is easier, particularly with magnification.
3. The dissection is quicker.
4. No retraction of the nerve ends occurs.
5. Nerve regeneration into the distal tubules occurs earlier.
6. Reexploration into an area of previously repaired blood vessels may be hazardous.
7. In partial nerve lacerations, orientation is particularly easier.
8. Electric stimulation as an aid to motor and sensory fascicular alignment may be used in the first 48 to 72 hours after injury. Direct electric stimulation on the motor fibers of the distal stump will elicit motor activity, and the patient will localize sensory bundles on stimulation of the proximal stump.

Some advantages of secondary repair are as follows:
1. The general condition of the patient may be improved.
2. The surgeon may be better rested and prepared.

3. The chance of infection is less.
4. Normal fasciculi are easier to identify in crushed or avulsed injuries.
5. The cell body may be more "primed" for regeneration of the axon if the delay is 5 to 21 days.[1]

CLOSING COMMENTS

Advancements in microneurosurgical techniques and equipment have made several types of nerve repair available to the surgeon. The choice of the optimal repair is still difficult, and, to paraphrase some recent conclusions of Robert Harris,[4] epineurial repair is better than perineurial repair except when perineurial repair is better than epineurial repair; direct repair is better than a nerve graft, except when a nerve graft is more suitable. The surgeon must assess the type of nerve injury and apply the most suitable timing and type of repair.

REFERENCES

1. Ducker, T.B.: Pathophysiology of peripheral nerve repair. In Omer, G.E., and Spinner, M., editors: Management of peripheral nerve problems, Philadelphia, 1980, W.B. Saunders Co.
2. Goldner, J.L.: Concepts of peripheral nerve repair with emphasis on management of small and large nerve gaps. In American Academy of Orthopaedic Surgeons: Symposium on Microsurgery, St. Louis, 1979, The C.V. Mosby Co.
3. Hakstian, R.W.: Funicular orientation by direct stimulation, J. Bone Joint Surg. **50A**:1178, 1968.
4. Harris, R.W.: American Academy of Orthopaedic Surgeons Instructional Course on Microsurgery, Las Vegas, Feb. 1977.
5. Hudson, A.R., Kline, D., Bratton, B., and Hunter, P.: Axonal growth at the suture line in nerve repair and regeneration: its clinical and experimental basis. In Jewett, D.L., and McCarroll, H.R., editors: Nerve repair and regeneration, St. Louis, 1980, The C.V. Mosby Co.
6. Jabaley, M.E., Wallace, W.H., and Heckler, F.R.: Internal topography of peripheral nerves: a current view, J. Hand Surg. **5**:1, 1980.
7. Millesi, H.: Interfascicular grafts for repair of peripheral nerves of the upper extremity, Orthop. Clin. North Am. **8**:387, 1977.
8. Millesi, H., Meissel, G., and Berger, A.: The interfascicular nerve grafting of the median and ulnar nerves, J. Bone Joint Surg. **54A**:727, 1972.
9. Sunderland, S.: Nerve and nerve injuries, Baltimore, 1979, Williams & Wilkins Co.
10. Tupper, J.W.: Fascicular nerve repair. In American Academy of Orthopaedic Surgeons: Symposium on Microsurgery, St. Louis, 1979, The C.V. Mosby Co.
11. Urbaniak, J.R., and Warren, F.H.: Application of microsurgical techniques in the care of the injured peripheral nerve. In American Academy of Orthopaedic Surgeons: Symposium on Microsurgery, St. Louis, 1979, The C.V. Mosby Co.

SECTION THIRTEEN   DUPUYTREN'S CONTRACTURE

Chapter 46 Persistent contracture of the little finger in Dupuytren's disease

Robert M. McFarlane

The topic of Dupuytren's disease is appropriate for inclusion in a volume on problems in hand surgery. In Dupuytren's disease it is more difficult to correct a contracture of the little finger than of one of the other fingers. It may be so difficult that the surgeon will accept incomplete correction of the contracture at the time of operation. Furthermore recurrence of contracture is most common in the little finger.

The little finger is different from the other fingers in Dupuytren's disease in at least two ways. First, it has a greater variety of joint contractures. Second, the cords that cause joint contracture are more frequently diseased in combination rather than alone.[3] Therefore these joint contractures and the patterns of diseased fascia that produce them need to be analyzed to appreciate the problem of persistent contracture.

TYPES OF JOINT CONTRACTURE IN THE LITTLE FINGER
Contracture at the metacarpophalangeal (MCP) joint alone

Contracture of just the MCP joint is caused by a pretendinous cord and is always fully correctable in the little as well as the other fingers. It is not a cause of persistent contracture.

Contracture at the proximal interphalangeal (PIP) joint alone

The little finger is unique in developing PIP joint contracture as a result of disease within the finger, with no connection between this tissue and disease in the palm (Fig. 46-1). The disease begins in a nodule in the proximal and/or middle segments, and the nodule becomes

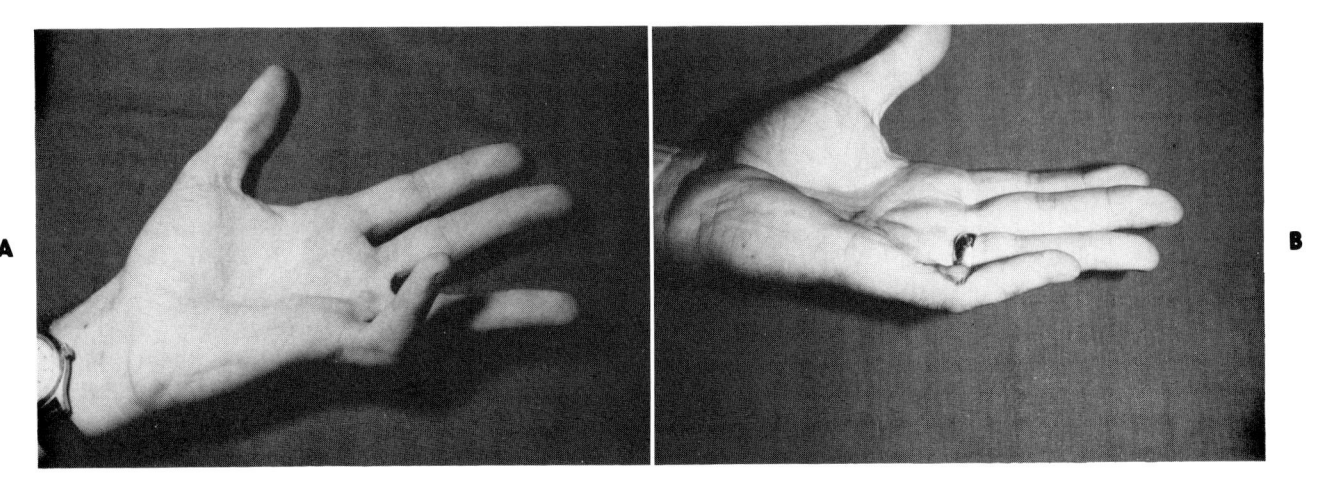

FIG. 46-1. A, Contracture of 55 degrees at PIP joint in 28-year-old man. There is no disease elsewhere. **B,** Fourteen years later there is still 20 degrees of contracture but no evidence of recurrence or extension of disease.

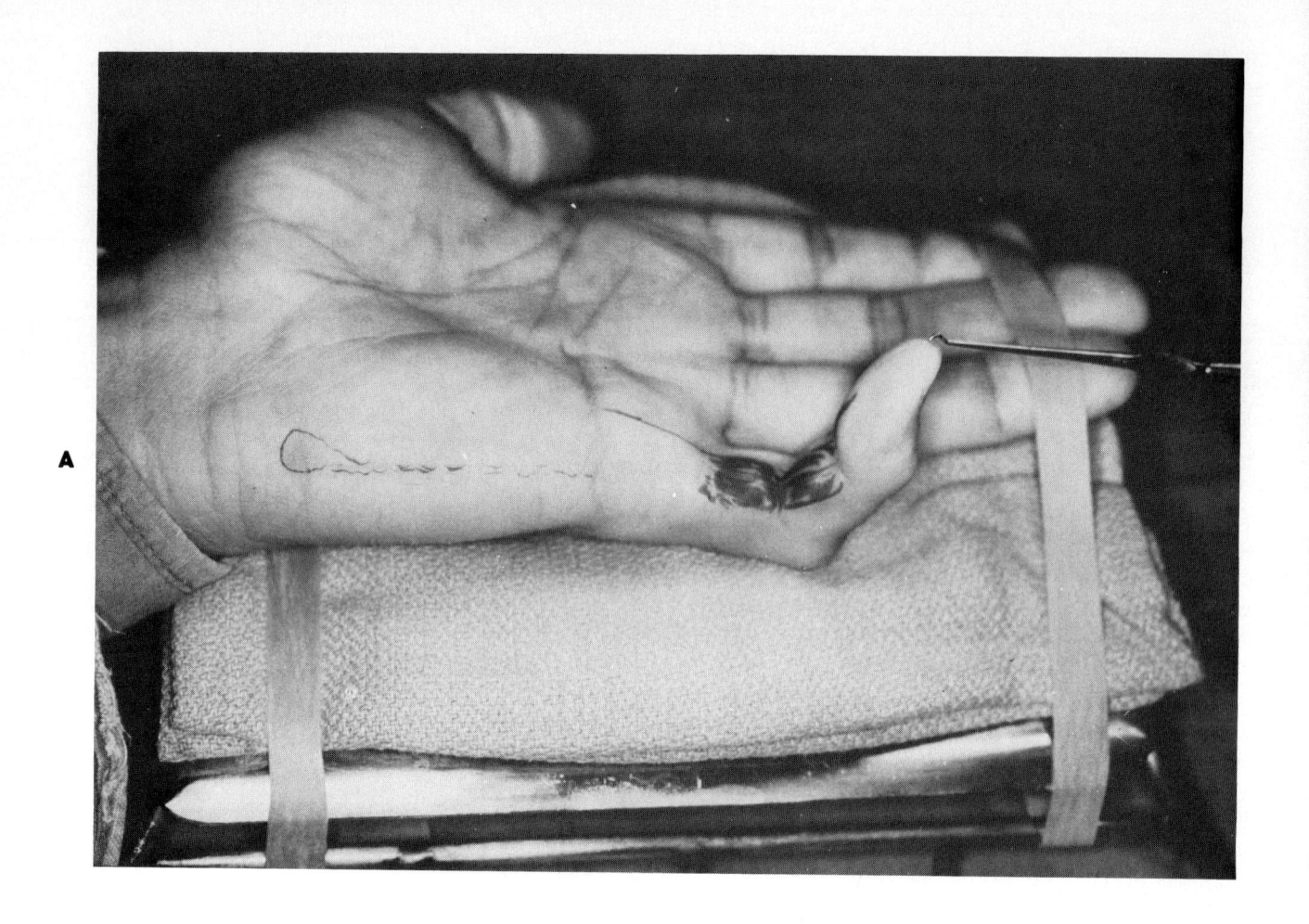

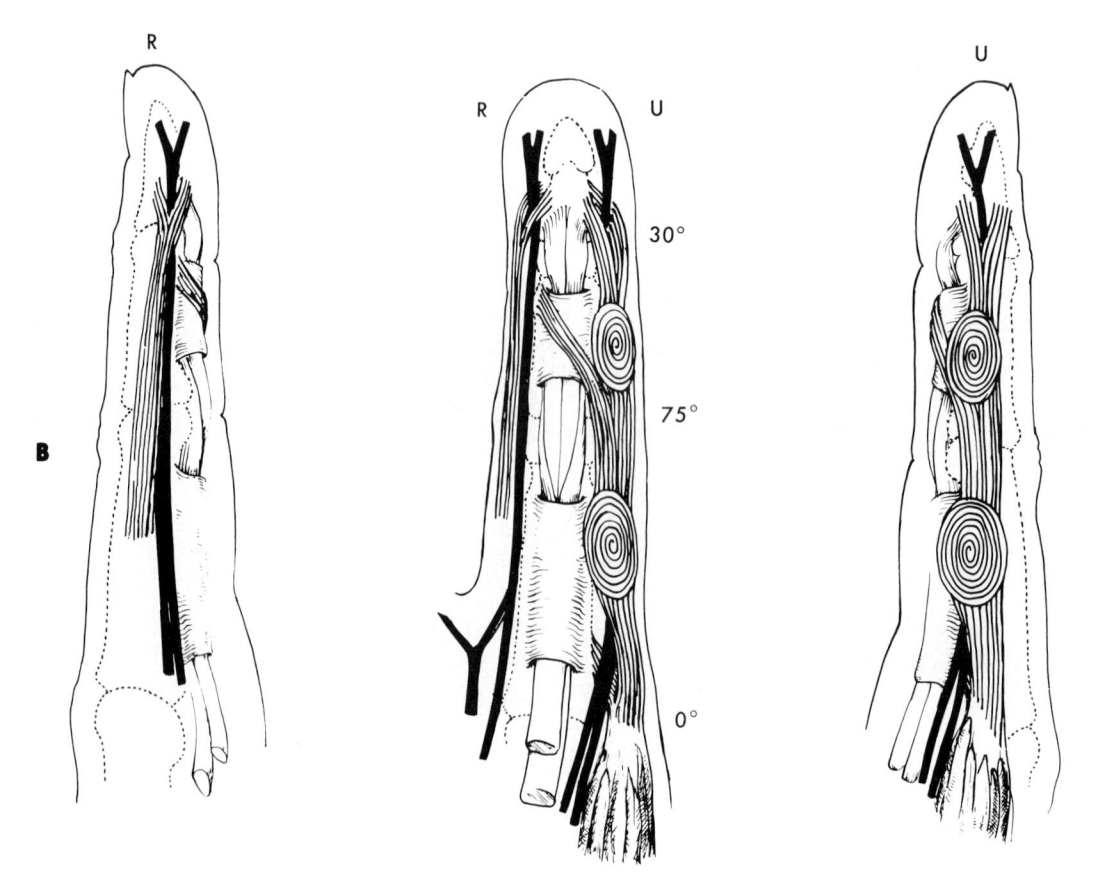

FIG. 46-2. For legend see opposite page.

CHAPTER 46 PERSISTENT CONTRACTURE OF THE LITTLE FINGER IN DUPUYTREN'S DISEASE

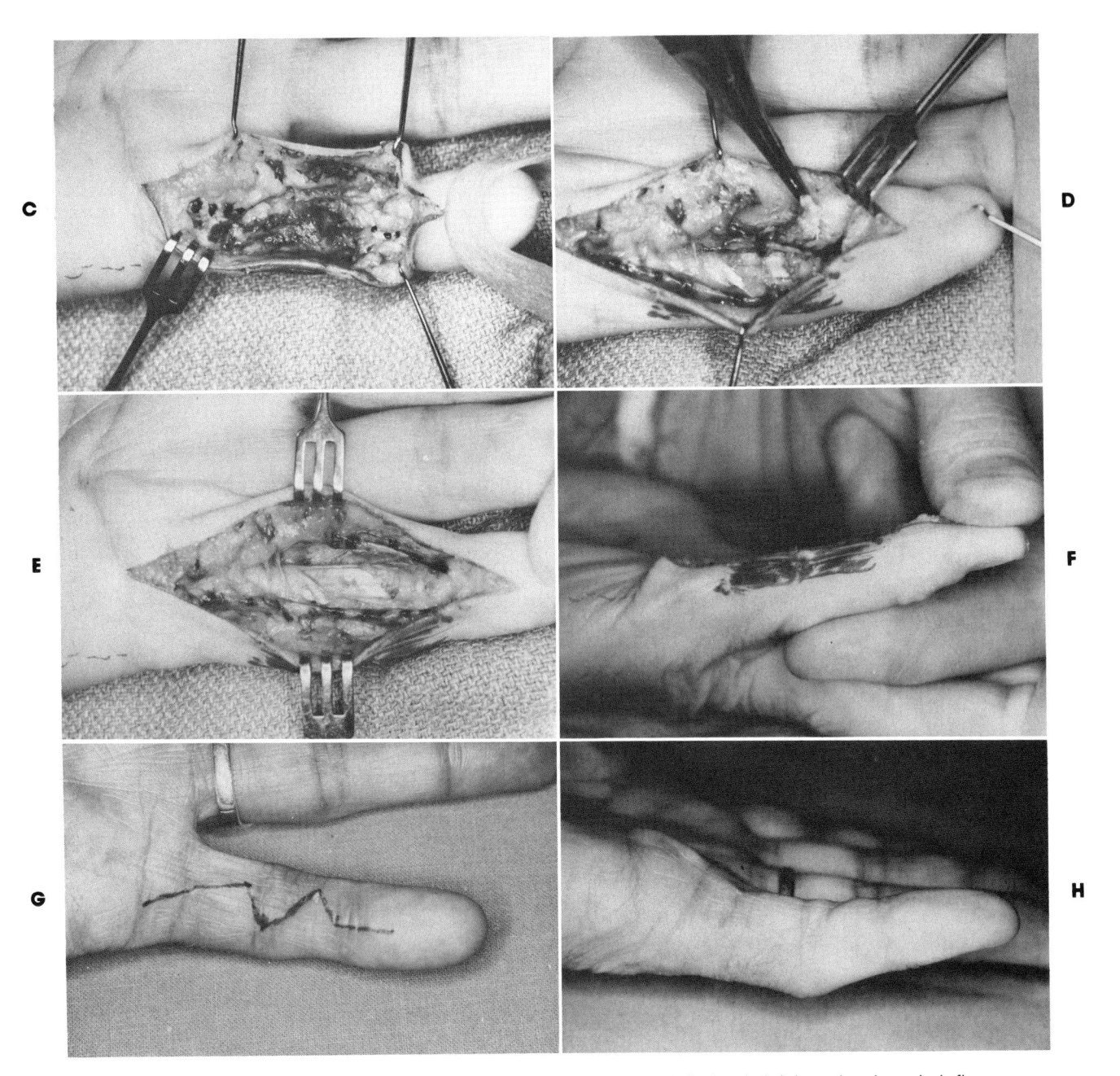

FIG. 46-2. This 69-year-old man had disease in both hands but only joint contractures in left little finger. **A,** There was 75 degrees of contracture at PIP joint and 30 degrees at distal interphalangeal (DIP) joint. **B,** Extent of disease on both sides of little finger and location of palpable nodules. There was no continuity of diseased tissue into palm. Disease on ulnar side *(U)* was essentially of lateral cord that began in tendon of abductor digiti minimi muscle and ended on distal phalanx. Fascia was attached to skin throughout its course but also attached to tendon sheath. It covered neurovascular bundle but did not displace it. Retrovascular cord was also present but was more apparent on radial side *(R)* of finger. **C,** Finger has been opened through midline incision. Neurovascular bundles are dotted and diseased fascia marked with ink. **D,** Disease on ulnar side has been removed. DIP joint is still flexed, but disease is being removed on radial side. **E,** Dissection has been completed, and tendon sheath has been incised over PIP joint. **F,** Both interphalangeal joints are easily straightened. **G,** Resulting scar, which includes a single Z-plasty. **H,** One year later he has 20 degrees of contracture at PIP joint.

SECTION 13 DUPUYTREN'S CONTRACTURE

FIG. 46-3. Example of isolated disease in little finger even though there is disease elsewhere in hand. This 68-year-old man had both hands operated on. **A,** Extent of disease in left hand: in little finger only PIP joint was contracted. **B,** Pattern of disease in little finger found at operation: it was spiral cord that originated in tendon of abductor digiti minimi muscle and attached to base of middle phalanx. Neurovascular bundle was displaced slightly toward midline. **C,** Finger has been opened by midline incision from palm *(left)* to beyond distal crease *(right)*. In this patient, skin flaps contain generous amount of fibrofatty tissue because diseased fascia (spiral cord) did not attach to skin. Ulnar digital nerve is marked by dots, and spiral cord is marked by ink just below nerve. Some fibers of abductor digiti minimi muscle are seen proximal to spiral cord. Fibrofatty tissue between neurovascular bundles, which is not diseased in this patient, is held by forceps. Termination of pretendinous cord is noted just proximal to tip of forceps. **D,** With tissue removed from between neurovascular bundles, spiral cord is seen more clearly. There is no disease on radial side of finger. **E** and **F,** Six months after operation, patient has full flexion and extension of fingers.

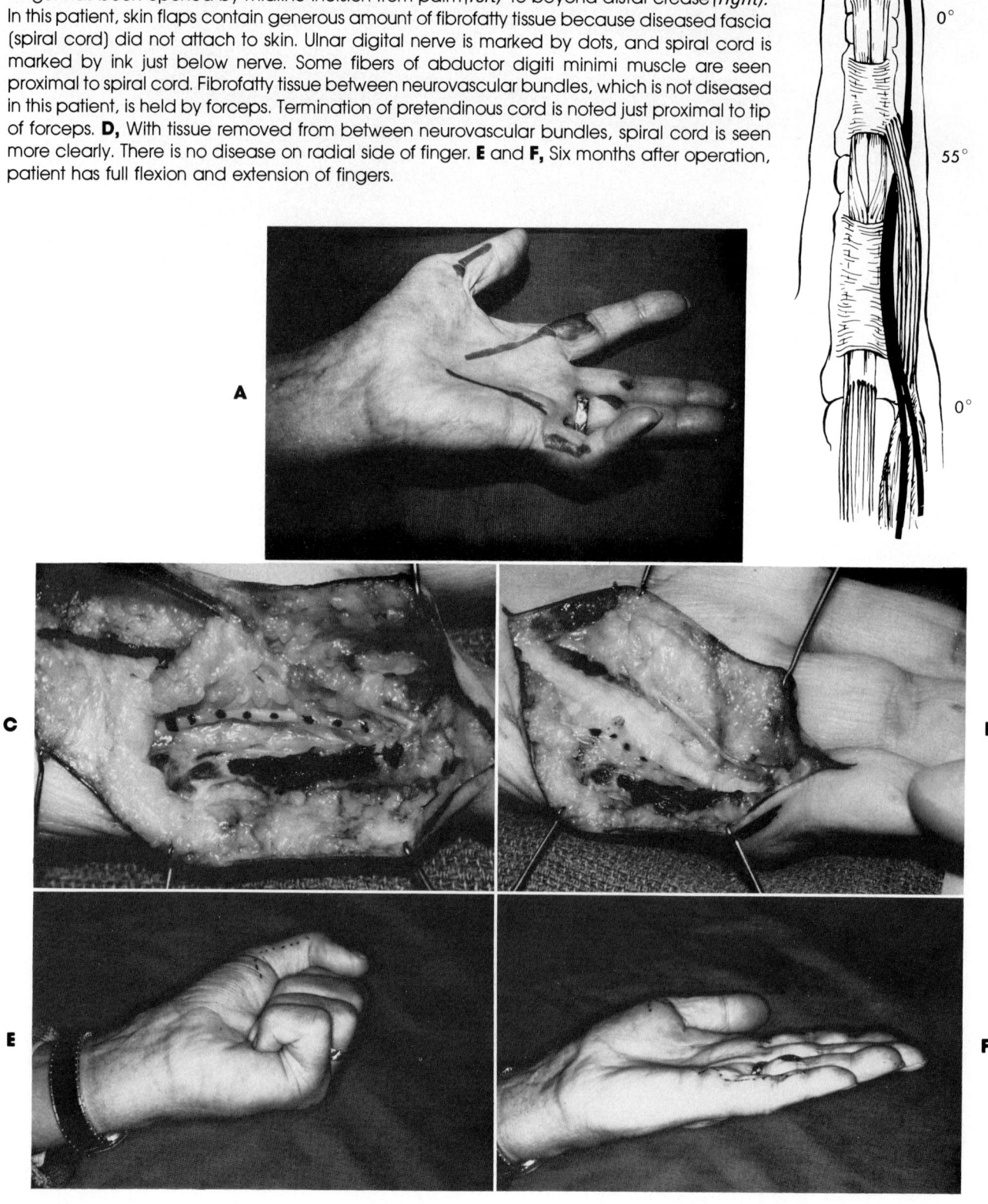

either a lateral or spiral cord. Usually a retrovascular cord is present as well[5] (Figs. 46-2 and 46-3).

Contracture at the distal interphalangeal (DIP) joint

On occasion the DIP joint can be flexed alone, but usually it is associated with a PIP joint contracture.[4] The contracture is caused by both the lateral and retrovascular cords, which terminate on the side of the distal phalanx. The diseased fibers intermingle with the terminal branches of the neurovascular bundle. All the fibers must be carefully identified and divided to correct the contracture. (See Fig. 46-2.)

Hyperextension at the DIP joint

Hyperextension at the DIP joint is not a joint contracture caused by Dupuytren's disease contracting Landsmeer's ligaments. Rather it is secondary and compensatory to a flexion contracture at the PIP joint. With the PIP joint held in flexion, forces similar to those that maintain a boutonniere deformity are applied to the DIP joint and result in hyperextension. Microscopic studies of Landsmeer's ligament do not reveal features of Dupuytren's disease. In fact Landsmeer's ligament is stretched rather than contracted in this state. Frequently at operation the hyperextended state is immediately corrected when the PIP joint contracture is corrected (Fig. 46-4).

Combinations of joint contractures

As in the other digits, it is not uncommon to have both MCP and PIP joints contracted in the little finger. However, the combination of cords that cause these contractures is more varied in the little finger (Fig. 46-5). In the other fingers the contracting cord is usually on one or the other side of the finger, but in the little finger, joint

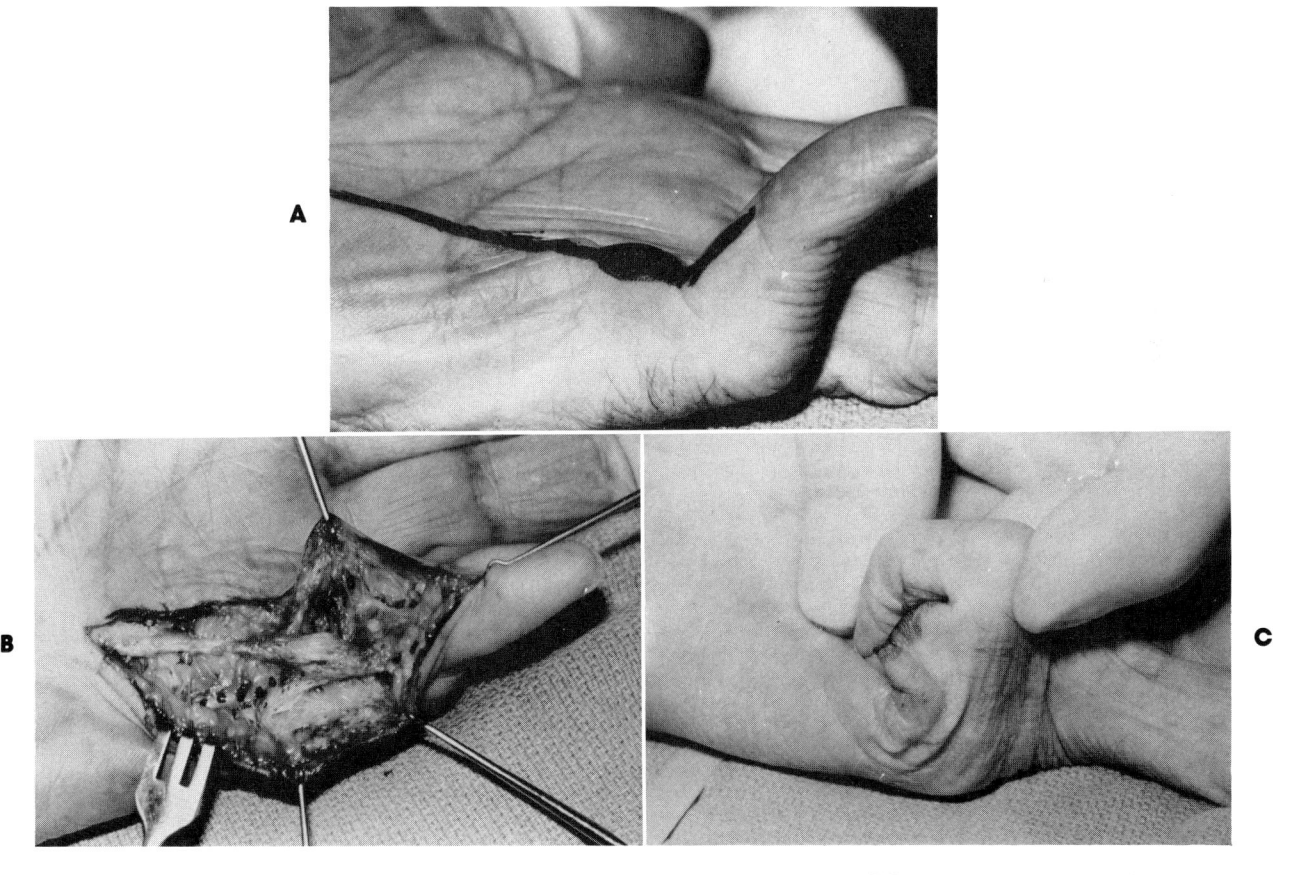

FIG. 46-4. A 59-year-old man with chronic pulmonary disease had PIP joint contracture and fixed hyperextension deformity at DIP joint. **A,** Appearance of finger before operation with palpable fascia marked. **B,** Disease involved pretendinous and central cord that attached to tendon sheath and bone at base of middle phalanx. There was no disease distal to this attachment. Note that incision extends beyond distal crease of finger and affords good exposure of middle segment of finger and DIP joint. **C,** There is full passive flexion at distal joint once disease has been removed.

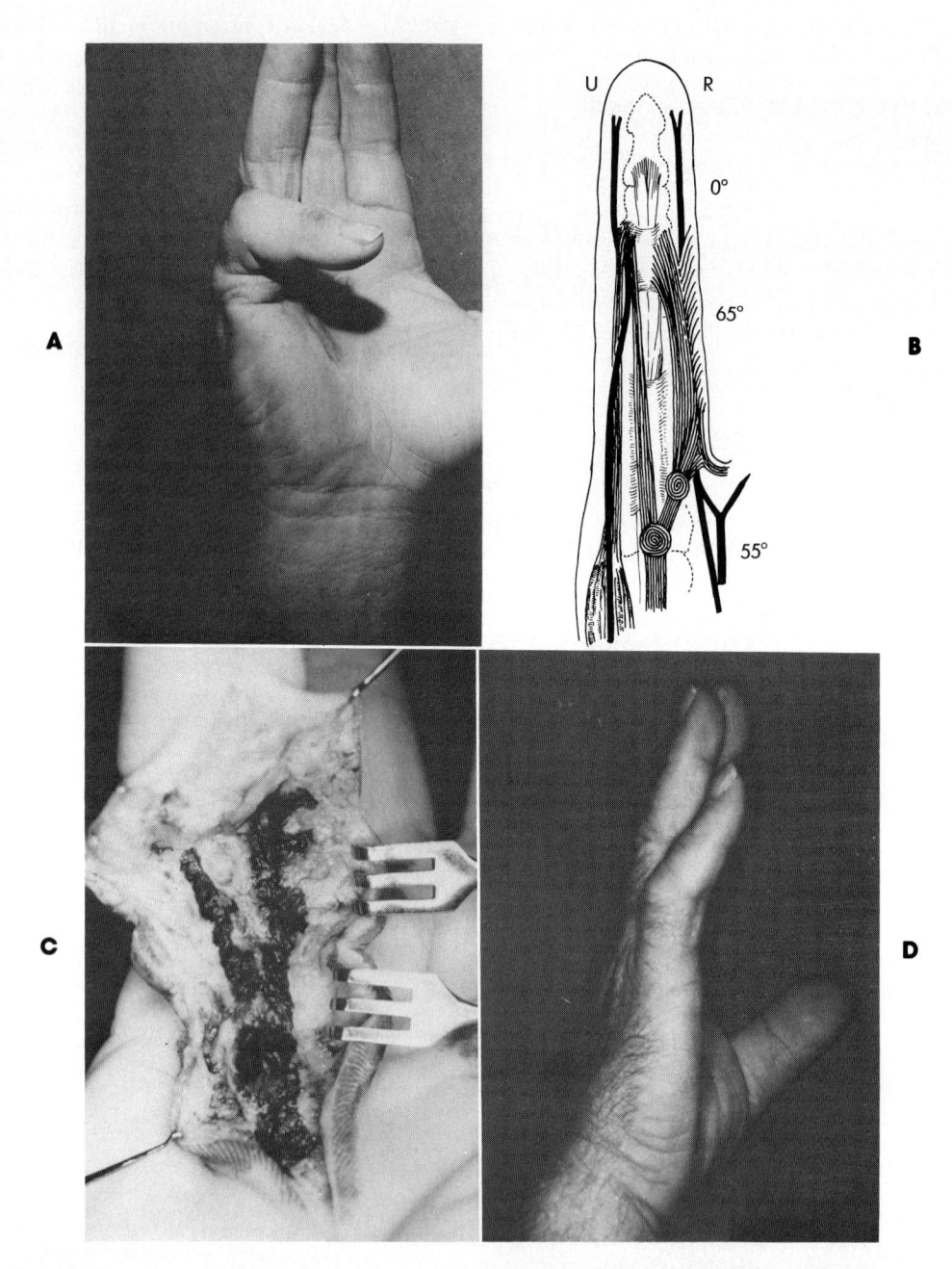

FIG. 46-5. Two examples of multiple cords causing joint contracture in little finger. **A,** A 56-year-old man with severe contracture at MCP and PIP joints. **B,** Cords that were found at operation: pretendinous cord ended in nodule and then became central cord that bifurcated. Ulnar part of central cord attached to side of middle phalanx together with spiral cord that originated in tendon of abductor digiti minimi muscle. Radial part of central cord blended with lateral cord, which began in natatory cord in web space. Disease is attached to skin throughout but also to tendon sheath over middle phalanx. **C,** Appearance of fascia at operation. **D,** One year after operation he had 30-degrees loss of extension of PIP joint.

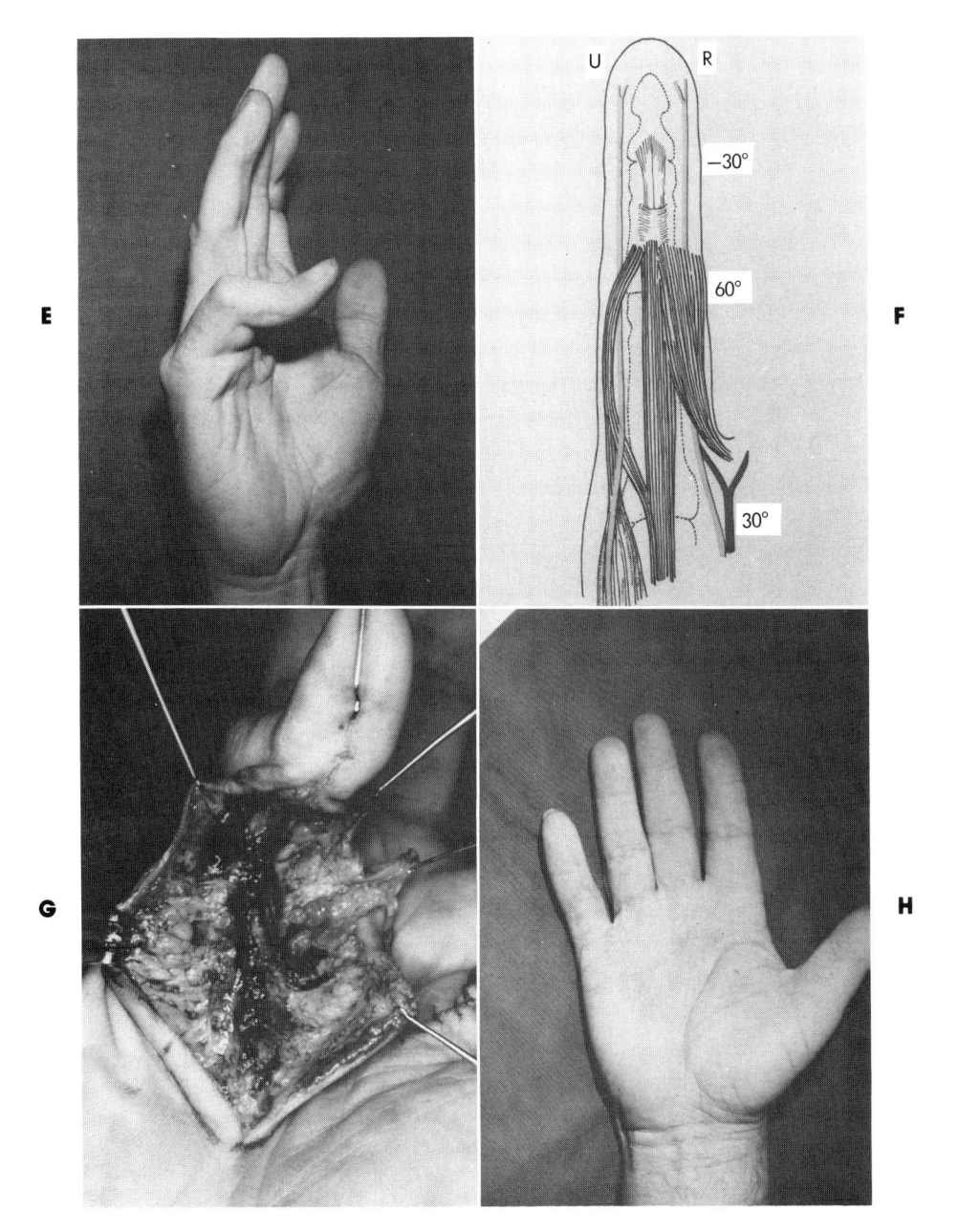

CHAPTER 46 PERSISTENT CONTRACTURE OF THE LITTLE FINGER IN DUPUYTREN'S DISEASE

FIG. 46-5, cont'd. E, A 51-year-old man with bilateral disease and previous operations in palm of each hand. Hyperextension deformity at DIP joint was fixed. **F,** Fascia found at operation: pretendinous cord continued into finger as central cord and attached to flexor tendon sheath at base of middle phalanx. Lateral cord on radial side was continuation of the natatory cord. Spiral cord on ulnar side originated from pretendinous cord as well as from tendon of abductor digiti minimi muscle and attached to bone and tendon sheath of middle phalanx. **G,** Appearance of fascia at operation. There was no evidence of disease to account for hyperextension deformity at DIP joint. Deformity was relaxed but not corrected by excision of diseased fascia. In retrospect, tenotomy of extensor tendon should have been performed. **H,** Appearance of the finger 1 year after operation. He still has 30 degrees of hyperextension at DIP joint but now has 60 degrees of flexion. PIP joint is still flexed to 30 degrees. (**B** and **C** from McFarlane, R.M.: Plast. Reconstr. Surg. **54**:31, 1974. © 1974 The Williams & Wilkins Co., Baltimore.)

SECTION 13   DUPUYTREN'S CONTRACTURE

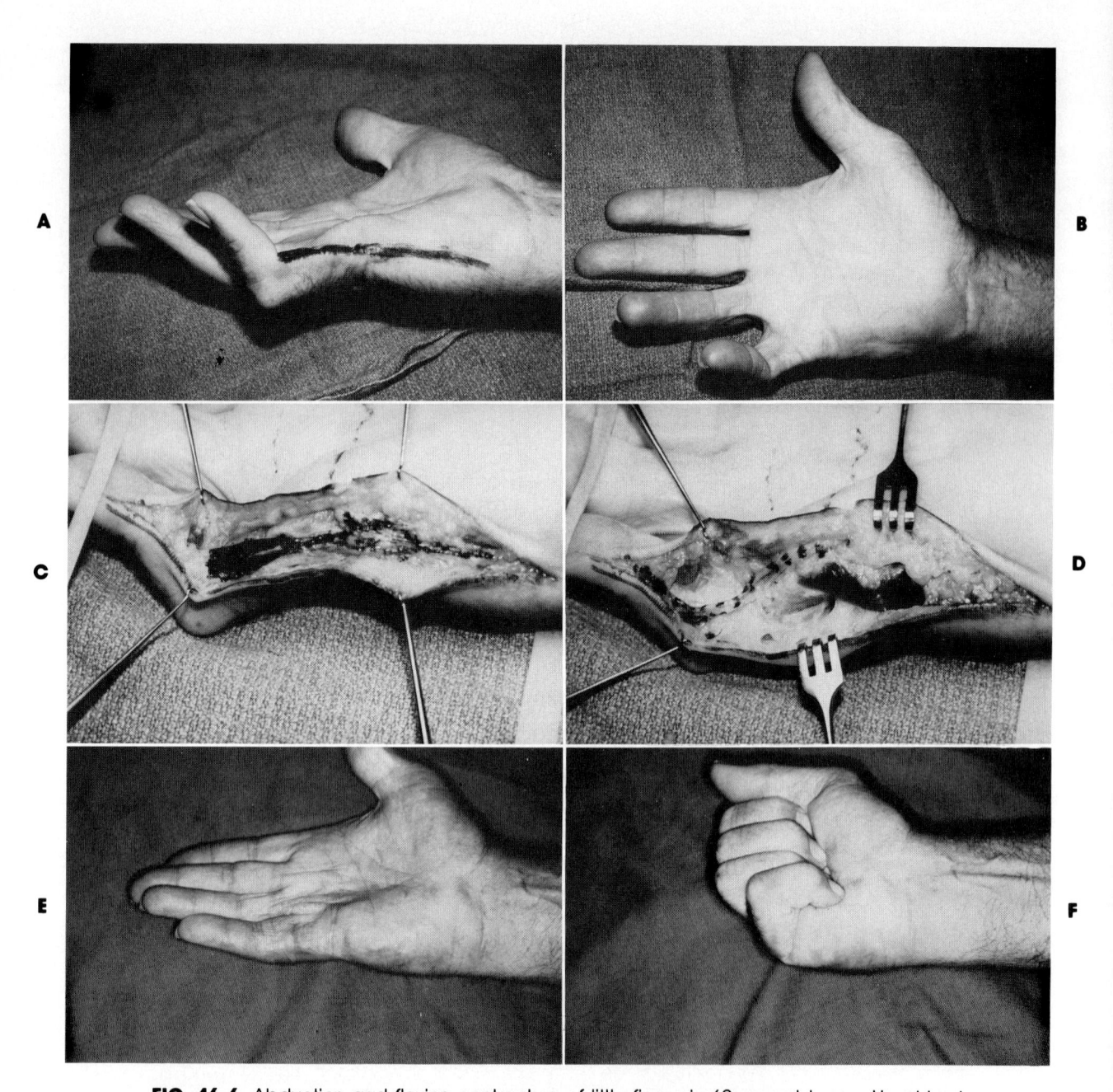

FIG. 46-6. Abduction and flexion contracture of little finger in 60-year-old man. Hand had been operated on previously but only in palm. **A,** PIP joint was flexed to 60 degrees. Palpable cord is marked. **B,** Little finger was slightly abducted and rotated at MCP joint. **C,** Diseased tissue is marked. It began proximally in hypothenar fascia and ended by attaching to bone and tendon sheath at base of middle phalanx. This is lateral cord because neurovascular bundle was not displaced. **D,** With lateral cord removed, abductor digiti minimi muscle has lost most of its tendinous attachment. Neurovascular bundle is dotted, and finger can be held straight. **E** and **F,** Six months after operation, patient has full flexion but lacks 30 degrees of extension at PIP joint.

contracture often is caused by disease on both sides of the finger. To this can be added either a flexion contracture at the DIP joint or a hyperextension deformity. Finally, the little finger can be abducted by a cord extending along the ulnar side of the hypothenar eminence (Fig. 46-6).

TREATMENT

The surgical treatment of Dupuytren's disease in the little finger is no different than elsewhere in the hand, but the surgeon must realize that full correction of the contracture is difficult, and all possible causes of contracture must be sought. If only the little finger is involved, I prefer a midline longitudinal incision that begins in the proximal aspect of the palm and ends distal to the distal crease of the finger. (See Figs. 46-3 and 46-4.) If the ring finger also is involved, I prefer to make a transverse incision in or near the distal crease of the palm and longitudinal incisions in the fingers, again extending beyond the distal crease of the fingers.

The skin flaps are reflected thin enough to leave all the diseased tissue behind. In some areas a generous amount of fatty subcutaneous tissue can be left on the skin (see Fig. 46-3, C), which ensures its later survival, whereas in other areas where the disease is intimately adherent to the skin, the skin flaps are dissected through the deep dermis. This thin skin still can survive if managed carefully. The flap should be reflected to about the midlateral line on each side. The use of a 4-power loupe facilitates the accuracy of this important dissection, permitting the skin flaps to be as thick as possible and yet ensuring that no diseased fascia is left attached to them.

If each neurovascular bundle is exposed the full length of the incision, the various cords that are causing the contracture will be identified in the process. It is unlikely that any diseased tissue will be left behind if it is removed in the following manner:

1. Remove the tissue from between the neurovascular bundles. (See Fig. 46-3, D.) This will remove the pretendinous cord in the palm and the central cord in the finger. It also will remove that portion of the spiral cord which is between the neurovascular bundles. The tissue will be attached firmly to the flexor tendon sheath and adjacent bone just distal to the PIP joint.

2. Remove all the tissue lateral to each neurovascular bundle. On the radial side the lateral cord may be diseased. If so, it will arise proximally in a natatory cord coming from the ring finger. The dissection should begin proximally to include the natatory cord and proceed distally as far as the disease is apparent. More often than not the disease can be followed to the side of the distal phalanx. On the ulnar side it is common for the diseased fascia to originate in the tendon of the abductor digiti minimi muscle and proceed distally as a spiral cord, a lateral cord, or both. (See Fig. 46-3, B.) To ensure complete excision of this tissue, the muscle fibers of the abductor digiti minimi should be identified and all the diseased tissue removed from this level distally.

3. Even though the PIP and DIP joints are fully corrected after the preceding steps, it is wise to examine the areas dorsal to the neurovascular bundles for fibers of the retrovascular cord. Even if the retrovascular tissue is not obviously diseased, it is best to remove it as a prophylactic measure. The retrovascular cord is the most common cause of failure to gain full correction at the time of operation, as well as the most common cause of recurrent contracture following operation. This cord is densest at the level of the PIP joint but can be dissected from the capsule of this joint easily if the neurovascular bundle is retracted. The cord extends distally and is a cause of contracture at the DIP joint, so it should be removed to this level. It is found with equal frequency on both sides of the finger, so both sides of the finger should be examined routinely.

4. If the PIP joint cannot be fully extended following adequate removal of the diseased fascia, the cause of the persistent contracture lies in foreshortening of the flexor tendon sheath of the capsular structures. It is a simple matter to incise the tendon sheath at the level of the PIP joint, and frequently gentle force will result in correction of the contracture. (See Fig. 46-2, E.) If this maneuver is not successful, the volar plate can be released, as described by Curtis,[1] where a slip of volar plate on either side is excised, thereby releasing the accessory collateral ligaments, or as suggested by Watson, Light, and Johnson,[6] where the check-rein ligaments of the volar plate are released. However, it may be good surgical judgment to accept as much as 15 degrees of flexion contracture. Inappropriate procedures on the PIP joint may prolong morbidity or result in permanent limitation of flexion, which is more disabling than a slight flexion contracture.

5. Flexion contracture at the DIP joint is more difficult to correct than one might expect. Usually the disease is on both sides of the joint and also is more lateral than volar. (See Fig. 46-2.) Therefore the terminal branches of the digital nerve and vessels must be dissected from the diseased tissue before it can be removed. In a recent analysis[2] of our results six patients had distal joint contracture, but none had full extension when examined 1 to 5 years after operation.

6. Hyperextension deformity at the DIP joint usually is corrected by correcting the PIP joint contracture. (See Fig. 46-4.) On only two occasions have I performed a tenotomy of the extensor tendon, but it is a useful procedure if required.

POSTOPERATIVE CARE

Since this problem was discussed at the Indianapolis Symposium on Difficult Problems in Hand Surgery (October 1978) I have intensified my regimen of postoperative splinting and have tried to impress on patients the need for prolonged splinting to obtain an optimal result. The operative dressing and splints are removed on the first or second day after operation, and a static dorsal extension splint is molded of thermoplastic material. The splint is worn most of the time but is removed according to the directions of the hand therapist for increasing periods to regain finger flexion. The sutures are removed between 10 and 14 days after operation, following which more emphasis is placed on regaining finger flexion. The splint is worn during the day as long as the finger has a tendency to contract. This is a variable period of up to 3 months. I advise the patients to wear a splint at least at night for 3 months. However, many patients do not do so simply because they are not concerned about a slight flexion deformity.

DISCUSSION

There appear to be three reasons for persistent contracture in the little finger. The first, and most important, is failure to remove all the diseased cords. It is not easy to identify all the diseased fascia in the little finger because so much may be present on both sides of the finger. Only by an orderly sequence of excision can one be ensured of removing all of it. It should be reemphasized that a common cause of persistent or recurrent contracture is failure to excise retrovascular tissue. It also should be apparent that adequate exposure is essential. The incision should extend beyond the distal crease of the finger so that the diseased fascia affecting both interphalangeal (IP) joints can be seen clearly.

The second cause of persistent contracture is lack of splinting in the postoperative period. Prolonged splinting is unnecessary if only the MCP joint or the PIP joint of one of the other fingers is involved. It is essential, however, to splint the PIP joint of the little finger for a prolonged period, perhaps as long as 3 months, if an optimal result is to be obtained.

The third cause of persistent contracture is unclear but is likely a result of the intrinsic anatomic relationships of the little finger. Given joints with equal severity and duration of flexion contracture, the correction of the contracture will be less complete in the little finger than in the ring or other fingers. A recent analysis showed that, only in the little finger, the amount of persistent contracture at the PIP joint is dependent on the severity of the contracture at the MCP joint.[2] The reason for this is unknown, but it supports the hypothesis that the little finger in Dupuytren's disease is unique. Furthermore it implies a relation between the two joints that is not immediately apparent but is likely on an anatomic basis.

REFERENCES

1. Curtis, R.M.: Capsulectomy of the interphalangeal joints of the fingers, J. Bone Joint Surg. **36A:**1219, 1954.
2. Legge, J.W.H., and McFarlane, R.M.: Prediction of results of treatment of Dupuytren's disease, J. Hand Surg. **5:** 608, 1980.
3. McFarlane, R.M.: Patterns of diseased fascia in the fingers in Dupuytren's contracture, Plast. Reconstr. Surg. **54:**31, 1974.
4. Millesi, H.: Uber die Beugekontraktur des distalen interphalangealgelenkes im rahmen einer Dupuytrenschen erkrankung, Brun's Beitr. Klin. Chir. **214:**399, 1967.
5. Thomine, J.M.: Le fascia digital—development et anatomie. In Tubiana, R., editor: La maladie de Dupuytren, ed. 2, Paris, 1972, L'Expansion Scientifique Française.
6. Watson, H.K., Light, T.R., and Johnson, T.R.: Checkrein resection for flexion contracture of the middle joint, J. Hand Surg. **4:**67, 1979.

Chapter 47 Treatment of Dupuytren's contracture by extensive fasciectomy through multiple Y-V–plasty incisions: short-term evaluation of 170 consecutive operations

H. Kirk Watson

The debate over technique in treating Dupuytren's contracture is far from resolved. Proponents exist for extensive fasciectomy,[12,22] partial fasciectomy,[2,7,16] fasciotomy,[9] skin grafting,[5,8] and open-palm techniques.[1,10] Additionally, amputation for severely affected digits is commonly mentioned.* Although the cause of Dupuytren's disease is not well understood, available evidence suggests that more complete fasciectomy or full-thickness skin grafting is associated with fewer recurrences.†

Simple fasciotomy is effective for immediate therapy but has a high recurrence rate.[13,15] In many published series the attempted wide excision of affected fascia led to unacceptably high initial complication rates.[18,22,23] These complications usually were secondary to hematoma, necrosis of the skin flaps, and prolonged edema and stiffness of the hand.

The purpose of this chapter is not to report long-term results or to prove the efficacy of extensive fasciectomy but rather to outline a surgical approach that allows wide exposure for radical fasciectomy, correction of contracture, easy closure, and minimal morbidity after operation. This chapter is a review of 170 consecutive operations for Dupuytren's contracture using a modification of the W-plasty closure described by Deming[4] in 1962.

CLINICAL MATERIAL

A total of 170 operations on 160 hands of 135 consecutive patients was performed from 1966 to 1977. Twenty-five patients underwent bilateral procedures, and a second operation was necessary in 10 hands during the time of this study, for a total of 170 operations. Eighteen hands had been operated on previously elsewhere. A patient was accepted as a candidate for operation if he or she felt that the degree of contracture interfered with his or her life-style either functionally (typically in men and more severe) or socially (typically in women and mild). Patients with simple palmar nodules were not treated unless they had associated stenosed tenosynovitis or common digital nerve symptoms. Angular contraction of the most affected joint was measured, and three categories were identified: mild, moderate, and marked.

With this classification 33 hands were identified as having mild contracture, 35 as moderate, and 67 as marked. Thirty-five were not measured but were recorded as "no," "mild," "moderate," or "marked" contracture.

TECHNIQUE

Nearly all patients are operated on while they are under general anesthesia. A zigzag incision is drawn on the palmar and digital skin with a surgical marking pen. The optimal number of flaps is four, extending from the proximal finger crease to the distal edge of the flexor retinaculum. Ninety-degree angles are ideal.[19] The incisions should center on or bisect any area where the skin is firmly attached to the diseased fascia. This minimizes the size of each undermined skin segment.

In severe contracture the palmar dissection is completed before the incisions are marked in the metacarpophalangeal (MCP) area.

MCP-area incisions are made, and MCP-area fascia is removed before finger incisions are marked. This progression facilitates proper placement of the zigzag incisions as the finger extends. The proximal finger crease is included entirely in a single flap. A rounded, elevated pouch of soft skin in the distal aspect of the palm between the fingers signifies that the digital nerve has been displaced into a spiral configuration around a band of fascia. Parallel incisions may be used to reach the most radial side of the palm. These two incisions should be as far from one another as the length of one side of a V-flap.

The radical fasciectomy is begun by lifting the overlying skin. The fascia then is transected in midpalm, while the underlying neurovascular structures are carefully protected. Dissection then progresses proximally and distally, concentrating on the vertical septa. As these are released, the entire fascia, including both longitudinal and transverse fibers, can be lifted free. The horizontal extension incisions (back cuts) that allow for the Y-V–pedicle advancement and concomitant skin length gain are not made until the end of the procedure.

---
*References 2, 6, 7, 11, 14, and 17.
†References 3, 5, 8, 22, and 24.

The diseased fascia in the finger is removed. This fascia typically ends in two bands lateral to the flexor sheath in the middle segment. Oblique thickening of the sheath across the proximal interphalangeal (PIP) joint area contributes to these bands distally and may restrict extension of the middle joint. Following excision of the fascia and thickened sheath, the check-reins may need to be released to obtain full extension.[20] The denser bands usually are central to the neurovascular structure, but tight fascia also lies laterally along the skin and must be separated from the skin and removed. On the ulnar side of the little finger a significant subcutaneous band is common. This band has strong attachments to the tendon of the abductor digiti minimi.

The finger joints are brought into full passive extension (180 degrees) in nearly every case. Skin grafting was required for closure in seven hands, of which three were reoperations. Three PIP joints had been operated on previously and, with fixed contractures, required arthrodesis. Amputation was necessary in only one reoperated finger. I feel strongly that better hand function results from arthrodesis than from amputation. Through a dorsal transverse incision enough bone is removed to allow adequate extension, and a concentric arthrodesis is performed.[21] No procedures are attempted on the volar aspect of these fingers because of the high incidence of trophic sequellae.

At closure the back cuts are made, beginning one after the other proximally and advancing the flaps. Often the back cut will fit the opposite flap better if made slightly proximal or distal to the V from which the flap was raised. No vessels are ligated or cauterized during the procedure, and the tourniquet is left inflated until the dressing is in place. The skin is closed using 5-0 monofilament stainless steel running and interrupted sutures.

The hands are dressed carefully in a bulky fluff compression dressing with the anteroposterior diameter of the dressing well in excess of the width of the metacarpal area. This transfers the circumferential dressing pressure from the sides of the index and the little metacarpals to the palm and dorsum of the hand. The bulky material is wrapped with bias-cut stockinette, and a dorsal plaster splint is applied over this to maintain immobilization. The fingers are in enough flexion to remove all tension from the skin. A second layer of bias-cut stockinette is applied over the plaster and the dressing reinforced with 2-inch adhesive tape. Once the dressing is completed, the tourniquet is deflated and fingertip circulation checked.

Usually patients are discharged on the day of the operation and seen again on the third or fourth day after operation. The dressing is then removed and wounds inspected. A light sterile dressing is applied and gentle, frequent use of the hand encouraged. A Joint Spring splint is applied for use through the night. This splint is replaced by the Joint Jack splint when sutures are removed. The patient uses the Joint Jack in 1-hour sessions during the day and through the night. Frequent observation is maintained well past the period of peak tissue reaction and until an improved and useful range of finger motion is demonstrated. If routine splinting has not accomplished this end, then serial plaster "pancake" splints are used volarly and dorsally to gain extension. Occasionally a web strap is necessary for one or two ½-hour sessions per day to gain passive flexion.

RESULTS

Long-term results, such as residual contractures and recurrent disease, are not covered in this chapter. Radical fasciectomies were used in all cases, demonstrating that extensive procedures can be done with this surgical approach.

In this series of 170 hand operations there were eight cases of superficial flap-tip necrosis. All healed within 3 weeks without need for secondary procedures. There were no cases of major wound dehiscence. There were no nerve or vascular problems beyond short-lived neurapraxia. No hematomas were noted beyond superficial ecchymoses, which resolved within a few days. There were two superficial infections, which responded promptly to antibiotics. Shoulder-hand syndrome, or "dystrophic" hand, is a diagnosis that could be applied to many hands following operation for Dupuytren's contracture. Eighty-seven patients were prescribed stress programs to prevent this type of problem.

DISCUSSION

The zigzag incision and the Y-V–closure are useful and have definite advantages over other techniques for the management of Dupuytren's contracture of the hand. Direct exposure of diseased fascia, both in the palm and in the fingers, is facilitated, and there is minimal disturbance to palmar skin circulation. The incision permits either radical or limited fasciectomy, depending on the indications or the preference of the surgeon. Exposure of the entire palmar fascia can be accomplished easily without circulatory embarrassment using parallel incisions with the option to extend into involved fingers. Added length of skin into the longitudinal axis without need for skin grafting is possible with allowance for full finger extension and for skin closure without tension.

With use of the W-closure, Z-plasties are seldom necessary. Nonetheless the option to use digital or palmar Z-plasty remains.

Maintaining the inflated tourniquet until the wound is closed and the dressing is applied is safe, and the operating time is significantly reduced. The anteroposterior orientation of the meticulously applied fluff compression dressing provides the necessary tamponade.

Early removal of the dressing on the third or fourth day after operation is safe, and early mobilization reduces morbidity from edema and joint stiffness. The judicious and early use of splints of progressively increasing force aids in restoration of full extension.

Radical resection of the transverse palmar fascia and fibrous tunnel system does not reduce healing time or the time of restoration of hand function.

SUMMARY

In 170 consecutive Dupuytren's operations the W-incision and flap advancement technique permitted radical fasciectomy, significant migration of skin into the longitudinal axis, and minimal postoperative morbidity.

REFERENCES

1. Ariyan, S., and Krizek, T.J.: In defense of the open wound, Arch. Surg. **111:**293, 1976.
2. Bruner, J.: Technique of selective aponeurectomy for Dupuytren's contracture. In Hueston, J.T., and Tubiana, R., editors: Dupuytren's disease, New York, 1974, Grune & Stratton, Inc.
3. Davis, J.E.: On surgery of Dupuytren's contracture, Plast. Reconstr. Surg. **36:**277, 1965.
4. Deming, E.G.: Y-V advancement pedicles in surgery for Dupuytren's contracture, Plast. Reconstr. Surg. **29:**581, 1962.
5. Gonzales, R.I.: Dupuytren's contracture of the fingers: a simplified approach to the surgical treatment, Calif. Med. **115:**25, 1971.
6. Homer, R.: Dupuytren's contracture: long term results after fasciectomy, J. Bone Joint Surg. **53B:**240, 1971.
7. Hueston, J.T.: Limited fasciectomy for Dupuytren's contracture, Plast. Reconstr. Surg. **27:**569, 1961.
8. Hueston, J.T.: The control of recurrent Dupuytren's contracture by skin replacement, Br. J. Plast. Surg. **22:**152, 1969.
9. Luck, J.V.: Dupuytren's contracture: a new concept of the pathogenesis correlated with surgical management, J. Bone Joint Surg. **41A:**635, 1959.
10. McCash, C.R.: The open palm technique in Dupuytren's contracture. In Hueston, J.T., and Tubiana, R., editors: Dupuytren's disease, New York, 1974, Grune & Stratton, Inc.
11. McFarlane, R.M., and Jamieson, W.G.: Dupuytren's contracture: the management of 100 patients, J. Bone Joint Surg. **48A:**1095, 1966.
12. McIndoe, A., and Beane, R.L.B.: The surgical management Dupuytren's contracture, Am. J. Surg. **95:**197, 1958.
13. Millesi, H.: The clinical and morphological course of Dupuytren's disease. In Hueston, J.T., and Tubiana, R., editors: Dupuytren's disease, New York, 1974, Grune & Stratton, Inc.
14. Moberg, E.: Three useful ways to avoid amputation in Dupuytren's contracture, Orthop. Clin. North Am. **4:**1001, 1973.
15. Rodrigo, J.J., Niebauer, J.J., Brown, R.L., and Doyle, J.R.: Treatment of Dupuytren's contracture: long term results after fasciotomy and fascial excision, J. Bone Joint Surg. **58A:**380, 1976.
16. Skoog, T.: Dupuytren's contracture: pathogenesis and surgical treatment, Surg. Clin. North Am. **47:**433, 1967.
17. Tubiana, R.: The principles of surgical treatment of Dupuytren's contracture. In Hueston, J.T., and Tubiana, R., editors: Dupuytren's disease, New York, 1974, Grune & Stratton, Inc.
18. Tubiana, R., Thomine, J.M., and Brown, S.: Complications in surgery of Dupuytren's contracture, Plast. Reconstr. Surg. **39:**603, 1967.
19. Watson, H.K., and Baker, G.: Relieving the skin shortage in Dupuytren's disease by advancing a series of triangular flaps: how to design and use them, Br. J. Plast. Surg. **33:**1, 1979.
20. Watson, H.K., Johnson, T.R., and Light, T.: Checkrein resection for flexion contracture of the middle joint, J. Hand Surg. **4:**67, 1979.
21. Watson, H.K., and Shaffer, S.R.: Concave-convex arthrodeses in joints of the hand, Plast. Reconstr. Surg. **46:**368, 1970.
22. Weckesser, E.C.: Results of wide excision of the palmar fascia for Dupuytren's contracture, Ann. Surg. **160:**1007, 1964.
23. Zachariae, L.: Extensive vs. limited fasciectomy for Dupuytren's contracture, Scand. J. Plast. Reconstr. Surg. **1:**150, 1967.
24. Zachariae, L.: Dupuytren's contracture: how limited should a limited fasciectomy be? Scand. J. Plast. Reconstr. Surg. **3:**145, 1969.

Chapter 48   Problems of Dupuytren's contracture

Harold E. Kleinert

Ian Leitch

David J. Smith, Jr.

Lawrence M. Lubbers

Dupuytren's contracture is a common disease among populations of Anglo-Saxon heritage. Hueston[8] estimated that in Australia 20% of the population over the age of 60 could be expected to show some evidence of this condition, whereas Ling[11] estimated that in Edinburgh 25% of men over 65 would be similarly affected. Despite its common occurrence and benign pathology, Dupuytren's contracture remains a major problem for the hand surgeon. Problems arise both from its tendency for inexorable progression, often despite seemingly adequate surgical treatment, and from the high morbidity associated with treatment, especially in cases of recurrent disease.

SURGICAL PROBLEMS
Intertrigo

Early cases of Dupuytren's syndrome, those with a simple palmar nodule and no associated deformity, present no real problem. However, patients with more advanced disease, possibly involving both hands, present numerous surgical problems. In some cases the contracture may even be severe enough to exclude surgical access to the volar aspect of the fingers and may be associated with skin maceration and intertrigo. The intertrigo is treated by the application of antibiotic dressings for several days prior to surgery. If necessary, definitive surgical excision may be preceded by percutaneous fasciotomy. Although this allows straightening of the fingers to improve surgical access, care must be taken to avoid digital nerves, which may be damaged easily.

Palmar fasciitis

Some conditions predispose a person to palmar fasciitis. For example, those with uncorrected adult syndactyly have a higher incidence of Dupuytren's contracture than does the normal population, possibly because of the increased amount of fibrous tissue between

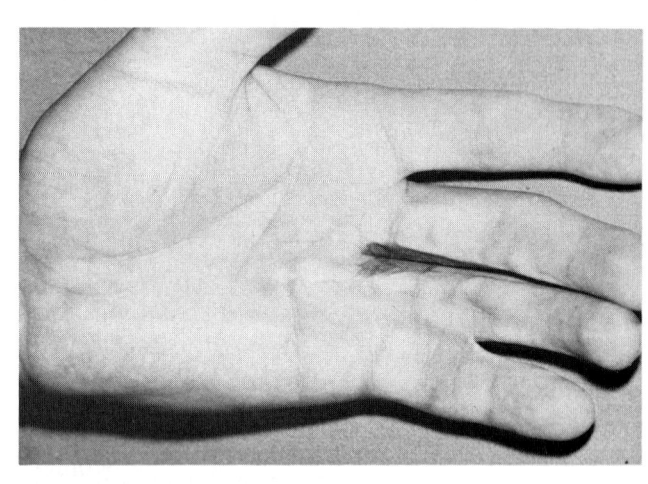

FIG. 48-1. Uncorrected adult syndactyly showing palmar fasciitis with marked longitudinal band of ring finger.

the unreleased digits (Fig. 48-1). In addition, ectopic sites of Dupuytren's disease should not be overlooked. Both plantar fasciitis and Peyronie's disease are difficult individual problems. Knuckle pads frequently antedate by years the appearance of palmar fasciitis and usually revolve spontaneously after palmar fasciectomy. Primary excision of the knuckle pad is difficult and should be undertaken only if the pads are symptomatic, e.g., painful after repeated injury. Complete excision is desired but seldom achieved because of intimate association with the extensor apparatus.

Postoperative hematoma

Some of the problems in Dupuytren's contracture are iatrogenic. The most common of these is postoperative hematoma. It is heralded by persistent pain and mild pyrexia in the early postoperative period and should be drained as soon as it is diagnosed. Hematoma occurred in 16% of cases reported by Tubiana[22] in 1974. Occasionally patients will have altered blood clotting function or rare factor deficiencies, be taking anticoagulants for coincidental medical diseases, or be chronic alcoholics with impaired prothrombin function. Preoperative questioning should identify most of these potential problem cases.

Attention to surgical detail will prevent most hematoma formation. Meticulous hemostasis following deflation of the tourniquet is mandatory, and use of the bipolar coagulator will minimize tissue necrosis. Suction drains may be a useful adjunct, but there is no substitute for meticulous hemostasis. Elimination of dead space is accomplished by suturing the flaps and applying a proper dressing. The most important aspect of the dressing is positioning the metacarpophalangeal joints in flexion, thus eliminating dead space by preventing elevation of the skin out of the palmar hollow.

The open-palm technique described by McCash[12] is the most reliable method of preventing hematoma. Following hemostasis the transverse palmar wound is left open, allowing blood and serum to drain freely. The mobilized skin flaps remain in their retracted position so that there is no tension on the skin, which already has compromised vascularity. Distal surgery is performed through separate finger incisions, which are closed without tension because of the relaxation of the palmar incision. The hand is splinted for 1 week and then active motion begun. Only a minimal scar is present 3 to 6 weeks later. In a series of 150 patients McCash[13] reported no hematomas. A few developed mild local infection, which responded to nitrofurazone dressings. A serous discharge was noted, which was thought to account for the remarkable freedom from edema, and postoperative pain was considerably reduced. Noble and Harrison[18] reported similar findings in a population of patients treated by several different surgeons.

Delayed healing

Delayed healing with or without skin necrosis is not an uncommon problem. Tubiana[22] reported healing problems in 5% of transverse palmar wounds, 20% of L-shaped wounds, and 10% of midline incisions with Z-plasty, whereas Honner, Lamb, and James[7] reported skin necrosis in 7% of their series of radical fasciectomies. Delayed healing significantly increases the amount of excess scar formation, which contributes to swelling, stiffness, and recurrent scar contracture. Devitalization of the skin flaps may be caused by an incorrect skin incision leaving narrowly based flaps, digital vessel injury, failure to replace devitalized skin at the time of the primary procedure, or suturing under too much tension. All these are potentially avoidable complications.

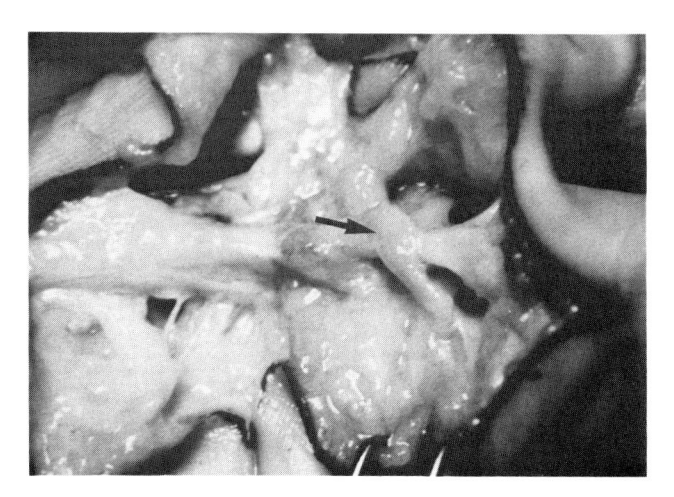

FIG. 48-2. Arrow emphasizes position of nerve overlying spiral cord.

Digital nerve injury

Digital nerve injury has been reported in 5% of patients by Honner and associates[7] and in 7% by Tubiana and Thomine.[23] The digital nerves usually are injured either in the palm as they emerge from the distal end of the transverse fibers of the flexor retinaculum or in the digits themselves. At the proximal interphalangeal (PIP) joint the fascia splits, with one band passing to a pretendinous insertion and the other to Cleland's fascia. The nerve may pass between these bands. It also may become twisted around the spiral cord, as described by McFarlane[14] (Fig. 48-2). Familiarity with these and other variants of pathologic anatomy should minimize the frequency of injury. When recognized, severed nerves should be sutured or grafted immediately.

Digital artery injury

Digital arteries are injured under similar circumstances but most frequently are damaged when the surgeon is operating on recurrent disease. Necrosis of skin flaps and indeed necrosis of all or part of the digit may result. In lesser degrees digital vessel damage will contribute to trophic changes, and, if there is concomitant injury of the digital nerves, the return of sensation after nerve suture will be poor. In long-standing contractures, reduction of the deformity may cause the digital nerves to undergo traction injury with demyelination and deterioration of function.

FLEXION DEFORMITIES

The insidious progression of Dupuytren's disease causes flexion deformities of varying degrees. There is no single underlying cause for the flexion contracture. It may range from problems with skin coverage to ad-

SECTION 13 DUPUYTREN'S CONTRACTURE

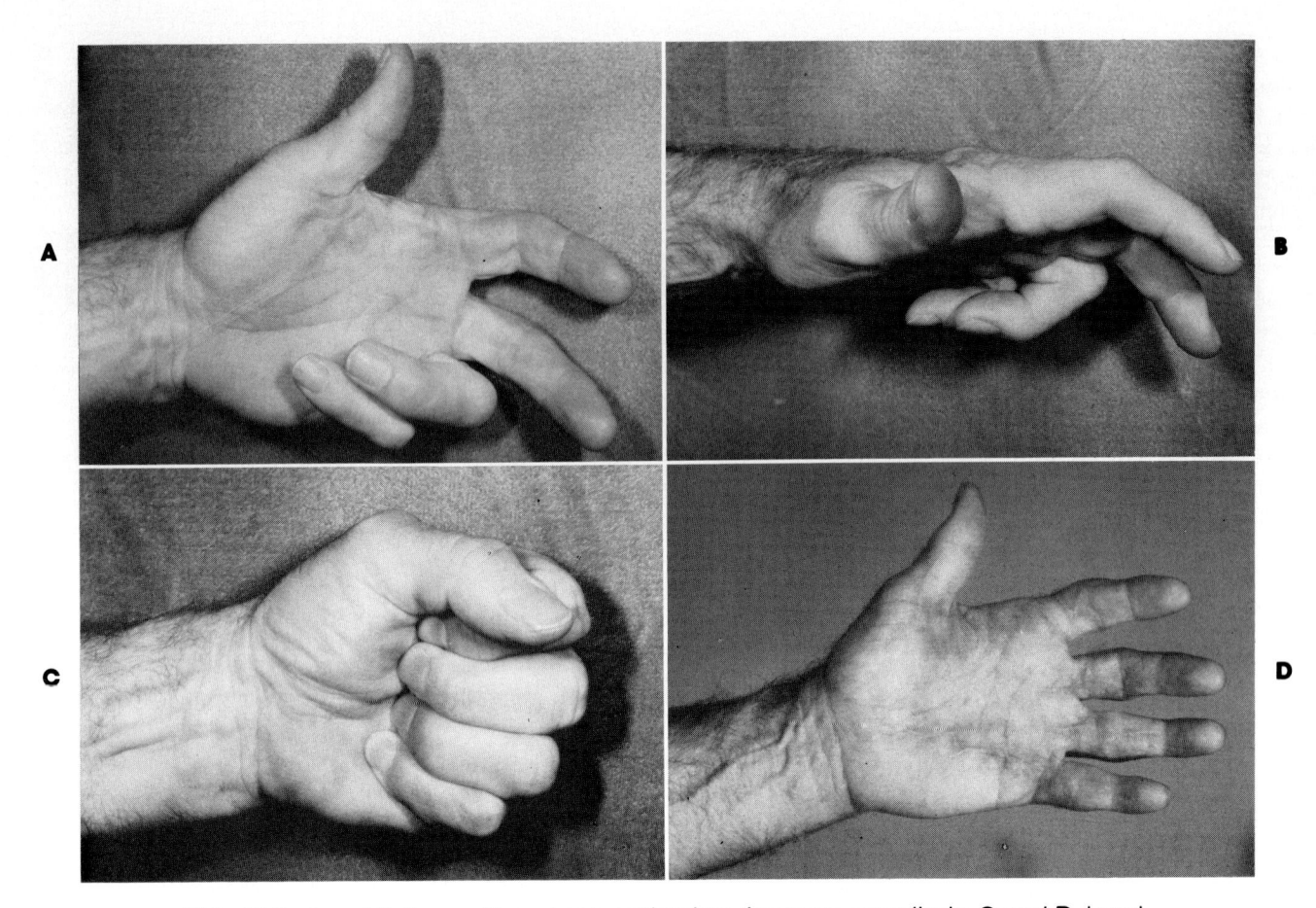

FIG. 48-3. A and **B,** Severe Dupuytren's contracture shown preoperatively. **C** and **D,** Longitudinal incision with Z-plasties incorporated allowed complete straightening without need for extra tissue.

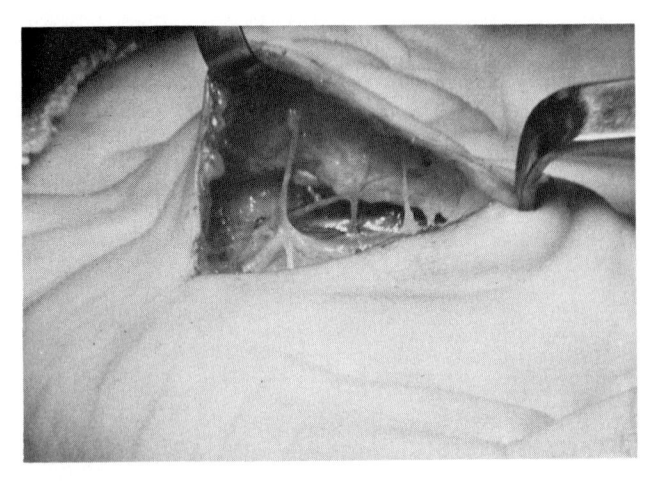

FIG. 48-4. Circulation to skin flaps is improved by maintenance of perforating vessels to skin.

herence of flexor tendons or loss of articular cartilage. To release the contracture, the underlying cause must be identified and corrected. Failure to do this will result in recurrent contracture even without recurrent disease.

Skin contracture

Shortage of palmar skin may produce an irreducible contracture. This may be a result of involvement of the skin by Dupuytren's tissue or, in recurrent cases, by scar contracture. Skin shortage caused by direct fascial invasion usually is best approached using a central longitudinal incision in the digits, which allows access to fascial cords and bands (Fig. 48-3). Careful dissection permits separation of nodules from the undersurface of the dermis, leaving the subdermal plexus intact (Fig. 48-4). After deflation of the tourniquet has allowed demonstration of adequate skin circulation, Z-plasties are fashioned to achieve sufficient skin lengthening to overcome the contracture. In some advanced cases and in recurrent cases with subdermal scarring and devitalized skin following even careful dissection there still may remain a primary skin shortage. If a suitable graft bed is available, a Wolfe graft taken from the groin or the inner aspect of the upper arm is the best solution. If there is exposed flexor tendon, bone, or joint after PIP joint and tendon sheath release, some form of pedicle flap will have to be employed.

Ordinarily small full-thickness defects can be covered by appropriately designed Z-plasties, but if the defect is larger, a cross-finger flap may be the easiest solution. A modified dorsal transpositional flap, as described by Harrison and Morris,[5] may cover the exposed structures, and, if necessary, a combination of flap plus full-thickness skin graft may be used. A distant pedicle flap (cross-arm, infraclavicular, subpectoral, or groin) occasionally may be necessary in larger defects involving more than one digit, but the postsurgical morbidity associated with immobilization of the hand makes this a poor choice.

Dense subcutaneous scar causing recurrent contracture is a problem because of the difficulty in contracture release, secondary loss of skin elasticity and circulation, and the ease with which the digital neurovascular bundles can be injured. This may result from inappropriately placed longitudinal incisions down the center of the finger. The method of treatment is the same as that for releasing any scar contracture, i.e., excision of the scar, recreation of the original defect, and introduction of sufficient healthy skin to overcome the shortage. In a longitudinal bridle scar with surrounding healthy skin, serial Z-plasties may be sufficient. If there is considerable peripheral scar or a larger central scar, the defect should be converted to a rhomboid shape, by extending the incision to the midlateral lines of the finger, and replaced by a Wolfe graft or, as previously discussed, by some form of pedicle flap.

Flexor tendon contracture

Hueston[8] reported uncorrectable contracture of the PIP joint in 26% of 112 patients operated on. We have found that it always has been possible to correct this flexion contracture but that this corrected state may not always persist into the postoperative period for various reasons. For example, contracted flexor muscles may cause a residual postoperative deformity even though passive extension is possible during surgery. Fixation of the PIP joint in extension by means of a transarticular Kirschner wire may be necessary for 1 or 2 weeks to allow the flexor muscle to accommodate to its new length. Dynamic extension splinting and later static extension night splinting also may be required to maintain this length.

Capsular and ligamentous contracture

Persistent flexion deformity may be a result of contracture of the fibrous flexion sheath, particularly when recurrence involves encasement of the digital neurovascular sheath and finger in a dense postsurgical scar. It may be necessary to relieve this contracture by incising the flexor sheath transversely. Care must be taken to preserve digital pulleys; otherwise bowstringing and loss of tendon excursion will result. In addition, adherent flexor tendons following previous surgery may require tenolysis and early active motion combined with dynamic splinting to achieve permanent mobilization.

Long-standing flexion contractures of the PIP joint may be associated with contractures of the volar plate, retinacular ligament, and accessory collateral ligaments. These will cause a deformity mimicking boutonniere deformity, and exploration of the PIP joint with release of the appropriate parts of the joint capsule may be required. Retinacular ligament shortening causing a boutonniere deformity has been described by Curtis.[1] The Dupuytren's cord inserts into the retinacular ligament, which pulls the lateral band volarly, flexing the PIP joint and extending the distal interphalangeal (DIP) joint. This occurs most commonly on the ulnar side of the small finger, where the spiral cord may firmly attach to the tendon of the abductor digiti minimi muscle (Fig. 48-5). Retinacular ligament release again will permit DIP joint flexion. A boutonniere deformity also may be produced by persistent tendon imbalance. Because of PIP joint flexion, there is a gradual stretching of the central slip of the extensor apparatus, allowing the lateral bands to subluxate volarly and resulting in a boutonniere deformity.

A mallet deformity may be caused by insertion of the spiral cord into the middle phalanx via Grayson's liga-

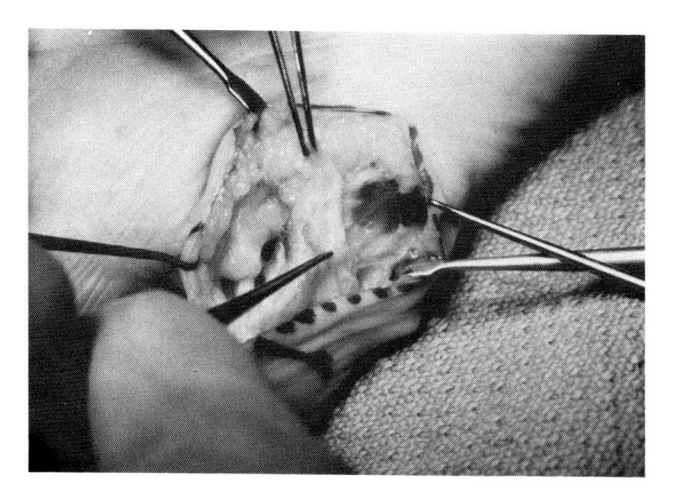

FIG. 48-5. Fibrous cord bridging digital nerve and inserting into tendon of abductor digiti minimi muscle.

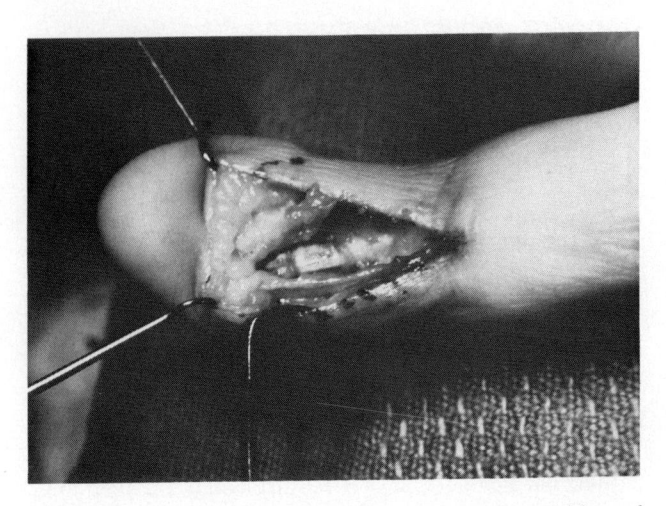

FIG. 48-6. Mallet deformity being released by division of fascia of distal phalanx.

ment with an extension through the lateral digital sheath to the fascia of the distal phalanx (Fig. 48-6). After release transarticular pinning probably will be required for 2 to 3 weeks and dynamic splinting thereafter.

Cartilage damage in the PIP joint

In cases of long-standing flexion contracture the dorsal two thirds of the head of the proximal phalanx comes into contact with the extensor tendon apparatus, removing the normal stimuli of joint surface pressure and function. The exposed articular cartilage of the proximal phalanx gradually is remodeled to fibrous tissue. After continued erosion of the cartilage to subchondral bone pits lined with granulation tissue, adhesions are formed between the extensor apparatus and this granulation tissue.[2,8] The loss of articular cartilage makes attempts to correct the joint contracture more difficult, and in this uncommon situation an arthrodesis can be considered. Use of the Harrison-Nicolle polypropylene intramedullary peg[5,6] is an effective and reliable method of arthrodesis in this situation.

It should be noted that we have not resorted to this method in any of our cases, since it always has been possible to straighten the PIP joint sufficiently. We believe that the difference between our experience and that of others in places such as the United Kingdom[11] and Australia[8] may be because of the more severe form of the disease seen in those countries.

RECURRENCES IN DUPUYTREN'S CONTRACTURE

Rank[19] noted that, in 85 hands of 50 patients reviewed 5 to 30 years after fasciectomy, 20% showed no recurrence, 45% developed extension of the disease, and 35% developed recurrence. Thirty percent of those with extension required further surgery, as did 60% of those with local recurrence. Recurrence is most frequent in the small finger and becomes less frequent in the more radially placed digits.[8] In addition, recurrence in the finger is more significant than recurrence in the palm, since it produces a flexion deformity more difficult to correct. Thus surgery should be designed to reduce the likelihood of recurrence in the digits.

Even when a radical palmar fasciectomy, as described by McIndoe and Beare,[16] was performed, only 49% of hands were disease free 5 to 25 years after surgery.[4] Secondary and tertiary surgery was required in two thirds of the remaining 51%. Extensive fasciectomy has more prophylactic value than does limited fasciectomy, since further multiple operations lead to successively poor results. The likelihood of poor wound healing increases with each operation, as does the formation of more postsurgical scar, both predisposing the patient to an earlier recurrence of contracture.

Recurrent flexion contractures cause even more difficult problems. Those contractures produced by fascial fibromatosis at the site of previous surgery must be differentiated from extension of the disease from new lesions occurring outside the area of previous surgery. In recurrent Dupuytren's contracture the overlying skin may be so adherent to the diseased tissue that dissection causes skin ischemia. Use of full-thickness skin grafts in this situation has led to the observation that, although further deposits of Dupuytren's contracture occurred in adjacent areas, none appeared beneath the skin graft. Removal of the involved volar skin of the palm or digit removes with it the mechanism or source of production of recurrent Dupuytren's contracture.[9] Because of this, Hueston[9] recommends excision of involved skin with Wolfe-graft replacement in recurrent cases. Simple fasciotomy in the palm, and again more distally, adequately releases the contracture, but the recurrence rate is high because the Dupuytren's band reestablishes continuity within the scar tissue bridge. Treating the Dupuytren's band in a manner similar to that used for a burn scar contracture, by division and insertion of a Wolfe graft, is advocated by Gonzalez.[3] In a 3-year follow-up analysis he has observed only one recurrence in 39 patients. Recently McGregor[15] has proposed that the Dupuytren's band be treated in the same manner as any contracting scar, by division of the scar and insertion of a partial thickness skin graft. He has used this principle in selected cases of extensive disease as a prophylaxis against recurrence in patients with a strong Dupuytren's diathesis. A transverse incision is made across the distal palmar crease, the bands are divided and well separated, and then the gutter is lined with a partial thickness skin graft. This procedure can be repeated in the first web space, the base of the thumb, or at the PIP joint. McGregor reports that, although the results are not conclusive because of the short follow-up time, there was re-

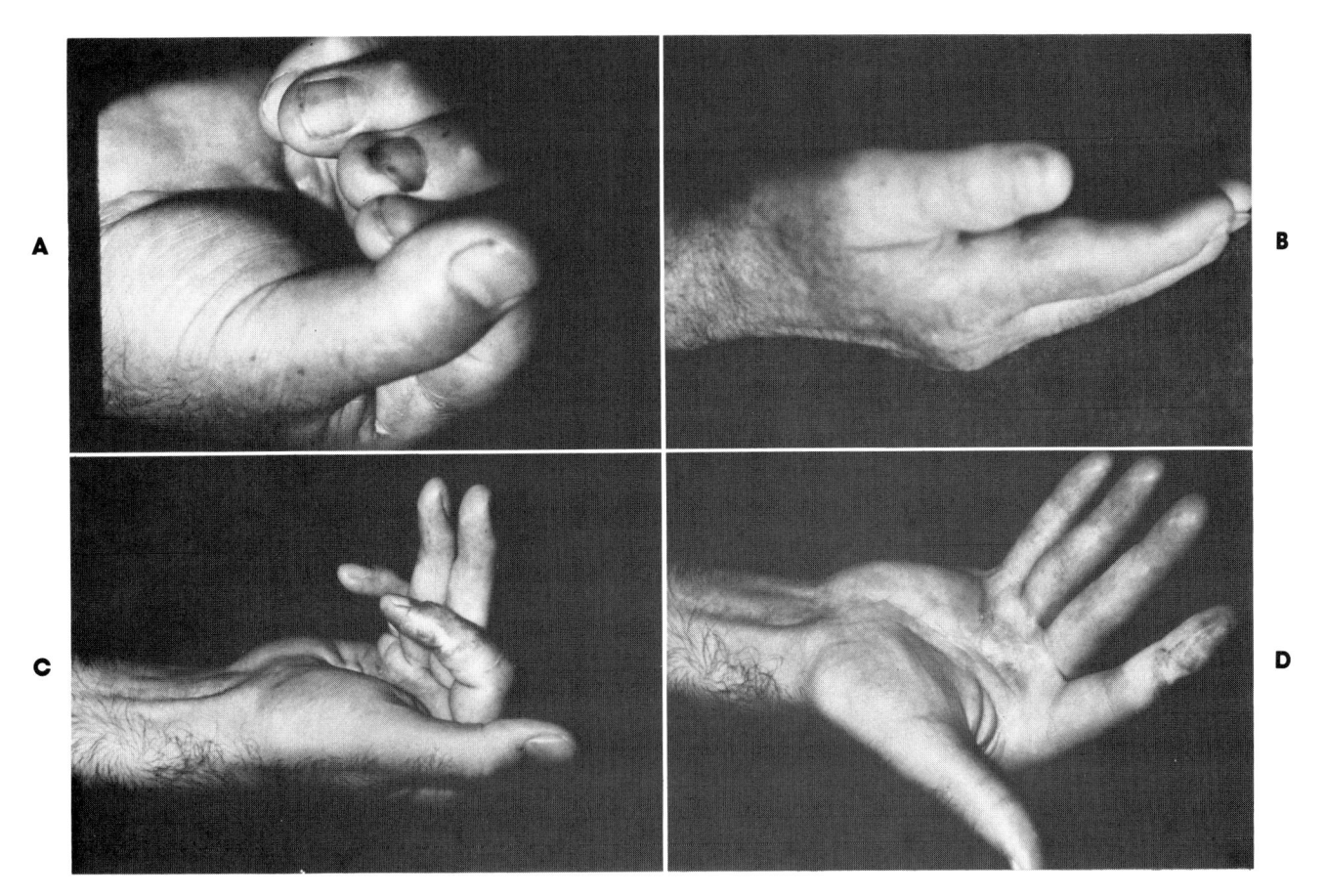

FIG. 48-7. A and **B,** Typical appearance of hand in posttraumatic sympathetic dystrophy. Hand is swollen. **C** and **D,** In another patient neither flexion nor extension is complete.

currence only when part of the skin graft was lost and reestablishment of continuity of bands occurred through a scar bridge.

Harrison and Morris[5] believe separation of the involved palmar and digital skin by insertion of normal skin and subcutaneous tissue breaks the continuity of Dupuytren's band and prevents recurrence at this site. They advocate the dorsal transpositional flap, whereas Moberg[17] uses a cross-finger flap.

POSTOPERATIVE COMPLICATIONS

Postoperative problems are usually self-limited. If a patient has pain associated with Dupuytren's contracture, it will be intensified postoperatively. The pain most often is caused by some concomitant disease such as cervical radiculitis or arthritis, and unless aware of this, both physician and patient will be unsatisfied even by complete release of the contracture.

Infrequently a swan-neck deformity is seen postoperatively. This may result either from excessive release of the PIP joint at surgery and during postoperative mobilization or from the intrinsic-plus deformity that develops after excessive interosseous compartment swelling. Usually it is self-limited, particularly if an extension block splint to the PIP joint is applied early. If the deformity is more severe and not correctable by passive means, Littler's procedure can be helpful.[21]

Postoperative swelling may be somewhat increased either by prolonged use of a tourniquet during dissection[24] or by widespread palmar and digital dissection. The accumulation of edema increases the risk of infection and fibrosis, thus endangering the various intricate gliding mechanisms.[20] Tourniquet edema may be significantly reduced by performing the dissection with the patient's hand elevated, thus reducing tourniquet time. If edema develops during wound closure, it can be minimized by leaving at least part of the transverse palmar incision open (McCash[12] technique). Postsurgical immobilization with the interphalangeal joint in flexion may allow a partial recurrence of flexion contracture from which it is difficult for the patient to mobilize.

Postoperative pain, stiffness, and swelling may be caused by posttraumatic sympathetic dystrophy (Fig. 48-7). In a series of 130 such cases following elective surgery 22% were patients who had undergone fasciectomies for Dupuytren's contracture.[10] Successful treatment of sympathetic dystrophy demands early recognition and early active motion. Therapy, including medication, transcutaneous nerve stimulation, and stellate ganglion blocks, is carried out as necessary.

SUMMARY

Surgery for Dupuytren's contracture remains fraught with hazards. Particularly, inadequate or poorly planned surgery may lead to even worse recurrent contractures. A thorough understanding of the pathologic anatomy and attention to surgical detail help to minimize these hazards. It is hoped that in the future the factors which cause progression of the disease will be identified so that it can be arrested before progression necessitates surgical intervention.

REFERENCES

1. Curtis, R.M.: Volar capsulectomy of the proximal interphalangeal joint. In Hueston, J.T., and Tubiana, R., editors: Dupuytren's disease, New York, 1974, Grune & Stratton, Inc.
2. Field, P.L., and Hueston, J.T.: Articular cartilage loss in long-standing flexion deformity of the proximal interphalangeal joint, Aust. N.Z. J. Surg. **40**:70, 1970.
3. Gonzalez, R.I.: Open fasciotomy and full-thickness skin graft in the correction of digital flexion deformity. In Hueston, J.T., and Tubiana, R., editors: Dupuytren's disease, New York, 1974, Grune & Stratton, Inc.
4. Hakstian, R.W.: Late results of extensive fasciectomy. In Hueston, J.T., and Tubiana, R., editors: Dupuytren's disease, New York, 1974, Grune & Stratton, Inc.
5. Harrison, S.H., and Morris, A.: Dupuytren's contracture: the dorsal transposition flap, Hand **7**:145, 1975.
6. Harrison, S.H., and Nicolle, F.V.: A new intramedullary bone peg for digital arthrodesis, Br. J. Plast. Surg. **27**:240, 1974.
7. Honner, R., Lamb, D.W., and James, J.I.P.: Dupuytren's contracture, J. Bone Joint Surg. **53B**:240, 1971.
8. Hueston, J.T.: Dupuytren's contracture, Baltimore, 1963, Williams & Wilkins Co.
9. Hueston, J.T.: Skin replacement in Dupuytren's contracture. In Hueston, J.T., and Tubiana, R., editors: Dupuytren's disease, New York, 1974, Grune & Stratton, Inc.
10. Kleinert, H.E., et al.: Post-traumatic sympathetic dystrophy, Orthop. Clin. North Am. **4**:917, 1973.
11. Ling, R.S.M.: The genetic factor in Dupuytren's disease, J. Bone Joint Surg. **45B**:709, 1963.
12. McCash, C.R.: The open palm technique in Dupuytren's contracture, Br. J. Plast. Surg. **17**:271, 1964.
13. McCash, C.R.: The open technique in Dupuytren's contracture. In Hueston, J.T., and Tubiana, R., editors: Dupuytren's disease, New York, 1974, Grune & Stratton, Inc.
14. McFarlane, R.M.: Patterns of the diseased fascia in the fingers in Dupuytren's contracture, Plast. Reconstr. Surg. **54**:31, 1974.
15. McGregor, E.A.: Personal communication, 1977.
16. McIndoe, A., and Beare, R.L.B.: The surgical management of Dupuytren's contracture, Am. J. Surg. **95**:197, 1959.
17. Moberg, E.: Three useful ways to avoid amputation in advanced Dupuytren's contracture, Orthop. Clin. North Am. **4**:1001, 1973.
18. Noble, J., and Harrison, D.H.: Open palm technique for Dupuytren's contracture, Hand **8**:272, 1976.
19. Rank, B.K.: Some observations on Dupuytren's contracture, J. Hand Surg. **3**:495, 1978.
20. Rank, B.K., Wakefield, A.R., and Hueston, J.T.: Surgery of repair as applied to hand injuries, ed. 4, Edinburgh, Scotland, 1973, Churchill Livingstone.
21. Thompson, J.S., Littler, J.W., and Upton, J.: The spiral oblique retinacular ligament (SORL), J. Hand Surg. **3**:482, 1978.
22. Tubiana, R.: The principles of surgical treatment of Dupuytren's contracture. In Hueston, J.T., and Tubiana, R., editors: Dupuytren's disease, New York, 1974, Grune & Stratton, Inc.
23. Tubiana, R., and Thomine, J.M.: Surgical treatment of Dupuytren's contracture: technique of fasciotomy and fasciectomy. In Hueston, J.T., and Tubiana, R., editors: Dupuytren's disease, New York, 1974, Grune & Stratton, Inc.
24. Ward, C.M.: Edema of the hand after fasciectomy with or without tourniquet, Hand **8**:179, 1976.

Chapter 49 Dupuytren's contracture: treatment by the open-palm technique

William B. Kleinman

Morbidity associated with the treatment of Dupuytren's contracture relates usually to small joint stiffness and a diminished total active arc of digital motion following surgery. Early postoperative complications such as hematoma formation, necrosis of skin edges or flaps with subsequent infection, or the severe pain associated with muscle spasm each may contribute to a less than optimal result.

FREE-SKIN GRAFTS VERSUS OPEN-PALM TECHNIQUE

The field is still quite controversial. Wound coverage following excision of diseased palmar or digital fascia has been performed by split- of full-thickness skin grafts,[6,9] V-Y- or Z-plasty incisions,[9,11,14] large dorsal rotation flaps,[7] open delayed suture,[17] and even amputation[15] in severely compromised cases. Howard[8] emphasized in his 1959 treatise on the subject that "prevention of postoperative stiffness" was the main problem, and that efforts in treatment should be directed toward minimizing this problem.

In 1964 McCash[12] proposed that the use of free-skin grafts (regardless of thickness) to cover palmar defects following excision of diseased palmar fascia was ineffective; he stated that serious effusion and hematoma formation could not be prevented by application of a skin graft and that applied free-skin graft had to be sutured to skin "reduced in vitality by disease and by the dissection." In addition to these two points, McCash claimed that application of a free-skin graft necessitated immobilization of the hand until the grafts could "take" to underlying tissues, usually 7 to 10 days; also, if the palmar fibromatosis involved the flexor tendon sheaths, thus exposing the flexor tendons following excision, free grafts could not effectively be applied to these gliding structures without failure.

Considering these inherent difficulties with palmar skin graft, McCash[12] proposed that the hand surgeon reconsider the four essential principles for the management of this disease, first recommended by Baron G. Dupuytren[4] in 1834. Dupuytren, the respected teacher and surgeon (who described the disease to which his name is affixed 10 years after it was described by Sir Astley Cooper), suggested (1) that all incisions be transverse and in the skin creases, (2) that longitudinal fascial bands responsible for joint contractures be divided, (3) that the fingers be treated in full extension between exercises for 4 weeks after surgery, and (4) that all wounds be left open and allowed to heal by granulation.

The open-palm technique in Dupuytren's contracture evolved using these principles. McCash[12] felt that postoperative complications could be eliminated if all wounds were left open following subtotal palmar or digital fasciectomy. McCash's principles of the open-palm technique are the following:

1. All incisions are made in transverse skin creases.
2. All incisions are closed primarily *except* the distal palmar crease.
3. Active exercises are begun after 7 days.
4. Metacarpophalangeal (MCP) joint extension splinting is used at night.
5. Only short hospitalization is necessary.
6. No prolonged physiotherapy is necessary.

DUPUYTREN'S VERSUS McCASH'S OPEN-PALM TECHNIQUE

Considerable differences are illustrated comparing Dupuytren's principles[4] of 1834 with McCash's open-palm technique[12] described more than 100 years later. With tourniquet control, safe anesthetics, and available antibiotics, postoperative morbidity has been drastically reduced. Dupuytren felt that diseased fascial cords responsible for tethering (holding the distal joints in flexion) could be simply cut by fasciotomy; no fascial excision was performed; all wounds were left open to heal by granulation and epithelialization. Tourniquet control, instituted in the early part of this century, now enables us to perform subtotal fasciectomies in bloodless fields; anesthetics are safe, and surgical efforts can be as aggressive as necessary. Our understanding of cellular enzymatic activity and the disease process in general is considerably better now than in 1834.

Nonetheless even today postoperative complications of hematoma, serious effusion and edema, infection, and persistent pain remain the most common causes for surgical failure and digital stiffness.* Skin dissected free from diseased underlying palmar fascia is marginal in quality, regardless of the technique used; normal elasticity is gone, and circulation at the skin edges or flap tips is poor.

The open-palm technique[12,13] eliminates hematoma, infection, graft slough, muscle spasm, and skin necrosis as postoperative complications. If incisions are made transversely in the palmar or digital creases, radial and ulnar circulation to the bridging skin ensures viability in the face of any undermining necessary for the excision of diseased palmar fascia. By leaving the transverse incisions wide open after full digital extension is achieved, one can eliminate risks of subcutaneous hematoma formation.

Postoperative digital stiffness following excision of diseased Dupuytren's tissue can be complicated by the length of time the hand is immobilized following surgery. A delay of 7 to 10 days necessary to ensure an adequate "take" of the graft to its recipient bed can further compromise the final function of the hand.

McCash[12,13] recommended that active motion begin as early as 7 days after subtotal fasciectomy. Using the principles he outlined, I have found no difficulties starting an active motion program for my patients as early as 3 to 5 days after surgery. Free drainage from the open wound prevents hematoma or seroma collection, thereby reducing postoperative edema. Absence of tension along a closed suture line eliminates the pain attributable to skin closure. These patients can be discharged from the hospital within 2 or 3 days after surgery to begin their exercise program in a relatively pain-free state. The bulky surgical dressing is removed in the office at approximately 5 days and replaced by a nonadherent light gauze dressing, which covers the wound but allows full range of motion.

Splinting in full MCP and interphalangeal (IP) joint extension between exercises and at night continues throughout the wound-healing process. The extension splinting greatly facilitates the home rehabilitation program.

Wounds treated by the McCash[12,13] open-palm technique heal in from 3 to 8 weeks, depending entirely on the size of the defect created at the time of surgery. Continuous use of extension splinting between exercises maintains tension along the proximal and distal margins of the wound, encouraging transverse linear closure rather than circular closure.

---

*References 1-3, 6, 7, 10, 12, and 16.

CHAPTER 49 DUPUYTREN'S CONTRACTURE: TREATMENT BY THE OPEN-PALM TECHNIQUE

CASE HISTORY

A 46-year-old right hand–dominant accountant had a 4-year history of progressive flexion contracture of his left hand secondary to Dupuytren's palmar fibromatosis (Fig. 49-1, *A*). After use of the open-palm technique (Fig. 49-1, *B*), healing began within 24 hours by slow contraction of wound edges. A rich vascular granulation bed completely filled the defect within 4 or 5 days of surgery. Biochemical and histologic studies suggest that a contractile actinomycin system in the cytoplasm of fibroblasts lining this granulation bed may have been responsible for putting tensile forces along the skin edges. In response to this stimulus, dermal elements formed at the edges of the open wound. Within 2 weeks of surgery (Fig. 49-1, *C*) wound edges were clean, and the patient was well into the active flexion program and extension splinting. Within 4 months of surgery a fine transverse scar is consistently found over the distal palmar crease, indistinguishable from a *per primam* closure (Fig. 49-1, *D*).

Work done in the mid-1950s by Gillman and Penn[5] suggests an actual regeneration of a single-cell layer of epithelium from the edges of the defect during this period rather than cellular division. Perhaps the potential for closure rests in the cut edges of the epithelium alone. To this day, the exact mechanism remains unknown.

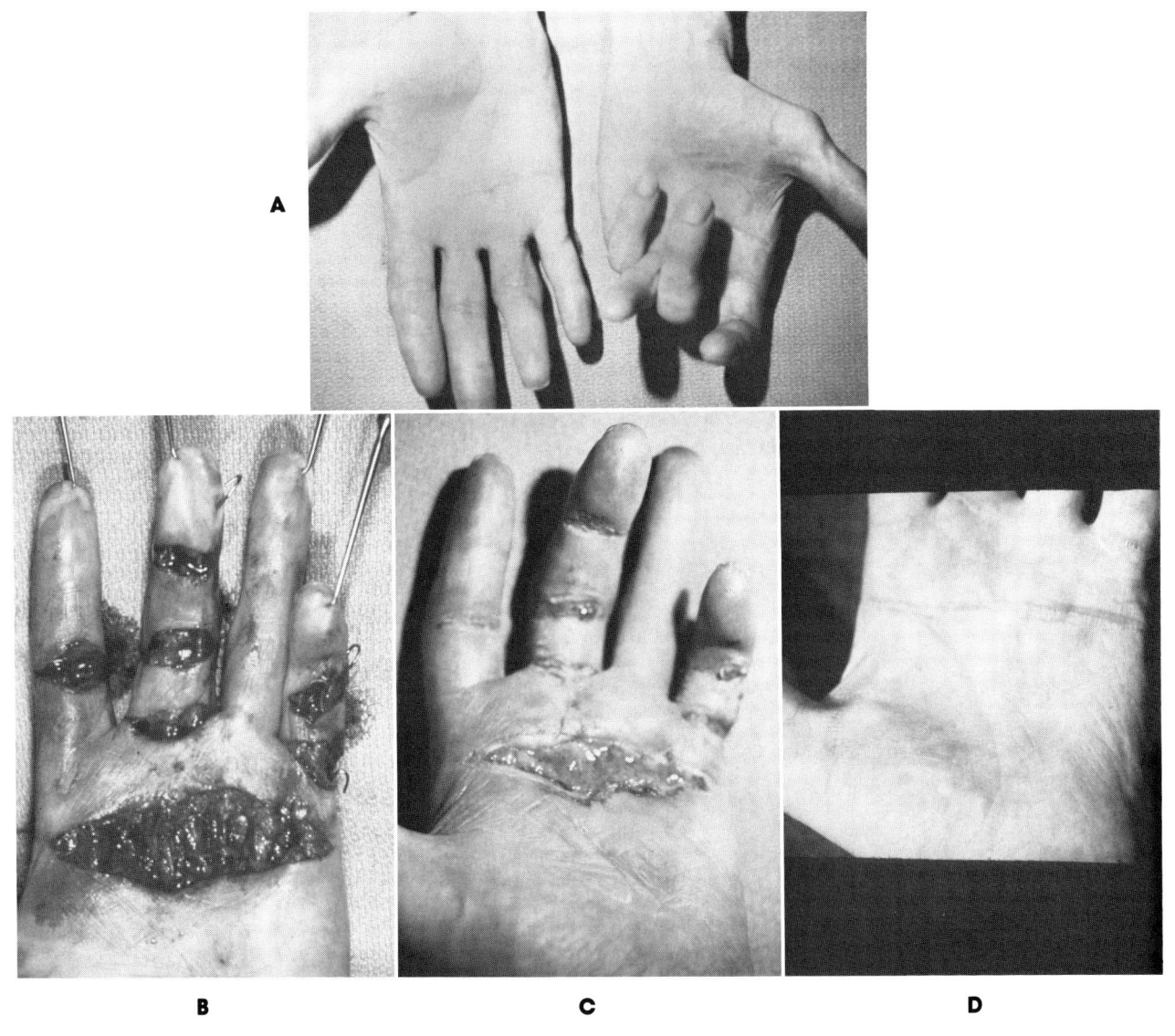

FIG. 49-1. A, Typical case of palmar fibromatosis and fixed flexion contractures involving fingers. **B,** Open-palm technique following excision of skin and diseased palmar fascia. **C,** Two weeks following program of active flexion and extension exercises and daily warm-water soaks. **D,** Four months following open treatment of Dupuytren's disease, healing is complete and scar indistinguishable from *per primam* closure.

SECTION 13 DUPUYTREN'S CONTRACTURE

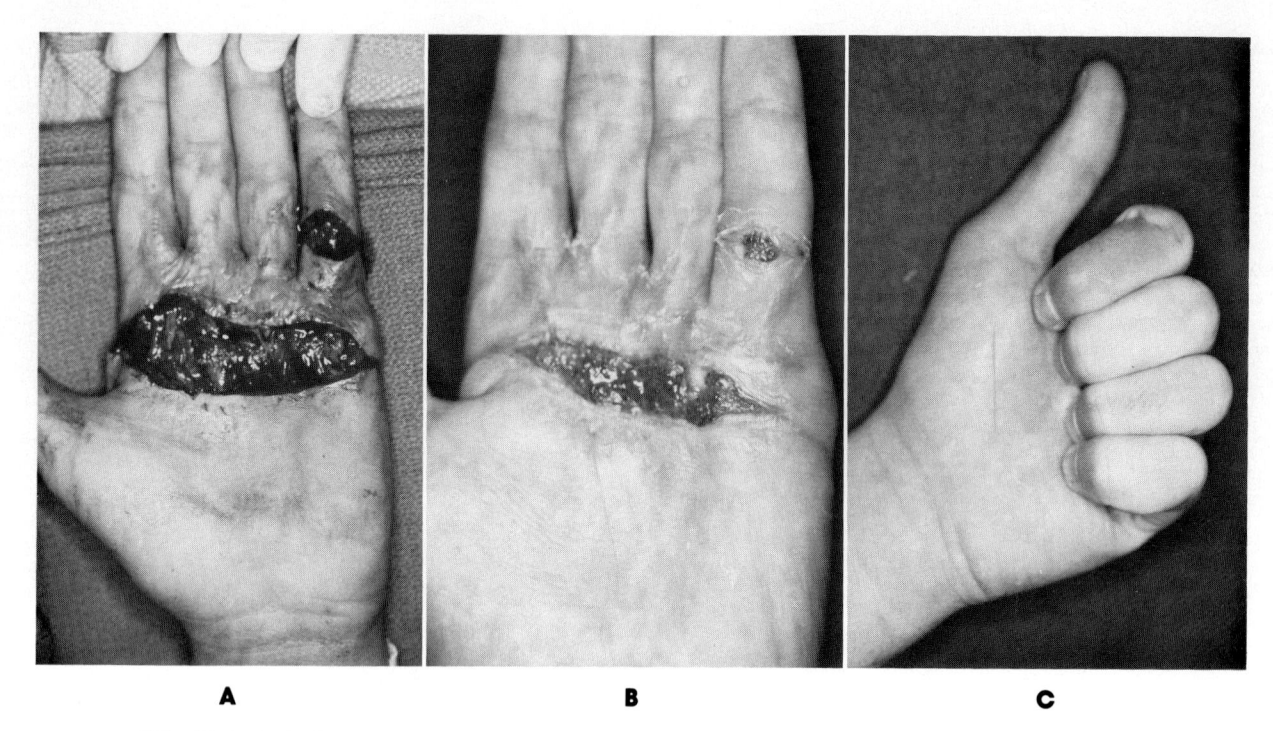

FIG. 49-2. A, A 47-year-old diabetic with necrotizing palmar fasciitis treated by wide excision of diseased skin and palmar fascia. After application of principles of McCash[12,13] open-palm technique, partial healing **(B)** and full range of motion **(C)** is seen at 6 weeks.

OTHER APPLICATIONS OF OPEN-PALM TECHNIQUE

The predominant application of the open-palm technique has been in the surgical management of Dupuytren's contracture. The same principle of treatment can be used effectively in other unrelated disease states involving palmar fascia. The hand of a 47-year-old securities analyst with diabetes mellitus and necrotizing palmar fasciitis was treated by wide excision of diseased skin and underlying fascia (Fig. 49-2, A). The principles of the open-palm technique were employed, and within 6 weeks the entire palm was healed and the range of motion full (Fig. 49-2, B and C).

SUMMARY

Use of the open-palm technique requires that the patient be wholeheartedly willing to cooperate in his or her own rehabilitation program. Without this cooperation, the benefits of early painless motion that the open-palm technique affords will be lost, and the result will be a stiff hand.

The most important aspect of this technique is that it affords free open drainage of blood and serious fluid in the early postoperative stages, eliminating the risk of hematoma formation. In addition, without tension along a suture line the early postoperative range of motion is painless, and rehabilitation progress is rapid.

The hand surgeon should be quite careful in selecting the well-motivated individual, predisposed to joint stiffness, in whom rapid mobilization is critical.

REFERENCES

1. Ariyan, S., and Krizek, T.J.: In defense of the open wound, Arch. Surg. **111**:293, 1976.
2. Beltran, J.E., Jimeno-Urban, F., and Yunta, A.: The open palm and digit technique in the treatment of Dupuytren's contracture, Hand **8**:73, 1976.
3. Briedis, J.: Dupuytren's contracture: lack of complications with the open palm technique, Br. J. Plast. Surg. **27**:218, 1974.
4. Dupuytren, G.: Permanent retraction of the fingers, produced by an affection of the palmar fascia, Lancet **2**:222, 1834.
5. Gillman, T., and Penn, J.: Reaction of granulation tissue in man to auto-Tiherschi, auto-dermal and humo-dermal pathology, Br. J. Plast. Surg. **6**:153, 1953.
6. Gonzalez, R.I.: Open fasciotomy and full thickness skin graft in the correction of digital flexion deformity. In Hueston, J.T., and Tubiana, R., editors: Dupuytren's disease, New York, 1974, Grune & Stratton, Inc.
7. Harrison, S.H., and Morris, A.: Dupuytren's contracture: the dorsal transposition flap, Hand **7**:145, 1975.

8. Howard, L.D., Jr.: Dupuytren's contracture: a guide for management, Clin. Orthop. **15**:118, 1959.
9. Hueston, J.T., and Tubiana, R., editors: Dupuytren's disease, New York, 1974, Grune & Stratton, Inc.
10. Kates, J., Burkhalter, W., and Mann, R.J.: Open palm open digit technique for Dupuytren's contracture, Presented at the Thirty-fourth Annual Meeting of American Society for Surgery of the Hand, San Francisco, 1979.
11. King, E.W., Bass, D.M., and Watson, H.K.: Treatment of Dupuytren's contracture by extensive fasciectomy through multiple Y-V–plasty incisions: short-term evaluation of 170 consecutive operations, J. Hand Surg. **4**:234, 1979.
12. McCash, C.R.: The open palm technique in Dupuytren's contracture, Br. J. Plast. Surg. **17**:271, 1964.
13. McCash, C.R.: The open palm technique in Dupuytren's contracture. In Hueston, J.T., and Tubiana, R., editors: Dupuytren's disease, New York, 1974, Grune & Stratton, Inc.
14. Matev, I.B.: Asymmetric Z plasty in the operative treatment of Dupuytren's contracture, Am. Dig. Orthop. Lit., first quarter, p. 11, 1970.
15. Moberg, E.: Three useful ways to avoid amputation in advanced Dupuytren's contracture, Orthop. Clin. North Am. **4**:1001, 1973.
16. Peacock, E.E., Jr.: Dupuytren's disease: controversial aspects of management, Clin. Plast. Surg. **3**:29, 1976.
17. Stone, M.M.: Open delayed suture for Dupuytren's contracture, Orthop. Rev. **7**:117, 1978.

Chapter 50 The proximal interphalangeal joint in Dupuytren's contracture

Thomas L. Greene

James W. Strickland

R. Fred Torstrick

Contracture of the proximal interphalangeal (PIP) joint of the finger is generally agreed to be the most difficult problem encountered in the surgical management of Dupuytren's disease. Several factors, including duration of the contracture, the type of palmar fascial involvement, shortening of the volar capsular structures, severity of contracture at the time of treatment, and the quality of the integument, may be responsible for the relatively high number of recurrent deformities following surgery. This chapter attempts to evaluate anatomic considerations, surgical techniques, and postoperative results and to indicate prognostic considerations based on the preoperative status of the affected PIP joint.

PATHOLOGIC ANATOMY

There exist several patterns of diseased fascia that can be responsible for contracture of the PIP joint.[5] The pretendinous band of the palmar fascia normally does not extend to the level of the PIP joint, whereas the pretendinous, or central, cord of diseases fascia often continues distally to insert about the flexor tendon sheath and bone over the middle phalanx (Fig. 50-1). The spiral cord, as its name implies, has a spiral course about the neurovascular bundle while passing from the palmar fascia into the digit. It usually arises from the pretendinous band, passing dorsal to the neurovascular bundle as it travels distally. While passing along the proximal

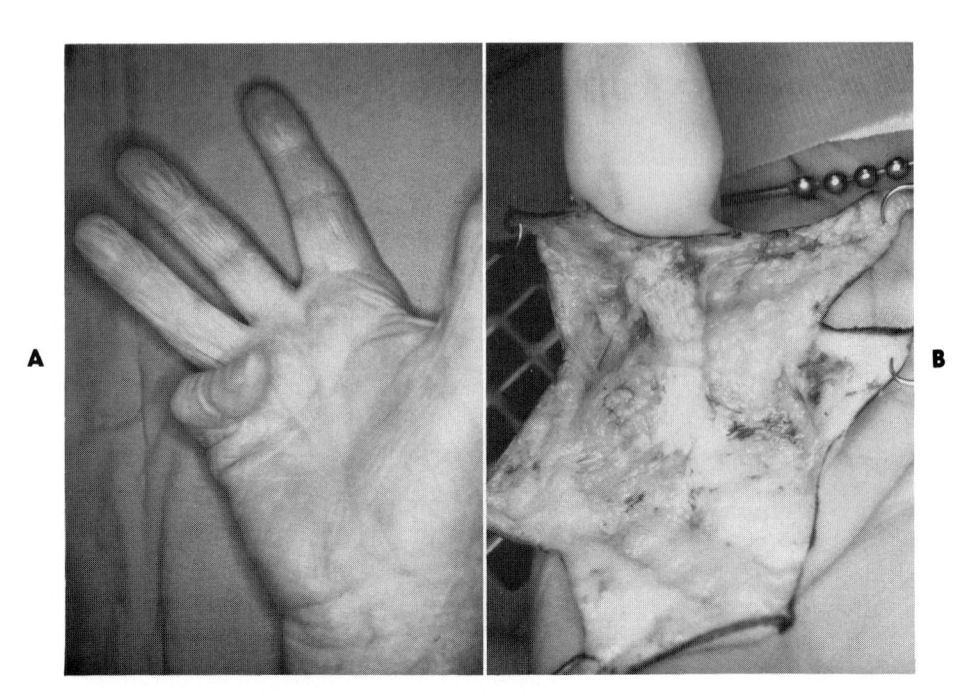

FIG. 50-1. A, Severe flexion deformity of PIP joint of small finger. **B,** Pretendinous cord of diseased fascia was responsible for this severe contracture.

phalanx, it again turns to lie volar to the digital nerve and artery to insert into Grayson's ligaments or the flexor tendon sheath over the middle phalanx. It is apparent that such a course renders the digital nerve and artery particularly susceptible to injury during the surgical dissection (Fig. 50-2).

Diseased fascia occasionally may be localized within the digit with an isolated cord arising from an intrinsic tendon, the volar plate of the metacarpophalangeal (MCP) joint, the deep transverse metacarpal ligament, or the base of the proximal phalanx (Fig. 50-3). The lateral digital sheet is a thin fascial structure normally lying between the lateral digital skin and the neurovascular bundles and passing to the volar and dorsal sides of the digit. Fibers of this sheet are also contributed by the natatory ligaments. This fascial sheet may form a cord that contracts the PIP joint, although it usually coexists with other contracting cords.

The volar plate of the PIP joint, anchored by its proximal extensions (the check-rein ligaments), may become shortened, often with concomitant shortening of the accessory collateral ligaments.[6]

In addition, the volar skin of the digit may be of poor quality because of direct involvement of the disease pro-

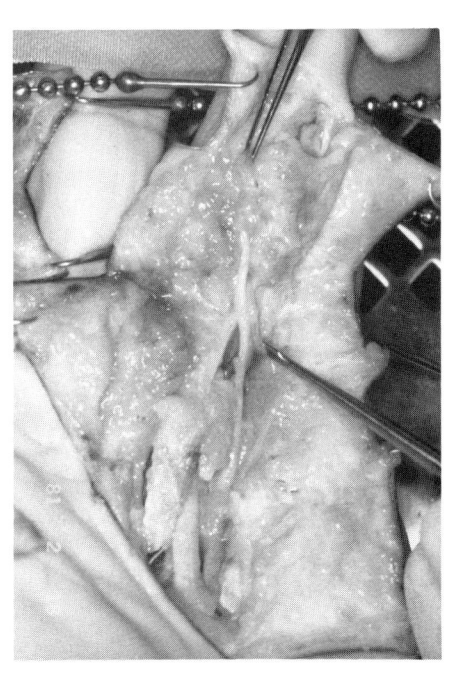

FIG. 50-2. Spiral cord, originating from pretendinous cord, is shown passing dorsal to neurovascular bundle (being held by retractor). It is volar to bundle again at PIP joint. Nerve has been displaced completely to midline of digit.

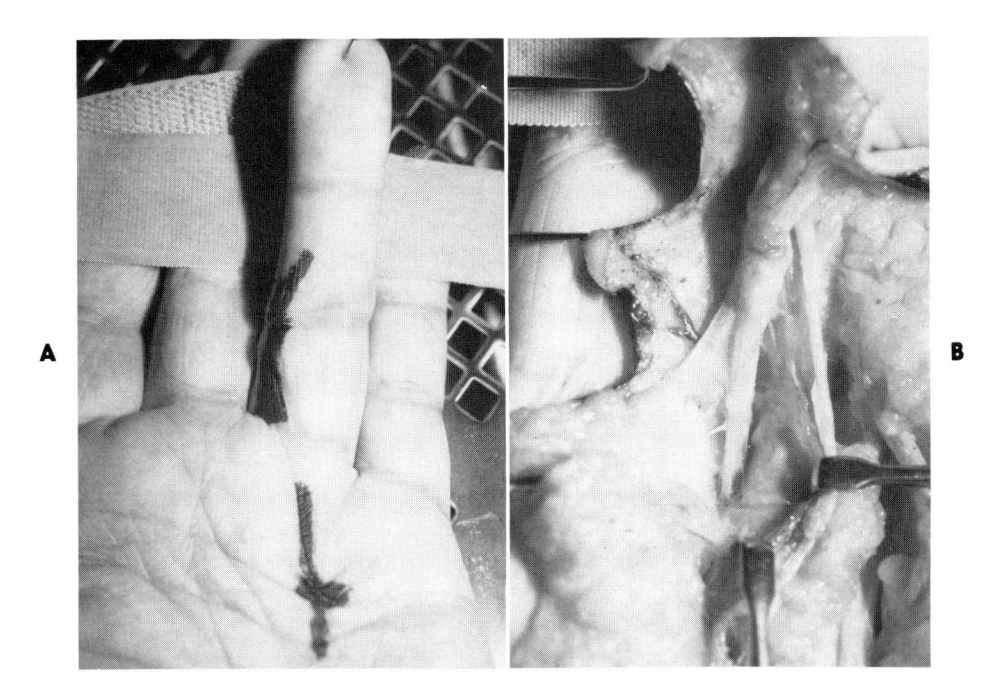

FIG. 50-3. A, Palpable pretendinous and digital cord of diseased fascia have been marked prior to skin incision. **B,** Flexion contracture of this PIP joint was caused solely by this digital cord. It originated from volar plate–deep transverse metacarpal ligament area deep within hand. It passed lateral and then volar to neurovascular bundle prior to inserting into flexor tendon sheath over middle phalanx.

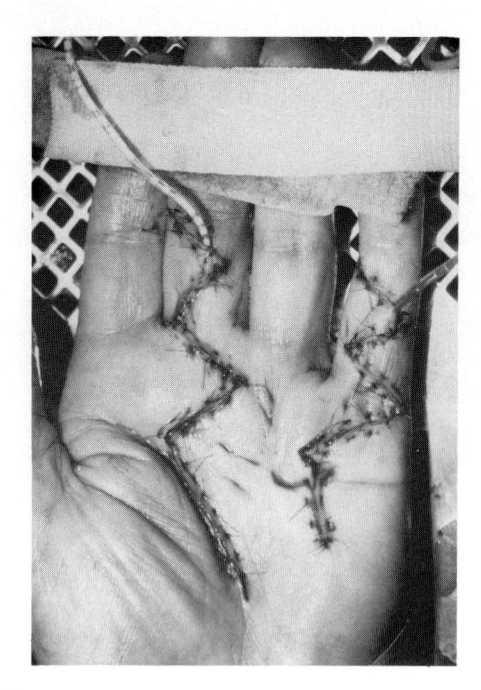

FIG. 50-4. Multiple zigzag incisions are used to identify and excise diseased palmar fascia and its extensions. Small suction drains made from 19-gauge intravenous catheters are used beneath each incision.

cess. Previous surgical scars also may lead to thin, firmly adherent skin, which can be a contracting influence at the PIP joint.

TREATMENT

The goal of treatment at the PIP joint is complete release of the flexion contracture and prevention of recurrence. Although this ideal is not always possible, every effort should be made to provide and maintain maximal correction.

A meticulous identification and excision of the offending fascial cords must be undertaken. We usually prefer short zigzag incisions centered over the palpable cords (Fig. 50-4). The flaps are thin enough to ensure removal of diseased fascia from the overlying skin. It is unusual to see flap necrosis if one is careful not to damage the base of the flap. Once all obviously diseased fascia is removed, the PIP joint frequently will have full passive extension. If it does not, attention must be directed to the volar plate, where the check-rein ligaments and volar fibers of the collateral ligaments are sequentially released until full passive extension is obtained.[7] On occasion it may be necessary to section the flexor sheath or perform a flexor tenolysis to obtain full motion.

After completion of fascial excision and joint release the tourniquet should be deflated to assess the vascularity of the digit, which may have been compromised by the rapid extension of the digit, particularly when the flexion contracture has been severe and long standing. If digital circulation is not adequate, it may be necessary to accept a less extended position to ensure viability of the distal aspect of the finger. Postoperative splinting may regain this loss of correction, but the prognosis for persistent deformity is probably worse.

Once the contracture has been corrected, an assessment of wound closure must be made. Usually the incisions are readily closed. A Y-V–plasty of the zigzag incision may facilitate closure if additional midline skin is needed.[2] For severe deformities or when extensively involved skin is excised, full-thickness skin graft coverage may be required.[1] Closure of the wounds over small suction drains minimizes the risk of hematoma formation with its attendant complications.[4] Active range of motion exercises are begun at 1 week postoperatively, alternating with static splinting of the involved joint in the corrected position. Passive range of motion is added at 2 weeks if needed. Splinting continues, at least part-time, for 3 to 6 months postoperatively.

RESULTS

Even though it is almost always possible to obtain correction of the PIP joint contracture at the operating table, correction has been more difficult to maintain, particularly long range (over 5 years).

In our experience one can expect to obtain initial correction by means of fascial excision and skin closure, including Z-plasty, Y-V–flap advancement, or skin graft, in 72% of PIP joints. The remaining 28% of joints will require a more extensive release of soft tissues, as previously described.

The ability to obtain long-term correction of flexion contractures of the PIP joints depends on many variables. The degree of initial contracture, age of the patient, number of digits involved, and number of joints affected all influence the long-term result. Legge and McFarlane[3] have found a flexion contracture of the metacarpophalangeal (MCP) joint of the small finger to be prejudicial to long-term correction of concomitant PIP joint contractures of that finger.

A retrospective review of the short- and long-term postoperative performance of the PIP joint was carried out by Torstrick, Hartwig, and Strickland, and the results are summarized in Tables 50-1 and 50-2.

Although those joints with the greatest preoperative contracture had the highest percentage of short-term improvement after fasciectomy, their long-term maintenance of this correction was the poorest. Conversely, those joints with the least preoperative contracture had a much less impressive short-term improvement but tended to not deteriorate on long-term analysis. From this study it would appear that PIP joints with an initial

Table 50-1. PIP joint contracture in Dupuytren's disease after fasciectomy

	Group A (0 to 29 degrees)	Group B (30 to 59 degrees)	Group C (60 degrees or more)	Total
Short-term (<1 year) results compared with preoperative status				
Number of joints	34	64	61	159
Improved	8	40	54	102
Percent of group	23	63	89	64
Average change (degrees)	+17	+28.4	+41.3	+34.3
Same (± 10 degrees)	19	22	4	45
Percent of group	56	34	6	28
Worse	7	2	3	12
Percent of group	21	3	5	8
Average change (degrees)	−25.7	−15.0	−16.7	−21.7
Long-term (>5 years) compared with short-term results				
Number of joints	6	14	12	32
Improved	1	0	1	2
Percent of group	16		8	6
Average change (degrees)	+15		+25	+20
Same (± 10 degrees)	5	11	5	21
Percent of group	84	79	42	66
Worse	0	3	6	9
Percent of group		21	50	28
Average change (degrees)		−46.6	−37.5	−40.5

Table 50-2. PIP joint contracture in Dupuytren's disease after fasciectomy

	Group A (0 to 29 degrees)	Group B (30 to 59 degrees)	Group C (60 degrees or more)	Total
Short-term (<1 year) results				
Number of joints	34	64	61	159
Average preoperative contracture (degrees)	17.1	43.5	70.5	48.2
Average postoperative contracture (degrees)	17.0	25.8	34.8	27.4
Average improvement				
Percent	+0.6	+40.7	+50.6	+43.2
Degrees	+0.1	+17.7	+35.7	+20.8
Long-term (> 5 years) results				
Number of joints	6	14	12	32
Average preoperative contracture (degrees)	20.0	40.0	66.7	46.3
Average short-term contracture (degrees)	11.7	18.9	30.4	21.9
Average long-term contracture (degrees)	7.5	27.5	47.9	31.4
Average long-term improvement from preoperative status				
Percent	+62.5	+31	+28	+32.2
Degrees	+12.5	+12.5	+18.8	+14.9
Average change from short-term results				
Percent	+35.9	−46	−58	−43.4
Degrees	+4.2	−8.6	−17.5	−9.5

contracture of 30 degrees or less can be expected to retain their postoperative correction, whereas 21% of those with a 30- to 60-degree contracture and 50% of those with a beginning deformity of 60 degrees or more will deteriorate significantly with time.

Although surgery for minimally contracted joints has a limited chance for complete correction, there is little tendency for these joints to worsen with time. Lasting correction of severe contractures has met with much less success. Surgical treatment of PIP joint contracture should be performed at the earliest possible time, possibly even in the presence of digital disease without contracture.

SUMMARY

The PIP joint contracture remains the most difficult problem in the care of Dupuytren's disease. The results continue to be disappointing in many cases, indicating not only our inability to correct deformities surgically but also our lack of understanding of the basic disease process. For the present, close attention to the pathologic anatomy, operative techniques, and postoperative rehabilitation offers the best chances for optimizing the results of surgery.

REFERENCES

1. Hueston, J.T.: Skin replacement in Dupuytren's contracture. In Hueston, J.T., and Tubiana, R., editors: Dupuytren's disease, ed. 2, New York, 1974, Grune & Stratton, Inc.
2. King, E.W., Bass, D.M., and Watson, H.K.: Treatment of Dupuytren's contracture by extensive fasciectomy through multiple Y-V–plasty incisions: short term evaluation of 170 consecutive operations, J. Hand. Surg. **4**:234, 1979.
3. Legge, M.B., and McFarlane, R.M.: Prediction of results of treatment of Dupuytren's disease, J. Hand Surg. **5**:607, 1980.
4. McFarlane, R.M.: Use of continuous suction after operation for Dupuytren's contracture, Br. J. Plast. Surg. **11**:301, 1959.
5. McFarlane, R.M.: Patterns of the diseased fascia in the fingers in Dupuytren's contracture: displacement of the neurovascular bundle, Plast. Reconstr. Surg. **54**:31, 1974.
6. McFarlane, R.M., and Jamieson, W.B.: Dupuytren's contracture, the management of 100 patients, J. Bone Joint Surg. **48A**:1095, 1966.
7. Watson, H.K., Johnson, T.R., and Light, T.: Checkrein resection for flexion contracture of the middle joint, J. Hand Surg. **4**:67, 1979.

Index

A

Abdominal pedicle flaps, 11
  in extensor tendon problems, 47, 48
  in first web space contracture, 37
Abrasion injuries of hand, 3-9
  avulsion injuries with, 3, 4
  dicing, 5
  extent and depth of damage in, 3, 8
  in rope burns, 6
  slicing, 7
Acid-fast disease in hand, 163-164
Acupuncture in painful neuroma, 321
Addiction to drugs in pain problems, 307, 322
Adduction contracture of first web space, 28-37
Adductor muscles; see specific muscles
Adhesions, tendon-bone
  biologic basis of, 140-141
  of extensor tendons, 141-142, 144, 313, 315, 318
  of flexor tendons, 78, 81-82, 83, 90-91, 140-141, 142, 143, 313, 318
  after phalangeal fractures, 140-141
  pharmacologic control of, 78
  tenolysis of, 140-144, 312-318; see also Tenolysis
Age of patients
  in boutonniere deformity and results of surgical treatment, 65-66
  in phalangeal fractures affecting digital function, 127, 141
Allen test in ulnar artery thrombosis, 255, 260, 263
Aminosalicylic acid in hand infections, 147
Amputation
  surgical
    in Dupuytren's contractures, 399, 400, 409
    in gangrene, 162
    indications for, 243
    in neglected infections, 149, 150
  traumatic
    flexor tendon problems in, 90-91
    of forearm, 267, 270
    of hand at wrist level, 266
    of index finger, 40-42, 248-250
    of little finger, 268
    local rotation flaps for, 40-42
    painful neuroma after, 319, 321, 325, 327, 328, 330
    and replantation, 243-252, 264-271; see also Replantation
    shearing type of, 264
    split-thickness skin grafts for, 12, 13, 40
    of thumb, 12, 16-17, 264-265, 269
    toe-to-hand transplants in, 12, 16-17, 20
    traction avulsion of upper extremity, 264-271
Analgesia
  in neuroma, transcutaneous electric stimulation for, 320-321, 325
  in reflex sympathetic dystrophy, 307
  in tenolysis, 98, 312-318
    postoperative, 312, 314, 317-318

Anastomosis, microvascular, in replantation; see Replantation
Anesthesia
  allowing patient participation
    in capsulotomy, 143
    in tenolysis, 98, 142, 143, 312-318
    in tenosynovectomy for flexor tenosynovitis, 203
  in painful neuroma, 321, 325
Annular pulleys of flexor tendons, 73, 74, 94-102
  anatomy of, 94, 96
  in digitorum profundus flexor tendon laceration, 87-88, 92-93
  key locations of, 98, 100, 102
  reconstruction of, 99, 100
  in tenolysis, 313-314
  in ulnar nerve palsy, 293, 296
Antibiotic therapy in hand infections, 157
  in human bites, 161
  in necrotizing fasciitis, 152
  in neglected infections, 149, 150
  in prosthesis implantation, 152
  in tenosynovitis, 158
Antituberculotic drug therapy, 147, 163, 164
Arteriography in ulnar artery thrombosis, 256, 257, 258, 260, 263
Arthritis
  boutonniere deformity in, 57, 60, 62, 205-209, 232, 233, 234, 236, 237
  first web space contracture in, 28
  mutilans, 207
  osteoarthritis, 173, 181, 183-188, 352, 377
  posttraumatic, of proximal interphalangeal joint, 112, 173-182
  psoriatic, 207
  rheumatoid, 157, 197-240; see also Rheumatoid arthritis
  silicone replacement arthroplasty in, 154-155, 173-188, 225-232
  tuberculous, 147, 148
  wrist arthrodesis in, 225-232, 336, 337, 339, 352, 353, 354
Arthrodesis
  capitate-hamate-lunate-triquetral, 336-337
  capitate-lunate, 335, 336
  in caput ulnae syndrome, 199, 202
  carpometacarpal, 335, 336, 337
    in chronic dislocation, 194
    for lateral pinch restoration after spinal cord injury, 278, 281
  in Dupuytren's contractures, 400, 406
  hamate-triquetral, 335, 337
  of interphalangeal joint of thumb
    in boutonniere deformity, 206, 207, 236
    for lateral pinch restoration after spinal cord injury, 279
    in swan-neck deformity, 211
    in ulnar nerve palsy, 293
  in Kienböck's disease, 337
  lunate-radial, 335, 337
  lunate-triquetral, 337

INDEX

Arthrodesis—cont'd
  of metacarpophalangeal joint of thumb
    in boutonniere deformity, 206, 207, 236
    in swan-neck deformity, 211
  in mycobacterial infections, 147
  of proximal interphalangeal joints
    posttraumatic, 38
    in rheumatoid arthritis, 234-236
  scaphocapitate-lunate, 336
  in scaphoid rotary subluxation, 336, 348
  scapholunate, 337
  in scapholunate dissociation, 348
  scapholunate-radial, 335, 337
  scaphoradial, 337
  trapeziometacarpal, 184
  triscaphe, 335, 336
  of wrist, 352-354
    in arthritis, 225-232, 336, 337, 339, 352, 353, 354
    complications of, 339
    contraindications to, 337-338
    indications for, 336, 337
    limited, 335-340
    position of, 352-353, 354
    postoperative management of, 338-339
    in radial clubhand, 358, 364
    technique of, 338, 353-354
Arthroplasty
  in caput ulnae syndrome, 199, 202
  of carpometacarpal joint in boutonniere deformity, 207-209
  of metacarpophalangeal joint
    in boutonniere deformity, 207
    in rheumatoid arthritis, 226-239
  in scaphoid fractures, 106
  silicone in; *see* Silicone implantation
  in swan-neck thumb deformity, 209-211, 212
  in trapeziometacarpal osteoarthritis, 183-188
    indications for, 185
    techniques of, 185
    with silicone replacement, 187
    without silicone replacement, 185-187
  of wrist, 352, 354
    in rheumatoid arthritis, 225-226, 227
Arthrosis, degenerative, of metacarpotrapezial joint, 169
Articulations, 167-195; *see also* specific joints
Asynchronous finger flexion in ulnar nerve palsy, 293-297
Atherosclerotic disease, hand infections in, 152
Avulsion injuries; *see also* Amputation, traumatic
  abrasion injuries with, 3, 4
  of nail matrix, 27
  of peripheral nerves
    group fascicular repair of, 382
    interfascicular nerve grafting of, 384
    nerve regeneration after, 380
  shearing amputation in, 264
  split-thickness skin grafts in, 4, 12, 13
  in traction avulsion amputations, 264-271
Axon(s) of peripheral nerves
  anatomy of, 379
  injury and regeneration of, 369, 380
Axonotmesis, 369

B

Bacterial infections, 147-159, 161-165
  gangrene in, 162
  in human bites of hand, 161

Bed of fingernails, 22
  injuries to, 22-24, 25
Bennett's fracture, 107-108, 111, 113
  osteoarthritis after, 185
  reduction of, 107-108
Biofeedback techniques in ulnar artery thrombosis, 260, 262
Biomechanical aspects
  of thumb axis joints, 169-172
  of wrist problems, 349-351
Bites
  dog, infection and loss of flexor tendon function after, 43
  human, hand infections in, 153, 161
  snake, toe-to-hand transplant after, 20
Blast injury in wrist region, extensor tendon problems in, 48
Blood vessels, 240-241; *see also* specific vessels
  of extensor pollicis longus tendon, 51-52
  of flexor tendons, 73, 94, 96
  in phalangeal fractures, injuries of, 130-131, 132
  of scaphoid, 105
  scoring system for assessment of, 247
  in traction avulsion amputations of upper extremity, 264-271
  in ulnar artery thrombosis, 253-263
  vein grafts in; *see* Vein grafts
Blowout injuries of peripheral nerves, repair of, 383, 384
Bone(s), 103-144
  fractures of; *see* Fractures and dislocations
  grafts with; *see* Bone grafts
  scoring system for assessment of, in digital injuries, 247
  tendon adhesion to, 140-144; *see also* Adhesions, tendon-bone
Bone grafts, 14
  iliac, 106, 353, 354
  in radial clubhand, 357, 358
  in scaphoid fracture, 106
  in ulnar nerve palsy, 294
  in wrist arthrodesis, 338, 339, 353, 354
Boutonniere deformity, 54-69
  anatomy of, 54-55, 62
  articular contractures in, 57, 59-60
  in Dupuytren's contractures, 405
  initial stage of, 57-59, 60
  pathogenesis of, 55-57
  posttraumatic, 38, 56, 57, 62, 66
  reducible, 57, 59, 60
  retinacular contractures in, 57, 59, 60, 405
  in rheumatoid arthritis, 57, 60, 62, 205-209, 232, 233, 234, 236, 237
  splinting in treatment of, 57, 59, 60, 64, 66-67
  surgical correction of, 57-60, 62-68, 207-209
    indications for, 64
    procedure in, 64
    results of, 64-68
Bouvier maneuver in ulnar nerve palsy, 293, 294
Bowler's thumb, 322
Boxer's fracture, 122-124
Brachial artery repair in traction avulsion amputation of forearm, 267, 270
Brachioradialis tendon transfers, 301
  after spinal cord injuries, 278, 279, 281, 283
Brand tendon transfer in ulnar nerve palsy, 296-297
Buerger's disease, 152
Bunnel safety-pin splint in boutonniere deformity, 67
Bupivacaine
  in postoperative pain after tenolysis, 312, 314, 317-318
  in reflex sympathetic dystrophy, 308
Burns
  boutonniere deformity from, 57, 60, 62

Burns—cont'd
　first web space contracture from, 28, 31
　local rotation flaps for, 38-42
　microvascular groin flap for, 18

C

Capener splint therapy in ulnar nerve palsy, 287, 291
Capitate in wrist arthrodesis, 335-337, 338, 339
　capitate-hamate-lunate-triquetral, 336-337
　capitate-lunate, 335, 336
　scaphocapitate-lunate, 336
Capsuloplasty of metacarpophalangeal joint in ulnar nerve palsy, Zancolli volar plate and, 293, 294-295
Capsulotomy after phalangeal fractures, 141, 143, 144
Caput ulnae syndrome, 199-202, 225, 232
Carbamazepine in painful neuroma, 320
Carpal bones; *see* specific bones
Carpal tunnel syndrome
　after Colles' fracture, 305, 309
　in flexor tenosynovitis at wrist, 203-204
　in rheumatoid arthritis, 203-204, 232
　surgical treatment of, 232, 322
Carpectomy, proximal row
　in caput ulnae syndrome, 201, 202
　in rheumatoid arthritis of wrist, 225
Carpi radialis
　brevis extensor muscle, 169, 190
　brevis extensor tendon transfer, 50
　　in spinal cord injury, 276, 278
　　in ulnar nerve palsy, 296-297
　flexor muscle, 169, 190
　flexor tendon transfer, 50
　longus extensor muscle, 169, 190
　longus extensor tendon transfer, 202
　　in caput ulnae syndrome, 202
　　in pollicis longus extensor tendon rupture, 52
　　in rheumatoid arthritis of wrist, 222, 225
　　in spinal cord injury, 279, 281, 283
　　in ulnar nerve palsy, 296-297
Carpi ulnaris
　extensor muscle, 190
　　in fifth metacarpal-hamate joint fractures, 109, 110
　extensor tendon
　　in caput ulnae syndrome, 199, 201, 202
　　repair of injuries to, 47-50
　　in rheumatoid arthritis of wrist, 221, 222, 225
　　tenosynovitis of, 199
　flexor muscle, 190
　flexor tendon transfer to wrist extensor, 50
Carpometacaral (CMC) joint
　anatomy of, 189-190
　arthritis of, 28
　arthrodesis of, 194, 335, 336, 337
　　for lateral pinch restoration after spinal cord injuries, 278, 281
　arthroplasty of, in boutonniere deformity, 207-209
　collapse of, in boutonniere deformity, 206, 207-209, 236
　dislocations and fracture-dislocations of, 189-195
　　acute dislocation of, 191-193
　　chronic dislocation of, 194
　　reduction of, 192-194
Carpus; *see* Wrist
Cartilage damage in proximal interphalangeal joint in Dupuytren's contractures, 406
Cast immobilization
　in Bennett's fractures, 107-108

Cast immobilization—cont'd
　in boutonniere deformity, 67
　in carpometacarpal dislocation, 192
　in metacarpal fractures, 120, 122, 124, 125
　in phalangeal fractures, digital performance after, 133, 135-137, 140
　of proximal interphalangeal joint fractures, 112-113
　in radial clubhand, 360, 364
　in scaphoid fracture, 105-106
　in scapholunate dissociation, 347
　in wrist arthrodesis, 338-339, 354
Causalgia, 305
Cell body of peripheral nerves
　anatomy of, 379
　in nerve regeneration, 380
Cellulitis, synergistic necrotizing, 162
Centralization of ulna in radial clubhand, 357-358, 359-360, 361, 364
Cerebrovascular accidents, reflex sympathetic dystrophy after, 305
Cervical spinal cord, 275-284
　eighth level of, 275-276, 282
　fifth level of, 275, 276
　injury of, restoration of lateral pinch after, 275-284
　muscles innervated by, 275, 276
　seventh level of, 275, 281-282, 283-284
　sixth level of, 275, 276-281, 283-284
Check-rein ligaments
　in boutonniere deformity, 60
　in phalangeal fractures, 143
Chest pedicle flap
　in abrasion injuries, 7, 8
　in first web space contracture, 37
Chlordiazepoxide in reflex sympathetic dystrophy, 307
Chlorpromazine in reflex sympathetic dystrophy, 307
Chordotomy, anterolateral, in painful neuroma, 322
Cigarette smoking and ulnar artery thrombosis, 262
Cineradiographic studies
　of rheumatoid wrist, 221
　in scapholunate dissociation, 345, 347
Claw hand deformity in ulnar nerve palsy, 285, 289, 290, 291
　simple and complicated, 293
　surgical correction of, 291, 293-294, 295
Clubhand, radial, 355-365
　radius replacement in, 357
　recurrence of, 360, 361
　soft tissue release in, 357, 364
　tendon transfers in, 360, 361, 364
　thumb reconstruction in, 360-361
　timing of treatments for, 359-360, 361, 364
　treatment objectives in, 355-357
　ulna centralization in, 357-358, 359-360, 361, 364
　ulnar osteotomy in, 357
　ulnar-oriented, 355, 356, 359
　wrist arthrodesis in, 358, 364
CMC joint; *see* Carpometacarpal (CMC) joint
Cold tolerance tests
　in painful neuroma, 319
　in ulnar artery thrombosis, 253, 254-255, 257
Collagen diseases, boutonniere deformity in, 57, 60
Colles' fractures
　pollicis longus extensor tendon rupture in, 51, 52
　reflex sympathetic dystrophy in, 305, 309
　tenolysis after, 316
Comminuted phalangeal fractures, digital performance after, 129, 130, 133, 135, 138, 144

INDEX

Compression
  of median nerve; see Carpal tunnel syndrome
  of ulnar nerve, 374-378
Concertina deformity, 341
Congenital disorders
  carpal bone fusion, 335
  cubitus valgus, 374
  radial clubhand, 355-365
  scaphoid bipartition, 106
Contractures
  in boutonniere deformity, 57, 59-60, 405
  in burns, microvascular groin flap in, 18
  Dupuytren's, 387-418; see also Dupuytren's contracture
  of first web space, 28-37
    causes of, 28
    cross-arm flap in, 35-37
    dorsal rotation flap in, 32-35
    four-flap Z-plasty in, 30-31
    free-skin grafting in, 31-32
    remote pedicle flaps in, 35-37
    simple Z-plasty for, 29
    splinting programs for, 28-29, 35, 37
  of little finger, persistent, in Dupuytren's contracture, 389-398
  of proximal interphalangeal joint in Dupuytren's contracture, 414-418
  of split-thickness skin grafts, 10
  Volkmann's, in ulnar nerve palsy, 296, 297
Corticosteroid therapy; see Steroid therapy
Costs
  of digital salvage, 250-251
  of phalangeal fracture treatment, 127
  of surgical management of rheumatoid hand, 224, 239
Cross-arm flaps, 11
  in Dupuytren's contracture, 405
  in first web space contracture, 35-37
Cross-finger flaps, 11
Cruciate pulleys of flexor tendons, 73, 74
  anatomy of, 94, 96
  reconstruction of, 100
  resection of, 97
  in surgical exploration of flexor system, 97-98
Crumpling deformity, 341
Crushing injuries
  of fingernails, 25
  first web space contracture in, 28, 33, 37
  fractures in, 126, 130
  local rotation flaps for digital defects in, 38-39
  painful neuroma after, surgical treatment of, 325, 327, 330
  patient neglect of, 150
  of peripheral nerves
    interfascicular nerve grafting in, 384
    nerve regeneration after, 380
  of proximal interphalangeal joint, 38, 173, 176, 178
  reflex sympathetic dystrophy after, 305
  split-thickness skin grafts for reconstructive procedures in, 12
Cubitus valgus deformity, congenital, 374
Cultures for diagnosis of hand infections, 152, 157, 161, 163

D

Debridement
  in fungal infections, 160
  in human bite infections, 161
  in mycobacterial infections, 147
  in necrotizing fasciitis, 152
  in neglected infections, 149

Debridement—cont'd
  in tenosynovitis, 159
Decompression of ulnar nerve, 375-378
Deformities
  boutonniere, 54-69; see also Boutonniere deformity
  of carpal bones, congenital fusion of, 335
  concertina, 341
  crumpling, 341
  cubitus valgus, 374
  eggcup, of metacarpophalangeal joints, 232
  mallet, 405-406
  radial clubhand, 355-365
  of scaphoid, congenital bipartition of, 106
  swan-neck, 209-211, 212-214; see also Swan-neck deformity
  in ulnar nerve palsy, 288, 290-291
    claw hand as, 285, 289, 290, 291, 293-294, 295
    surgical treatment of, 293-297
  of wrist, static and dynamic forces in, 349-351
  zigzag, 341
Degenerative diseases
  of thumb, 155, 169-172
  of wrist, arthrodesis in, 336, 337, 339
Deltopectoral flap, 11, 16-17
Diabetes mellitus, hand infections in, 151, 152
Diazepam
  in reflex sympathetic dystrophy, 307
  in tenolysis, 313
Dicing injuries, 5
Digit(s); see Finger(s)
Digital artery
  injuries of
    in Dupuytren's contracture surgery, 403, 415
    in traction avulsion amputations, repair of, 264-265, 268, 269, 270
  transverse communicating branches of, 74, 94, 96
Digital nerve injuries, 90, 305
  in Dupuytren's contracture surgery, 402, 403, 415
  epineurial repair of, 382
  fascicular repair of, 383
  interfascicular nerve grafting of, 383
Digiti minimi extensor tendon
  function after injury of, 49
  transfer of
    in hand reconstruction, 301
    in ulnar nerve palsy, 289, 296
Digitorum communis extensor tendon
  adhesion of, after phalangeal fractures, 140-141
  reestablishing function of, in hand reconstruction, 301
  tendon grafts into, 49
  tenodesis of, after spinal cord injury, 279
Digitorum profundus flexor tendon, 74, 75, 96
  adhesion of
    after phalangeal fractures, 140-141, 142
    tenolysis in, 81, 90-91, 140-141, 142
  bowstringing of, 76
  laceration of
    in phalangeal fractures, digital performance after, 131
    reconstruction procedure in, 77, 87-88, 92-93, 301
  in quadraregia syndrome, 301-302
  ruptured at wrist in rheumatoid arthritis, 204
  zone I injuries of, 87-88
  zone II injuries of, 90-93
Digitorum superficialis flexor tendon, 74, 96
  adhesion of
    after phalangeal fractures, 140-141
    tenolysis in, 81, 141, 142

Digitorum superficialis flexor tendon—cont'd
  in boutonniere deformity, 62
  free tendon grafting with, 79
  in phalangeal fractures, injuries of, digital performance after, 131
  ruptured at wrist in rheumatoid arthritis, 204
  surgical repair of, 75, 77
  transfer of, 50, 79, 301
    in radial clubhand, 360, 361
    in ulnar nerve palsy, 289, 296
  zone II injuries of, 90-93
DIP joint; see Distal interphalangeal (DIP) joint
Dislocations; see Fractures and dislocations
Dissociation, scapholunate, 216-218, 222, 225, 341-348, 350
Distal interphalangeal (DIP) joint
  contracture of little finger at, 393, 397
  fractures of, digital performance after, 128
  hyperextension of
    in boutonniere deformity, 54-69
    in little finger, 393, 398
  in rheumatoid arthritis, 233, 234
Distant pedicle flaps
  in abrasion injuries, 7, 8
  advantages and disadvantages of, 11, 16
  in Dupuytren's contractures, 405
  in extensor tendon problems, 47, 48
  in first web space contracture, 35-37
Dog bite complications, digital rotation flap in, 43
Doppler mapping in ulnar artery thrombosis, 258, 260
Dorsal rotation flap in first web space contracture, 32-35
Dorsalis pedis flap, 19
Drainage of hand infections, 157
  in neglected infections, 149
  in tenosynovitis, 158
Drug therapy; see also specific drugs
  for adhesion control during tendon healing, 78
  antibiotic; see Antibiotic therapy in hand infections
  antituberculotic, 147, 163, 164
  hand infections related to, 157, 160
  for pain
    addiction to, 307, 322
    in capsulotomy, 143
    in flexor tenosynovitis of fingers, 203
    in neuroma, 320, 321, 325, 329
    in reflex sympathetic dystrophy, 307, 308
    in tenolysis, 98, 142, 143, 312-318
    in tenosynovectomy, 203
    in trapeziometacarpal osteoarthritis, 183
  steroid; see Steroid therapy
  in ulnar artery thrombosis, 253, 260
Drummer boy's palsy, 52
Duchenne's sign in ulnar nerve palsy, 290
Dupuytren's contracture, 387-418
  capsular and ligamentous contractures in, 405-406
  digital artery injury in surgery for, 403, 415
  digital nerve injury in surgery for, 402, 403, 415
  fasciectomy in, 406, 407-408, 416-418
    with multiple Y-V–plasty incisions, 399-401
  flexor tendon contractures in, 405
  hematoma in, postoperative, 402-403, 409, 410, 412, 416
  intertrigo in, 402
  of little finger, 406, 416
    persistent, 389-398
    treatment of, 397-398
  mallet deformity in, 405-406
  open-palm technique in treatment of, 403, 409-413

Dupuytren's contracture—cont'd
  palmar fasciitis in, 402, 412
  postoperative care in, 398, 400, 401, 402-403, 407-408, 409-410, 412
  problems of, 402-408
  proximal interphalangeal joint in, 389-393, 398, 405, 414-418
    cartilage damage of, 406
    treatment of, 416-418
  recurrence of, 399, 406-407, 416-418
  skin contracture and shortage in, 404-405
  wound healing in, postoperative, 403, 409, 410, 411, 416
Dupuytren's open-palm technique, 409-410
Dystrophy, reflex sympathetic, 305-311

E

Eggcup deformity of metacarpophalangeal joints, 232
Eikenella corrodens, 159, 161
Elbow
  dislocation of, 374, 377
  innervation of muscles of, 275, 276
  traction avulsion amputation of forearm at, 267, 270
  ulnar neuropathy at, 374-378
Electric stimulation
  after peripheral nerve repair, 384
  in neuroma-in-continuity evaluation, 370-373
  transcutaneous
    in painful neuroma, 320-321, 325
    in reflex sympathetic dystrophy, 307
Electromyography
  in ulnar artery thrombosis, 255-257
  in ulnar neuropathy, 375
Endoneurium, anatomy of, 379
Enterobacteriaceae infections, 152
Epicondylectomy in ulnar neuropathy, 376-377
Epinephrine in painful neuroma, 321
Epineurial repair of peripheral nerves, 381-382
Epineurium of peripheral nerves
  anatomy of, 380
  in repair procedures, 381-382
Escherichia coli infection, gangrene in, 162
Ethambutol in hand infections, 164
Exercise programs
  after carpometacarpal dislocation, 192
  postoperative
    in boutonniere deformity, 59, 60
    in caput ulnae syndrome, 202
    in Dupuytren's contractures, 400, 401, 403, 405, 409, 410, 411, 412, 416
    in flexor tendon problems, 78, 82, 88, 90-91, 203
    in painful neuroma, 322
    patient compliance with, 90-91, 128, 141, 143, 144
    in phalangeal fractures, 135-137, 140, 143, 144
    in silicone implant arthroplasty, 176
    in tenolysis, 312, 314-318
    in tenosynovitis, 158, 159, 203
    in wrist arthrodesis, 339, 354
  in reflex sympathetic dystrophy, 307
  in ulnar nerve palsy, 287
Extension-block splint in proximal interphalangeal joint fractures, 112-113
Extensor hood of fingers, anatomy of, 54
Extensor tendon problems, 45-69; see also specific tendons
  in abrasion injuries, 8
  adhesion to bones of, 141-142, 144, 313, 315, 318
  artificial silicone rubber tendons in, 50
  in boutonniere deformity, 54-69

Extensor tendon problems—cont'd
  direct repair of, 47, 48, 52
  in fractures, 50, 51-52, 131, 139, 141-142, 144
    digital performance after, 131, 139, 144
  and spontaneous regeneration in, 47, 48
  tendon grafts in, 47-50, 52, 202
  tenolysis in, 141-142, 144, 313, 315, 318
  tenosynovitis in rheumatoid arthritis, 199
  of wrist and fingers, 47-50
Extrinsic test in ulnar nerve palsy for classification of claw hand deformity, 293, 294

F

Fascicular repair of peripheral nerves, 381, 382-383
Fasciculus of peripheral nerves
  anatomy of, 379
  in repair procedures, 381, 382-383
Fasciectomy in Dupuytren's contractures, 406, 407-408, 416-418
  with multiple Y-V–plasty incisions, 399-401
Fasciitis
  necrotizing, 150-152, 162, 412
  palmar, in Dupuytren's contractures, 402, 412
Fasciodermadesis in ulnar nerve palsy, 294
Fasciodermal sling in ulnar nerve palsy, 377
Fasciotomy in Dupuytren's contracture, 399
Felon, 149
Fentanyl in tenolysis, 98, 312-313
Fibula bone grafts in radial clubhand, 357, 358
Financial considerations
  in digital salvage, 250-251
  in phalangeal fracture treatment, 127
  in surgical management of rheumatoid hand, 224, 239
Finger(s); see also specific fingers
  avulsive amputation of, 12
  in boutonniere deformity, 54-68
  extensor tendon problems of, reconstruction in, 47-50
  flexor tendons of
    severance of, 73-85
    tenosynovitis in, 203
  fractures of; see Fractures and dislocations
  joints of; see specific joints
  local rotation flaps for injuries of, 38-44
    in burns, 38-42
    in crushing injury, 38-39
    in dog bite complications, 43
  pulp temperature test of, in painful neuroma, 319
  salvage of, 243-252; see also Replantation, digital
  in ulnar nerve palsy, asynchronous flexion of, 293
Fingernails, 22-27
  anatomy of, 22
  bed of, 22
    grafts of, 27
    injuries to, 22-24, 25
  fold of, 22
    injuries to, 24-25
  grafts of, 27
  matrix of
    avulsion of, 27
    injury to, 22-24
  physiology of, 22
  as splints, 22-23, 25, 26, 27
  subungual hematoma of, 22
  in tuft fractures, 26
First web space contractures, reconstruction of, 28-37
Flaps; see Grafts and flaps

Flexor tendons, 71-102; see also specific tendons
  in abrasion injuries, 6
  adhesion to bones, 78, 81-82, 83, 90-91, 140-141, 142, 143, 313, 318
    pharmacologic control of, 78
    tenolysis of, 81-82, 83, 90-91, 140-144, 313, 318
  contracture of, in Dupuytren's disease, 405
  in dog bite complications, 43
  healing of, intrinsic capability of, 73
  nourishment of, 73, 94
  in phalangeal fractures, 131, 139, 140-144
  pulley system of, 73-75, 94-102; see also Pulley system of flexor tendons
  repair of, 75, 77
    postoperative management of, 78
  severed in finger, functional recovery after, 73-85
  sheath of, 74
  silicone implantation in, 79-81, 83, 87, 93, 94, 95
  suture techniques for, 75, 77, 82
  in tendon grafts, 43, 50, 76, 78-80, 82-83, 87-88, 92-93, 98-100
  tenosynovitis of
    in rheumatoid arthritis, 203-204
    septic, 158-159
  vincular system of, 73, 94, 96
  zone I problems of, 86-88
  zone II problems of, 78, 88-93
Forearm
  innervation of muscles of, 275, 276
  in radial clubhand, 355-365
  reconstruction of extensor system of, 47-52
  traction avulsion amputation of, 267, 270
Foreign material retained and infections, 152-155
Fractures and dislocations, 103-144
  arthritis after, 112, 173-182
  Bennett's fracture, 107-108, 111, 113, 185
  boutonniere deformity after, 56, 57, 66
  boxer's fracture, 122-124
  of carpometacarpal joints, 189-195
  Colles' fracture, 51, 52, 305, 309, 316
  complications of, 137-138
  in crushing injuries, 126, 130
  digital performance after, 126-139, 140-144
  of distal interphalangeal joint, 128
  of elbow, 374, 377
  extensor tendon problems in, 50, 51-52, 131, 139, 141-142, 144
  of index finger, 115-117, 120-121
  metacarpal, 107-108, 111, 113, 114-125
  of metacarpal-hamate joint, 108-111, 113
  of metacarpophalangeal joint, 115-117
  mobilization of joints after, 135-137, 140, 143, 144
  phalangeal, 126-144; see also Phalangeal fractures
  of proximal interphalangeal joint, 111-113, 128, 173, 174, 176, 177
  of radius, dorsal subluxation of carpus in, 351
  reflex sympathetic dystrophy after, 305, 309
  of scaphoid, 105-106
    nonunion of, 106, 337-338, 349-350
  silicone implant arthroplasty after, 173, 174, 176, 177
  soft tissue injuries in, 130-131, 132, 138, 139, 191-192, 305
  tendon-bone adhesions after, 140-144
  of tuft, 26
  ulnar neuropathy in, 374, 377
  wrist arthrodesis after, 336, 337
Free-skin grafting
  in Dupuytren's contracture, 409
  in first web space contracture, 31-32

Free-tendon grafting, 76, 78-80
Froment's sign
  prevention of, 277, 293
  in ulnar nerve palsy, 289, 290, 293
Full-thickness skin grafts, 11
  in Dupuytren's contractures, 405, 406, 409, 416
  in first web space contracture, 31-32
Functional activities of hand, 300
  grasping, 285, 293-297, 300, 318
  pinching, 275-284, 285, 291-293, 300, 301
  for placement, 300
  and prefunctional activities, 300
  tendon transfers for, 300, 301
Fungal infections of hand, 157, 160
Funiculus of peripheral nerves, 379
Fusobacterium infections, 152

G

Gangrene, infectious, 162
Gout, 157
Grafts and flaps, 10-21
  abdominal pedicle flaps, 11, 37, 47, 48
  in abrasion injuries, 309
  bone grafts; *see* Bone grafts
  chest pedicle flaps, 7, 8, 37
  cross-arm flaps, 11, 35-37, 405
  cross-finger flaps, 11
  deltopectoral flaps, 11, 16-17
  for digital defects, 38-44
  in Dupuytren's contracture, 399, 400, 405, 406-407, 409-410, 416
    open-palm technique compared with, 409
  in fingernail injuries, 27
  in first web space contractures, 28-37
  full-thickness skin grafts, 11
    in Dupuytren's contractures, 405, 406, 409, 416
    in first web space contracture, 31-32
  groin flaps, 11, 18-19, 37, 405
  local flaps, 11, 32-35, 38-44
  microvascular composite tissue transplants, 11, 20
  nerve, 14
    interfascicular, 383-384, 385
  neurovascular island flaps, 11, 14-17
  palmar flaps, 11
  split-thickness grafts, 10; *see also* Split-thickness skin grafts
  tendons in; *see* Tendon transfers
  thenar flaps, 11
  veins in; *see* Vein grafts
Granuloma, swimming pool, 164
Grasp function of hand
  for large objects, 300
  in spinal cord injuries, procedure to provide, 277
  after tenolysis, exercises strengthening, 318
  in ulnar nerve palsy, 285, 293-297
Grind test in trapeziometacarpal osteoarthritis, 183
Grinding injury, split-thickness skin grafts in, 19
Groin flaps, 11, 18
  in Dupuytren's contracture, 405
  in first web space contracture, 37
  microvascular, 18-19
Guanethidine, tourniquet-controlled limb perfusion of, in reflex sympathetic dystrophy, 308
Gunshot wounds of peripheral nerves, fascicular repair of, 383
Guyon's canal, ulnar artery thrombosis in, 258-260

H

Hamate
  in fifth metacarpal-hamate joint fractures, 108-111, 113
  in wrist arthrodesis, 335, 336-337, 339
    capitate-hamate-lunate-triquetral, 336-337
    hamate-triquetral, 335, 337
Healing
  in Dupuytren's contracture, 403, 409, 410, 411, 416
  of extensor tendons, spontaneous, 47, 48
  of flexor tendons, intrinsic capability for, 73
  of scaphoid fractures, delayed union or nonunion in, 106, 337-338, 349-350
Heart disease, ischemic, reflex sympathetic dystrophy in, 305
Hematoma
  in Dupuytren's contracture, postoperative, 402-403, 409, 410, 412, 416
  subungual, 22
Hemorrhage in pollicis longus extensor tendon sheath, 51-52
Horner's sign in reflex sympathetic dystrophy, 308
Hydrocortisone therapy in hand infections, 160, 164
Hypnosis in painful neuroma, 321
Hypothenar hammer syndrome, 253

I

Iliac bone grafts, 106
  in wrist arthrodesis, 353, 354
Immunocompromised patients, hand infections of, 157, 160
Index finger
  fractures and dislocations of
    in metacarpal epiphysis, 120-121
    in metacarpophalangeal joint, 115-117
  microvascular composite tissue transplant from foot restoring sensation and function of, 20
  pollicization of, in radial clubhand, 361
  silicone implant arthroplasty of proximal interphalangeal joint of, in rheumatoid arthritis, 174, 178
  snake bite of, 20
  tendon transfers restoring movement of, in ulnar nerve palsy, 289
  traumatic amputation of, 40-42
    and replantation, 248-250
Indicis proprius extensor tendon transfer
  in pollicis longus extensor tendon rupture, 52, 202
  in ulnar nerve palsy, 296
Infections, 145-165; *see also* specific organisms
  bacterical, 147-159, 161-165
    acid-fast, 163-164
  boutonniere deformity after, 64
  diagnosis of, 152, 157, 161, 163
  in dog bites, 43
  in Dupuytren's contracture, postoperative, 403, 410
  fasciitis, 150-152, 162, 402, 412
  first web space contracture with, 28
  in forearm replantation, 267, 270
  foreign material retention causing, 152-155
  fungal, 157, 160
  gangrene in, 162
  in human bites, 153, 161
  mycobacterial, 147-148, 163-164
  patient neglect of, 149, 150
  split-thickness skin grafts in prevention of, 19
  systemic disease complicating, 152
  tenosynovitis, 158-159, 160, 199, 203-204
Informing patients about digital salvage, obligation of surgeon in, 251
Injuries; *see* Trauma
Innovar anesthesia in tenolysis, 98, 312-313, 318

Interfascicular nerve grafting, 383-384, 385
Interosseous muscles, first dorsal, 169
  contracture of, 28
Interphalangeal (IP) joint
  arthrodesis of, in thumb
    in boutonniere deformity, 206, 207, 236
    in spinal cord injuries for lateral pinch restoration, 279
    in swan-neck deformity, 211
    in ulnar nerve palsy, 293
  in boutonniere deformity, 205-209, 236
  distal; *see* Distal interphalangeal (DIP) joint
  proximal; *see* Proximal interphalangeal (PIP) joint
  in ulnar nerve palsy, 285, 287, 290, 291
    asynchronous motion of, 293-297
Intertrigo in Dupuytren's contractures, 402
Intrinsic–intrinsic plus test in boutonniere deformity, 55, 57, 59, 60
IP joint; *see* Interphalangeal (IP) joint
Isoniazid, 147

J

Jeanne's sign, 289, 290
Joint(s), 167-195; *see also* specific joints
  arthritis of, 173-182, 197-240; *see also* Arthritis
  assessment of, in digital injuries, 247
  exercise programs for motion of; *see* Exercise programs
  fractures of, 107-113
  silicone implant arthroplasty in, 173-182
Joint Jack splint
  in boutonniere deformity, 67
  in Dupuytren's contracture, postoperative, 400
  in ulnar nerve palsy, 287

K

Kessler sutures in flexor tendon repair, 75, 77, 82
Kienböck's disease, limited wrist arthrodesis in, 337
Kirschner wire fixation
  in Bennett's fracture, 108
  in boutonniere deformity, 58, 60, 64
  in carpometacarpal dislocation, 193
  in first web space contracture, 34
  in metacarpal-hamate joint fractures, 109, 110
  in phalangeal fractures, 134-135, 136
  of proximal interphalangeal joint
    in Dupuytren's contracture, 405
    in fractures, 111
  in scaphoid fractures, 106
  in scapholunate dissociation, 347
  in wrist arthrodesis, 338, 354
Klebsiella infection, 162

L

"Laborer" philosophy in hand reconstruction, 300
Lacerations
  boutonniere deformity in, 64
  of digitorum profundus flexor tendon
    in phalangeal fractures, digital performance after, 131
    reconstruction of, 77, 87-88, 92-93, 301
  first web space contracture in, 28, 31
  of forearm, extensor tendon problems in, 48
  of nail bed, 22-24, 25
  in zone I of flexor tendons, 87-88
  in zone II of flexor tendons, 90-93
Landsmeer's ligament in hyperextension at distal interphalangeal joint, 393

Lateral bands, 54
  in boutonniere deformity, 55-57, 62
Lateral pinch restoration after spinal cord injury, 275-284
Lidocaine
  in painful neuroma, 321
  in reflex sympathetic dystrophy, 308
  in tenolysis, 98, 313
Ligaments; *see also* specific ligaments
  in Dupuytren's contractures, 405-406
  in scapholunate dissociation, reconstruction of, 347-348
Little finger
  abrasion injuries of, 6, 8
  Dupuytren's contracture of, 406, 416
    combinations of joints in, 393-397
    at distal interphalangeal joint, 393, 397
    at metacarpophalangeal joint, 389, 398, 416
    persistent, 389-398
    at proximal interphalangeal joint, 389-393, 398
    recurrence of, 406
    treatment of, 397-398
  hyperextension at distal interphalangeal joint of, 393, 398
  metacarpal fractures of, 108-111, 113, 122-125
  silicone implant arthroplasty for posttraumatic arthritis of proximal interphalangeal joint of, 174, 177
  traction avulsion amputation and replantation of, 268
  in ulnar neuropathy, 288-289, 374-375
Local flaps
  advantages and disadvantages of, 11
  for digital defects, 38-44
  for first web space contracture, 32-35
Long finger
  abrasion injury of, 8
  burns of, 18, 38-41
  dog bite of, 43
  local rotation flaps for injuries of, 38-41, 43
  tendon transfers restoring function of, in ulnar nerve palsy, 289
Lumbrical bar splints in ulnar nerve palsy, 286, 287, 291, 294
Lunate
  in Kienböck's disease, 337
  motion with scaphoid, 335
  in scapholunate dissociation, 216-218, 222, 225, 341-348, 350; *see also* Scapholunate dissociation
  silicone prosthesis for, 152
  in wrist arthrodesis, 335-337, 338, 339
    capitate-hamate-lunate-triquetral, 336-337
    capitate-lunate, 335, 336
    lunate-radial, 335, 337
    lunate-triquetral, 337
    scaphocapitate-lunate, 336
    scapholunate, 337
    scapholunate-radial, 337

M

McCash open-palm technique, 409-410
Mallet deformity in Dupuytren's contracture, 405-406
Massage of painful neuromas, 321, 325
Masse's sign in ulnar nerve palsy, 290
Matrix of fingernails, injuries of, 22-24, 27
MCP joint; *see* Metacarpophalangeal (MCP) joint
Median nerve
  communication with ulnar nerve, 285
  compression of; *see* Carpal tunnel syndrome
  injuries of
    in carpometacarpal joint dislocation, 192
    epineurial repair of, 382

Median nerve—cont'd
  injuries of—cont'd
    group fascicular repair of, 382
    interfascicular nerve grafting in, 383, 384
    reflex sympathetic dystrophy in, 305, 309
  painful neuroma of, 322
  paralysis of
    contracture of first web space in, 28
    with ulnar nerve palsy, 290, 295, 296-297
Mepivacaine hydrochloride
  in painful neuroma, 321
  in reflex sympathetic dystrophy, 308
Metacarpal fractures, 114-125
  displaced without dislocation, 118-119
  epiphyseal, 120-121
  of fifth metacarpal, 122-125
    at joint with hamate, 108-111, 113
  of first metacarpal, 107-108, 111, 113
  reduction of, 114-125
Metacarpal-hamate joint fracture, 108-111, 113
Metacarpophalangeal (MCP) joint
  in boutonniere deformity, 205-209, 236
    arthrodesis in, 206, 207, 236
    silicone implant in, 207
  contracture of little finger at, 389, 398, 416
  eggcup deformity of, 232
  fracture-dislocation of, 115-117
  local flap for coverage of injury in area of, 14
  loss of extension at, treatment of, 47-50
  in rheumatoid arthritis, 225-239
  in swan-neck deformity, arthrodesis in, 211
  traction avulsion amputation of thumb at, 264-265, 269
  in ulnar nerve palsy, 285-297
    asynchronous motion of, 293-297
    capsuloplasty of, 293, 294-295
    in splinting therapy, 294
    in surgical procedures, 294-295
Metacarpotrapezial joint
  degenerative disease of, 169-172
  muscles acting on, 169
Microvascular problems, 241-271
  composite tissue transplants for, 11, 18, 19, 20
  in digital salvage, 20, 243-252
  in ulnar artery thrombosis, 253-263
  in upper extremity replantation, 264-271
Middle finger; see Long finger
Mimocausalgia, 305
Motivation of patients; see Patient considerations
Mycobacterial infections, 147-148, 163-164
Myelinated nerves, anatomy of, 379

N

Nails, 22-27; see also Fingernails
Necrotizing hand infections
  cellulitis, synergistic, 162
  fasciitis, 150-152, 162
Neglected conditions
  in carpometacarpal dislocation, 194
  in hand infections, 149, 150
Neoplasia, reflex sympathetic dystrophy in, 305
Nerve(s), 367-385; see also specific nerves
  action potential recordings of, in neuroma-in-continuity evaluation, 370-373
  blocking procedures
    in painful neuroma, 320, 322, 325

Nerve(s)—cont'd
  blocking procedures—cont'd
    in reflex sympathetic dystrophy, 307-308
  conduction velocity of
    in neuroma-in-continuity, 370
    in ulnar neuropathy, 375
  grafts of, 14
    interfascicular, 383-384, 385
  injuries of; see Trauma, of nerves
  neuromas of, 319-331, 369-373; see also Neuromas
Neurapraxia, 369
Neurectomy in painful neuroma, 322, 325, 327-330
Neuroleptanalgesics (NLA) and local anesthesia in tenolysis, 98, 312-318
Neurolysis in neuroma-in-continuity, 369-370
Neuromas, 319-331, 369-373
  abnormal generator theory of, 319
  acupuncture in, 321
  amputation and, 319, 321, 325, 327, 328, 330
  artificial synapse theory of, 319
  case histories of, 326-330
  differential localization of, 319
  drug therapy in, 320, 321, 325
  electric stimulation in
    for evaluation, 370-373
    for pain relief, 320-321, 325
  electrophysiology of, 319
  fascicular repair in, 383
  fiber dissociation theory of, 319
  functional activity of extremity in, 322, 324
    restoration of, 320, 322
  hypnosis in, 321
  in-continuity, 322, 326, 369-373
  inspection and palpation of, 369
  local anesthetic injections in, 321, 325
  neurolysis of, external and internal, 369-370
  painful, 319-331
    compared with nonpainful, 319, 324
  percussion of, 321, 325
  prevention of, 321-322, 324
  silicone capping of nerve end in, 325
  transposition of intact, 325, 327, 328
Neurorrhaphy of peripheral nerves, 90, 369, 379-385; see also Peripheral nerve repairs
Neurotmesis, 369
Neurotomy in painful neuroma, 322
Neurovascular island flaps, 11, 14-17
Night bracing in radial clubhand, 360, 364
Nonunion of scaphoid fractures, 106, 337-338, 349-350
Numbness complaints in ulnar artery thrombosis, 255

O

Obligation of surgeon in digital salvage, 251
Oblique ligament, anterior, 107
Oblique phalangeal fractures, digital performance after, 144
Open-palm technique in Dupuytren's contracture treatment, 403, 409-413
Opponens muscle of thumb, 169
Osteoarthritis
  postmenopausal, 183-187
  silicone implant arthroplasty in, 173, 181, 183-188
  of trapeziometacarpal joint, comparison of operative procedures for, 183-188
  ulnar neuropathy in, 377
  wrist arthrodesis in, 352

INDEX

Osteoporosis in reflex sympathetic dystrophy, 305, 307
Osteotomy of ulna in radial clubhand, 357

P

Pain problems, 303-331
  in caput ulnae syndrome, 199
  drug therapy for; see Drug therapy, for pain
  in Dupuytren's contracture, postoperative, 407, 410
  in flexor tenosynovitis of finger, 203
  in neuromas, 319-331
  in posttraumatic arthritis, silicone implant arthroplasty for, 176, 181
  in quadraregia syndrome, 301-302
  in reflex sympathetic dystrophy, 305-311
  in tenolysis, 98, 142, 143, 312-318
  in trapeziometacarpal osteoarthritis, 183-187
  in ulnar artery thrombosis, 253-254
    on cold exposure, 254-255
Palmar arch, superficial
  anatomy of, 258-259
  in ulnar artery thrombosis, assessment of blood flow in, 260-262, 263
Palmar flaps, 11
Palmaris longus tendon grafts, 49, 80
  in digitorum profundus flexor tendon laceration, 87
  in trapezial resection arthroplasty, 185, 187
Palsy
  drummer boy's, 52
  median nerve, 28
    ulnar nerve palsy with, 290, 295, 296-297
  radial, 50
  Saturday night, 322
  ulnar nerve, 28, 285-299, 374
Pantrapezial degenerative joint disease, 155, 171
Paralysis; see also Palsy
  median nerve, 28
  in spinal cord injury, restoration of lateral pinch in, 275-284
Paronychia, 149
Patient considerations
  in carpometacarpal dislocation management, 194
  in digital salvage, 243, 250-251
  in Dupuytren's contracture rehabilitation, 412
  in exercise programs, postoperative, 90-91, 128, 141, 143, 144, 312
  in laborer philosophy of hand reconstruction, 300
  in lateral pinch restoration after spinal cord injury, 275
  in neglected infections, 149, 150
  in phalangeal fractures, digital performance after, 127-128, 141, 143, 144
  in reflex sympathetic dystrophy, psychiatric guidance for, 307
  in rheumatoid arthritis with surgical management, 224-225, 239
  in ulnar nerve palsy treatment, 293-294
  in wrist arthrodesis position, 353, 354
Pedicle flaps, distant; see Distant pedicle flaps
Penicillins in hand infections, 157, 161
Percussion of painful neuromas, 321, 325
Perineurium of peripheral nerves
  anatomy of, 379
  in repair procedures, 382, 385
Peripheral nerve repairs, 90, 369, 379-385
  anatomy of, 379-380
  electric stimulation after, 384
  epineurial, 381-382, 385
  equipment for, 380
  fascicular, 381, 382-383
  group fascicular, 381, 382
  interfascicular nerve grafting, 381, 383-384, 385
  nerve regeneration after, 380, 384

Peripheral nerve repairs—cont'd
  in neuromas, 324, 325, 326, 369
  primary or secondary, 384-385
  suture line in, 380, 383
Phalangeal fractures, 126-144
  capsulotomy after, 141, 143, 144
  closed reduction of, 133
  comminuted, 129, 130, 133, 135, 138, 144
  complications of, 137-138, 140-144
  digital performance after, 126-139, 140-144
  displacement of, 129, 137-138
  joint involvement in, 129-130
  patient factors affecting recovery in, 127-128, 141, 143, 144
  stability of, 129
  tendon injuries in, 130-131, 132, 138, 139
  tenolysis after, 140-144
  total active motion after, 127, 143-144
  types of, 129, 144
Phalangization technique in first web space contracture, 29
Pharmacotherapy; see Drug therapy
Phialophora gougerotii, 160
Physical therapy; see Exercise programs
Pinch function of hand, 300, 301
  after spinal cord injury, 275-284
  in ulnar nerve palsy, 285, 291-293
PIP joint; see Proximal interphalangeal (PIP) joint
Placement function of hand, 300
Plantaris tendon grafts, 49
  in pulley reconstruction, 99, 100
  in ulnar nerve palsy, 296-297
Plethysmography, digital, in ulnar artery thrombosis, 254-255, 257-258, 260, 262
Pollicis adductor muscle, 107, 169
  in Bennett's fracture, 107
  in boutonniere deformity, 205, 207
  contracture of, 28
  loss of, 300-301
  in pinching, 300
  restoring power of, 300-301
  in ulnar nerve palsy, 290, 291
    tendon transfers replacing head of, 291, 292, 293
Pollicis brevis extensor muscle, 169
  in boutonniere deformity, 205
Pollicis brevis extensor tendon
  rupture of, thumb deformities in, 211
  transfer of, 52
Pollicis brevis flexor muscle, 169
Pollicis brevis flexor tendon in ulnar nerve palsy, 290
  tendon transfers replacing deep head of, 291-293
Pollicis longus abductor muscle, 169
Pollicis longus abductor tendon, 107
  in Bennett's fracture, 107, 108
  tenodesis of, after spinal cord injury, 279
Pollicis longus extensor muscle, 169
Pollicis longus extensor tendon
  anatomy and function of, 51
  in boutonniere deformity, 205, 206, 207
  rupture of, 51-52, 202, 211
  tendon transfers supplementing power of, 291-293
Pollicis longus flexor muscle, 169
Pollicis longus flexor tendon
  repair of, 14
  rupture of
    in rheumatoid arthritis, 204
    thumb deformities in, 211

Pollicis longus flexor tendon—cont'd
  tenodesis of, for thumb flexion after spinal cord injury, 276-278
Pollicization of index finger in radial clubhand, 361
Postmenopausal osteoarthritis of trapeziometacarpal joint, 183-187
Postoperative management
  of boutonniere deformity, 59, 60
  in Dupuytren's contractures, 398, 400, 401, 407-408, 409-410, 411, 412, 416
    hematoma in, 402-403, 409, 412, 416
  exercise programs in; see Exercise programs, postoperative
  in flexor tendon repairs, 78, 90
  of phalangeal fractures, 133, 135-137, 140, 143, 144
  in silicone implant arthroplasty, 176
    tenolysis, 314-318
    analgesia in, 312, 314, 317-318
  in wrist arthrodesis, 338-339, 354
  functional activities of hand, 300
  operative preparation for tenolysis, 312
  styloid recess in rheumatoid arthritis of wrist, 218, 220
Pronator teres tendon transfer, 50
  for lateral pinch restoration in spinal cord injuries, 281, 283
Propranolol in reflex sympathetic dystrophy, 308
Prosthesis
  in fingernail injuries, 23, 25
  infections after implantation of, 152, 154-155
  for lunate, 152
  for scaphoid, 106, 152, 336
  for scaphoradial joint, 337
  silicone implants as; see Silicone implantation
  in tendon grafting, 50, 152
    in flexor tendon problems, 79-81, 83
  for trapezium, 152, 155
Proteus infection, 162
Proximal interphalangeal (PIP) joint
  arthrodesis of
    in crushing and burn injury, 38
    in rheumatoid arthritis, 234-236
  in boutonniere deformity, 54
    postoperatively, 64-68
  crushing injury of, 38, 173, 176, 178
  in Dupuytren's contracture, 389-393, 398, 405, 414-418
    cartilage damage in, 406
    pathologic anatomy of, 414-416
    treatment of, 416-418
  fractures and dislocations of, 111-113, 173, 174, 176, 177
    digital performance after, 128
    internal fixation of, 111, 112-113
  posttraumatic arthritis of, 112, 173-182
  pulleys surrounding, 97
  in rheumatoid arthritis, 232-236
  silicone implant arthroplasty of, 173-182
  swan-neck deformity of, 232-234, 237
  in ulnar nerve palsy, 290, 291, 296
Pseudocysts of radius in rheumatoid arthritis of wrist, 216-218, 222
Psoriatic arthritis, 207
Psychiatric guidance in reflex sympathetic dystrophy, 307
Psychological factors affecting postoperative rehabilitation, 312
Pulley system of flexor tendons, 73-75, 82, 83, 87-88, 92-93, 94-102
  anatomy of, 94, 96
  annular, 73, 74, 94-102; see also Annular pulleys of flexor tendons
  in bowstringing of tendon, 76, 97, 98-100, 101
  cruciate, 73, 74, 94, 96, 97-98, 100
  in digitorum profundus flexor tendon laceration, 87-88, 92-93
  reconstruction of, 75, 76, 82, 83, 98-100
    five-pulley system in, 100, 102

Pulley system of flexor tendons—cont'd
    four-pulley system in, 95, 100
    two-pulley system in, 100
  in rheumatoid arthritis, 203
  tendon forces on, 97
  in tenolysis procedures, 142, 143, 313-314

Q

Quadraregia syndrome, 301-302
Quadriga syndrome, 88
Quadriplegia after spinal cord injury, restoration of lateral pinch in, 275-284

R

Radial artery repair in avulsive amputation of hand, 13, 266, 270
Radial nerve injuries, 305
  epineurial repair of, 382
  painful neuroma after, 322, 324, 326, 329
Radial palsy, tendon transfer in, 50
Radiocapitate ligament, 342, 343, 344
  in rheumatoid arthritis of wrist, 216, 217, 219
Radiocarpal subluxation, ulnar translatory, 351
Radiocarpal synovectomy
  in caput ulnae syndrome, 199, 200
  in rheumatoid arthritis of wrist, 222
Radiodigital artery clot proximal to anastomosis in thumb replantation, 265, 270
Radiodigital nerve graft, 14
Radiographic examination
  of carpometacarpal dislocation, 190, 191
  of metacarpal fractures, 110-111, 118, 119, 120-121, 122-125
  of metacarpophalangeal joint fracture-dislocation, 115, 116
  of metacarpotrapezial degenerative joint disease, 169, 170
  of phalangeal fractures, 132, 133
  of proximal interphalangeal joint fractures, 112
  of radial clubhand, 355, 356
  of rheumatoid wrist, 216-218, 219, 221
  of scaphoid fracture, 105
  of scapholunate dissociation, 345, 346-347
  of trapeziometacarpal osteoarthritis, 183, 186
  of ulnar neuropathy, 375
Radiolunate ligament in rheumatoid arthritis of wrist, 218, 219
Radioscapholunate ligament, deep, 341-344
  in rheumatoid arthritis of wrist, 216-218
Radioulnar joint
  subluxation of, 351
  synovectomy of, 222
Radioulnocarpal complex
  in caput ulnae syndrome, reconstruction of, 199, 201
  normal, 199
  in rheumatoid arthritis of wrist, 199
Radius
  in clubhand deformity, 355-365
  fractures of, 351
  pseudocysts of, in rheumatoid arthritis of wrist, 216-218, 222
  in wrist arthrodesis, 335, 337, 338, 339
    lunate-radial, 335, 337
    scapholunate-radial, 335, 337
    scaphoradial, 337
Ranvier nodes, anatomy of, 379
Raynaud's disease, 152
Reconstruction of hand
  laborer philosophy of, 300
  tendon transfer problems in, 300-302

INDEX

Reflex sympathetic dystrophy, 305-311
  classification of, 305
  diagnosis of, 307
  pathogenesis of, 307
  stages of, 305-307
  treatment of, 307-309
Regeneration
  of finger extensors, spontaneous, 47, 48
  of peripheral nerves, 369, 380
Remote pedicle flaps; see Distant pedicle flaps
Replantation
  digital, 12, 243-252
    contraindications to, 243, 248, 249
    function after, 243-244, 250
    of index finger, 248-250
    indications for, 243
    of little finger, 268
    of multiple digits, 244-247
    patient considerations in, 243, 250-251
    scoring system for preoperative assessment of, 247
    of single digit, 248-250
    split-thickness skin grafts in, 12, 13
    of thumb, 244, 264-265, 269
  of forearm at elbow, 267
  of hand at wrist, 266
  of upper extremity, 264-271
Resection arthroplasty in trapeziometacarpal osteoarthritis, 183-188
Reserpine, intraarterial, in ulnar artery thrombosis, 260
Retinacular system of hand
  anatomy of, 54-55, 94
  in boutonniere deformity, 55-57, 59, 62, 405
  in Dupuytren's contracture, 405
  repositioning of, in rheumatoid arthritis, 222, 225
  trauma of, 97
Rheumatoid arthritis, 157, 197-240
  boutonniere deformity in, 57, 60, 62, 205-209, 232, 233, 234, 236, 237
  caput ulnae syndrome in, 199-202, 225, 232
  carpal tunnel syndrome in, 203-204, 232
  contraindications to surgery in, 224
  distal interphalangeal joints in, 233, 234
  extensor tenosynovitis in, 199
  flexor tenosynovitis in, 203-204
  indications for surgery in, 224, 232
  metacarpophalangeal joints in, 225-239
  multiple-level deformities in, surgical management of, 224-240
  proximal interphalangeal joints in, 232-236
  radiographic findings in, 216-218, 219, 221
  silicone implant arthroplasty in, 173, 181, 225-232
  staging of reconstructive procedures in, 236-239
  swan-neck deformities in, 209-211, 212-214, 232-234, 237
  tendon ruptures in, 52, 204
  thumb deformities in, 205-215, 236
  of wrist, 199-202, 216-223, 353, 354
Rifampin, 164
Ring finger
  abrasion injury of, 8
  flexion contracture of, after burn, 18
  local rotation flap for coverage of, 38
  in ulnar neuropathy, 374-375
Rolling finger flexion, 293
Rope-burn injuries, 6

Rotation flaps
  for contracture of first web space, 32-35
  for digital defects, 38-44

S

Safety pin splints
  in boutonniere deformity, 67
  in ulnar nerve palsy, 287, 291
Saturday night palsy, 322
Scaphocapitate-lunate arthrodesis, 336
Scaphoid
  anatomy of, 169, 341-344
  blood supply of, 105
  congenital bipartition of, 106
  dissociation from lunate, 216-218, 222, 225, 341-348, 350; see also Scapholunate dissociation
  fractures of, 105-106
    delayed union of, 106
    diagnosis of, 105
    healing time of, 105
    management of, 105-106
    nonunion of, 106, 337-338, 349-350
  prosthesis for, 106, 152, 336
  in rheumatoid arthritis of wrist, 216-218, 219, 221, 222
  rotary subluxation of, 336, 341-348
  in wrist arthrodesis, 335-337, 338, 348
    scaphocapitate-lunate, 336
    scapholunate, 335, 337
Scapholunate dissociation, 341-348, 350
  anatomy of, 341-344
  diagnosis of, 345-347
  mechanism of injury in, 344-345
  in rheumatoid arthritis of wrist, 216-218, 222, 225
  treatment of, 222, 225, 347-348
Scapholunate ligaments, 341, 342, 343
Scapholunate-radial arthrodesis, 335, 337
Scaphoradial joint, 337
Scaphotrapezial joint
  degenerative disease of, 169-172
  muscles acting on, 169
Schwann sheath, anatomy of, 379
Self-care goals
  in restoration of lateral pinch after spinal cord injuries, 275
  and wrist arthrodesis position, 352, 353
Shearing amputations compared with traction avulsion amputations, 264
Shoulder-hand syndrome, 305
  in Dupuytren's contracture, postoperative, 400
Signs; see Tests and signs
Silastic prosthesis
  in fingernail injuries, 23, 25
  for scaphoid combined with limited wrist arthrodesis, 336
  in scaphoradial joint degenerative disease, 337
Silicone implantation
  in boutonniere deformity, 207
  complications of, 176, 179-180, 181
    infections as, 152, 154-155
  in extensor tendon problems, temporary use of, 50
  in flexor tendon problems, 79-81, 83, 94, 95
    in laceration of digitorum profundus flexor tendon, 87, 93
  in fracture complications, 173, 174, 176, 177
  for lunate prosthesis, 152
  in osteoarthritis, 173, 181
    trapeziometacarpal, 183-188
  in painful neuroma, 325

Silicone implantation—cont'd
  in posttraumatic arthritis of proximal interphalangeal joint, 173-182
  in rheumatoid arthritis, 173, 181, 225-232
  for scaphoid prosthesis, 152
  in swan-neck deformity, 209-211, 212
  in tendon grafting, 50, 152
  for trapezium prosthesis, 152, 155
Skin problems, 1-44
  assessment of, in digital injuries, 247
  in Dupuytren's disease, contracture and shortage of, 404-405
  in fractures, digital performance after, 130-131, 132
  grafts and flaps for; see Grafts and flaps
Small finger; see Little finger
Smoking and ulnar artery thrombosis, 262
Snakebite, toe-to-hand transplant after, 20
Soft tissue injuries
  in carpometacarpal dislocation, 191-192
  in phalangeal fractures, 130-131, 132, 138, 139
  reflex sympathetic dystrophy after, 305
Soft tissue interpositional arthroplasty in swan-neck thumb deformity, 209
Soft tissue release in radial clubhand, 357, 364
Spinal cord injury, restoration of lateral pinch in, 275-284
Spiral phalangeal fractures, digital performance after, 128-129, 135
Splinting
  in boutonniere deformity, 57, 59, 60, 64, 66-67
  in carpometacarpal dislocation, 192
  in Dupuytren's contracture, postoperative, 398, 400, 403, 409, 410, 411, 416
  in fingernail injuries, 22-23, 25, 26, 27
  in first web space contracture, 28-29, 35, 37
  in flexor tendon problems, 78
    in tenosynovitis, 158
    in zone II injuries, postoperative, 90
  in human bite infections, 161
  in painful neuroma, 322
  patient compliance with, 128
  in phalangeal fractures, 133, 143, 144
  in proximal interphalangeal joint fractures, 112-113
  in radial clubhand, 359-360, 364
  in silicone implant arthroplasty, postoperative, 176
  in trapeziometacarpal osteoarthritis, 183
  in ulnar nerve palsy, 286, 287, 291, 294
  in wrist arthrodesis, postoperative, 338, 339, 354
Split-thickness skin grafts
  in abrasion injuries, 4, 5, 8
  advantages and disadvantages of, 10, 11
  in crushing injuries, 12
  in first web space contracture, 31-32
  in grinding injury, 19
  in infection prevention, 19
  in nail matrix avulsion, 27
  in necrotizing fasciitis, 151
  in traumatic amputation, 12, 13, 40
Sprain of wrist, pollicis longus extensor tendon rupture in, 52
Staphylococcal infections, 149, 150, 151
  gangrene in, 162
  in human bites, 161
  in tenosynovitis, 158-159
Steinmann pin fixation of rheumatoid wrist, 226, 227, 229
Stellate ganglion blocks
  in painful neuroma, 321
  in reflex sympathetic dystrophy, 307-308
  in ulnar artery thrombosis, 260

Steroid therapy
  in flexor tenosynovitis of finger, 203
  in hand infections, 157, 160
  in inflammatory arthrosis, 320
  in painful neuroma, 325, 329
  in reflex sympathetic dystrophy, 308
Stiles-Bunnell tendon transfer, modified, in ulnar nerve palsy, 296
Streptococcal infections, 150-152
  gangrene in, 162
  in human bites, 161
Streptomycin, 147
Stress testing for cold tolerance
  in painful neuroma, 319
  in ulnar artery thrombosis, 253, 254-255, 257
Styloidectomy in scaphoid fractures, 106
Subluxation
  radiocarpal, ulnar translatory, 351
  of radioulnar joint, 351
  of scaphoid
    scapholunate dissociation in, 341-348
    wrist arthrodesis in, 336
  of ulnar nerve, 374
  of wrist, dorsal, 351
Subungual hematoma, 22
Sural nerve as donor for interfascicular nerve grafting, 383
Sutures
  in flexor tendon repairs, 75, 77, 82
  in peripheral nerve repairs, 380, 383
Swan-neck deformity, 209-211, 212-214
  in Dupuytren's contracture, postoperative, 407
  in rheumatoid arthritis, 209-211, 212-214, 232-234, 237
Swimming pool granuloma, 164
Sympathectomy
  in painful neuroma, 320
  in reflex sympathetic dystrophy, 308-309
  in ulnar artery thrombosis, 253, 260, 262
Sympathetic dystrophy, posttraumatic, 305-311
  in Dupuytren's contractures, postoperative, 407-408
Synovectomy
  radiocarpal
    in caput ulnae syndrome, 199, 200
    in rheumatoid arthritis of wrist, 222
  radioulnar, in rheumatoid arthritis of wrist, 222
Synovial fluid in flexor tendon nutrition, 73
Synovitis in mycobacterial infections, 147, 148

T

Tantalum as nail substitute, 23
Tendinitis, calcific, 157
Tendon(s), 45-102; see also specific tendons
  adhesion to bones, 140-144, 312-318
  assessment of, in digital injuries, 247
  extensor, 45-69
  flexor, 71-102
  in phalangeal fractures, 130-131, 132, 138, 139, 140-144
  in rheumatoid arthritis, 52, 199, 203-204
Tendon transfers, 273-302
  in boutonniere deformity, 207
  in caput ulnae syndrome, 202
  diameter of material for, 98-100
  in extensor tendon problems, 47-50, 52, 202
  in flexor tendon problems, 43, 78-81, 82-83, 87-88, 92-93
    in digitorum profundus laceration, 87-88, 92-93
    free grafts in, 76, 78-80
    in pulley reconstruction, 76, 98-100

INDEX

Tendon transfers—cont'd
  in flexor tendon problems—cont'd
    tenolysis after, 82, 83
  in hand reconstruction, 300-302
  palmaris longus tendon in, 49, 80, 87, 185, 187
  plantaris tendon in, 49, 99, 100, 296-297
  in radial clubhand, 360, 361, 364
  silicone prosthesis in, 50, 152
  in spinal cord injuries for lateral pinch restoration, 275-284
  in trapezial resection arthroplasty, 185, 187
  in ulnar nerve palsy, 288-297
    for grasp strength, 296-297
    for pinch restoration, 291-293
    with motors available, 295
    with motors not available, 294-295
Tenodesis in ulnar nerve palsy, 294
Tenolysis, 312-318
  assessment of tendon quality in, 314
  in Colles' fracture, 316
  of extensor tendons, 141-142, 144, 313, 315, 318
  of flexor tendons, 81-82, 83, 90-91, 140-144, 313, 318
    digitorum profundus, 81, 90-91, 140-141, 142
  incision for, 313
  indications for, 312
  neuroleptanalgesics and local anesthesia allowing patient participation in, 98, 312-318
  in phalangeal fractures, 140-144
  postoperative management of
    analgesia in, 312, 314, 317-318
    exercise in, 312, 314-318
  preoperative preparation for, 312
  pulley system in, 142, 143, 313-314
  surgical technique of, 313-314
  tourniquet technique in, 313
Tenorrhaphy of digitorum profundus flexor tendon, 90, 92
Tenosynovectomy
  in caput ulnae syndrome, 199, 200
  in flexor tenosynovitis, 203, 204
Tenosynovitis
  chronic, fungal infection in, 160
  extensor, in rheumatoid arthritis, 199
  flexor, 158-159
    in finger, 203
    in rheumatoid arthritis, 203-204
    at wrist, 203-204
Tenotomy of extensor tendons in boutonniere deformity, 58, 59, 60
Tests and signs
  Allen test, 255, 260, 263
  of cold tolerance
    in painful neuroma, 319
    in ulnar artery thrombosis, 253, 254-255, 257
  Duchenne's sign, 290
  extrinsic test in claw hand deformity classification, 293, 294
  Froment's sign, 277, 289, 290, 293
  grind test in trapeziometacarpal osteoarthritis, 183
  Horner's sign in reflex sympathetic dystrophy, 308
  intrinsic–intrinsic plus test in boutonniere deformity, 55, 57, 59, 60
  Jeanne's sign in ulnar nerve palsy, 289, 290
  Masse's sign in ulnar nerve palsy, 290
  of pollicis longus extensor tendon integrity, 51
  retinacular-plus test in boutonniere deformity, 55
  Tinel's sign, 255, 375
  in ulnar nerve palsy, 288, 289, 290, 293, 294
  Wartenberg's sign in ulnar nerve palsy, 288, 290
Thenar flaps, 11

Thermography
  of normal hand, 256, 257
  in painful neuroma, 319
  in ulnar artery thrombosis, 256, 257, 260
Thromboangiitis obliterans, 152
Thrombosis
  in radiodigital artery proximal to anastomosis after traction avulsion amputation, 265, 270
  ulnar artery, 253-263
Thumb
  amputation of, traumatic, 12
    replantation of, 264-265, 269
    toe transplant in, 12, 16-17
  arthritis disabilities of, 205-215, 236
    types of, 205
  arthrodesis of
    of carpometacarpal joint, 335, 336
    of interphalangeal joint, 206, 207, 211, 236, 279, 293
    of metacarpophalangeal joint, 206, 207, 211, 236
  Bennett's fracture of, 107-108, 111, 113, 185
  biomechanical model of, 169-172
  boutonniere deformity of, 205-209, 236; see also Boutonniere deformity
  bowler's, 322
  degenerative diseases of, 155, 169-172
  lacerations of flexor surface of, 7
  neurovascular island flap for injury of, 14
  in radial aplasia, reconstruction of, 360-361
  salvage of, 244
  swan-neck deformity of, 209-211, 212-214
  in tendon ruptures, 211
  tendon transfers restoring function of, after spinal cord injuries, 275-284
Tinel's sign
  in ulnar artery thrombosis, 255
  in ulnar neuropathy, 375
Toenail grafts, 27
Toe-to-hand transplants
  after snakebite of index finger, 20
  in thumb amputation, 12, 16-17
Tolazoline hydrochloride in ulnar artery thrombosis, 260
Tourniquet techniques
  in Dupuytren's contracture surgery, 400-401, 403, 407, 409, 416
  in reflex sympathetic dystrophy for control of guanethidine limb perfusion, 308
  in tenolysis, 313
Traction avulsion amputations, 264-271; see also Amputation, traumatic
Transplantation, toe-to-hand, 12, 16-17, 20
Transposition
  of neuroma in surgical treatment of painful neuroma, 325, 327, 328
  of ulnar nerve, 377-378
Transverse phalangeal fractures, 129, 130, 133, 134-135
  digital performance after, 144
Trapeziometacarpal joint osteoarthritis, comparison of operative procedures for, 183-188
Trapezium
  anatomy of, 169
  arthroplasty of, in swan-neck deformity, 209, 211
  in osteoarthritis, 184-187
  silicone prosthesis for, 152, 155
  in wrist arthrodesis, 335, 336, 338
Trapezoid in wrist arthrodesis, 336
Trauma
  abrasion in, 3-9

Trauma—cont'd
  amputation in; see Amputation, traumatic
  arthritis after, 173-182
  of blood vessels, 247
    in avulsion amputations of upper extremity, 13, 264-271
    in digital injuries, 243-252
    in Dupuytren's contracture surgery, 403, 415
    in phalangeal fractures, 130-131, 132
    radial artery, 13, 266, 270
    ulnar artery, 13, 253, 260, 266, 270
  boutonniere deformity after, 38, 56, 57, 62, 66
  in burns; see Burns
  carpometacarpal dislocations in, 189-195
  crushing; see Crushing injuries
  dicing, 5
  digital salvage after, 243-252
  of extensor tendons, 47-52
  of fingernails, 22-27
  first web space contracture in, 28-37
  of flexor tendons, functional recovery after, 73-85
  in fractures, 103-144; see also Fractures and dislocations
  grafts and flaps for, 10-21, 38-44; see also Grafts and flaps
  grinding, 19
  of gunshot wounds, 383
  infections after, 150, 153, 158-159
  in lacerations; see Lacerations
  of nerves
    assessment of, 247
    axonotmesis in, 369
    in carpometacarpal dislocation, 191-192
    digital nerve, 90, 305, 382, 383, 402, 403, 415
    in Dupuytren's contracture surgery, 402, 403, 415
    median nerve, 192, 305, 309, 382, 383, 384
    nerve regeneration after, 380
    neurapraxia in, 369
    and neuroma formation, 319, 322, 324, 325, 326-331, 369-373
    neurotmesis in, 369
    in phalangeal fractures, 131, 132
    radial nerve, 305, 322, 324, 326, 329, 382
    reflex sympathetic dystrophy after, 305, 309
    types of repairs in, 379-385
    ulnar nerve, 192, 285, 305, 374-378, 382, 384
  patient neglect of, 149, 150, 194
  in scapholunate dissociation, 344-345
  scoring system for assessment of, 247
  of spinal cord, restoration of lateral pinch after, 275-284
  of tendons, adhesion formation in, 140-144, 312-318; see also Adhesions, tendon-bone
  of wrist, 344-345, 349
Triamcinolone acetonide, percutaneous injections of, in painful neuroma, 321
Triangular fibrocartilage in rheumatoid arthritis of wrist, 218, 220
Triangular ligament, 54
  in boutonniere deformity, 62
Trifluoperazine in reflex sympathetic dystrophy, 307
Triggering of finger in flexor tenosynovitis, 203-204
Triquetrum
  in limited wrist arthrodesis, 335-337, 339
    capitate-hamate-lunate-triquetral, 336-337
    hamate-triquetral, 337
    lunate-triquetral, 337
  in rheumatoid arthritis of wrist, 218, 220, 221
Triscaphe arthrodesis, 335, 336
Tuberculosis of hand, 147-148, 163
Tuft fractures, 26

U

Ulna
  in caput ulnae syndrome, 199-202
  in radial clubhand
    centralization of, 357-358, 359-360, 361, 364
    osteotomy of, 357
  in rheumatoid arthritis of wrist, radiographic changes of, 216-218, 219
  subluxation of, 351
  in wrist arthrodesis, 337
Ulnar artery
  injuries of, 253, 260
    in traction avulsion amputation of hand, 13, 266, 270
  thrombosis of, 253-263
    anatomy and pathophysiology of, 258-260
    clinical syndrome of, 253
    differential diagnosis of, 260
    historical background on, 253
    signs and symptoms of, 253-255, 262
    special studies in, 255-260
    treatment of, 260-262
    ulnar nerve in, 255, 257, 260
Ulnar ligament, deep, 107
Ulnar nerve, 374-378
  anatomy of, 374
  classification of disorders of, 375
  communication with median nerve, 285
  compression of, 374-378
  conservative treatment of disorders of, 375
  decompression of, 375-378
  diagnosis of disorders of, 285-287, 374-375
  at elbow, neuropathy of, 374-378
  injuries of, 285, 374-378
    in carpometacarpal dislocation, 192
    combined epineurial and group fascicular repair of, 382
    interfascicular nerve grafting in, 384
    in palmar branch, 305
  palsy of, 285-299, 374
    asynchronous finger flexion in, 293-297
    contracture of first web space in, 28
    digital abduction and adduction in, 288-289
    grasp strength in, 285, 293-297
    median nerve palsy with, 290, 295, 296-297
    partial, 289
    pattern of involvement and deficit of, 285
    pinch strength in, 285, 291-293
    sensory loss in, 288
    splinting therapy in, 286, 287, 291, 294
    tendon transfers in, 287-297
  subluxation of, 374
  transposition of, 377-378
  in ulnar artery thrombosis, 255, 257, 260
Ulnocarpal ligament complex in rheumatoid arthritis of wrist, 218
Unmyelinated nerves, anatomy of, 379

V

Valleix's phenomena, 374
Vascular system; see Blood vessels
Vein grafts
  mechanical occlusion of, at fracture site, 269, 270
  in replantation of traction avulsion amputation, 264-271
  in ulnar artery thrombosis, 253, 260, 262
Vincular system of flexor tendons of fingers, 73, 74, 94, 96
Volar intercalated segment instability (VISI) pattern, 350-351
Volkmann's contracture in ulnar nerve palsy, 296, 297

INDEX

W

Wallerian degeneration, 380
Wartenberg's sign in ulnar nerve palsy, 288, 290
Web space, first, contracted, reconstruction of, 28-37; see also Contractures, of first web space
Weilby technique of pulley reconstruction, 93
Wolfe grafts in Dupuytren's contractures, 405, 406
Wound healing; see Healing
Wrist, 333-365
   anatomy of, 221-222, 335-336, 341-344, 349
   arthrodesis of, 335-340, 352-354; see also Arthrodesis, of wrist
   arthroplasty of, 352, 354
      in rheumatoid arthritis, 225-226
   biomechanical aspects of, 349-351
   extensor tendon problems of, reconstruction in, 47-50
   flexor tenosynovitis at, 203-204
   injuries of, 344-345, 349
   in radial clubhand, 355-365
   in radioulnar joint subluxation, 351
   rheumatoid arthritis of, 216-223
      caput ulnae syndrome in, 199-202
      factors in deformity of, 218-222
      radiographic findings in, 216-218, 219, 221
      surgical management of, 222, 225-232, 353, 354
   in scaphoid nonunion, 337-338, 349-350

Wrist—cont'd
   in scapholunate dissociation, 341-348, 350
   in spinal cord injuries, tendon transfer for extension improvement, 276, 278
   subluxation of, 351
   traction avulsion amputation of hand at, 266
   in volar instability, 350-351
Wynn Parry splints in ulnar nerve palsy, 286, 287, 294

Y

Y-V flap advancement in Dupuytren's contracture, 416
Y-V–plasty incisions, multiple, extensive fasciectomy through, in Dupuytren's contracture, 399-401

Z

Zancolli lasso procedure in ulnar nerve palsy, 296
Zancolli volar plate capsuloplasty in ulnar nerve palsy, 293, 294-295
Zigzag deformity, 341
Zigzag incisions in Dupuytren's contracture surgery, 399, 400, 401, 416
Z-plasty procedures
   in Dupuytren's contracture, 405, 409, 416
   in first web space contracture
      four-flap, 30-31
      simple, 29